MW00835485

EMERGENCY MEDICINE

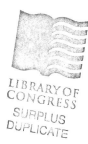
LIBRARY OF
CONGRESS
SURPLUS
DUPLICATE

EMERGENCY MEDICINE

BOARD REVIEW

EDITED BY

Danielle D. Campagne, MD, FACEP

VICE CHIEF, DEPARTMENT OF EMERGENCY MEDICINE

ASSOCIATE PROFESSOR OF CLINICAL EMERGENCY MEDICINE

UNIVERSITY OF CALIFORNIA, SAN FRANCISCO, SCHOOL OF MEDICINE

FRESNO, CA

Lori Weichenthal, MD, FACEP, RYT

ASSISTANT DEAN OF GRADUATE MEDICAL EDUCATION

ASSISTANT PROGRAM DIRECTOR, EMERGENCY MEDICINE

PROFESSOR OF CLINICAL EMERGENCY MEDICINE

UNIVERSITY OF CALIFORNIA, SAN FRANCISCO, SCHOOL OF MEDICINE

FRESNO, CA

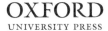

OXFORD
UNIVERSITY PRESS

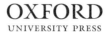

OXFORD
UNIVERSITY PRESS

Oxford University Press is a department of the University of Oxford. It furthers
the University's objective of excellence in research, scholarship, and education
by publishing worldwide. Oxford is a registered trade mark of Oxford University
Press in the UK and certain other countries.

Published in the United States of America by Oxford University Press
198 Madison Avenue, New York, NY 10016, United States of America.

© Oxford University Press 2019

All rights reserved. No part of this publication may be reproduced, stored in
a retrieval system, or transmitted, in any form or by any means, without the
prior permission in writing of Oxford University Press, or as expressly permitted
by law, by license, or under terms agreed with the appropriate reproduction
rights organization. Inquiries concerning reproduction outside the scope of the
above should be sent to the Rights Department, Oxford University Press, at the
address above.

You must not circulate this work in any other form
and you must impose this same condition on any acquirer.

Library of Congress Cataloging-in-Publication Data
Names: Campagne, Danielle D., editor. | Weichenthal, Lori, editor.
Title: Emergency medicine : board review / edited by Danielle D. Campagne, Lori Weichenthal.
Other titles: Emergency medicine (Campagne)
Description: New York, NY : Oxford University Press, [2019]
Identifiers: LCCN 2018029069 | ISBN 9780190852955 (pbk.)
Subjects: | MESH: Emergency Medicine | Emergencies | Examination Questions
Classification: LCC RC86.9 | NLM WB 18.2 | DDC 616.02/5076—dc23
LC record available at https://lccn.loc.gov/2018029069

This material is not intended to be, and should not be considered, a substitute for medical or other professional advice.
Treatment for the conditions described in this material is highly dependent on the individual circumstances. And, while this
material is designed to offer accurate information with respect to the subject matter covered and to be current as of the time it
was written, research and knowledge about medical and health issues is constantly evolving and dose schedules for medications
are being revised continually, with new side effects recognized and accounted for regularly. Readers must therefore always
check the product information and clinical procedures with the most up-to-date published product information and data sheets
provided by the manufacturers and the most recent codes of conduct and safety regulation. The publisher and the authors make
no representations or warranties to readers, express or implied, as to the accuracy or completeness of this material. Without
limiting the foregoing, the publisher and the authors make no representations or warranties as to the accuracy or efficacy
of the drug dosages mentioned in the material. The authors and the publisher do not accept, and expressly disclaim, any
responsibility for any liability, loss or risk that may be claimed or incurred as a consequence of the use and/or application of
any of the contents of this material.

1 3 5 7 9 8 6 4 2

Printed by Sheridan Books, Inc., United States of America

CONTENTS

PREFACE

Preparing for your Emergency Medicine Boards can be a very stressful time. It is the culmination of many years of hard work in college, medical school, and an emergency medicine residency. You have taken a new job out on your own, and now you need to study for "The Boards." Our goal was to take the information given from the American Board of Emergency Medicine (ABEM) about the Qualifying Exam and create a user-friendly exam preparation book.

We understand that finding time to study is hard. That is why this book is all question based. The nearly 1000 questions are board-style with detailed explanations and many tables, figures, and images to support your learning. The questions are tailored to be high yield and hit on commonly tested themes. Each question also has a "test-taking tip" to help you better navigate standardized examinations. The book is broken up into sections (cardiac emergencies, toxicologic emergencies, etc.), and the number of questions is weighted similarly to how they are weighted on the actual examination. The different sections allow you to focus on areas that may be more problematic for you and spend less time on areas in which you excel.

The book is also very useful to the practicing emergency physician who is studying for the ConCert exam and for emergency medicine residents preparing for the in-service exam. Reviewing questions and answers will help you brush up on commonly tested topics and prepare you for taking a standardized examination.

CONTRIBUTORS

Janak Acharya, MD
Medical Director, American Ambulance and Skylife
Assistant Clinical Professor of Emergency Medicine
University of California, San Francisco, School of Medicine
Fresno, CA

Leah Bauer, MD
Resident Physician
University of California, San Francisco
Fresno, CA

Deena Bengiamin, MD
Assistant Program Director
Director, Medical Student Clerkship
Assistant Professor of Emergency Medicine
University of California, San Francisco, School of Medicine
Fresno, CA

Rimon Bengiamin, MD, RDMS
Medical Director, CRMC Emergency Department
Director, Emergency Medicine Ultrasound Fellowship
Associate Clinical Professor of Emergency Medicine
University of California, San Francisco, School of Medicine
Fresno, CA

Amy Briggs, MD
Resident Physician
Los Angeles County+USC Medical Center
Los Angeles, CA

Kurt Brueggeman, MD
Assistant Clinical Professor of Emergency Medicine
University of California, San Francisco, School of Medicine
Fresno, CA

Brandon Chalfin, MD
Hospice and Palliative Care Fellow
University of California, San Francisco, School of Medicine
Fresno, CA

Carolyn Chooljian, MD
Director, Ultrasound Resident Education and Credentialing
Clinical Professor of Emergency Medicine
University of California, San Francisco, School of Medicine
Fresno, CA

Desiree Crane, DO
Volunteer Clinical Faculty
University of California, San Francisco, School of Medicine
Fresno, CA

Michael A. Darracq, MD, MPH, FACEP
Associate Professor of Clinical Emergency Medicine
Toxicology Faculty
University of California, San Francisco, School of Medicine
Fresno, CA

Brenna Jane McCarney Derksen, MD
Resident Physician
University of California, San Diego
San Diego, CA

Scott DeShields, MD, JD
Associate Clinical Professor of Emergency Medicine
Director of Quality Improvement
Medical Director of Risk
University of California, San Francisco, School of Medicine
Fresno, CA

Sukhjit Dhillon, MD
Resident Physician
University of California, San Francisco
Fresno, CA

Nelson Diamond, MD
Resident Physician
University of California, San Francisco
Fresno, CA

Seth Eidemiller, MD
Resident Physician
University of California, San Francisco
Fresno, CA

Nicholas Gastelum, MD
Ultrasound Fellow
University of California, San Francisco, School of Medicine
Fresno, CA

Anjali Gupta, MD
Emergency Medicine and Minor Injury Clinic
Kaiser Permanente
Assistant Clinical Professor
University of California, San Francisco
San Francisco, CA

Jordan Harp, MD
Resident Physician
University of California, San Francisco
Fresno, CA

Shawn Hersevoort, MD, MPH
Director of Integrated Psychiatry
Assistant Clinical Professor of Psychiatry
University of California, San Francisco, School of Medicine
Fresno, CA

Lily Hitchner, MD
Resident Physician
University of California, San Francisco
Fresno, CA

Danielle Holtz, MD
Resident Physician
University of California, San Francisco
Fresno, CA

Stephen Hurwitz, MD
Director of Consultation–Liaison Psychiatry
Community Regional Medical Center
Associate Clinical Professor of Psychiatry
University of California, San Francisco, School of Medicine
Fresno, CA

Whitney Johnson, MD
Resident Physician
University of California, San Francisco
Fresno, CA

Michael Kukurza, MD
Resident Physician
University of California, San Francisco
Fresno, CA

Xian Li, MD
Clinical Instructor of Emergency Medicine
Education Fellow
University of California, San Francisco, School of Medicine
Fresno, CA

Janelle Lee, MD
Resident Physician
University of California, San Francisco
Fresno, CA

Miranda Lewis, MD
Resident Physician
University of California, San Francisco
Fresno, CA

Fernando Macias, MD
Parkmedic Program Faculty
Base Hospital Medical Director
Assistant Clinical Professor of Emergency Medicine
University of California, San Francisco, School of Medicine
Fresno, CA

Leann Manis, MD
Resident Physician
University of California, San Francisco
Fresno, CA

Jannifer Matos, PA-C
PA Resident
University of California, San Francisco
Fresno, CA

James McCue, MD
Resident Physician
University of California, San Francisco
Fresno, CA

Adrienne Quinn, MPH
MD Candidate 2018
Keck School of Medicine
University of Southern California
Los Angeles, CA

Rene Ramirez, MD
Director, Emergency Scribe Program
Assistant Clinical Professor of Emergency Medicine
University of California, San Francisco, School of Medicine
Fresno, CA

John Ramos, MMS, PA-C
Assistant Professor
Dominican University of California
San Raphael, CA

Steven Riccoboni, MD
Clinical Instructor of Emergency Medicine
University of California, San Francisco, School of Medicine
Fresno, CA

Michelle Storkan, MD
Parkmedic Program Faculty
Medical Director, Two Cities Marathon
Clerkship Director, Wilderness Medicine Medical Student
    Elective
Clinical Instructor of Emergency Medicine
University of California, San Francisco, School of Medicine
Fresno, CA

Caleb Sunde, MD
Resident Physician
University of California, San Francisco
Fresno, CA

Stephen Thornton, MD
Associate Professor and Director of Toxicology
Department of Emergency Medicine
University of Kansas
Kansas City, KS

Vaishal Tolia, MD, MPH, FACEP
Associate Clinical Professor
Emergency Department Medical Director
Director of Observation Medicine, Care Coordination, and
    Integration
Department of Emergency Medicine
Department of Internal Medicine, Division of Hospital
    Medicine
University of California, San Diego
San Diego, CA

Megan Tresenriter, MD
Resident Physician
University of California, San Diego
San Diego, CA

Susan Woodmansee, MD, JD, FACEP
Clinical Instructor of Emergency Medicine
University of California, San Diego
School of Medicine
Fresno, CA

Fred Wu, MHS, PA-C
Program Director
Emergency Medicine PA Residency
University of California, San Diego
Fresno, CA

EMERGENCY MEDICINE

1.

SIGNS AND SYMPTOMS

Danielle Holtz

1. A 35-year-old male presents to the emergency department (ED) with progressively worsening right arm pain, swelling, and redness for 3 days. He reports injecting heroin into the area a few days before symptom onset. Associated symptoms include nausea, vomiting, and diffuse myalgias. He denies fever or numbness/tingling in his extremity. Vital signs are all within normal limits. Pertinent labs include white blood cell (WBC) count 36,000/μL, Na 130 mmol/L, and glucose 160 mg/dL. On exam, he is writhing in pain, and the area is tense, swollen and indurated beyond the borders of the erythema and appears as shown in Figure 1.1. What is the best next step in management?

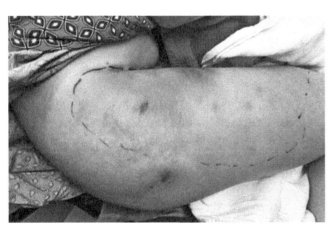

Figure 1.1 Upper extremity.

    A. Admit to medicine team for IV antibiotics
    B. Consult surgery
    C. Perform bedside incision and drainage (I&D)
    D. Order a computed tomography (CT) scan of the right lower extremity

2. A 2-year-old male is brought in by his mother after a choking episode that occurred 1 hour before arrival. At the time, he was playing on the floor alone while his mother was cooking. Vital signs are normal. He continues to intermittently cough and is drooling. His lungs are clear to auscultation bilaterally, and there is no stridor or cyanosis. His chest radiograph is shown in Figure 1.2. What is best next step in management?

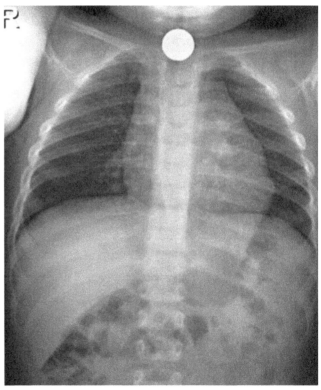

Figure 1.2 Chest radiograph.

    A. Induce vomiting with ipecac
    B. Notify child protective services
    C. Endoscopy
    D. Discharge home with follow-up with pediatrician

3. A 53-year-old male presents to the ED with a chief complaint of rash. A photo of the rash is shown in

Figure 1.3. Which of the following is the best next step in management?

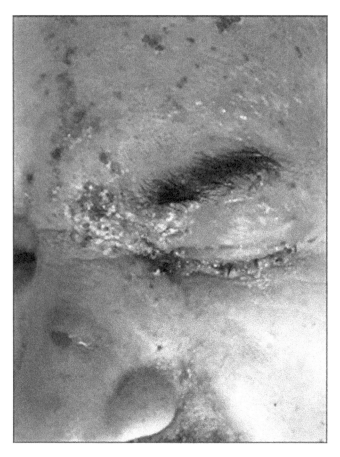

Figure 1.3 Face with rash.

A. Administer topical steroids
B. Administer cephalexin
C. Dermatology consult
D. Fluorescein exam of the eye

4. A 21-year-old female presents with lower abdominal pain and vomiting for 3 days. Her temperature is 39° C, heart rate (HR) is 130 beats/min (bpm), and BP 90/60 mm Hg. She is actively vomiting. Her entire lower abdomen is tender to palpation without rebound or guarding. Pelvic exam reveals thick yellow vaginal discharge, cervical motion tenderness, and bilateral adnexal tenderness. She is sexually active with several male partners and has an intrauterine device for contraception. A pregnancy test is negative. She has a documented history of anaphylaxis to penicillin. Which of the following antibiotics should be used in this case?

A. Ceftriaxone IM and doxycycline PO
B. Clindamycin IV and gentamicin IV
C. Vancomycin IV
D. Ceftriaxone IM and metronidazole PO

5. A 42-year-old obese female presents to the ED with dyspnea on exertion, bilateral lower extremity edema, and headaches for the past 2 weeks. Her BP is 220/110 mm Hg, and her HR is 105 bpm. She is afebrile. She has no known medical history. Chest radiograph reveals mild cardiomegaly and pulmonary vascular congestion, and her brain natriuretic peptide is 200 pg/mL, but her lungs are clear. Her electrocardiogram (EKG) is normal, and troponin is negative. She has no focal neurologic deficits. What is the best next step in management?

A. Lasix
B. Pregnancy test
C. Echocardiogram
D. Head CT scan

6. A 62-year-old male is brought in by ambulance for chest pain. He describes the pain as substernal pressure that radiates to his back. He received aspirin and nitroglycerin from emergency medical services and is now chest pain free. His vital signs are normal. He does not have any known medical problems but has not seen a physician for many years. His troponin at 6 hours after symptom onset is negative, and his EKG is shown in Figure 1.4. Which of the following is best next step in management?

A. Admit for serial troponin and cardiology consult for cardiac catheterization
B. Activate the catheterization lab immediately for intervention
C. Treadmill stress test
D. Repeat troponin and if negative discharge home

7. A 21-year-old female is brought in by ambulance after a motor vehicle collision. She complains of right arm pain. Her radiograph is shown in Figure 1.5. Injury to which of the following is most commonly associated with this type of fracture?

A. Median nerve
B. Ulnar nerve
C. Brachial artery
D. Radial nerve

8. A 23-year-old male presents after an alleged assault. He complains of left eye pain and blurred vision. He has extensive facial trauma, including a large left periorbital contusion. The left eye is proptotic with subconjunctival hemorrhage. The intraocular pressures are 35 mm Hg in the left eye and 10 mm Hg in the right eye. What is the best next step in management?

A. Anterior chamber paracentesis
B. Lateral canthotomy

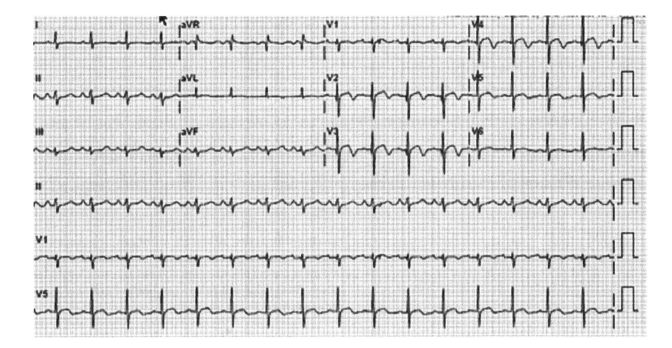

Figure 1.4 Electrocardiogram.

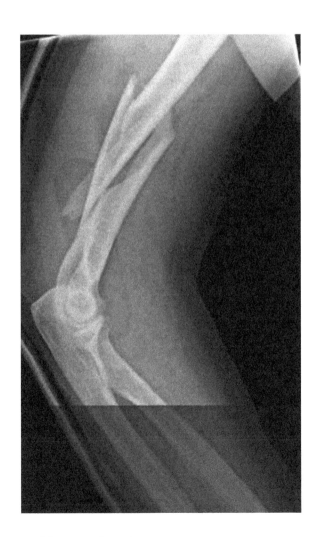

Figure 1.5 Humerus radiograph.

C. Maxillofacial CT with orbits

D. Topical timolol to left eye

9. A 21-day-old male is brought in by his mother because of poor feeding. The baby was delivered at home with the assistance of a doula, but the mother did not receive any prenatal care. He is breastfed but can only feed for a few minutes before he becomes tired and sweaty. He has yet to return to his birth weight. He is afebrile by rectal temperature, and his oxygen saturation is normal. There are no retractions. A holosystolic murmur is appreciated at the left lower sternal border, and the liver is palpable below to the costal margin. Which of the following diagnoses is most likely?

A. Tetralogy of Fallot

B. Tricuspid atresia

C. Total anomalous pulmonary venous return

D. Ventricular septal defect

10. A 46-year-old male presents with rectal pain and bleeding after a bowel movement. He has had external hemorrhoids before but states that he has never had pain like this before. He does not have any medical problems or take any medications. On exam, he appears very uncomfortable and you see a hemorrhoid with a bluish-purple color to the exposed vein. What is the best next step in management?

A. Sitz baths and stool softeners

B. Bedside excision

C. Needle aspiration

D. Emergent surgical consultation

11. A 30-year-old female is involved in a rollover motor vehicle crash at freeway speeds. She was unrestrained and ejected from the vehicle. On arrival, her BP is 80/40, HR is 130 bpm, and she is screaming in pain. Breath sounds are equal bilaterally. There are multiple abrasions and extensive bruising noted to the lower abdomen and hips, and the pelvis is unstable. She has two large-bore IV lines in place, and fluids are infusing. What is the best next step in management?

A. Abdomen/pelvis CT

B. Placement of a pelvic binder

C. Chest and pelvis radiograph

D. Embolization by interventional radiology

12. A 49-year-old female presents with pain, swelling, and redness of the left index finger. She works at an animal shelter and was bitten by a cat 3 days ago on that finger. She has also had fevers, vomiting, and some mild paresthesias in that finger. There is tenderness to palpation along the flexor tendon and severe pain with movement of the index finger. A photo of her hand is shown in Figure 1.6. What is the best next step in management?

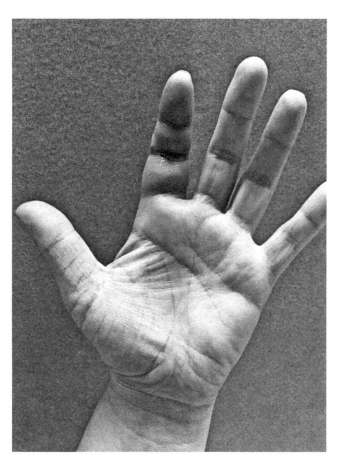

Figure 1.6 Finger.

A. Admit to medicine for IV antibiotics

B. Bedside incision and drainage in the ED, discharge home

C. Hand surgery consult

D. Discharge home with oral antibiotics

13. A 29-year-old male surgery resident presents to the ED with right wrist pain after tripping down the stairs on his way home from a 30-hour shift. He landed on his outstretched right arm. He has limited range of motion in the wrist but no obvious deformity, numbness, or tingling. His radial pulse is 2+, and his digits are warm and well perfused. He has focal tenderness over the anatomic snuffbox and significant pain with axial loading of the thumb. His wrist and hand radiographs are negative for fracture or dislocation. Which of the following is the best next step in management?

A. Place thumb spica splint and follow up in 7 to 10 days for repeat radiographs

B. Discharge home without further intervention

C. CT of the wrist

D. ACE wrap to wrist for comfort

14. A 19-year-old female presents to the ED after smashing her middle finger in a door. She reports significant pain in the distal phalanx of the middle finger and is noted to have a large subungual hematoma. The nail plate and surrounding folds are intact. There is no fracture or dislocation noted on radiograph. Despite pain medication, she complains of severe throbbing pain. Which of the following is the most appropriate management?

A. Apply finger splint and discharge home

B. Nail trephination

C. Removal of the nail

D. Digital block for comfort and discharge home

15. A 33-year-old female presents with a chief complaint of vaginal pain. On exam, she is noted to have swelling and significant tenderness to a fluid collection that is at the 4-o'clock position on the labium majora without overlying cellulitis. She has never had a similar problem in the past. She denies vaginal discharge, dysuria, fevers, nausea, or vomiting. A pregnancy test is negative, and her vital signs are normal. What is the most appropriate course of action in this case?

A. Discharge home on oral antibiotics

B. Bedside I&D with placement of Word catheter

C. CT scan of the pelvis with contrast

D. Surgical marsupialization

16. A 29-year-old female presents with a "bump" on her eyelid. She noticed it a week ago, but it is not very painful. She does not wear contacts and has never had anything like this before. Her vision is normal. One exam, you see a small bump at the eyelid margin (Figure 1.7). How should this problem be managed?

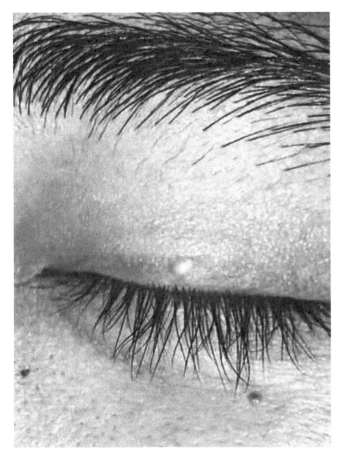

Figure 1.7 Eyelid.

A. IV antibiotics
B. Oral antibiotics
C. Warm compresses
D. Urgent ophthalmology consultation

17. A 13-year-old male is brought in by helicopter after a high-speed motor vehicle collision. He was restrained in the back middle seat of the car. He complains primarily of low back pain and is noted to have a step-off in his lumbar spine with significant midline tenderness. He is moving all extremities, and his sensation is intact. His lumbar spine CT is shown in Figure 1.8. What other injury is classically associated with this type of fracture?

A. Diaphragm rupture
B. Bowel perforation

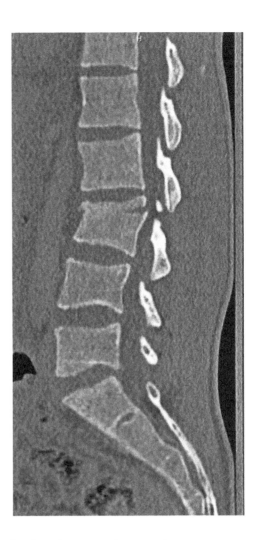

Figure 1.8 Lumbar spine computed tomography.

C. Cervical spine fracture
D. Hip dislocation

18. A 3-year-old female is brought in by her mother with anal pruritus. Her mother states that the girl is constantly scratching herself, but she has noticed that it is much worse at night. She has no other complaints and appears healthy with normal vital signs. Which of the following is true about the condition that is most likely affecting this child?

A. It may present with vaginal discharge in young girls
B. Children may go to group child care without worry about spread to other children
C. The first-line treatment is ivermectin
D. A definitive diagnosis can be made with a stool sample

19. A 59-year-old female with a history of breast cancer presents with leg pain. Her exam is remarkable for a swollen and blueish-colored lower extremity. She has faint distal pulses in her foot, her sensation is intact, and she can wiggle her toes. You are working in a rural hospital that does not have any subspecialty coverage. There is a storm that has grounded all helicopters in the area, and the nearest tertiary care center is 6 hours away by ground. What is the best next step in management?

A. Transfer the patient to the tertiary care center
B. Administer thrombolytics
C. Administer IV antibiotics
D. Apply a compression stocking

20. A 36-year-old female is brought in by ambulance after sustaining a gunshot wound to the left lower leg in a drive-by shooting. She is in severe pain and writhing around the gurney. The primary and secondary survey are completed, and there are no other injuries identified. Her vital signs are stable. She is sent to radiology for tests, and when she returns, her lower leg is very tense. Which of the following is the earliest sign of compartment syndrome?

A. Absent distal pulses
B. Pallor
C. Paralysis
D. Paresthesias

21. A 47-year-old previously healthy woman is brought in by her daughter who states she has been acting strange for several days. She cannot seem to focus, and everyday tasks that she could previously complete with ease are now much more difficult. She has also been unsteady on her feet. The daughter is not aware of any recent falls or trauma. All her vital signs are normal, including a rectal temperature. A noncontrast head CT is done, and the scan is shown in Figure 1.9. Which other finding is most likely to be present?

A. Left-sided hemiparesis
B. Hyporeflexia
C. Anisocoria
D. Urinary incontinence

22. A 5-year-old male is brought in by ambulance from an urgent care center in respiratory distress. He had presented there with his mother for a barky cough and difficulty breathing. Stridor was noted by the urgent care provider, and he was given racemic epinephrine and dexamethasone, but he did not improve. His vital signs include temperature 40.2 °C, HR 140 bpm, respiratory rate (RR) 42 breaths/min, and oxygen saturation 89% on room air. He appears toxic and exhibits deep intercostal retractions as well as stridor. Auscultation of his lungs reveals equal but diminished breath sounds and faint transmitted upper airway noise. What is the best next step in management?

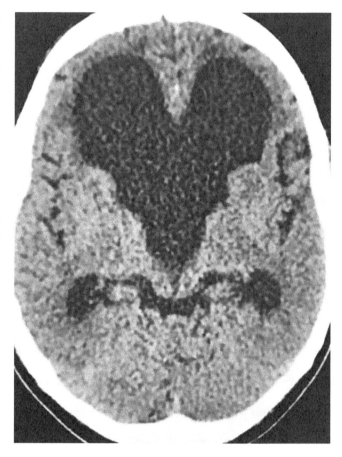

Figure 1.9 Head computed tomography.

A. Continue racemic epinephrine
B. Aggressive suctioning and oxygen using high-flow nasal cannula
C. Noninvasive bilevel positive airway pressure ventilation
D. Intubation

23. A 22-year-old female is sent to the ED by her primary care doctor because of concern for appendicitis. The patient reports right lower quadrant pain that has been worsening over 2 days. She has associated fevers, chills, nausea, and vomiting. A pregnancy test done by her doctor was negative. She appears uncomfortable, and her right lower quadrant is quite tender on exam. She has moderate right adnexal tenderness but no cervical motion tenderness or significant vaginal discharge on pelvic exam. A CT of the abdomen/pelvis is normal, and the appendix was visualized. What is the best next step in management?

A. Urgent general surgery consultation
B. Pelvic ultrasound
C. Discharge home
D. Admit for serial abdominal exams

24. A 34-year-old female is brought in by police after a domestic dispute. She reports being punched multiple times in the face by her husband. There was no loss of consciousness. She reports jaw pain and has tenderness and swelling over the body of the mandible on the right side. She is able to open her mouth fully. There is no blood in the mouth, malocclusion, or other evidence of dental trauma. She is able to break a tongue blade with her teeth. There is no evidence of trauma to the nose or orbits. What is the best next step in management?

A. Panorex
B. Maxillofacial CT scan
C. Discharge with resources for domestic violence
D. Plain film facial series

25. A 12-year-old male presents to the ED with bleeding from a "growth" on his hand. The mother states that he has had it for several weeks, and it bleeds very easily. She has been able to stop the bleeding at home previously but not today. It has been bleeding for the past 2 hours and has nearly soaked through a kitchen towel. The lesion looks like a dark blood blister. The child appears healthy with normal vital signs. You attempt to control the bleeding with direct pressure, but the bleeding worsens. What is the best next step in management?

A. Silver nitrate cautery
B. Bedside excision of the lesion
C. Cryotherapy with liquid nitrogen
D. Emergent dermatology consultation

26. You are working the night shift in a small rural ED. A 19-year-old male presents with right ear pain and swelling after a boxing match earlier in the day. The ear is shown in Figure 1.10. Which of the following is the most appropriate course of action?

A. Immediate needle aspiration or I&D
B. Apply pressure dressing
C. Apply ice, follow up with primary doctor
D. Transfer for urgent ear, nose, and throat specialist consult

27. A 29-year-old male presents with daily headaches for the past 3 weeks. He describes sharp, stabbing pain behind his left eye that occurs several times a day for short periods of time and is associated with lacrimation. He had a similar bout of headaches 6 months ago that lasted for 2 weeks. On exam, he is agitated and restless, his left eye exhibits conjunctival injection, and the left side of his face is sweating. He is started on high-flow oxygen, and his headache completely resolves. Which of the following treatments is most appropriate for this patient after discharge?

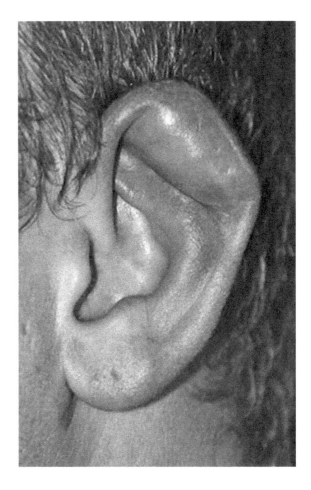

Figure 1.10 Ear.

A. Nonsteroidal antiinflammatory drugs (NSAIDs)
B. Verapamil
C. Lithium
D. Botulinum toxin injections

28. A 36-year-old female presents to the ED with pain in the left side of her neck and head as well as right arm weakness. She reports that the pain started after she went to a chiropractor for an "adjustment" a few days ago, and she noted the weakness last night. On exam, she has objective weakness in the right arm as well as left-sided ptosis and miosis. The remainder of her exam is unremarkable. Her vital signs are normal. A noncontrast CT of the head does not show any abnormalities. What is the most appropriate next step in management?

A. Cerebral angiography
B. Tissue plasminogen activator (tPA)
C. High-dose prednisone
D. CT angiography of the neck

29. A 57-year-old female with a history of chronic obstructive pulmonary disease (COPD) is brought in by ambulance for shortness of breath. She has diminished

breath sounds with diffuse wheezing and accessory muscle use. Noninvasive positive pressure ventilation is started with significant improvement. An hour later, you are notified by nursing that the patient is in severe respiratory distress. She has new onset of jugular venous distention, and her BP is 74/40 mm Hg. Breath sounds are still diminished but are louder on the left. An emergent chest radiograph is taken and shown in Figure 1.11. She suddenly becomes unresponsive and you are unable to find a pulse. In addition to standard advanced cardiac life-saving, what other step should be taken in this case?

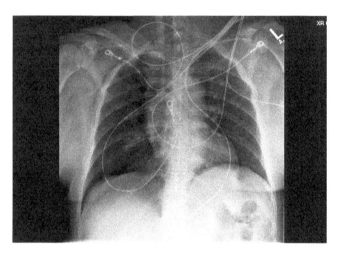

Figure 1.11 Chest radiograph.

A. Administer tPA
B. Needle decompression of the right chest
C. Immediate placement of a right chest tube
D. Intentional right main-stem intubation

30. A 55-year-old female presents with a right-sided headache that has been worsening over the past 3 days. On exam, she exhibits tenderness over the right temporal area but no focal neurologic deficits or meningeal signs. Her vital signs are normal. She later mentions that she has noticed pain with chewing. Labs are unremarkable with the exception of an elevated erythrocyte sedimentation rate (ESR). Which other detail may be elicited from the history in this patient?

A. Urinary incontinence
B. Bilateral shoulder pain
C. Abdominal pain
D. Peripheral neuropathy

31. A 37-year-old male with HIV presents with fevers, chills, and cough productive of thick yellow sputum with occasional streaks of blood. He is noncompliant with his antiretroviral medications, and his most recent CD4 count was 150. He appears ill, and his vital signs include a temperature of 38.8° C, HR of 124 bpm, RR 28 breaths/min, room air oxygen saturation of 92%, and BP of 96/48 mm Hg. Which of the following is the most likely cause of his symptoms?

A. *Streptococcus pneumoniae*
B. Tuberculosis
C. *Pneumocystis jirovecii*
D. *Staphylococcus aureus*

32. A 16-year-old female presents to the ED with joint pain. The pain started in her left knee a few days ago, then spread to her right knee and left wrist. She appears ill and has a fever. She has several lesions that are grey pustules on her extremities, as shown in Figure 1.12. Which of the following tests is most likely to confirm the probable diagnosis?

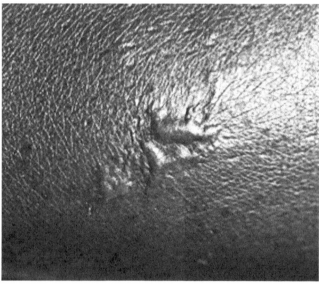

Figure 1.12 Lesion.

A. Blood cultures
B. Darkfield microscopy
C. Cervical and pharyngeal cultures
D. Synovial fluid cultures

33. A 4-year-old male is brought in by his parents for fever and rash that have been ongoing for the past week. The parents are concerned he may have "pink eye" because both his eyes appear bloodshot. The rash is maculopapular and fairly diffuse. There is erythema and desquamation noted on the palms and soles. His oral exam is as shown in Figure 1.13, with extremely red and dry cracked lips. There are no tonsillar exudates. Which of the following treatments is indicated for this condition?

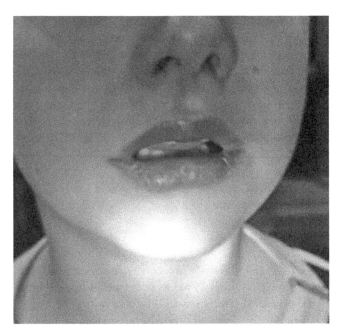

Figure 1.13 Lips.

A. Amoxicillin
B. Aspirin
C. Vitamin B$_{12}$
D. Corticosteroids

34. A 63-year-old female presents with a chief complaint of facial pain. She describes sharp pain in the right side of her face that worsens with chewing or talking. She has also noted that pain is triggered by cold weather. She denies headache, vision changes, or recent trauma. On exam, sensation is intact in all distributions of the face. Which of the following is considered first line treatment for this condition?

A. Corticosteroids
B. NSAIDs
C. Surgical intervention
D. Carbamazepine

35. A 43-year-old female presents to the ED complaining of rash, vomiting, headache, and fatigue. She is febrile and lethargic. Her skin exam is remarkable for a nonblanching purpuric rash. The pertinent lab results include WBC 10.1 × 10³/microliter, hemoglobin 7.8 g/dL, platelets 10,000/mm³, schistocytes on peripheral smear, creatinine 1.5 mg/dL, total bilirubin 1.9 mg/dL (direct bilirubin 0.2 mg/dL). Her head CT is normal. Which of the following is the best next step in management?

A. Lumbar puncture
B. Hematology consultation for plasma exchange

C. Platelet transfusion
D. IV immunoglobulin

36. A 22-year-old male is brought in by ambulance after sustaining a stab wound to the neck in a bar fight. His vital signs are stable, and his Glasgow Coma Scale (GCS) score is 15. There is a 5-cm laceration to the right side of his neck between the thyroid cartilage and the angle of the mandible that violates the platysma. There is minimal active bleeding, a small nonexpanding hematoma, and some subcutaneous emphysema. He does not exhibit stridor or voice change. Which of the following is the most appropriate course of action?

A. Emergent surgical exploration in the operating room
B. Bedside exploration in ED
C. CT angiography of the neck
D. Endoscopy

37. A 57-year-old female presents with left-sided facial droop that she noted when she woke up approximately 1 hour ago. She denies any extremity weakness, numbness, tingling, dysphagia, or dysphonia. Her vital signs are normal. Her physical exam is remarkable for left-sided facial droop that includes both the upper and lower face. Which other finding may be associated with the most likely diagnosis?

A. Decreased hearing in the left ear
B. Inability to open the left eye completely
C. Loss of taste
D. Anisocoria

38. A 42-year-old male with history of Crohn's disease status post ileostomy presents with pain and bleeding from his ostomy. On exam, you see intestine that is pink and normal-looking protruding into his bag. His abdomen is soft, nondistended, and nontender. What is the best next step in management?

A. Attempt bedside reduction
B. Emergent surgical consultation
C. Discharge home with outpatient follow-up
D. Apply an abdominal binder

39. A 38-year-old male is brought in by ambulance with burns after an explosion in a methamphetamine lab. He has partial-thickness burns over most of his face, including his lips, but not inside his mouth. There is no soot in his mouth or nose, his airway is patent, he denies shortness of breath or voice change, and his lungs are clear to auscultation. Which of the following should be done next?

A. Fluorescein exam of the eyes
B. Intubation

C. Start fluid resuscitation using the Parkland formula
D. Place a nasogastric tube

40. A 47-year-old male presents to the ED with nausea, vomiting, generalized weakness, and lethargy. Labs reveal hypernatremia and hypokalemia. Physical exam is remarkable for an obese man with thin extremities, a rounded face, purple striae on his abdomen, and a large fatty deposit in the upper back. Which of the following acid-base disturbances is most likely to be present?

A. Metabolic acidosis
B. Metabolic alkalosis
C. Respiratory acidosis
D. Respiratory alkalosis

41. A 20-year-old female presents with the oral lesions shown in Figure 1.14. Which feature can help distinguish oral herpetic lesions from aphthous ulcers?

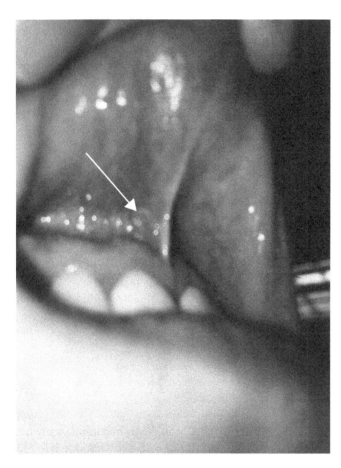

Figure 1.14 Mouth ulcer.

A. Pain
B. Prodromal burning sensation
C. May be precipitated by trauma
D. Lesions on the hard palate

42. A 9-year-old male is brought in by his parents because of swelling in his neck. The parents noticed it this morning, but it does not seem to be bothering the patient. Parents deny any fevers, voice changes, or difficulty swallowing or breathing. The patient has normal vital signs and appears healthy. During the exam of the oropharynx, you note a midline mass that moves when the patient sticks out his tongue. Which of the following is the most likely diagnosis?

A. Branchial cleft cyst
B. Lymphangioma
C. Thyroglossal duct cyst
D. Lymphoma

43. A 24-year-old female presents with severe headache. She reports that she is 15 weeks pregnant by her last menstrual period with her first child but has not yet had an ultrasound or any prenatal care. She has no known medical problems. Her vital signs include BP 170/110 mm Hg, HR 102 bpm, RR 18 breaths/min, and temperature 37.5° C. Her serum β-human chorionic gonadotropin (β-hCG) is 140,000. She has no focal neurologic deficits or meningeal signs. Her lower extremities are edematous, but her lungs are clear to auscultation. The uterine fundus is palpable at the umbilicus. A bedside ultrasound shows heterogeneous material in the uterus but no definite intrauterine pregnancy. What is the most likely diagnosis?

A. Ectopic pregnancy
B. Empty sac pregnancy
C. Missed abortion
D. Molar pregnancy

44. A 13-year-old female presents with pain and swelling of her finger that has been worsening for 3 days (Figure 1.15). The swelling started on the nailbed and has stayed

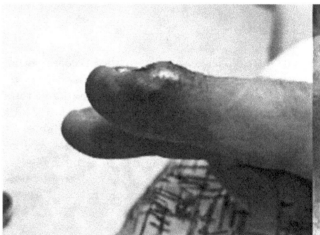

Figure 1.15 Finger.

localized to the side of the finger. What is the best next step in management?

A. Bedside incision and drainage
B. Consult a hand surgeon
C. Discharge with warm water soaks
D. Nail removal

45. A 52-year-old male presents with a painful penile rash. He denies urethral discharge, dysuria, or testicular pain. He is monogamous with his wife of 20 years. Physical exam reveals an uncircumcised penis with an inflamed, erythematous glans covered in small red papules and a small amount of exudate. The patient reports this is the third time he has had such a rash, and it has resolved previously with a cream he was prescribed. Which of the following is the best next step in management?

A. Discharge with clotrimazole cream
B. Discharge with trimethoprim-sulfamethoxazole
C. Point-of-care glucose test
D. Culture of exudate

46. A 41-year-old male presents with hand pain. He was working with a high-pressure paint gun when he accidentally sprayed his left middle finger. The middle finger is mildly edematous and has a small puncture mark near the distal interphalangeal joint. Which of the following is the best treatment option for this patient?

A. Discharge home if radiograph is negative for fracture
B. Emergent surgical consultation for debridement
C. Update tetanus, irrigate, and discharge home with oral antibiotics
D. Admit to medicine for IV antibiotics

47. A 41-year-old male is brought in by ambulance for fever and altered mental status for 1 day. His only medical problem is schizophrenia for which he takes haloperidol. His vital signs include BP 174/110 mm Hg, HR 136 bpm, RR 32 breaths/min, and temperature of 42° C. He is diaphoretic, agitated, and confused. Widespread muscle rigidity is noted. There is no clonus or hyperreflexia. Which of the following is the best next step in management?

A. Diphenhydramine
B. Antipyretics
C. Cyproheptadine
D. Lorazepam

48. A 17-year-old male presents after an alleged assault with a laceration that goes through the top border of his lateral upper lip. Which of the following is the best choice for anesthesia to facilitate laceration repair?

A. Local infiltration through the wound margins
B. Infraorbital nerve block
C. Mental nerve block
D. Topical application of lidocaine

49. A 33-year-old male presents to the ED as part of a mass casualty incident after a bombing at a political rally. He was thrown several feet by the blast. He has no burns or external signs of trauma other than a perforated left tympanic membrane. He denies loss of consciousness, his GCS is 15, he has no focal neurologic deficits, his lungs are clear bilaterally, and his abdomen is nontender. He states that he feels fine and wants to leave. At a minimum, which of the following diagnostic studies should be obtained?

A. Chest radiograph
B. Head CT
C. Cervical spine radiographs
D. Abdominal/pelvic CT

50. A 36-year-old female is brought in by ambulance for shortness of breath that started 1 hour before arrival. She is noted to have swollen lips and tongue, stridor, and labored breathing. She has no wheezing, rash, abdominal pain, nausea, or vomiting. Her vital signs include BP 156/92 mm Hg, HR 110 bpm, RR 34 breaths/min, and SpO$_2$ 97% on a non-rebreather mask. There is no improvement with intramuscular epinephrine or IV diphenhydramine, and she is emergently intubated. A family member arrives and reports that the patient's mother has had a similar presentation in the past. What is the best next step in management?

A. Start an epinephrine drip
B. Administer fresh frozen plasma
C. Administer C1 esterase inhibitor
D. Administer corticosteroids

51. A 41-year-old female with history of psoriasis presents to the ED with a rash over most of her body that spares the mucous membranes. She just moved to the area and has not yet established care with a dermatologist. She had gone to a walk-in clinic for a psoriasis flare and was given a medication. Since starting the medication, the rash is now much worse. Which of the following was likely prescribed?

A. Prednisone
B. Clobetasol ointment
C. Cephalexin
D. Topical tacrolimus

52. A 28-year-old male presents with right testicle pain that has been worsening over the past 2 days. He denies any trauma, penile discharge, dysuria, fever, vomiting,

or abdominal pain. Physical exam reveals a swollen and tender right testicle without any overlying skin changes or penile discharge. Prehn's sign is positive. He is afebrile and appears healthy with normal vital signs. Doppler ultrasound is performed and shows increased flow to the right testicle. Which of the following is the best next step in management?

A. Emergent urology consultation
B. Outpatient treatment with ceftriaxone and azithromycin
C. Outpatient treatment with levofloxacin
D. Admission for IV antibiotics

53. A 17-day-old female is brought in by her mother for cough for 3 days and respiratory distress for the last hour. Her rectal temperature is 37.5° C, and she is tachypneic with intercostal retractions, diffuse rales, and a staccato cough. A chest radiograph does not show any focal consolidation. She was born at home at about 37 weeks' gestation, and her mother did not have any prenatal care. What is the most likely organism responsible for her condition?

A. *S. aureus*
B. *Chlamydia trachomatis*
C. Influenza A
D. *Pseudomonas*

54. A 27-year-old female with von Willebrand's disease presents with heavy vaginal bleeding. She reports that she has soaked through two large menstrual pads an hour for the past 3 hours. Her pregnancy test is negative. Pelvic examination reveals heavy bleeding from the os with several large clots in the vaginal vault. Labs include hemoglobin of 8.2 g/dL and platelets of 175×10^3/microliter. Which of the following treatments will be the most effective in this case?

A. Platelet transfusion
B. Factor VIII concentrate
C. Desmopressin
D. Cryoprecipitate

55. A 3-year-old male is brought in by his stepfather with right leg pain. The stepfather reports that the child fell while running around the house and now refuses to bear weight on his right leg. In the ED, he will not move the leg or bear weight, and he cries when his lower leg is touched. He has a strong pedal pulse in the right foot, and his sensation appears to be intact. His compartments are soft. His radiograph is shown in Figure 1.16. Which of the following is the best next step in this case?

A. Urgent consult to orthopedics

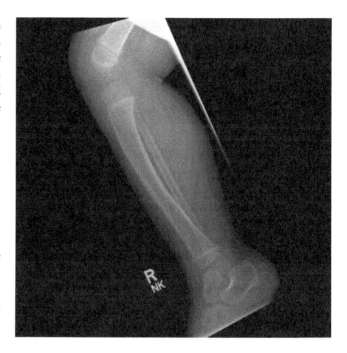

Figure 1.16 Tibia-fibula radiograph.

B. Long leg splint and discharge home with outpatient orthopedics follow-up
C. Perform skeletal survey and notify child protective services of suspected abuse
D. Discharge home with reassurance

56. A 59-year-old female presents with right eye pain and blurred vision for 2 days. She denies foreign body sensation, discharge, headache, fever, or vomiting. She does not wear contact lenses. On exam, there is conjunctival injection and both direct and consensual photophobia. The intraocular pressure is 18 in the left eye and 20 in the right eye. There is no uptake of fluorescein. Her visual acuity is 20/20 in the left eye and 20/80 in the right eye. There is cell and flare noted on slit lamp examination of the right eye. Which of the following medications is most appropriate to administer in the ED?

A. Scopolamine drops
B. Timolol drops
C. Gentamicin drops
D. Prednisolone drops

57. A 31-year-old female presents with right wrist pain that has been gradually worsening over 3 weeks. She denies trauma. The pain is making it difficult for her to hold her baby. Examination of the wrist reveals point tenderness and mild swelling over the radial styloid as well as significant worsening of the pain with ulnar deviation of the wrist. Her sensation is intact to light touch in all distributions of the hand and she has a

strong radial pulse. Which of the following is the best next step in management?

A. Arthrocentesis of the right wrist
B. Volar splint worn at night and NSAIDs
C. Thumb spica splint and NSAIDs
D. Right wrist radiograph

58. A 39-year-old female presents with chest pain, shortness of breath, and diaphoresis for 1 hour. Her vital signs are BP 189/110 mm Hg, HR 105 bpm, RR 24 breaths/min, SpO_2 97% on room air, temperature 37.2° C. On exam, she is diaphoretic, appears distressed, and is clutching her chest. Her heart sounds are regular with a mid-systolic click. You notice that she is so tall that her feet hang off the end of the gurney and that she has long slender fingers. The EKG shows sinus tachycardia with signs of left ventricular hypertrophy, but no ST or T wave changes. What is the best next step in management for this patient?

A. CT angiogram of the aorta
B. Emergent consult to cardiology for left heart catheterization
C. CT pulmonary angiogram
D. D-dimer

59. A 4-year-old female presents with the rash shown in Figure 1.17. Per the mother, the patient had a high fever for the past 3 days with associated mild cough and rhinorrhea. She has not had a fever today, and the rash just appeared shortly before arrival to the ED. She is fully immunized and appears healthy and playful. Her rash is generalized with blanching red macules and papules. Which of the following is the most likely cause of her rash?

A. Rubella
B. Varicella-zoster
C. Human herpesvirus 6
D. Rubeola

60. An 18-month-old boy is brought to the ED by ambulance after his mother caught him biting an electrical cord. He sustained facial burns as shown in Figure 1.18. There is no active bleeding. He is crying vigorously but is without other signs of trauma and appears healthy. Development of which of the following is a concern for this patient?

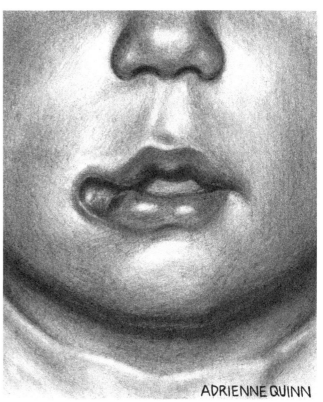

Figure 1.18 Lip burn.

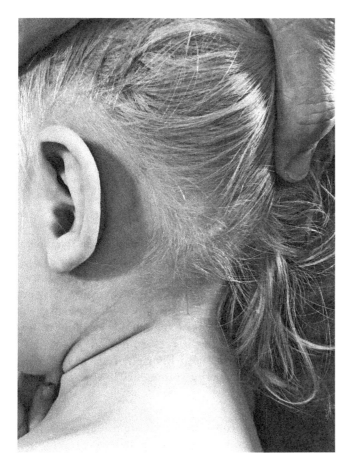

Figure 1.17 Rash.

A. Delayed labial artery bleeding
B. Rhabdomyolysis
C. Hyperkalemia
D. Seizures

61. A 49-year-old female presents with left knee pain after a fall. She tripped while walking her dog and struck her flexed knee against the edge of a cement curb. There are no open wounds noted. Her knee radiograph is shown in Figure 1.19. Which of the following features, if present, would be most helpful in determining whether this patient could be safely managed nonoperatively?

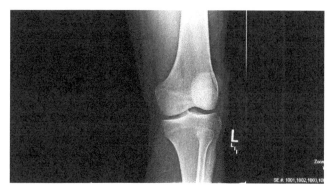

Figure 1.19 Knee radiograph.

A. Ability to bear weight
B. Ability to fully extend the knee
C. Ability to fully flex the knee
D. Lack of significant hemarthrosis

62. A 34-year-old female presents with severe headache, left eye pain, and double vision. She was recently treated for a sinus infection but otherwise has no medical problems. She denies any trauma. She is ill appearing with a high fever. The left eye is proptotic with chemosis, conjunctival injection, and eyelid edema. The left pupil is nonreactive to light. Which of the following additional findings is most likely to be present in this patient?

A. Decreased sensation over left side of chin
B. Inability to abduct the left eye
C. Upper and lower left-sided facial droop
D. Deviation of the mandible with mouth opening

63. A 6-year-old male presents to the ED with right knee pain and swelling for 2 days. He refuses to bear weight. He has associated fever and vomiting. His mother denies any recent trauma. His knee is hot to the touch, and he has severe pain with mild passive motion. Labs reveal leukocytosis and an elevated C-reactive protein (CRP). Which of the following statements is true regarding the most likely diagnosis in this case?

A. Blood cultures are positive in the majority of cases

B. *Streptococcus* is the most common causative organism
C. Right knee radiograph is likely to be diagnostic
D. Synovial fluid cultures are negative in approximately one-third of cases

64. A 55-year-old male presents with altered mental status and left-sided weakness. He is unable to provide any history, but chart review reveals he has history of hypertension and atrial fibrillation for which he takes lisinopril and apixaban. He does not move his left arm or leg even with painful stimuli. His BP is 210/140 mm Hg, and his HR is 65 bpm. A CT of his head is shown in Figure 1.20. Which of the following is the most appropriate treatment?

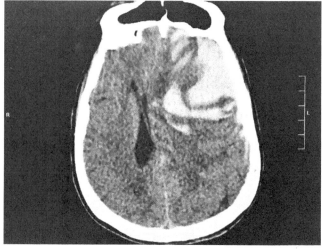

Figure 1.20 Head computed tomography.

A. Protamine sulfate
B. Prothrombin complex concentrates
C. Idarucizumab
D. Fresh frozen plasma

65. A 15-year-old male presents with fever, headache, malaise, myalgias, and testicular pain. He denies dysuria, penile discharge, or rash and is not sexually active. He recently immigrated from Haiti. On exam, you note facial swelling that is bilateral, mostly localized over the parotid glands and tender to palpation. His abdomen is soft and nontender, but his scrotum is edematous and mildly erythematous, and his right testicle is tender. Which of the following statements is true regarding this condition?

A. Sterility is a common complication
B. Aseptic meningitis is a rare complication
C. It is a leading cause of deafness in the developing world

D. All cases should be treated with systemic antibiotics

66. A 22-year-old male presents with blurred vision in his right eye after a boxing match. He denies eye pain, headache, loss of consciousness, or vomiting. He has some periorbital edema and ecchymosis, but his extra-ocular movements are intact. His left pupil is 5 mm, round, and reactive. His right pupil is 2 mm, round and minimally reactive. There is no fluorescein uptake, and the globe appears intact. His visual acuity is 20/30 in the left eye and 20/200 in the right eye, and he endorses monocular diplopia with the right eye. His intraocular pressures are 18 in the right eye and 17 in the left eye. An ocular ultrasound of his right eye is done and shows a circular structure free-floating in the globe.
What is the most likely diagnosis?

A. Retinal detachment
B. Traumatic iritis
C. Vitreous hemorrhage
D. Lens dislocation

67. A 27-year-old female who is 29 weeks pregnant presents after a motor vehicle collision. She is complaining of abdominal pain, and a seat belt sign is noted across her abdomen. Which of the following is the most sensitive indicator of placental abruption?

A. Retroplacental hematoma on ultrasound
B. Uterine irritability measured by tocometry
C. Vaginal bleeding
D. Maternal hemodynamic instability

68. A 34-year-old obese female presents with progressively worsening headaches over the past 3 weeks. She denies fever, numbness, weakness, or gait disturbance. She appears uncomfortable and is holding her head in her hands but is afebrile with normal vital signs. Her neck is supple, and she has no focal neurologic deficits. Her fundoscopic exam shows papilledema. A CT of the head is unremarkable. Lumbar puncture is performed in the left lateral decubitus position, and the opening pressure is noted to be 32. The fluid is clear, and laboratory analysis is normal. What is the major complication of this condition if not treated appropriately?

A. Uncal herniation
B. Permanent visual loss
C. Deafness
D. Hydrocephalus

69. A 31-year-old male with history of schizophrenia is brought in on an involuntary psychiatric hold. He is disheveled, and his thoughts are disorganized. He has not been taking his psychiatric medications for quite some time and appears to be responding to internal stimuli. He is combative and given an intramuscular injection of haloperidol. Shortly thereafter, he is noted to have unusual facial grimacing. Which of the following medications should be administered?

A. Lorazepam
B. Benztropine
C. Cyclobenzaprine
D. Amantadine

70. A 41-year-old male presents with skin lesions on his arm. He initially noticed a reddish-purple papule and assumed that he had been bitten by an insect while working outdoors at his job as a landscaper. He did not think much of it until he developed painless nodules that spread proximally up his arm and later ulcerated. The lesions have now started draining serous fluid. He appears healthy with normal vital signs. Which of the following is the most appropriate treatment for this patient?

A. Surgical consultation for debridement
B. Wet to dry dressing changes until resolution
C. Oral itraconazole
D. Oral trimethoprim-sulfamethoxazole

71. A 62-year-old male presents after a syncopal episode that occurred while jogging. He was assisted to the ground by a friend who was jogging alongside him, and he did not hit his head. Immediately before the fall he complained of chest pain. He is now alert and oriented, and his chest pain has resolved. His vital signs are normal. On exam, he is a fit man who appears younger than his stated age. Auscultation of his chest reveals a normal rate and regular rhythm with a systolic murmur heard best at the right second intercostal space. His lungs are clear bilaterally. His abdomen is soft, nondistended, and nontender, and he does not have any peripheral edema. He has never smoked, and he has no known medical problems. Labs including a complete blood count (CBC), chemistry panel, and troponin are unremarkable, and his chest radiograph is normal. He denies family history of heart disease. His EKG is shown in Figure 1.21. Which of the following is the most likely diagnosis?

A. Aortic stenosis
B. Pulmonary embolism
C. Acute coronary syndrome
D. Wolff-Parkinson-White syndrome

72. A 71-year-old female with history of hypertension, congestive heart failure, and atrial fibrillation presents

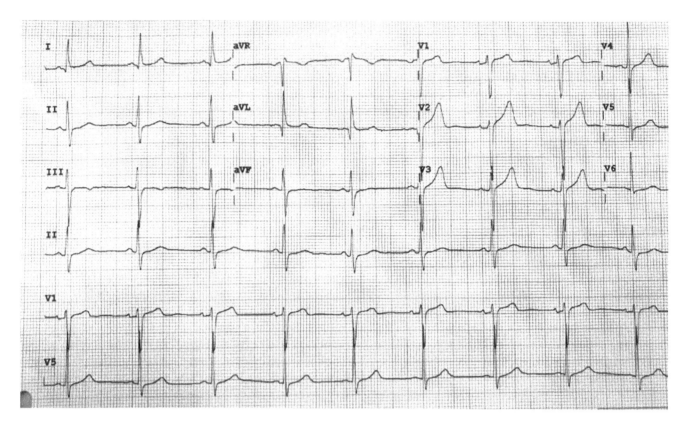

Figure 1.21 Electrocardiogram.

with abdominal pain and vomiting that started 1 hour ago. The pain is poorly localized but severe. She is writhing around on the bed. On exam, her abdomen is soft and nondistended with mild generalized tenderness but no guarding. She has an irregularly irregular heart rhythm, and her lungs are clear to auscultation. Pertinent labs include WBC 18, hemoglobin 11.2, platelets 240, Na 140, K 4.1, Cl 102, CO_2 15, blood urea nitrogen 30, creatinine 1.2, glucose 92, and lactate 4.2. CT of the abdomen and pelvis shows multiple areas of small bowel thickening but is otherwise unremarkable. What is the best next step in management?

A. Start antibiotics and admit to medicine
B. Start antibiotics and consult general surgery
C. Attempt to control pain and discharge home
D. Consult gastroenterology

73. A 48-year-old female presents with left wrist pain that has been worsening over the past month. The pain interferes with her work as a medical transcriptionist and worsens at night. She reports numbness and tingling in her hand as well. You are concerned about carpal tunnel syndrome. Which of the following would be the most useful to confirm your suspicions?

A. Positive Tinel test
B. Positive Phalen maneuver

C. Two-point discrimination in index and middle fingers
D. Weakness with wrist extension

74. A 7-month-old female is brought in by ambulance with her mother after she reportedly stopped breathing. Per the mother, she was changing the infant's diaper when she appeared to stop breathing for approximately 30 seconds. She did not exhibit any cyanosis or loss of consciousness. She had not been fed for more than 2 hours before the episode, but she typically feeds without any difficulty and does not arch her back or have excessive spitting up after feeds. The patient does not have any medical problems and was born at term by vaginal delivery without complication. She has normal vital signs, including a core temperature, and appears healthy without any abnormalities noted on exam. The mother states that the patient was at her usual state of health before this event and has not recently been ill. Her immunizations are up to date. There is no family history of sudden cardiac death. After a period of 4 hours of observation in the ED, the patient's condition has not changed, and she has tolerated a bottle feed without complication. Which of the following is the best next step in management of this patient?

A. Obtain CBC, chemistry panel, and CRP
B. Recommend a home cardiopulmonary monitoring system

C. Admit for observation with cardiopulmonary monitoring

D. Reassure the mother and discharge the patient home with return precautions and next-day follow-up

75. A 31-year-old male presents with thoracic back pain progressively worsening over the past 3 days. He is now unable to walk and is having difficulty urinating. Today he developed diffuse myalgias, chills, and neck stiffness. He denies any trauma. His oral temperature is 38.8° C, HR is 128 bpm, and BP is 104/68 mm Hg. Exam reveals midline tenderness over the entire thoracic spine, weakness in both lower extremities, diminished patellar reflexes, weak rectal tone, and track marks. Which of the following is the best diagnostic test for this patient?

A. CT of the thoracic spine with contrast

B. Magnetic resonance imaging (MRI) of the thoracic spine with contrast

C. MRI of the cervical, thoracic, and lumbar spine with contrast

D. Lumbar puncture

76. A 21-year-old male presents with left shoulder pain after reaching up for an object on the top shelf of his closet. He reports feeling a clunk when his arm was extended. His shoulder appears squared off and he cannot range it. He denies any direct trauma. His shoulder radiograph is shown in Figure 1.22. Which of the following is most commonly associated with this injury?

A. Radial nerve neuropraxia with wrist drop

B. Axillary nerve neuropraxia with diminished sensation over the deltoid

C. Axillary artery injury

D. Brachial plexus injury

77. A 37-year-old male presents with rectal pain and diarrhea for 2 days. He endorses painful bowel movements with a constant feeling of rectal fullness but denies any obvious rectal bleeding. His social history is pertinent for receptive anal intercourse. On exam, he has significant tenderness with digital rectal examination, but there are no apparent anal fissures, hemorrhoids, or areas of fluctuance. His vital signs are normal aside from a HR of 110 bpm. You are concerned about perirectal abscess and obtain a CT scan. The scan does not reveal any abscesses but is suggestive of proctitis. Which of the following treatment regimens should be initiated?

A. Oral clindamycin

B. Intramuscular ceftriaxone and oral doxycycline

C. IV vancomycin

D. Oral metronidazole and ciprofloxacin

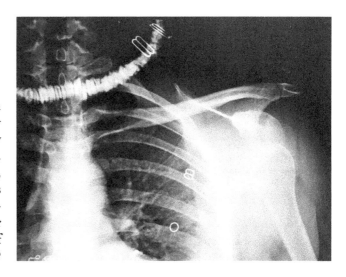

Figure 1.22 Shoulder radiograph.

78. A 15-day-old male presents with lethargy and vomiting for 12 hours. He is ill appearing and tachycardic and has a distended, tense abdomen. His core temperature is normal. The mother shows you a blanket that is covered in bright green emesis. In addition to resuscitation, which of the following is the best next step in management?

A. Obtain surgical consultation

B. Abdominal ultrasound

C. CT of the abdomen

D. Air-contrast enema

79. A 42-year-old female presents from her primary care doctor's office for a supratherapeutic international normalized ratio (INR) and rectal bleeding. The patient takes warfarin for right lower extremity deep vein thrombosis. Her INR was 12 at her physician's office and is confirmed on repeat testing. She reports bloody stools for 3 days and had a large grossly bloody bowel movement in the ED. She is hemodynamically stable at this time. She is given vitamin K and fresh frozen plasma. During the transfusion, the patient develops acute shortness of breath, and her oxygen saturation drops to 85%. A chest radiograph shows bilateral pulmonary infiltrates with a normal cardiac silhouette. She has no history of cardiac disease. Aside from stopping the transfusion, which of the following will most likely be a part of this patient's management?

A. Aggressive diuresis

B. IV antibiotics

C. Intubation

D. Steroids

80. A 59-year-old male presents with a painless lesion on his hand. It has an eschar in the center and a raised

red rim. He first noticed a pruritic papule in the area that evolved into the lesion. He has no other complaints and appears healthy with normal vital signs. He is visiting from West Africa, where he manufactures handmade leather drums for a living. Which of the following is the most appropriate treatment for his condition?

A. Ciprofloxacin
B. Surgical consultation for emergent debridement
C. High-dose IV penicillin
D. Plasmapheresis

81. A 67-year-old female with history of both COPD and congestive heart failure presents with shortness of breath. She is tachypneic and hypoxic and has diminished but coarse breath sounds bilaterally. The etiology of her shortness of breath is uncertain, and the radiology technician is tied up taking care of a trauma patient. A bedside ultrasound of her lungs is performed and is shown in Figure 1.23. This finding is most suggestive of which of the following causes for her shortness of breath?

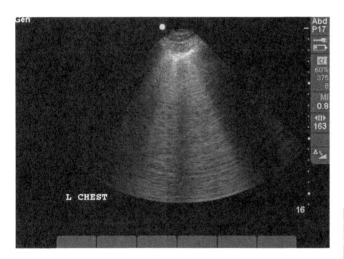

Figure 1.23 Ultrasound of chest.

A. Pneumothorax
B. Pulmonary edema
C. Bronchospasm
D. Pulmonary embolism

82. A 5-day-old male neonate is brought in by his mother for redness and purulent drainage around the umbilical stump. The mother had very limited prenatal care, and the baby was born at home without assistance. On exam, the umbilical stump has surrounding erythema and edema. According to the mother, the neonate has been breastfeeding well and has had normal urine output. He is afebrile by rectal temperature and vigorous with a strong suck. Which of the following is the most appropriate management for this patient?

A. Discharge home with instructions to apply rubbing alcohol to stump
B. Discharge home with oral trimethoprim-sulfamethoxazole
C. Start broad-spectrum IV antibiotics and admit
D. Perform bedside incision and drainage of the umbilical stump

83. A 38-year-old male with sickle cell disease presents with a chief complaint of eye pain. He denies any recent trauma and has no other complaints. His vision remains intact. A photo of the eye is shown in Figure 1.24. Which of the following medications should be avoided in this patient?

A. Timolol
B. Acetazolamide
C. Cyclopentolate
D. Prednisolone drops

84. A 32-year-old male presents with a fracture of the right tibia after a fall from a ladder. The patient tells the orthopedist that he sometimes has an "irregular heartbeat." You are handed an EKG by the patient's nurse that was ordered by the orthopedist for preoperative clearance. The EKG is shown in Figure 1.25. If the patient were to suddenly develop a wide-complex

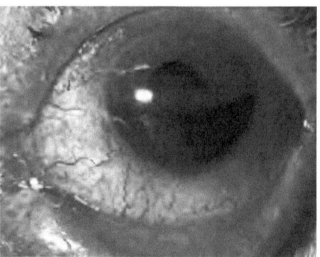

Figure 1.24 Eye.

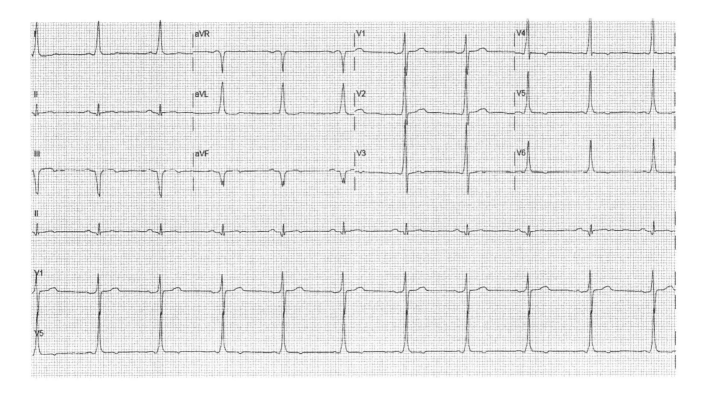

Figure 1.25 Electrocardiogram.

tachycardia while in the ED, which of the following medications would be most appropriate?

A. Metoprolol
B. Diltiazem
C. Digoxin
D. Procainamide

85. A 32-year-old G3P2 female at 39 weeks' gestation presents in active labor. On initial inspection of the perineum you see the umbilical cord coming out of the introitus. Which of the following is the best next step in management?

A. Attempt to reduce the cord immediately
B. Instruct the mother to push immediately
C. Elevated the presenting part and consult obstetrics-gynecology immediately for emergency cesarean delivery
D. Perform the Gaskin maneuver

ANSWERS

1. ANSWER: B

This presentation is concerning for necrotizing fasciitis. Necrotizing fasciitis is a rapidly progressing life-threatening infection. The next step in management is surgical consultation for debridement. Broad-spectrum IV antibiotics should also be started as soon as possible, and blood cultures should be collected. Bedside incision and drainage (I&D) is not appropriate. If a computed tomography (CT) scan were to be done, it would show soft tissue gas, but CT should not delay surgical consultation or administration of IV antibiotics.

These infections are usually polymicrobial in origin. Patient risk factors for this include diabetes, immunosuppression, alcoholism, and IV drug abuse.

Mortality approaches 100% in true necrotizing infections if treated with antibiotics alone, rather than surgical debridement plus antibiotic therapy.

Test-taking tip: There are few indications for emergent surgical consultation that cannot wait for imaging, and it is worth familiarizing yourself with these for the "best next step in management" questions.

2. ANSWER: C

This child swallowed a coin that is now lodged in his esophagus, with some degree of obstruction given the drooling. Coins in the esophagus will generally present on anteroposterior view, while those in the trachea will display on lateral view. Coins at the cricopharyngeus muscle (level of C6) in children generally do not pass and should be removed. In asymptomatic children, coins in the mid to lower esophagus may be observed for 24 hours with repeat radiographs to evaluate for passage. If there is any suggestion that the object ingested was a button battery, it must be removed immediately because perforation can occur in as little as 6 hours. Button batteries classically display a "double-ring sign" on the radiograph. Other indications for emergent endoscopy include ingestion of sharp or elongated objects, ingestion of more than one magnet, evidence of perforation or airway compromise, or ingestion that occurs more than 24 hours before presentation. Vomiting should not be induced because it may result in aspiration. There is no indication of abuse, and therefore child protective services do not need to be involved.

Test-taking tip: The image in this question is the key to the answer. Coins are face up (horizontal) in the esophagus and vertical (on edge) in the trachea.

3. ANSWER: D

This rash is consistent with herpes zoster, commonly known as shingles. Shingles presents with a vesicular rash in a dermatomal distribution. In this patient, the infection involves the ophthalmic distribution of the trigeminal nerve. This puts the patient at high risk for developing herpes ophthalmicus. Involvement of the nasociliary nerve manifests with lesions on the tip or sides of the nose (as seen here) and is known as Hutchinson's sign. Hutchinson's sign is highly suggestive of ocular involvement. This patient should have a fluorescein exam to evaluate for corneal lesions.

Topical steroids are not indicated for the treatment of herpes zoster. Cephalexin is a first-generation cephalosporin commonly used to treat skin infections such as cellulitis but is not indicated for the treatment of shingles. A dermatology consult may be ordered at some point but is not emergent.

Test-taking tip: This image is a classic picture of herpes zoster. It is one you need to know.

4. ANSWER: B

This patient most likely has pelvic inflammatory disease (PID). The most common cause of PID is sexually transmitted infection, particularly gonorrhea and/or chlamydia. However, polymicrobial infections also occur. The outpatient regimen typically includes a single intramuscular dose of ceftriaxone followed by oral doxycycline for 14 days. However, this patient may be too sick for outpatient treatment given her unstable vital signs and active vomiting. Additionally, she has had anaphylaxis to penicillin. She will therefore require parenteral antibiotics and should not be given cephalosporins. The best regimen in this case would be IV clindamycin and gentamicin. Vancomycin does not cover the usual pathogens associated with PID. Metronidazole is used for trichomoniasis and bacterial vaginosis and may be added if the wet mount is suggestive of these infections, but a combination of ceftriaxone and metronidazole does not provide coverage for chlamydia, which is essential in the management of PID.

Test-taking tip: The key to this question is knowing the treatment of PID for a penicillin-allergic patient. You can rule out answers A and D because ceftriaxone is a close relative to penicillin.

5. ANSWER: B

This patient is a female of childbearing potential with classic findings of preeclampsia. A pregnancy test should be performed, and if positive, obstetrics-gynecology should be consulted and treatment promptly initiated. If the pregnancy test is negative, the patient likely has hypertensive emergency with new-onset congestive heart failure. In that case, Lasix and an echocardiogram would be indicated. A CT of the head may be included in the workup of hypertensive emergency if there are focal neurologic deficits, signs of encephalopathy, hypertensive retinopathy, or elevated intracranial pressure.

Test-taking tip: Hypertension in a patient of childbearing age is pregnancy related until proved otherwise.

6. ANSWER: A

The EKG demonstrates changes seen in Wellens' syndrome and is highly suggestive of a proximal left anterior descending artery occlusion. The Wellens' pattern is characterized by deep T wave inversions, or biphasic T waves, in V_1–V_4, sometimes extending to V_5–V_6. Wellens' pattern is classically seen when the patient is chest pain free, and the EKG may normalize when the pain returns. Serial troponin levels are often normal. Patients with Wellens' syndrome should be admitted for cardiology evaluation and early catheterization, but emergent intervention is not required. Given that this patient most likely has critical stenosis of his left anterior descending (LAD) artery, he should *not* undergo stress testing because this may result in an acute myocardial infarction or cardiac arrest. Finally, discharging home is not advised as he is at high risk for having an ST elevation myocardial infarction within the next month.

Test-taking tip: This is a "you know it or don't" kind of question. If you don't know it, choose an answer and move on. You can perhaps mark it for review when you are done at the end of the test. Don't, however, let these kinds of questions get you stuck and waste your time. Review high-risk EKGs like Wellens' syndrome before the exam.

7. ANSWER: D

While all of the listed structures can be injured with humeral shaft fractures, injury to the radial nerve is the most common, particularly when the fracture involves the distal third of the humerus. Depending on the severity, radial nerve injury may manifest as full wrist drop, weak wrist extension, or numbness over the dorsum of the hand between the thumb and index finger. Median nerve injury would result in inability to oppose the thumb and small finger, flex the thumb, and flex the distal and proximal interphalangeal joints of the index finger as well as sensory loss over the volar surfaces of the thumb, index, and middle fingers and the dorsal surface of the middle and distal phalanges of the index and middle fingers. Injury to the brachial artery would result in decreased or absent pulses distally. Finally, if the ulnar nerve were injured, the patient would be unable to hold a piece of paper pinched between the thumb and radial side of the index finger (thumb adduction) and would have diminished sensation over the volar aspect of the small finger and the dorsal surface of the distal phalanx of the small finger.

Test-taking tip: While it is important clinically to be familiar with all possible complications of a particular type of fracture, exams will often test you on the most common.

8. ANSWER: B

The most likely diagnosis in this patient is retrobulbar hematoma. This may occur after trauma to the face or ocular surgery. The buildup of pressure from the hematoma behind the eye increases intraocular pressure and results in pain, proptosis, vision changes, and restricted extraocular movements. If the pressure is not relieved, it may result in permanent vision loss due to ischemia of the optic nerve and/or occlusion of the central retinal artery. The best treatment option is surgical decompression, but lateral canthotomy should be performed at the bedside in the ED if there is any delay in obtaining ophthalmology consultation.

Anterior chamber paracentesis is rarely performed in the ED but may be used to treat elevated intraocular pressure from acute angle closure glaucoma, uveitis, or hyphema. It would not be indicated for a retrobulbar hematoma. A maxillofacial CT with orbits would confirm the diagnosis of retrobulbar hematoma (Figure 1.26) as well as evaluate for other facial trauma, but the diagnosis is

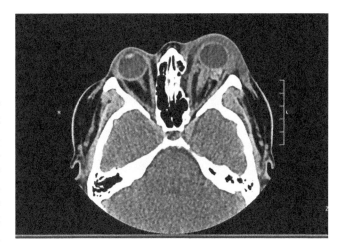

Figure 1.26 Maxillofacial computed tomography.

clinical, and decompression should not be delayed to obtain imaging. Finally, timolol is a topical β-blocker that is used to lower intraocular pressure in glaucoma. It may be used as an adjunct in retrobulbar hematoma but is not a definitive treatment and would not be the best next step in the management of this patient.

Test-taking tip: You can eliminate A because this is not a procedure that emergency medicine physicians perform. Also, you can tell by the question stem that this is not glaucoma, so you can eliminate D and narrow you choices down to two.

9. ANSWER: D

This child is exhibiting signs of congenital heart disease, specifically sweating and difficulty with feeding, failure to thrive, and hepatomegaly. The most likely diagnosis in this case is ventricular septal defect (VSD) as evidenced by the holosystolic murmur at the left lower sternal border.

Hepatomegaly results from congestion of the liver from backup of venous blood due to heart failure. Remember that in infants and children, fluid overload from heart failure generally results in hepatomegaly and ascites rather than the extremity edema seen in adults. All of the other answer choices are types of cyanotic congenital heart diseases and therefore should present with cyanosis and hypoxia. Cyanosis is not typically seen in VSD until later in childhood or adolescence if it has gone uncorrected, resulting in right-to-left shunting known as Eisenmenger's complex.

Remember the cyanotic congenital heart diseases include the "five Ts":

- Tetralogy of Fallot
- Truncus arteriosus
- Tricuspid atresia
- Transposition of the great vessels
- Total anomalous pulmonary venous return.

Test-taking tip: Even if you are unsure of the answer, look for patterns. For example, in this question, all of the answer choices are types of congenital heart disease, but all except one are cyanotic heart diseases; therefore the one answer that does not fit the pattern is likely correct.

10. ANSWER: B

This patient is suffering from a thrombosed external hemorrhoid. This can be very painful, and significant relief can be achieved with bedside excision. This is done by administering local anesthetic, making an elliptical incision, and removing the clot. Needle aspiration and incision and drainage are ineffective because they will not remove the entire clot and may lead to rebleeding or skin tag formation. Sitz baths and stool softeners may be appropriate management for nonthrombosed external hemorrhoids in addition to analgesics. Patients with hemorrhoids may be referred to a surgeon as an outpatient to consider hemorrhoidectomy, but this is typically not emergent unless the patient has thrombosed or gangrenous internal hemorrhoids.

Test-taking tip: You can eliminate D immediately because you know that hemorrhoids are not surgical emergencies.

11. ANSWER: B

This patient is presenting after major trauma with unstable vital signs and a physical exam suggestive of pelvic fracture. The pelvic radiograph may reveal an open book pelvis as seen in Figure 1.27. She is most likely hemorrhaging as the result of vascular injury from pelvic fracture fragments. A pelvic binder should be placed immediately in an attempt to temporarily tamponade the bleeding. Remember that hemorrhage control is part of the "C" in the "ABCs" of advanced trauma life support. When pelvic fracture is suggested by the physical exam in an unstable patient, the binder should be placed before obtaining the chest and pelvis radiographs that are adjuncts to the primary survey. If pelvic fractures are confirmed on the radiographs, the patient should undergo emergent embolization by interventional radiology, if available, or emergent surgical intervention to control the bleeding after the binder is placed as a temporizing measure. This patient is too unstable to go for a CT scan at this moment.

Test-taking tip: This question paints the picture of a very unstable trauma patient. You can eliminate A (CT scan) because the patient is too unstable to go to the scanner initially.

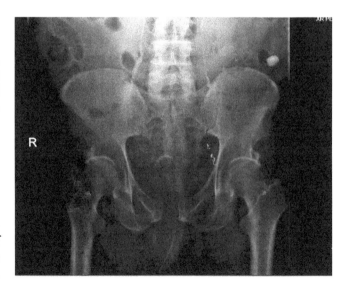

Figure 1.27 Pelvis radiograph.

12. ANSWER: C

This case is concerning for flexor tenosynovitis. The classic findings of flexor tenosynovitis are known as the Kanavel signs and include: digit held in partial flexion, pain with passive extension, tenderness along flexor tendon sheath, and fusiform swelling of the digit.

A hand surgeon should be consulted emergently for potential surgical drainage and debridement. Patients should also be started on IV antibiotics with coverage for staphylococci and streptococci and, in this case in particular, coverage for pathogens associated with cat bites such as *Pasteurella* and anaerobes. Antibiotics should be given parenterally, but antibiotics alone are insufficient. If untreated, tenosynovitis may result in tendon necrosis or need for amputation. If you do not have a hand surgeon at your hospital, this patient will need to be transferred.

Test-taking tip: You do not need the image to know that the patient in the question stem has tenosynovitis. You can eliminate A and D because you wouldn't want to send this person home and the medicine service is not the appropriate place for a surgical patient.

13. ANSWER: A

This presentation is concerning for scaphoid fracture given the snuffbox tenderness and pain with axial loading of the thumb. Although not visualized on the radiographs, scaphoid fracture must be considered because approximately 15% of scaphoid fractures are missed on initial plain films, and these fractures are at high risk for avascular necrosis (AVN). Options for management of occult scaphoid fractures include immobilization in a thumb spica splint with repeat plain films in 7 to 10 days or immediate advanced imaging. This particular patient is a surgery resident who would be unable to work if immobilized, and therefore advanced imaging is likely a better option. However, the gold standard imaging modality is magnetic resonance imaging (MRI), which has a sensitivity of nearly 100%. If negative, he would not require immobilization and could return to work immediately. Discharge home without any further workup or splinting would be inappropriate, and ACE wrap is not sufficient to immobilize the wrist.

Test-taking tip: Complications of missed scaphoid fractures are so severe (AVN and scapholunate advanced collapse) that you can narrow your choices to two by eliminating B and D right away.

14. ANSWER: B

This patient is presenting with a traumatic subungual hematoma. Blood beneath the nail in large enough quantities can be very painful and should be at least partially evacuated. Because there is no damage to the nail or surrounding folds, complete nail removal is not necessary. Trephination can be completed, with significant pain relief in most cases. In cases with damage to the nail or folds, the entire nail should be removed, and the nail bed should be repaired primarily with sutures. Applying a finger splint will not relieve the patient's pain. Digital block will temporarily relieve the pain, but it does not address the underlying problem.

Test-taking tip: This is a bread-and-butter emergency medicine case of a subungual hematoma. You can eliminate A and D as options because you would not splint a finger that is not broken, and a block would not fix the underlying problem. This narrows your choices down to B and C.

15. ANSWER: B

This patient most likely has a Bartholin gland abscess. The Bartholin glands are located at the four- and eight-o'clock positions around the vaginal vestibule. If they become infected, an abscess may form that requires drainage. The usual organisms are vaginal flora, including anaerobes, but abscesses may also be caused by sexually transmitted infections such as gonorrhea and chlamydia. A Word catheter is often inserted after I&D and is left in place for 6 to 8 weeks to allow formation of a fistula to promote drainage. After successful I&D, antibiotics are typically not required, and antibiotics alone without I&D would not provide adequate treatment. A CT scan of the pelvis with contrast may be done in cases of cellulitis to the perineum to rule out a necrotizing infection such as Fournier's gangrene, but this is unlikely in this patient. Surgical marsupialization to form a permanent fistula may be required in patients with recurrent Bartholin gland abscesses but would not be indicated in this case.

Test-taking tip: It is important to recognize from the question stem that this is a Bartholin gland abscess and *not* a necrotizing infection. Then you can quickly rule out A and C because the abscess will need drainage but a CT is not needed.

16. ANSWER: C

The photo shows a chalazion, which results from obstruction of a meibomian gland. It is usually painless but may be painful in some cases. There also may be slight erythema of the overlying skin, but antibiotics are generally not required in the absence of cellulitis. The first-line treatment is warm compresses. It may be difficult to distinguish from an internal hordeolum, but the treatment is the same.

Test-taking tip: Like most photographs on this test, you do not need to look at the photo to be able to get the question correct. The noncellulitic appearance and the short duration are clues to the diagnosis.

17. ANSWER: B

The CT scan shows an L3 Chance fracture. This type of fracture typically occurs after a flexion-distraction injury, for example, during a motor vehicle collision in which the patient is restrained with a lap belt without shoulder belt. It results in injury to all three columns of the spine and is therefore an unstable fracture. There is a high incidence of intraabdominal injuries associated with Chance fractures, particularly duodenal injuries. In addition to evaluating for intraabdominal pathology, an emergent neurosurgical consultation should be obtained. Although any of the other answer choices could be present after a motor vehicle collision, they are not classically associated with Chance fractures.

Test-taking tip: This is a "you know it or don't" kind of question. If you don't know it, choose an answer and move on. You can perhaps mark it for review when you are done at the end of the test.

18. ANSWER: A

This is a classic description of infestation with *Enterobius vermicularis,* commonly known as pinworms. The pinworm eggs are spread through fecal-oral transmission or through shared items such as clothing or bedding. The eggs hatch in the duodenum, and mature females migrate to the perineum where they deposit more eggs, which result in pruritus. The patient can then spread the eggs to others, particularly household members or caregivers and other children at group child care or preschool. In young girls, the eggs may be deposited in the vulva and result in vulvovaginitis. The child's first presentation of pinworms may be with vaginal discharge. The definitive test for pinworms is the "Scotch tape test" in which a piece of tape is placed on the perineum while the patient sleeps and evaluated in the morning by microscopy for eggs or adult worms. A stool sample may not be adequate. Pinworms are treated with albendazole, mebendazole, or pyrantel pamoate. Ivermectin is used for a variety of parasites but not for pinworms.

Test-taking tip: This is a classic presentation of pin worms. Review classic presentations of common things before the exam.

19. ANSWER: B

This question describes phlegmasia cerulea dolens, a painful blue leg caused by massive iliofemoral occlusion due to deep venous thrombosis (DVT). It is commonly associated with malignancy. If the venous pressure becomes high enough to impede arterial flow, or if arterial spasm occurs, the leg may become white, a condition known as phlegmasia alba dolens (or "milk leg"). Patients should be promptly evaluated by a vascular surgeon to consider thrombectomy if possible. When timely consultation is not available, thrombolytics should be started because this is a limb-threatening condition. While the decision is being made to escalate to more aggressive therapies, the patient should be started on unfractionated heparin, even before obtaining imaging if there is a high pretest probability. Transferring to the tertiary care center without giving thrombolytics may result in loss of limb and is not advised. Antibiotics do not play a role in the management of DVT. The application of a compression stocking would worsen the condition by raising venous pressure even more. In fact, any constrictive clothing or dressings should be removed from these patients.

Test-taking tip: From the description of a blue lower extremity, you can ascertain that this is a limb-threatening condition. You can rule out C and D and narrow down your choice because antibiotic and compression stockings are not limb saving.

20. ANSWER: D

Acute compartment syndrome is a complication of trauma that is both life-threatening and limb-threatening. Elevated pressure within the fascial compartments results in ischemia that may produce necrosis and permanent nerve injury. It should be suspected in trauma patients with tense extremities. Of the possible answer choices, paresthesias are the earliest sign of compartment syndrome. Pallor and pulselessness are late findings when the pressure has risen to a level high enough to impede arterial flow. Paralysis is also a late finding. Other signs that are often present in compartment syndrome include pain out of proportion to exam and pain with passive stretch of the involved muscle groups. Suspected compartment syndrome should prompt an emergent consultation with either an orthopedic or general surgeon depending on the mechanism of injury and other associated injuries.

The Five P's of Compartment Syndrome

- Pain out of proportion
- Paresthesia
- Paralysis
- Pallor
- Pulselessness

Test-taking tip: All of the answers are associated with compartment syndrome, but paresthesias happen first.

21. ANSWER: D

This patient is most likely suffering from normal pressure hydrocephalus (NPH). The classic triad in this condition is altered mental status, unsteady gait, and urinary incontinence, often referred to as "wet, wobbly, and wacky." Asymmetric neurologic deficits are not common. Hyperreflexia may be present rather than hyporeflexia. Anisocoria may be suggestive of uncal herniation, which is unlikely in NPH. Management of NPH typically involves shunting. A trial of lumbar puncture to evaluate for clinical response may be done before surgical intervention, but these decisions will be made in conjunction with a neurosurgeon. The CT scan shown in Figure 1.9 shows enlarged lateral ventricles.

Test-taking tip: You can eliminate A because lateralizing signs are not common in NPH.

22. ANSWER: D

The most likely diagnosis in this case is bacterial tracheitis. The clinical picture appears similar to croup with stridor and barky cough, but patients with bacterial tracheitis are very ill, typically have a high fever, and are in significant respiratory distress. Work of breathing may be improved when supine. A life-threatening upper airway obstruction may occur, and there should be a low threshold to intubate children suspected of having this condition. Radiographs may show a narrowed and irregular trachea but are not required to make the diagnosis. Bronchoscopy should be performed because it can be both diagnostic and therapeutic, with removal of thick secretions from the airway. If the suspected diagnosis is croup, continued use of racemic epinephrine would be reasonable, but it is unlikely to benefit this patient. Suctioning and supplemental oxygen would be appropriate for bronchiolitis but not bacterial tracheitis. Finally, noninvasive ventilation is unlikely to be sufficient for this patient and does not allow for bronchoscopy.

Test-taking tip: The question stem describes a toxic-appearing child in respiratory distress who is not improving with croup treatment. The next step regardless of the underlying condition would be intubation.

23. ANSWER: B

A young female with lower abdominal pain should raise concern for both abdominal and pelvic pathology. The differential includes appendicitis, ectopic pregnancy, ovarian cyst, tubo-ovarian abscess, ovarian torsion, endometriosis, and pelvic inflammatory disease, among others. Although the CT was normal, pathology involving the female reproductive organs is often missed on CT and may be better visualized with pelvic ultrasound. This is particularly true of ovarian torsion. The most consistent finding in those with ovarian torsion is an ovarian cyst larger than 4 cm. Doppler flow should be evaluated and compared with the contralateral ovary. Absence of arterial flow is a late finding but has a 100% positive predictive value. The torsion is often intermittent, and therefore the ultrasound may be normal depending on the timing of the study. If your pretest probability for torsion was very high, an urgent gynecology consult should be obtained even if the ultrasound is negative. Urgent general surgery consultation is not indicated at this point because a potential pelvic etiology needs to be addressed first. Discharge home without further evaluation of the reproductive organs is not appropriate. Admission for serial exams may be the ultimate disposition depending on the remainder of the ED course, but the pelvic ultrasound should be obtained before making a disposition decision.

Test-taking tip: Remember for questions asking for the "best next step in management," multiple answers may seem reasonable, but one choice is more urgent or more correct than the others.

24. ANSWER: C

This patient complains of mandibular pain after blunt trauma to the face, but her exam is reassuring, and it is unlikely that she has a fracture. Exam findings suggestive of mandibular fracture include asymmetry of the jaw, malocclusion, trismus, intraoral hematoma, and numbness of the lower lip or chin from injury to the mental nerve. The tongue blade test is commonly used to evaluate for possible mandibular fracture. The patient is asked to bite down on a tongue blade on the affected side. The examiner then twists the blade, asking the patient to attempt to break the blade between his/her teeth. If the patient opens his/her mouth because of pain, the test is positive and further imaging should be done to assess for mandibular fracture. If the patient can break the tongue blade, it is unlikely that the mandible is fractured, and imaging is not indicated. This test has been shown to have a 96% sensitivity. Both Panorex and maxillofacial CT can be used for suspected mandibular fractures. If there is concern for other facial trauma, CT should be obtained. If it appears to be an isolated mandibular injury, panorex is likely sufficient. A plain film facial series is rarely ordered because it is not sensitive for facial fractures.

Test-taking tip: Even if you are unsure of the answer, look for patterns. For example, in this question, all of the answer choices are types of imaging except for one. Therefore, the one answer that does not fit the pattern is likely correct.

25. ANSWER: A

The lesion is a pyogenic granuloma, a benign vascular tumor typically found on the extremities or face. The term "pyogenic granuloma" is a misnomer because it is neither infectious nor granulomatous. These lesions tend to be very friable and will bleed with even minor trauma. Patients may present with brisk bleeding from lesions that they are unable to stop themselves. As with most sources of bleeding, the initial step is to hold direct pressure. If this is unsuccessful, as it was in this case, silver nitrate will usually stop the bleeding, but it should not be used on the face because of the risk for scarring.

Ultimately, the lesion should be removed and sent to pathology to rule out malignancy, but this is better done by a dermatologist than at the bedside in the ED. While liquid nitrogen cryotherapy has been used in the past, it is not recommended because it often requires multiple treatments to be successful. Additionally, liquid nitrogen is not readily available in many EDs. The patient should be referred to a dermatologist for definitive management, but it does not need to be emergent.

Test-taking tip: You can initially eliminate D and C and narrow the options because there is rarely ever an emergent dermatologic condition. Also, liquid nitrogen is not a readily available treatment in the ED.

26. ANSWER: A

This photo demonstrates an auricular hematoma. If the blood is not evacuated, it will result in a deformity of the auricle known as "cauliflower ear." Small hematomas may be aspirated with a 20-gauge needle, whereas larger hematomas may require I&D. In both cases, a pressure dressing should be applied after the hematoma is evacuated to prevent reaccumulation and therefore reduce the risk for deformity. Pressure dressing alone is not appropriate. Urgent ear, nose, and throat specialist consultation is not required in this case. For hematomas that have been present for more than 1 week at the time of presentation, the patient should be referred to a surgeon as an outpatient.

Test-taking tip: It is important to know when a procedure can be done by an emergency physician versus when a patient should be transferred for higher level of care.

27. ANSWER: B

This patient appears to be suffering from cluster headaches. The classic presentation of cluster headaches is a man in his 20s or 30s with unilateral headache localized around one eye that lasts minutes to hours and occurs several times a day. The pain may be associated with ipsilateral conjunctival injection, lacrimation, facial sweating, miosis, ptosis, or nasal congestion. Patients are typically restless and agitated and may be pacing back and forth. Although it can occur in women, this is the only type of headache that occurs more frequently in males than females. Treatment of acute cluster headache is with high-flow oxygen. Upon discharge, the patient should be given a trial of verapamil because this is the drug of choice for prevention of cluster headaches. The patient may also be given a prednisone taper while waiting for verapamil to reach steady state, though data on the effectiveness of glucocorticoids are limited. It is unlikely that nonsteroidal antiinflammatory drugs (NSAIDs) alone will be sufficient for cluster headaches. Lithium has been used for cluster headaches but generally only in chronic, refractory cases because of the narrow therapeutic index. There are no data to support the use of botulinum toxin for cluster headaches.

Test-taking tip: This is a "you know it or don't" kind of question. If you don't know it, choose an answer and move on. You can perhaps mark it for review when you are done at the end of the test.

28. ANSWER: D

This presentation is concerning for carotid artery dissection with subsequent stroke. Carotid dissection can occur after even minor trauma to the neck from a motor vehicle collision, sports injury, or chiropractic manipulation and is one of the causes of stroke in young people. It may present with neck pain and headache with associated ipsilateral Horner's syndrome and contralateral weakness as seen here. The diagnosis can be confirmed with CT angiography of the neck. An alternative approach would be to use magnetic resonance angiography, but it is usually more time-consuming and not available at many hospitals. Cerebral angiography can be used to diagnose aneurysms or large vessel occlusions that may be amenable to neurointervention but is not the first imaging modality used for suspected carotid dissection. Giving tissue plasminogen activator (tPA) is also not indicated because this patient presented outside the window. High-dose prednisone would be indicated for multiple sclerosis or cerebral vasculitis but is not involved in the treatment of carotid dissection.

Test-taking tip: Neurologic symptoms in a patient status post chiropractor is carotid artery dissection until proved otherwise.

29. ANSWER: B

The chest radiograph is not needed in this case to answer the question correctly.

This patient initially presented with a chronic obstructive pulmonary disease (COPD) exacerbation but developed a right-sided tension pneumothorax after she was started on noninvasive positive pressure ventilation. Patients with COPD are prone to subpleural blebs that may rupture, thereby resulting in pneumothorax. This is even more likely to occur during positive pressure ventilation. Tension pneumothorax may present with decreased or absent breath sounds, jugular venous distention, tracheal deviation to the opposite side, and hypotension or cardiac arrest. The first step in suspected tension pneumothorax should always be needle decompression. This may be done in a variety of ways, but commonly a 10-gauge needle is placed in either the second intercostal space in the midclavicular line or the fourth intercostal space in the anterior axillary line. A rush of air should be heard when the pleura is punctured, and ideally, the patient's condition will improve. This must always be followed by placement of a chest tube because the needle decompression is only a temporizing measure. While placement of a chest tube is indicated, in the case of cardiac arrest resulting from tension pneumothorax, there should be no delay in decompressing the chest while setting up for tube thoracostomy. Administering tPA is not appropriate in this case a her cardiac arrest is less likely to have resulted from a massive pulmonary embolus. Although this patient should be intubated, intentional placement of the endotracheal tube in the right main-stem bronchus will not solve this patient's problem.

Test-taking tip: It is important to know not only how to diagnose and manage common conditions but also how to identify and treat complications of those conditions.

30. ANSWER: B

The most likely diagnosis in this case is temporal arteritis, also called giant cell arteritis. It is a type of vasculitis characterized by temporal headache, fatigue, fever, jaw claudication, visual disturbances, and elevated erythrocyte sedimentation rate (ESR). The examiner should be able to elicit tenderness when palpating the temporal artery. It may also be associated with polymyalgia rheumatica, another inflammatory condition that causes pain in the neck, shoulders, and pelvic girdle muscles with associated stiffness, particularly in the morning. The treatment for both conditions is high-dose steroids. The gold standard for the diagnosis of temporal arteritis is a temporal artery biopsy. The other answer choices are not classically associated with temporal arteritis.

Test-taking tip: This is a "you know it or don't" kind of question. If you don't know it, choose an answer and move on. You can perhaps mark it for review when you are done at the end of the test.

31. ANSWER: A

S. pneumoniae is the most common cause of community-acquired pneumonia. While people with HIV/AIDS are at risk for developing specific infections as a result of their immunocompromised state, they are still susceptible to the usual pathogens that infect immunocompetent people. Therefore, statistically speaking, the most likely organism to cause community-acquired pneumonia in an HIV patient is still *S. pneumoniae*. Immunocompromised patients are at higher risk for tuberculosis, but the question stem does not provide specific clues to this diagnosis. The streaks of blood in the sputum may occur with pneumonia and do not necessarily imply tuberculosis. *Pneumocystis jirovecii* (PCP) typically occurs in patients with CD4 counts less than 200 and is considered an AIDS-defining illness. The serum lactate dehydrogenase level is usually elevated, and the chest radiograph may show diffuse interstitial infiltrates. The treatment is trimethoprim-sulfamethoxazole, with corticosteroids if the patient's arterial partial pressure of oxygen is 70 or less, or the alveolar-arterial gradient is 35 or greater. *S. aureus* is another common cause of community-acquired pneumonia but is not as common as *Streptococcus*.

Test-taking tip: Remember that even special patient populations are susceptible to the same pathogens and conditions as healthy patients.

32. ANSWER: C

The skin lesions and migratory arthralgias are characteristics of disseminated gonococcal infection. This condition is much more common in females than males, possibly because of delayed diagnosis of the initial mucosal infection given that females are more likely to be asymptomatic than males. Joint pain may be isolated to a single joint and manifest as septic arthritis, or it may be migratory as seen here. The skin lesions are described as gray pustules as seen in the photo.

Patients may be ill appearing and bacteremic. Cultures of the cervix, urethra, rectum, and pharynx should be collected and are positive in up to 75% of cases. Blood and synovial fluid cultures are only positive 10% to 50% of the time. Patients with disseminated gonococcal infection should be hospitalized for antibiotic therapy, and the drug of choice is ceftriaxone.

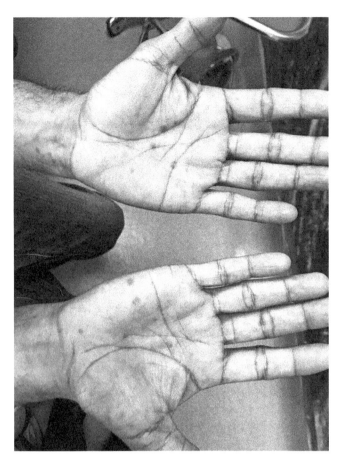

Figure 1.28 Syphilis rash on palms.

Darkfield microscopy may confirm the diagnosis of syphilis, which is not described by this case, and the rash with syphilis is nontender flat papules involving the palms and soles of the feet. See Figure 1.28.

33. ANSWER: B

The combination of findings described in the question stem is suggestive of Kawasaki disease. This condition generally affects children younger than 5 years. The criteria for diagnosis include a fever for at least 5 days, plus at least four of the following: rash, bilateral nonpurulent conjunctivitis, inflammation of the lips and oral mucosa (beefy red and cracked lips, strawberry tongue), erythema and/or swelling of the hands and feet (particularly the palms and soles) with desquamation after 1 to 2 weeks, and cervical lymphadenopathy that is often unilateral.

Patients may develop pericarditis, myocarditis, or coronary artery aneurysms, with the most feared complication being sudden death. Treatment for Kawasaki disease includes IV immunoglobulin and aspirin to prevent the development of coronary artery aneurysms. Some of the signs and symptoms of Kawasaki disease overlap with those of scarlet fever, including rash, desquamation, and strawberry tongue. However, the palms and soles are typically spared in scarlet fever. Amoxicillin may be used to treat scarlet fever but would not be indicated for Kawasaki disease. Glossitis may be explained by a vitamin B_{12} deficiency, but the remainder of the signs and symptoms would not be. Finally, corticosteroids should be avoided because they may actually increase the likelihood of developing coronary artery aneurysms.

Test-taking tip: This question is asking for the treatment of Kawasaki disease. You can eliminate A and C initially because Kawasaki disease is a virus and not helped by antibiotics or vitamins.

34. ANSWER: D

This patient is most likely suffering from trigeminal neuralgia. This painful condition is often debilitating. Patients experience attacks of sharp pain or "electric shocks" that primarily affect the V_2 distribution of the trigeminal nerve, though may affect any of the three branches. The pain is often worsened with talking or chewing. Allodynia is common, and pain may be triggered by touching the face, shaving, or even a gust of wind. First-line treatment for trigeminal neuralgia is with anticonvulsants, generally carbamazepine or gabapentin.

Corticosteroids would be indicated for suspected giant cell (temporal) arteritis. This condition is generally characterized by unilateral headache, vision changes, jaw claudication, and an elevated ESR and, if left untreated, can result in permanent blindness. NSAIDs are not likely to be very helpful in this condition. A variety of surgical interventions are available for trigeminal neuralgia but are generally reserved for cases refractory to medical management.

Test-taking tip: This is a "you know it or don't" kind of question. If you don't know it, choose an answer and move on. You can perhaps mark it for review when you are done at the end of the test.

35. ANSWER: B

This patient most likely has thrombotic thrombocytopenic purpura (TTP). This hematologic condition is caused by reduced activity of ADAMTS13, an enzyme that cleaves von Willebrand factor multimers, resulting in widespread thrombus formation. It is classically characterized by the pentad of microangiopathic hemolytic anemia, thrombocytopenia, neurologic symptoms, renal dysfunction, and fever, though few patients present with the full pentad. Other associated symptoms may include abdominal pain, nausea, vomiting, fatigue, and generalized weakness. It is more common in women, typically presents in the fourth or fifth decade of life, and is almost always fatal if left untreated.

The differential for TTP is vast, including sepsis, central nervous system infections, disseminated intravascular coagulation, HELLP syndrome, and systemic lupus erythematosus. During the initial workup, patients may be given broad-spectrum antibiotics empirically, including meningitis coverage, until the diagnosis is ascertained. The first-line treatment is plasma exchange, and a hematologist should be consulted as soon as possible to initiate therapy. Glucocorticoids and rituximab are also commonly used and, when combined with plasma exchange, have been shown to improve outcomes. Lumbar puncture is not safe in this patient because of severe thrombocytopenia. Platelet transfusion should be avoided in TTP except in cases of severe, life-threatening bleeding or intracranial hemorrhage because transfusion may actually worsen the patient's condition. Finally, IVIG is used to treat immune thrombocytopenia (ITP), an acquired thrombocytopenia due to antibody-mediated platelet destruction, but is not commonly used for TTP.

Test-taking tip: You can eliminate A as an answer choice because low platelets are a contraindication to lumbar puncture. Deciphering between ITP and TTP treatment is the crux of this question.

36. ANSWER: C

This patient has a zone II penetrating neck injury. As with any trauma, the ABCs should be assessed first, and if there is any evidence of current or impending airway compromise, the patient should be intubated. Bleeding should be controlled with direct pressure if possible. If the patient is unstable, he should be taken to the operating room for exploration immediately.

For stable patients, if the wound does *not* violate the platysma, it is typically safe to observe the patient as significant injury is unlikely. If it does violate the platysma, the patient should be assessed for hard and soft signs of neck injury.

The hard signs include expanding or pulsatile hematoma, bruit or thrill, obvious arterial bleeding, shock unresponsive to fluids, pulse deficit, hemoptysis, air bubbling from the wound, and stridor.

The soft signs include nonexpanding hematoma, hypotension responsive to fluids, hoarse voice, subcutaneous emphysema, dysphagia, and odynophagia. Patients with hard signs of neck injury should be taken emergently for surgical exploration. As a general rule, penetrating neck injuries should not be explored in the ED. Patients with only soft signs who are hemodynamically stable should undergo CT angiography of the neck to characterize injuries. If there is any suggestion of injury to the aerodigestive tract on the CT, the next step would be endoscopy. If there is evidence

of vascular injury, the patient should be taken either for surgical exploration or to interventional radiology for formal angiography and repair.

Test-taking tip: Hard and soft signs in penetrating neck injury are a commonly tested topic and therefore worth memorizing and reviewing before the test.

37. ANSWER: C

The most likely diagnosis in this case is Bell's palsy, also called idiopathic facial paralysis. This is a lower motor neuron paresis affecting one side of the face. It is characterized by ipsilateral findings of facial droop, hyperacusis, diminished taste, and inability to fully close the eye. This can be differentiated from a central cause of facial droop such as ischemic stroke by the involvement of the upper face (forehead). A patient with facial droop from stroke should still be able to raise the eyebrows, unlike this patient.

Treatment of Bell's palsy is controversial, but there is some evidence to suggest treatment with prednisone and acyclovir given that the cause is thought to be inflammation of the nerve because of viral illness. An ear exam should be done to evaluate for Ramsay Hunt syndrome, a herpes zoster outbreak involving the ear or external auditory canal that also causes unilateral facial paralysis.

Test-taking tip: This question is trying to confuse you between Bell's palsy and stroke. Try to remember that involvement of the forehead is key to the diagnosis of Bell's palsy.

38. ANSWER: A

This patient is presenting with a stomal prolapse at his ostomy site (see Figure 1.29). This may be caused by weak abdominal muscles, increased intra-abdominal pressure, or issues with the construction of the ostomy. When prolapsed, the stoma may become edematous or bleed because of the friability of the tissue. If perfusion is compromised, the stoma may become ischemic with a dusky or purple appearance. In this case, the stoma appears pink and well perfused, and therefore, the best next step is to attempt bedside reduction. Place the patient flat or in slight Trendelenburg position. Granulated sugar or a cold compress may be applied to the stoma to reduce edema and facilitate reduction. If the reduction is successful, the patient can be discharged to follow up with his surgeon as soon as possible. If there is any concern for ischemia, or if the stoma is not reducible, emergent surgical consultation would be the best choice.

Discharging without reduction or surgical consultation would be inappropriate because the bowel may become

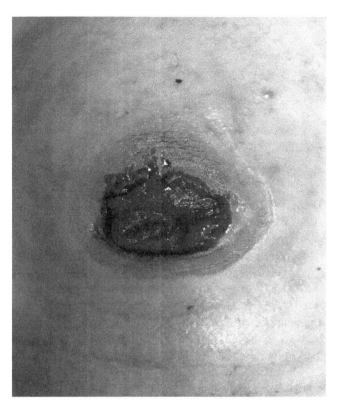

Figure 1.29 Stoma.

ischemic if it remains prolapsed. Finally, an abdominal binder with a prolapse overbelt may be applied after successful reduction but would not be useful before reduction.

Test-taking tip: A nondusky, pink, and well-perfused intestine can easily have reduction attempted in the ED. Answer C can be excluded because discharge without reduction is not an option.

39. ANSWER: A

It is important to remember that every patient with burns to the face should have a fluorescein eye exam to rule out corneal burns. Burns to the cornea or anterior chamber may cause permanent vision loss and, if identified, should prompt urgent ophthalmology consult and treatment with topical antibiotics.

There should be a low threshold to intubate patients with burns to the face, neck, or chest, but this patient is not exhibiting signs of impending airway compromise. The Parkland formula is one option for guiding fluid resuscitation in patients with partial- and/or full-thickness burns but is generally not used for patients with less than 15% total body surface area (TBSA) burns. Finally, a nasogastric tube is often required in patients with burns greater than 20% TBSA owing to the high incidence of ileus in these patients.

Test-taking tip: You can easily eliminate B and C because the patient's burns are not extensive, and the patient does not have respiratory distress.

40. ANSWER: B

Cushing's syndrome results from excessive glucocorticoids. Hypernatremia results from increased absorption of sodium in the kidney. Hypokalemia and metabolic alkalosis are caused by increased urinary loss of potassium and hydrogen ions. Patients with Cushing's syndrome are generally obese with round faces and thin extremities, and they may have a "buffalo hump" between the shoulder blades.

Test-taking tip: This is a "you know it or don't" kind of question. If you don't know it, choose an answer and move on. You can perhaps mark it for review when you are done at the end of the test.

41. ANSWER: D

Aphthous ulcers and oral herpetic lesions are sometimes difficult to distinguish; however, unlike herpes, aphthous ulcers almost never occur on the hard palate or gingiva. Both are painful, may have a prodromal burning sensation before ulcer formation, and may be precipitated by local trauma.

Aphthous ulcers may be treated with topical anesthetics and triamcinolone dental paste. Management of oral herpetic lesions is typically supportive with local anesthetics. Primary herpes infections in adults may be treated with oral antivirals. Episodic therapy with oral antivirals may also be considered for recurrences of oral herpes, particularly with patients who have a reliable prodrome.

Test-taking tip: This is a "you know it or don't" kind of question. If you don't know it, choose an answer and move on. You can perhaps mark it for review when you are done at the end of the test.

42. ANSWER: C

The neck mass described is a thyroglossal duct cyst. It is characterized by the presence of a fluctuant mass in the midline of the neck that moves with swallowing or tongue protrusion. They are generally painless but may be painful if infected. There is a small risk for malignant transformation, and therefore the cyst should be removed electively.

A branchial cleft cyst is another type of congenital neck mass and is most commonly found anterior to the sternocleidomastoid near the angle of mandible. They too are generally painless but may become painful if infected. Branchial cleft cysts may also rupture, resulting in formation of a draining sinus. Similar to thyroglossal duct cysts, they should be removed with elective surgery.

Lymphangiomas, also known as cystic hygromas, result from obstructed lymphatic drainage and most commonly occur in the neck along the jugular lymphatic chain. They may become very large, resulting in compression of the airway. Lymphoma must be on the differential for neck masses in both children and adults. It most commonly occurs in the anterior triangle of the neck, but it should not move with tongue protrusion like a thyroglossal duct cyst would.

Test-taking tip: Because the mass is described as midline, you can eliminate D and B because those both present as lateral masses.

43. ANSWER: D

The most likely diagnosis in this case is a molar pregnancy, a type of gestational trophoblastic disease. It is a neoplasm composed of trophoblastic cells of the placenta that produce β-human chorionic gonadotropin (β-hCG), typically in levels >100,000 in the serum. Bedside ultrasound may show a "snowstorm" or "cluster of grapes" appearance to the uterus (Figure 1.30), and on physical exam, the uterine size is greater than the estimated gestational age. This diagnosis should be suspected in women presenting with signs of preeclampsia before 20 weeks' gestation. Molar pregnancies are treated with dilation and curettage. While a positive β-hCG with the absence of an intrauterine pregnancy on ultrasound often signifies an ectopic pregnancy, the additional details of this case point toward a molar pregnancy. An empty sac pregnancy, previously known as blighted ovum or anembryonic pregnancy, occurs when embryonic

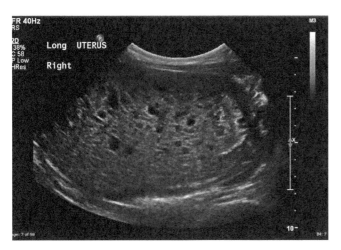

Figure 1.30 Ultrasound of uterus.

development stops at a very early stage. It is characterized by a gestational sac greater than 25 mm without a yolk sac or embryonic pole. A missed abortion occurs when an embryo or fetus dies in utero before 20 weeks' gestation but the pregnancy is retained. Women report that they no longer "feel pregnant" because of resolution of pregnancy symptoms such as nausea, vomiting, and breast tenderness.

Test-taking tip: You can narrow down your choices by the ultrasound finding of no intrauterine pregnancy. This reduces your choice to D or A.

44. ANSWER: A

The photo shows a paronychia, an infection along the nail fold. It may occur after nail biting or a manicure. In the early stages of infection before there is significant purulence, this may be treated with warm soaks and/or oral antibiotics. However, the infection depicted has progressed to abscess formation, and it should be opened with bedside I&D to increase the likelihood of successful treatment. This procedure is performed using a digital block and an incision parallel to the nail fold under the eponychium. If the abscess has progressed under the nail, a portion of the nail should be removed to facilitate complete drainage; however, removal of the entire nail is not necessary in most cases. The role of antibiotics after drainage is controversial. Most abscesses will resolve with drainage and warm soaks.

Test-taking tip: This question requires the picture to answer. With the infection seen, you can eliminate C and B because it is not serious enough to need a hand surgeon and is not simple enough to be discharged home without I&D.

45. ANSWER: C

The rash described is consistent with candidal balanitis, a fungal infection of the glans of the penis. See Figure 1.31 for an example of balanitis. This patient has had recurrent episodes of candida and should be screened for diabetes. His wife should also be tested for vulvovaginal candidiasis and treated if indicated to prevent reinfection. Topical antifungal creams and good personal hygiene are usually sufficient to eradicate the infection. While clotrimazole cream will most likely treat the candida in this patient, the better option for the "best next step" is to screen for diabetes. Oral antibiotics are useful for cellulitis but would not be indicated for this fungal infection. Finally, a culture of exudate will likely confirm the diagnosis of candida but is not necessary because this diagnosis can usually be made clinically.

Test-taking tip: This question is not asking for treatment but asking for the "next" best management step. So

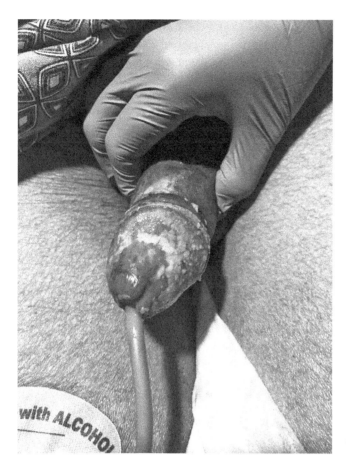

Figure 1.31 Balanitis.

(Photo courtesy of Jessica Mason, MD, UCSF-Fresno.)

even though A is a treatment of balanitis, the next best step is C.

46. ANSWER: B

High-pressure injection injuries can be quite misleading. Immediately after the injection, the exam may be fairly unremarkable with only minor swelling or a small puncture mark as seen here. However, the injected substance often spreads along the fascial planes, resulting in much more extensive damage beneath the skin than what can be seen externally. With time, ischemia may result from venous outflow obstruction or arterial compression. Additionally, depending on what is injected, the substance itself may damage the tissues. High-pressure injection injuries should be treated with emergent debridement. Imaging should be obtained to rule out fracture, antibiotics should be started, and tetanus should be updated if needed, but these alone are insufficient without debridement.

Test-taking tip: This is a "you know it or don't" kind of question. If you don't know it, choose an answer and move on. You can perhaps mark it for review when you are done at the end of the test.

47. ANSWER: D

This patient appears to be suffering from neuroleptic malignant syndrome (NMS) induced by haloperidol. This condition is a complication of antipsychotic use and is characterized by muscle rigidity, fever, autonomic instability, and altered mental status. It is more likely to occur after the initiation of therapy but may occur even in patients who have been on a stable regimen for years. Laboratory abnormalities that may be seen include leukocytosis, elevated creatinine kinase, transaminitis, electrolyte disturbances, metabolic acidosis, and elevated blood urea nitrogen and creatinine. Treatment is mostly supportive and includes stopping the offending agent. Benzodiazepines may be given to treat agitation and decrease sympathetic activity. Diphenhydramine should not be given because it may potentiate the effects owing to its anticholinergic properties. Cooling measures should be used for fever, but there is no role for antipyretics given that the elevated temperature is not driven by the hypothalamus. Although many of the signs and symptoms overlap with serotonin syndrome, rigidity is seen in NMS, whereas hyperreflexia and clonus are seen in serotonin syndrome. Cyproheptadine is used to treat serotonin syndrome but does not have a role in the treatment of NMS (Table 1.1).

Test-taking tip: Review the differences between NMS and serotonin syndrome before the exam. The muscle rigidity is the key to the diagnosis in this question.

Table 1.1 COMPARISON OF NEUROLEPTIC MALIGNANT SYNDROME, SEROTONIN SYNDROME, AND MALIGNANT HYPERTHERMIA

SYNDROME	PHYSICAL EXAM FINDING	TREATMENT	MEDICATION TRIGGERS
Neuroleptic malignant syndrome	Febrile Rigid ("lead pipe rigidity")	Paralysis and cooling	Antipsychotics, Withdrawal of dopaminergic drugs
Serotonin syndrome	Febrile Clonus	Benzodiazepine Cyproheptadine	Selective serotonin reuptake inhibitors, tramadol, monoamine oxidase inhibitors (MOIs), cocaine
Malignant hyperthermia	Febrile Muscle rigidity	Dantrolene	Inhaled anesthetics

48. ANSWER: B

Repair of lip lacerations involving the vermillion border must be done carefully to ensure a good cosmetic result. To achieve adequate realignment of the vermillion border, it is important to avoid any distortion of the anatomy. This is best accomplished with an infraorbital nerve block to provide anesthesia to the upper lip. Local infiltration through the wound margins will most definitely distort the anatomy and make repair of the vermillion border nearly impossible. A mental nerve block would provide anesthesia to the lower lip but not the upper lip. Finally, topical application of LET (lidocaine, epinephrine, tetracaine) may not provide sufficient anesthesia to facilitate the repair and would be inferior to infraorbital nerve block.

Test-taking tip: You can narrow down your choices by eliminating C because the laceration is on the upper lip and also D because topical anesthetics are not as good as subcutaneous.

49. ANSWER: A

Perforation of the tympanic membrane after an explosion is a sign of blast injury and should prompt further evaluation for other injuries. Blast injuries primarily affect hollow organs, most commonly the lungs. A chest radiograph should be obtained for anyone with evidence of blast injury to evaluate for pulmonary contusion, pneumothorax, hemothorax, pneumomediastinum, or subcutaneous emphysema. Bowel injuries are also a concern but may be occult and have a delayed presentation. While unlikely in this patient, an upright chest radiograph may also show free air under the diaphragm to suggest bowel perforation. This patient has a benign abdomen at this time but may develop signs of injury later and should be provided with strict return precautions on discharge. A CT of the abdomen and pelvis is not yet indicated. A CT of the head is unnecessary in this patient who is neurologically intact with no evidence of direct trauma to the head. Although there is no mention of a spinal exam in the question stem, the patient denies any neck pain and does not have any focal neurologic deficits; thus cervical spine radiographs are likely low yield.

Test-taking tip: This is a "you know it or don't" kind of question. If you don't know it, choose an answer and move on. You can perhaps mark it for review when you are done at the end of the test.

50. ANSWER: C

This presentation is concerning for hereditary angioedema, a rare autosomal dominant disease caused by a deficiency of C1 esterase inhibitor. It is characterized by edema of the upper airway, trunk, extremities, and gastrointestinal tract and may mimic anaphylaxis. However, it is not associated with rash and does not improve with typical anaphylaxis treatments such as epinephrine, steroids, or antihistamines. Intubation may be required if the airway is obstructed. The first-line treatment in hereditary angioedema is C1 esterase inhibitor. Bradykinin-2 receptor antagonists or kallikrein inhibitors may also be used. If these treatments as not available, fresh frozen plasma can be used as a second-line option.

Test-taking tip: Because hereditary angioedema does not respond to normal anaphylaxis treatment, you can eliminate A and D right from the start narrowing your option down to two.

51. ANSWER: A

This patient was most likely prescribed a systemic steroid such as prednisone. Systemic steroids should not be prescribed in psoriasis because they are known to cause both rebound and pustular psoriasis. Clobetasol ointment is commonly used for psoriasis and should improve, not worsen, symptoms. Cephalexin is an antibiotic commonly used for cellulitis but would not typically be prescribed for psoriasis. Topical tacrolimus is sometimes used off-label for the treatment of psoriasis and, like topical corticosteroids, should improve symptoms rather than worsen them.

Test-taking tip: This is a "you know it or don't" kind of question. If you don't know it, choose an answer and move on. You can perhaps mark it for review when you are done at the end of the test.

52. ANSWER: B

This patient most likely has epididymitis given the testicular pain, positive Prehn's sign, and increased Doppler flow to the affected side on ultrasound. Prehn's sign is positive if elevation of the testicle relieves the pain. Epididymitis may be difficult to distinguish from testicular torsion on physical exam; however, in torsion, the Doppler flow to the affected side should be reduced, whereas in epididymitis, it should be increased.

Epididymitis in young men (<35 years of age) is typically caused by gonorrhea or chlamydia, and therefore a single dose of intramuscular ceftriaxone combined with oral azithromycin is an appropriate choice for this patient. In patients older than 35 years, epididymitis is more commonly caused by *Escherichia coli,* and therefore levofloxacin would be a better option in this population. Patients should follow up with urology, but this is not emergent and can be done as an outpatient. In patients who are afebrile, do not appear toxic, and have stable vital signs, admission is generally unnecessary. Patients should be advised to wear underwear that supports the scrotum to improve pain.

Test-taking tip: This question is getting at the treatment of epididymitis in a patient younger than 35 years. Because the patient does not appear toxic, you can eliminate A and D from the start.

53. ANSWER: B

This case describes *C. trachomatis* pneumonia. This condition is rare in the developed world because of screening and treatment during pregnancy, but it still occurs in infants born to mothers without adequate prenatal care. Affected neonates are often afebrile and classically have a "staccato cough" with diffuse rales. *S. aureus* may cause pneumonia in infants and children, but these patients typically have rapidly progressing symptoms and are febrile and toxic appearing. *S. aureus* pneumonia occurs more commonly after influenza infection and may be complicated by pulmonary abscesses. It is less likely that she has influenza given lack of fever and the description of the staccato cough that is classically associated with *Chlamydia* pneumonia. *Pseudomonas* is not a common cause of pneumonia in infants, but it should be considered in older children with cystic fibrosis because it carries a high risk for morbidity and mortality in this group. In general, chest radiographs are frequently nondiagnostic in infants with respiratory conditions.

Test-taking tip: Familiarize yourself with buzzwords (i.e., "staccato cough") because they are commonly tested on the boards.

54. ANSWER: B

Von Willebrand's disease is the most common inherited bleeding disorder, affecting approximately 1% of the population. The two essential roles of von Willebrand factor are to assist in platelet adhesion and to bind factor VIII to protect it from degradation. In von Willebrand's disease, the von Willebrand factor is either defective or deficient.

Cutaneous and mucosal bleeding may occur, particularly epistaxis, gingival bleeding, gastrointestinal bleeding, and menorrhagia. Unlike hemophilia, hemarthrosis is rare in von Willebrand's disease. The platelet count and prothrombin time/international normalized ratio should be normal, but bleeding time is prolonged. For cases of severe bleeding from von Willebrand's disease, factor VIII

concentrate is the first-line treatment. For mild bleeding or in patients with known type 1 von Willebrand's disease, desmopressin may be used. Desmopressin stimulates the release of von Willebrand factor from endothelial cells. Platelet transfusion is typically reserved for refractory cases. Cryoprecipitate contains von Willebrand factor but is not recommended because of the risk for viral transmission except in the setting of life-threatening bleeding when factor VIII is not available.

Test-taking tip: This is a "you know it or don't" kind of question. If you don't know it, choose an answer and move on. You can perhaps mark it for review when you are done at the end of the test.

55. ANSWER: B

The radiograph shows a nondisplaced, spiral fracture of the distal tibia, commonly known as a toddler's fracture. While spiral fractures in children should typically raise concern for nonaccidental trauma, this particular fracture is common among ambulatory children up to 6 years of age from minor accidental trauma such as a ground-level fall. These fractures may be difficult to identify on radiographs, and an oblique view may be helpful. Management includes a long leg splint and close outpatient orthopedics follow-up. Children should remain non–weight bearing until cleared by orthopedics. A skeletal survey and child protective services report are not necessary in the absence of other signs of trauma.

Test-taking tip: You can eliminate D because there is fracture on the radiograph, so discharge with reassurance is not an option. Also, A can be eliminated because this fracture is nonoperative, so orthopedics is not needed urgently.

56. ANSWER: A

The condition described is anterior uveitis or iritis. Signs and symptoms include eye pain, ciliary flush, photophobia that may be both direct and consensual, and decreased vision. Slit lamp examination will reveal cell and flare in the anterior chamber and in some cases a hypopyon. Cycloplegics such as scopolamine, homatropine, or cyclopentolate can be used to relax the ciliary muscle, which relieves pain from ciliary spasm. Timolol drops would be used for glaucoma, but the intraocular pressures are normal in this patient. Gentamicin drops can be used for corneal abrasion, but this is unlikely without fluorescein uptake. Finally, prednisolone drops are used for anterior uveitis but should not be given without ophthalmology consultation.

Test-taking tip: You can narrow down your choices by removing C (no infection or abrasion) and B (no glaucoma with normal pressures).

57. ANSWER: C

This patient has de Quervain's tenosynovitis with pain along the tendon sheaths of the abductor pollicis longus and the extensor pollicis brevis. As with most tendinopathies, this is typically an overuse injury and may occur in new parents from holding an infant for long periods of time. The diagnosis should be suspected in patients with tenderness and mild edema over the radial styloid and may be confirmed with a positive Finkelstein's test. This test is positive if the patient experiences worsening of his or her pain with ulnar deviation of the wrist while the thumb is held in the palm by the other fingers. The patient should be immobilized with a thumb spica splint, and NSAIDs can be used for pain.

Arthrocentesis is not necessary in this case because the presentation is not consistent with septic arthritis or gout. A volar splint worn at night is the correct treatment for carpal tunnel syndrome rather than de Quervain's tenosynovitis. Carpal tunnel syndrome is a peripheral mononeuropathy that presents with pain and numbness/tingling in the distribution of the median nerve that is often worse at night. It is the result of compression of the median nerve as it travels through the carpal tunnel, and the diagnosis can be confirmed with nerve conduction studies. It may be managed conservatively with bracing or may require surgical release. De Quervain's tenosynovitis is a clinical diagnosis; therefore radiographs are not indicated, especially given the lack of trauma.

Test-taking tip: This is a "you know it or don't" kind of question. If you don't know it, choose an answer and move on. You can perhaps mark it for review when you are done at the end of the test. You can eliminate A because it is not a septic joint.

58. ANSWER: A

The description of this patient's body habitus is suggestive of Marfan's syndrome. Marfan's is a connective tissue disorder characterized by tall stature, arachnodactyly, and hyperextensibility of joints. Marfan's is also associated with mitral valve prolapse, which produces a mid-systolic click on auscultation of the heart as seen here. Patients with Marfan's are at much higher risk for developing aortic disease, including aortic root aneurysm and aortic dissection. This presentation is concerning for aortic dissection, and therefore a CT angiogram of the aorta would be the best next step in management. While pulmonary embolism (PE) is also on the differential and should be ruled out, dissection is more likely; thus CT angiogram of the aorta would be more appropriate. A D-dimer is unlikely to be useful in this patient. If it is negative, this is not necessarily reassuring in a patient who appears in distress on exam, and it is unlikely to change management. When there is concern for both aortic dissection and PE, the CT angiogram of the aorta will still provide decent visualization of the pulmonary vasculature, but a CT pulmonary angiogram does not adequately visualize the entire aorta because of the timing of the contrast bolus. While the patient should also be assessed for coronary artery disease as a cause of her chest pain and distress, the EKG is not suggestive of the need for emergent cardiology consult, and the possibility of aortic dissection needs to be excluded in this high-risk patient before even considering anticoagulation or catheterization.

Test-taking tip: There are certain disease associations you cannot forget. One of those is Marfan's syndrome with aortic problems.

59. ANSWER: C

This presentation is classic for roseola, a common childhood illness caused by human herpesvirus 6. Roseola typically affects children aged 6 months to 3 years and is characterized by high fever for 3 to 5 days, followed by a rash for 1 to 2 days that appears after defervescence. Children often appear healthy and remain active, though they may be fussy when the fever is high. Associated symptoms may include cough or rhinorrhea but are often mild. Roseola is often confused with other exanthems such as those of rubeola or rubella. Rubeola is more commonly known as measles. It begins with a prodrome of "three Cs" with cough, coryza, and conjunctivitis, in addition to fever and malaise. This is followed by a descending maculopapular rash that first appears on the head and face, spreading down throughout the body, but sparing the palms and soles. Koplik spots, small white lesions on the buccal mucosa, are pathognomonic for measles and may occur before the cutaneous rash, but they are not present in all cases. Children with measles may develop serious complications, including encephalitis and death.

Rubella, commonly known as German measles, starts with a prodrome of fever, malaise, and sore throat. This is followed by a descending maculopapular rash that may be similar to that of the measles rash. Rubella is often associated with posterior auricular and suboccipital lymphadenopathy, which along with a history of inadequate immunization may help make the diagnosis. Finally, varicella-zoster is the virus responsible for chickenpox. This vesicular rash begins on the trunk, spares the palms and soles, and is characterized by lesions in different stages of healing.

Test-taking tip: Child rashes are very testable on standard exams, so brush up on the major viral rashes in young children.

60. ANSWER: A

This child sustained an electrical burn to his lips. There may be little to no bleeding on initial presentation because of vasospasm, thrombosis, and eschar formation. However, serious bleeding from the labial artery develops in up to 10% of these patients and may not occur until 5 to 14 days later. Parents should be educated on this potential complication as well as how to control bleeding on discharge. Unlike other types of electrical burns, it is uncommon for children to develop systemic complications such as rhabdomyolysis, hyperkalemia, or seizures after isolated oral burns.

Test-taking tip: This is a "you know it or don't" kind of question. If you don't know it, choose an answer and move on. You can perhaps mark it for review when you are done at the end of the test.

61. ANSWER: B

The radiograph shows a nondisplaced patella fracture. This is typically caused by a direct blow to the patella, as seen in this scenario. These fractures are often managed nonoperatively if the extensor mechanism remains intact, depending on the type of fracture and the degree of displacement. If this patient can fully extend her knee, she can likely be discharged in a knee immobilizer with outpatient orthopedics follow-up.

Patients with nondisplaced patellar fractures can often still bear weight, but inability to bear weight is not generally used to determine management because the level of pain that is tolerated by patients can be highly variable. Ability to flex the knee is not as useful as the ability to extend the knee when making management decisions for patella fractures. Finally, hemarthrosis may occur, and if large, may require aspiration for pain relief; however, it is not as helpful as the evaluation of the extensor mechanism when determining the management of this patient.

Test-taking tip: This is a "you know it or don't" kind of question. If you don't know it, choose an answer and move on. You can perhaps mark it for review when you are done at the end of the test.

62. ANSWER: B

The most likely diagnosis in this case is cavernous sinus thrombosis. This condition is rare but generally occurs from spread of infection from the face, sinuses, or teeth. Patients are ill appearing and may have lethargy, headache, vision changes, fever, or vomiting. It is initially unilateral but may extend to opposite sinus resulting in bilateral findings, which may include eyelid edema, proptosis, restricted extraocular movement, or fixed gaze, nonreactive pupils. Multiple cranial nerves travel through the cavernous sinus, including cranial nerves III, IV, and VI and the V_1 and V_2 branches of cranial nerve V. Any of these nerves may be affected by cavernous sinus thrombosis; however, cranial nerve VI is most likely to be affected because it lies free in the sinus. A cranial nerve VI palsy would result in an inability to abduct the left eye.

Sensation of the chin and the motor input to the muscles of mastication are both controlled by the V_3 branch of cranial nerve V, which does not pass through the cavernous sinus; therefore choices A and D are incorrect. Upper and lower facial droop is caused by a lower motor neuron lesion to cranial nerve VII, which also does not travel through the cavernous sinus and therefore would not be affected in this case. The management of cavernous sinus thrombosis includes CT of the head and orbits, blood cultures, antibiotics, and consultation with both ophthalmology and neurology.

Test-taking tip: This question is basically testing what nerves pass through the cavernous sinus. You can eliminate A and D because the V_3 branch of cranial nerve V does not go through the sinus.

63. ANSWER: D

This presentation is concerning for septic arthritis of the knee. Patients with septic arthritis generally have acute joint pain, swelling, erythema, limp or refusal to bear weight, severe pain with range of motion, and fever and may look toxic. This condition should be taken very seriously and treated promptly and aggressively, given the risk for permanent joint damage. As such, there should be a low threshold to perform arthrocentesis in suspected cases.

A complete blood count, C-reactive protein (CRP), and blood cultures are also typically collected. Leukocytosis and an elevated CRP favor the diagnosis but are nonspecific. Blood cultures are negative in more than half of the cases, and synovial fluid cultures are negative in approximately one-third of cases. The most common organism is *S. aureus,* though *Streptococcus, Haemophilus influenzae, Neisseria gonorrhoeae,* and multiple gram-negative bacilli have also been implicated. Radiographs should be taken to evaluate for joint effusion and possible osteomyelitis and to exclude fracture but are often nondiagnostic. Orthopedics should be consulted as soon as possible for drainage, and the patient should be started on antibiotics.

Test-taking tip: The case description is classic for septic joint, so you can narrow your choices down by eliminating C because septic joint is not seen on radiograph.

64. ANSWER: B

This patient has a large intraparenchymal hemorrhage and is taking apixaban, a direct factor Xa inhibitor. Bleeding is a risk of all anticoagulants and is classified as either major or minor. Major bleeding includes significant blood loss requiring transfusion or bleeding into an enclosed space such as intracranial bleeding or compartment syndrome. Major bleeding is an indication for reversal of anticoagulation.

Apixaban does not currently have a specific reversal agent. Given this severe, life-threatening bleeding, reversal should be attempted with prothrombin complex concentrates (PCCs). These infusions contain clotting factors 2, 9, and 10 and may include factor 7, and they can generally be used for bleeding associated with any of the factor Xa inhibitors as well as warfarin. Protamine sulfate is the reversal agent for heparin and would therefore not be useful in this case. Idarucizumab is the reversal agent for the direct thrombin inhibitor dabigatran. Fresh frozen plasma, as well as vitamin K, can be used to reverse warfarin.

Test-taking tip: It is necessary to brush up on reversal agents for different anticoagulants.

65. ANSWER: C

This case describes a patient with mumps. This is a viral condition that is rare in developed countries owing to vaccinations but still commonly occurs in the developing world. Signs and symptoms may include fever, malaise, myalgias, headache, parotitis, and orchitis. It remains a leading cause of acquired deafness in developing countries. Aseptic meningitis is common but usually mild. Mumps should be considered in the evaluation of a patient with aseptic meningitis even in the absence of parotitis or orchitis, particularly if the patient is not fully immunized. Sterility is a very rare complication. Treatment is supportive with NSAIDs and fluids, and the condition is usually self-limited.

Test-taking tip: This is a "you know it or don't" kind of question. If you don't know it, choose an answer and move on. You can perhaps mark it for review when you are done at the end of the test.

66. ANSWER: D

The ocular ultrasound shows a lens dislocation. This typically occurs after trauma from stretching of the zonule fibers that hold the lens in place. The lens may become subluxated or completely dislocated. It may be painless and results in blurred vision and monocular diplopia. Lens dislocation may be associated with hyphema or acute angle closure glaucoma, though these are not described here. Retinal

detachment may also occur after ocular trauma but is classically associated with flashing lights and on ultrasound appears as a bright echogenic line floating above the rest of the retina that remains attached. This line may move if the patient moves his or her eyes side to side. Traumatic iritis would present with eye pain, photophobia, and ciliary flush, in addition to decreased vision, and would not produce the ultrasound findings shown. A vitreous hemorrhage can be traumatic but is more commonly associated with diabetes and presents with sudden onset of decreased vision with loss of the red reflex. On ultrasound, hyperechoic material may be seen filling the vitreous chamber but may require the gain to be increased to adequately visualize it.

Test-taking tip: You can eliminate B because the patient does not have consensual light pain. You can also eliminate C because vitreous hemorrhage does not usually happen in trauma. This narrows your options down by half.

67. ANSWER: B

Placental abruption occurs when the placenta is separated from the uterine wall before delivery. This may occur spontaneously or after trauma. Risk factors include advanced maternal age, hypertension/preeclampsia, smoking, cocaine abuse, and oligohydramnios. It often presents with painful vaginal bleeding, though contained abruptions do occur, and these present without vaginal bleeding. The most sensitive findings for abruption are uterine irritability as demonstrated by greater than three contractions per hour as well as fetal distress. A reassuring fetal heart tracing has a 100% negative predictive value for adverse outcomes. Therefore, it is crucial to start cardiotocodynamometry as soon as possible. Ultrasound may show a retroplacental hematoma, but this finding is specific, not sensitive. Maternal hemodynamic instability may or may not occur depending on the severity of the abruption.

Test-taking tip: This is a "you know it or don't" kind of question. If you don't know it, choose an answer and move on. You can perhaps mark it for review when you are done at the end of the test.

68. ANSWER: B

This is a classic description of idiopathic intracranial hypertension (IIH), also known as pseudotumor cerebri. This condition primarily occurs in obese women 20 to 44 years of age. Symptoms include headaches, tinnitus, and vision changes. Exam should reveal papilledema but no focal neurologic deficits. The diagnosis is confirmed by elevated opening pressure on lumbar puncture. Hydrocephalus is not a feature. Treatment may include acetazolamide, serial lumbar punctures, shunt placement, or optic nerve fenestration. Obese patients should be encouraged to lose weight. If left untreated, permanent visual loss and total blindness may occur. Although many patients experience tinnitus, deafness does not occur. Uncal herniation can develop from a variety of conditions that increase intracranial pressure, but it is not known to be a complication of IIH.

Test-taking tip: This is a "you know it or don't" kind of question. If you don't know it, choose an answer and move on. You can perhaps mark it for review when you are done at the end of the test.

69. ANSWER: B

The facial grimacing is most likely a type of dystonic reaction induced by haloperidol. Acute dystonia is characterized by involuntary muscle spasm, most commonly in the face and neck. It may manifest as facial grimacing, trismus, dysarthria, abnormal tongue movements, torticollis, or prolonged upward eye deviation (oculogyric crisis). Rarely, laryngospasm may occur, and this can be life-threatening. Dystonia typically occurs shortly after initiation of therapy or an increase in dosage and may recur even after the offending agent is stopped. Dystonic reactions can be treated with either benztropine or diphenhydramine. None of the other answer choices are indicated.

Test-taking tip: This is a "you know it or don't" kind of question. If you don't know it, choose an answer and move on. You can perhaps mark it for review when you are done at the end of the test. You know you need an anticholinergic to treat dystonia, so you have to know that benztropine is an anticholinergic.

70. ANSWER: C

The lesions shown are consistent with sporotrichosis, a cutaneous fungal infection caused by *Sporothrix schenckii*. Patients are exposed to the fungus through a site of injury from a thorn, barb, or pine needle; therefore it is more common in those who work around plants such as landscapers or berry harvesters and among patients who garden as a hobby. It is classically associated with rose thorns on board exam questions. A purple or red papule forms at the site of inoculation approximately 1 to 10 weeks later and may be confused for an insect bite. The fungus can then travel along the lymphatic system, forming additional nodules as it moves proximally. These nodules later ulcerate and drain serous fluid. The lesions are painless, which can help distinguish them from bacterial infections, which are generally painful. The treatment of choice is oral itraconazole, and treatment may be required for several

months. Typically, it is not necessary to perform surgical debridement. Wet to dry dressings will not address the underlying infection. Finally, trimethoprim-sulfamethoxazole is used for bacterial infections but would not be appropriate treatment for this fungal infection.

Test-taking tip: You can eliminate A because this rash does not sound life-threatening and does not need a surgeon. Deciphering whether it is a fungal rash or bacterial is hard. But hints that it is *not* bacterial are that it is painless and is not red.

71. ANSWER: A

The most likely diagnosis in this case is aortic stenosis. This diagnosis should be considered when a patient presents with exertional syncope, particularly if there is an associated crescendo-decrescendo systolic murmur. It may also present with exertional chest pain without syncope. The EKG shows evidence of left ventricular hypertrophy, which develops to force blood out of the left ventricle through a narrowed aortic valve.

There is no delta wave or shortening of the PR interval to suggest Wolff-Parkinson-White syndrome, though this condition can also cause syncope. Both PE and acute coronary syndrome (ACS) can result in chest pain and syncope, especially with exertion; however, this patient does not appear to have risk factors for these conditions aside from age. He exercises and appears to be in good physical condition, has never smoked, and does not have any medical conditions that predispose him to PE or ACS. Additionally, the EKG does not show evidence of ischemia and heart strain. The troponin should be trended to further evaluate for the possibility of ACS; however, the exertional syncope coupled with the systolic murmur makes aortic stenosis the most likely diagnosis, and an echocardiogram should be obtained.

Test-taking tip: Exertional syncope with a systolic murmur is aortic stenosis until proved otherwise.

72. ANSWER: B

This presentation is most concerning for mesenteric ischemia. This condition typically occurs in older adults, and risk factors include atrial fibrillation, prior myocardial infarction, valvular disease, cardiomyopathy, diabetes, hypertension, smoking, and prior thromboembolic events, including pulmonary embolism, deep venous thrombosis, mural thrombi, or ischemic stroke. The superior mesenteric artery is most affected because of its large caliber, and the jejunum is most frequently involved. It typically presents with severe, poorly localized abdominal pain that is out of proportion to the exam. As it progresses, patients may become hemodynamically unstable and develop bloody stools or signs of peritonitis. The most frequently used imaging modality is CT, which may show a variety of findings depending on the degree of ischemia, including bowel wall thickening, mesenteric stranding, pneumatosis intestinalis, or free intraperitoneal air and/or fluid. Lactate is an important marker that should be ordered in any patient with suspected mesenteric ischemia. One study showed an elevated lactate to be 100% sensitive in mesenteric ischemia, though it is not specific. Patients with suspected mesenteric ischemia should be started on IV antibiotics to cover intestinal flora and should have an emergent general surgery consult. This is true even in cases in which the patient's presentation is consistent with ischemia but the imaging is not necessarily diagnostic given the high risk for morbidity and mortality if not treated promptly. Starting antibiotics and admitting to medicine may be an appropriate choice for certain types of enteritis and colitis, but this patient needs to be seen by a surgeon as soon as possible. Consulting a gastroenterologist is not indicated at this point in this patient's workup because mesenteric ischemia is a surgical problem.

Test-taking tip: Mesenteric ischemia is a life-threatening disease. You can rule out C because a patient with pain out of proportion should never go home.

73. ANSWER: C

This patient's presentation is consistent with carpal tunnel syndrome, a mononeuropathy of the median nerve that is caused by compression of the nerve as it passes through the carpal tunnel. The median nerve supplies sensation to the palmar aspect of the thumb, index finger, middle finger, and radial half of the ring finger as well as the dorsal aspect of the index finger, middle finger, and radial half of the ring finger. Patient with carpal tunnel syndrome often experience paresthesias in this distribution, and two-point discrimination is one of the most useful tests to diagnose the condition. The Tinel test and Phalen maneuver have also been used in the diagnosis of carpal tunnel syndrome but are neither sensitive nor specific. The Tinel test involves tapping over the median nerve and is positive if this produces paresthesias. To perform the Phalen maneuver, the patient holds the dorsal surfaces of the hands together with the wrists flexed, and it is positive if this causes paresthesias. Finally, wrist extension is a function of the radial nerve, not the median nerve, and should therefore be preserved in carpal tunnel syndrome.

Test-taking tip: You can narrow down your choices by eliminating D because wrist extension is due to the radial (not medial) nerve.

74. ANSWER: D

The scenario describes a brief resolved unexplained event (BRUE). A BRUE is defined as an unexplained event that occurs in an infant younger than 1 year, lasts for less than 1 minute before the infant returns to baseline, and involves any of the following: cyanosis, pallor, apnea or irregular breathing, hypertonia or hypotonia, or an altered level of consciousness. To be classified as a BRUE, the child must be otherwise asymptomatic with a normal physical exam and normal vital signs. If an explanation for the event can be identified, then by definition, it cannot be called a BRUE. Patients presenting with a BRUE must be risk-stratified to determine the best management. A BRUE is considered low risk if the patient is older than 60 days and was born at 32 weeks' gestation or later with a postconceptual age of at least 45 weeks; if it is the patient's first event; and if there was never any cardiopulmonary resuscitation initiated by a trained health professional. Low=risk BRUEs can be managed with a period of brief observation with cardiopulmonary monitoring in the ED, and if there are no concerning findings, the patient can be discharged home with next-day follow-up with the pediatrician. There is no need for laboratory studies or admission for monitoring, and home cardiopulmonary monitoring systems are not recommended.

Test-taking tip: This is a "you know it or don't" kind of question. If you don't know it, choose an answer and move on. You can perhaps mark it for review when you are done at the end of the test.

75. ANSWER: C

The most likely diagnosis in this patient is a spinal epidural abscess. It is implied that he is an IV drug abuser given the track marks, and in this setting, a fever, midline back pain, neurologic deficits, and urinary retention are highly suggestive of a spinal epidural abscess. The best imaging modality to confirm the diagnosis is MRI with contrast. In this case, given that he has neck stiffness, tenderness involving the entire thoracic spine, and findings suggestive of lumbar involvement, MRI of the entire spine should be completed to evaluate the full extent of the abscess. An MRI of only the thoracic spine may miss part of the abscess, and it is also possible to have noncontiguous abscesses simultaneously. A CT scan may be done at institutions that do not have MRI to evaluate for cord impingement or osseous involvement but is not the imaging modality of choice and may miss an abscess. Finally, although the presentation may mimic meningitis, a lumbar puncture should never be performed in patients with suspected epidural abscess because it could cause further spread of the infection or seeding of the spine.

Test-taking tip: You can eliminate D and A right away because lumbar puncture is contraindicated in anyone you suspect has an epidural abscess, and CT is not the best test.

Test-taking tip: Take note that the question stem gave information that the patient has receptive anal intercourse. This is a huge clue to treat this patient for STIs.

76. ANSWER: B

This patient has an anterior shoulder dislocation. Of the choices listed, neuropraxia of the axillary nerve is the most commonly associated injury. This results in diminished sensation over the deltoid that is transient. The motor function of the axillary nerve may also be affected, resulting in weakness with shoulder abduction and external rotation.

The radial nerve, axillary artery, and brachial plexus can all be injured as well, but these are rarer. Axillary artery injury is more likely to occur among older adults, particularly with an associated humerus fracture, and may present with absent distal pulses. Neurovascular function should be documented before and after reduction in all patients. Other common injuries associated with anterior shoulder dislocations include the Hill-Sachs deformity, a compression fracture of the posterolateral aspect of the humeral head, as well as the Bankart lesion, a fracture of the anteroinferior aspect of the glenoid. These should be noted, but there is no specific intervention indicated in the ED for such injuries. Patients should be referred to orthopedics as an outpatient after successful reduction in the ED.

Test-taking tip: Anterior shoulder dislocation is very common. We do not really see any complications from this injury, so look for the least serious complication listed.

77. ANSWER: B

This patient has proctitis, and given his history of receptive anal intercourse, the etiology is most likely a sexually transmitted infection (STI). Proctitis is also commonly associated with radiation treatment for pelvic and lower gastrointestinal tumors, but there is no mention of this in the patient's history. The most common organisms associated with proctitis include gonorrhea and chlamydia, and thus he should be treated for both with intramuscular ceftriaxone and oral doxycycline. He should also be tested for syphilis, herpes, and HIV if there are any findings suggestive of these conditions, which he is also at risk for developing. Proctitis can less commonly be caused by other enteric organisms, many of which would also be covered by doxycycline. Treatment with clindamycin alone does not provide adequate STI coverage. Treatment with vancomycin is not indicated in this patient. Finally, oral metronidazole and ciprofloxacin are commonly used to treat gastrointestinal conditions, including many causes of diarrhea, but this combination does not cover the most likely organisms.

78. ANSWER: A

Bilious emesis in a neonate is a surgical emergency until proved otherwise. Causes of bilious emesis in the neonate include necrotizing enterocolitis (NEC), malrotation with midgut volvulus, duodenal atresia, and meconium ileus. In cases of bilious emesis, a pediatric surgeon should be involved as soon as possible, and surgical consultation should not be delayed to obtain imaging studies. Gastrointestinal obstruction can result in ischemic bowel in these cases, and delaying treatment can have serious and potentially life-threatening implications.

Imaging may be indicated but should be ordered in conjunction with the surgeon. Abdominal ultrasound would be the imaging modality of choice for pyloric stenosis and appendicitis in infants and children but is not likely to provide a definitive diagnosis for the etiology of bilious emesis. A CT scan of the abdomen would likely reveal the cause; however, given the risk for radiation, potential for allergic reactions to contrast, need for sedation, and delay to treatment, it would not be the best next step in this case. Air-contrast enema is both diagnostic and therapeutic in intussusception but should not be done in patients with signs of shock, peritonitis, or signs of perforation on plain film. Those patients require emergent surgical intervention. Intussusception is rare in neonates.

Test-taking tip: The questions describes a very sick 15-day-old. You can eliminate B, C, and D because all of that imaging takes time to complete and delay definitive treatment by a surgeon.

79. ANSWER: C

This patient is experiencing transfusion-related acute lung injury (TRALI), a potentially fatal transfusion reaction. This condition occurs within 6 hours of a transfusion of any type of blood product and by definition must be characterized by hypoxemia and pulmonary infiltrates on radiograph. Hypotension and fever are also common. Treatment is primarily supportive. The transfusion should be stopped immediately, and any remaining blood product should be returned to the blood bank for further analysis.

Patients should be started on supplemental oxygen initially, but there should be a low threshold to intubate these patients because most cases will ultimately require mechanical ventilation. The pulmonary edema of TRALI is noncardiogenic in nature, and aggressive diuresis should be avoided because many of these patients will develop hemodynamic instability, which can be exacerbated by diuresis. Antibiotics do not play a role in the management of TRALI because it is not an infectious process.

Test-taking tip: Be familiar with the indications for transfusion and the complications that can arise with a transfusion.

80. ANSWER: A

This presentation is concerning for cutaneous anthrax. While rare in developed nations, outbreaks still occur in developing countries where infected animals are common. Most exposures occur from contact with cattle, goats, or sheep or their products such as hides or wool. Spores deposit in the skin and form painless lesions that ultimately turn into eschars. Systemic involvement may occur. Up to 20% of cases of cutaneous anthrax are fatal if not treated. Ciprofloxacin has been used for first-line therapy. Debridement should not be performed on cutaneous anthrax because it can cause dissemination. High-dose IV penicillin has been used for systemic anthrax but does not play a role in uncomplicated cutaneous anthrax. Plasmapheresis is not indicated.

Test-taking tip: The clues of travel from Africa and contact with animals (patient makes leather drums) are clues to the diagnosis of anthrax.

81. ANSWER: B

The ultrasound shows B lines, vertical streaks of artifact extending from the pleural line to the bottom of the screen that resemble comet tails and move with respiration. This finding is characteristic of pulmonary edema and suggests that this patient's shortness of breath is at least in part related to her congestive heart failure. The diagnosis of pneumothorax can be made on ultrasound by a lack of lung sliding when examining the pleural line. Diagnosis of pneumothorax can be assisted by using M-mode. A stratosphere sign, also known as barcode sign, is suggestive of pneumothorax, whereas a seashore sign makes pneumothorax less likely. There are no reliable findings on ultrasound that suggest bronchospasm. A dilated right ventricle on ultrasound is characteristic of pulmonary embolism. The identification of B lines on ultrasound may result in the proper treatment being initiated sooner for this patient.

Test-taking tip: In this question the ultrasound image is key to the diagnosis. You can eliminate D because there are no hints in the question in regard to PE.

82. ANSWER: C

This presentation is consistent with omphalitis, an infection of the umbilical stump. It is uncommon in developed countries given the fairly sterile conditions during most hospital deliveries; however, it is still seen in home births in which the umbilical cord is cut with a nonsterile object, or in certain cultures in which foreign substances, including animal feces, are sometimes rubbed on the stump. The infection is typically polymicrobial and should be taken very seriously because potential complications include sepsis, necrotizing fasciitis, hepatic abscess, portal vein thrombosis, peritonitis, and death. Discharge home with oral antibiotics is not appropriate. Cultures of both the purulent drainage and blood should be collected, and broad-spectrum IV antibiotics should be initiated as soon as possible.

Some drainage from the umbilicus may be normal in the absence of erythema, swelling, tenderness, or systemic signs. Some providers advocate the application of alcohol locally around the stump to keep the area clean and enhance drying, but there is no evidence to support this practice. Bedside I&D should not be performed in the ED, and if there is any concern for abscess formation or necrotizing infection, a pediatric surgeon should be consulted.

Test-taking tip: This can be a life-threatening condition in a neonate. You can eliminate choices A and B because they both involve discharge home, which is not a viable option in this case.

83. ANSWER: B

The image demonstrates a hyphema, a collection of red blood cells in the anterior chamber of the eye. Hyphemas may occur from trauma or may be spontaneous in patients with sickle cell disease or in those taking certain medications such as anticoagulants or antiplatelet agents. Complications of hyphema include increased intraocular pressure, vision impairment, rebleeding, corneal staining, and formation of peripheral anterior synechiae.

An ophthalmologist should be consulted for all hyphemas; however, depending on the size and other factors, many hyphemas can be managed as an outpatient. The patient's ultimate disposition should be determined by the ophthalmologist in the absence of other injuries or illness. Management includes lowering intraocular pressure and preventing rebleeding. Patients with sickle cell are at higher risk for these complications. The head of the bed should be elevated to 45 degrees to promote settling of the red blood cells in the anterior chamber, thereby preventing occlusion of the trabecular meshwork. Topical β-blockers, mannitol, and carbonic anhydrase inhibitors have all been used to lower intraocular pressure in patients with a hyphema.

However, in this patient with sickle cell disease, a carbonic anhydrase inhibitor such as acetazolamide should not be given because this medication lowers the pH in the anterior chamber, promoting further sickling of the blood cells. The sickle cells obstruct the trabecular meshwork and increase intraocular pressure. Cyclopentolate, a cycloplegic medication, is used to dilate the pupil in hyphema. This reduces stress on the iris vessel that caused the bleeding, thereby reducing the risk for rebleeding. Finally, topical glucocorticoids such as prednisolone also reduce the risk for rebleeding and should be given.

Test-taking tip: This is a "you know it or don't" kind of question. If you don't know it, choose an answer and move on. You can perhaps mark it for review when you are done at the end of the test.

84. ANSWER: D

The EKG shows delta waves and a short PR, which are consistent with a diagnosis of Wolff-Parkinson-White syndrome. This condition is caused by an accessory pathway from the atria to the ventricles that bypasses the AV node and predisposes patients to a variety of supraventricular tachydysrhythmias. Treatment of wide-complex tachycardia with any AV nodal blocking agent can worsen the tachycardia by promoting further conduction through the accessory pathway and may result in ventricular fibrillation. Therefore, β-blockers, calcium channel blockers, and digoxin must all be avoided in Wolff-Parkinson-White syndrome with wide-complex tachycardia.

The treatment of choice is procainamide, a class Ia antiarrhythmic agent. If procainamide is unsuccessful at converting the patient back to sinus rhythm or if the patient is hemodynamically unstable, synchronized cardioversion can also be used.

Test-taking tip: Wolff-Parkinson-White syndrome, along with other unique EKG findings like Brugada's and Wellens' syndromes, are commonly tested on standardized exams.

85. ANSWER: C

The question describes an umbilical cord prolapse, a life-threatening emergency for the fetus because of potential cord compression. The safest way to manage this condition is to elevate the presenting fetal part by placing one hand inside the vagina. This position should be maintained until emergent cesarean delivery is performed, including during transport and preparation in the operating room. No attempt should be made to reduce the cord or deliver vaginally because these may worsen cord compression and result in death of the fetus.

The Gaskin maneuver is used for shoulder dystocia and has no role in cord prolapse. The Gaskin maneuver is performed by placing the mother on all fours to open the pelvis wider and use gravity to deliver the shoulders.

Test-taking tip: Cord prolapse is an obstetric emergency, and vaginal delivery is not recommended. You can eliminate B and D immediately because you will not proceed with vaginal delivery.

2.

GASTROINTESTINAL EMERGENCIES

Sukhjit Dhillon, James McCue, Steven Riccoboni, and Caleb Sunde

1. A 54-year-old female with history of congestive heart failure (CHF), cirrhosis, and diabetes is brought in by emergency medical services (EMS) for evaluation of altered mental status. Her family reported that she had numerous episodes of coffee-ground emesis, and they found her to be somnolent and disoriented. Initial vital signs are heart rate (HR) 98 bpm, blood pressure (BP) 104/54 mm Hg, So_2 98% on room air, respiratory rate (RR) 16 breaths/min, and temperature 36.1° C. The patient is somnolent but awakens easily. She is oriented to person only. Exam is notable for a distended abdomen and flapping tremors of bilateral hands. Abnormal labs include white blood cell (WBC) count 4.1, hemoglobin (Hgb) 12.2, platelets 78, Na 131, blood urea nitrogen (BUN) 53, creatinine 1.3, glucose 210, aspartate aminotransferase (AST) 63, ammonia 127. Which of the following is the most common precipitating factor of hepatic encephalopathy?

   A. Infection
   B. Upper gastrointestinal (GI) bleed
   C. Dehydration
   D. Hypoxia

2. A cirrhotic patient is evaluated for gradually worsening altered mental status. A family member notifies you that that patient had stopped taking a certain medication several days ago because of subsequent increased frequency of bowel movements. Which best describes this medication's main mechanism of action?

   A. Alteration of gut flora
   B. Decreased bacterial production of NH_3
   C. Increased conversion of NH_3 to NH_4^+
   D. Decreasing renal reabsorption

3. A 37-year-old male presents to the emergency department (ED) for evaluation of fever and right upper quadrant (RUQ) pain. The patient had recently been hospitalized for management of multiple abdominal stab wounds complicated by peritonitis. Presently the patient is febrile and tachycardic. An abdominal computed tomography (CT) scan reveals an intrahepatic fluid collection with surrounding edema. Which of the following lab values will most likely be elevated?

   A. AST
   B. Alanine aminotransferase (ALT)
   C. Alkaline phosphatase
   D. Serum bilirubin

4. A 45-year-old male returns from abroad after spending several months in rural India. Shortly after returning he experiences gradually worsening RUQ pain, sweats, and fever. Workup in the ED reveals a mild leukocytosis, elevations in alkaline phosphatase and transaminases, and a cystic intrahepatic cavity on ultrasound. Which of the following statements comparing pyogenic liver abscesses and amebic liver abscesses is TRUE?

   A. Pyogenic abscesses often resolve with a regimen of oral antibiotics, such as metronidazole
   B. Aspiration of amebic abscesses most commonly reveals a predominance of trophozoites and polymorphonuclear cells
   C. All amebic abscesses require surgical drainage for complete resolution
   D. Amebic abscesses are at higher risk for rupture than pyogenic abscesses

5. A 63-year-old female with history of hepatitis C cirrhosis presents for evaluation of worsening abdominal pain, distention, and yellowing of her eyes. The patient states she had fluid taken out her abdomen one time in the past, several years ago. Vital signs are HR 74 bpm, BP 134/80 mm Hg, RR 14 breaths/min, So_2 100%, and temperature 37.1° C. Exam is remarkable for a distended, nontender abdomen with positive fluid wave and scleral icterus. Which of the following statements regarding hepatocellular carcinoma is TRUE?

A. Characteristic ultrasound findings reveal well-defined, cystic mass
B. Hypocalcemia may be secondary to bone metastases or paraneoplastic syndrome
C. Hepatocellular cancer classically presents as hepatomegaly and jaundice
D. Cutaneous manifestations include dermatomyositis and porphyria cutanea tarda

6. A 42-year-old woman complaining of severe RUQ pain, nausea, and vomiting undergoes ultrasound of the RUQ. The ultrasound findings in Figure 2.1 are consistent with which of the following?

A. Cholelithiasis
B. Acute calculous cholecystitis
C. Acute acalculous cholecystitis
D. Choledocholithiasis

7. A 38-year-old male presents with constant RUQ pain, nausea, and vomiting. Exam is notable for fever, RUQ tenderness, and a positive Murphy's sign. Abnormal labs include WBC 14.3, alkaline phosphatase 280, AST 52, ALT 56, and total bilirubin 0.9. Ultrasound reveals a thickened gallbladder wall and pericholecystic fluid. Which of the following is the best management?

A. Draw peripheral blood cultures and start IV antibiotics
B. Arrange for emergent endoscopic retrograde cholangiopancreatography (ERCP)
C. General surgery consult for urgent cholecystectomy

D. PO challenge and arrange outpatient surgical follow-up

8. A patient presents with RUQ abdominal pain and jaundice. Labs are notable for WBC 6.7, alkaline phosphatase 130, ALT 73, AST 51, lipase 98, and total bilirubin 4.3. Ultrasound of the RUQ reveals multiple small stones in the gallbladder with a wall thickness of 0.2 cm as well as a rounded echogenic focus in the common bile duct measuring 1 cm. Which of the following is the most appropriate definitive management?

A. General surgery consult for emergent cholecystectomy
B. Arrange for ERCP
C. Administer broad-spectrum IV antibiotics
D. Obtain a hepatobiliary iminodiacetic acid (HIDA) scan to confirm gallstone location

9. A patient presents to the ED with worsening RUQ pain 1 week after having undergone elective cholecystectomy for symptomatic cholelithiasis. The patient reports fever, chills, and nausea and denies vomiting, diarrhea, or constipation. Initial vital signs are HR 94 bpm, BP 124/74 mm Hg, So$_2$ 98% on room air, RR 12 breaths/min, and temperature 38.6° C. On exam, the patient exhibits mild abdominal distention, RUQ tenderness without rebound or guarding. Surgical incisions are well approximated without discharge or erythema. Heart and lung sounds are unremarkable. Notable labs include WBC 12.4, Hgb 13.7, platelets 356, ALT 24, AST 18, alkaline phosphatase 112, total bilirubin 1.6,

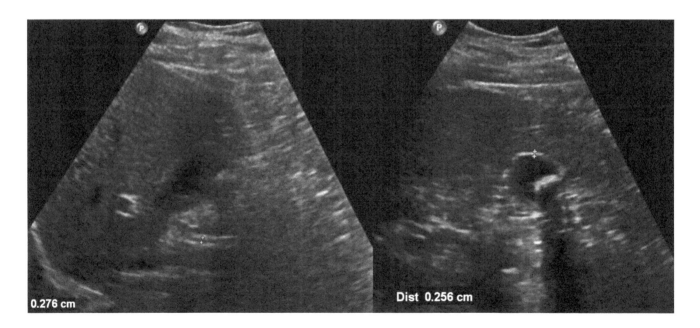

Figure 2.1 Ultrasound of the right upper quadrant.

and lipase 23. An abdominal ultrasound is obtained that shows a common bile duct of 1 cm and a complex fluid collection in the gallbladder fossa. Which of the following diagnoses is most likely?

A. Postoperative ileus
B. Postoperative bile leak
C. Retained common bile duct stone
D. Right lower lobe pneumonia

10. A 43-year-old female presents with RUQ abdominal pain, nausea, and vomiting that started after eating a hot dog at the local fair. On ultrasound, there are gallstones visualized. What is the most sensitive ultrasound finding in acute cholecystitis?

A. Positive sonographic Murphy's sign
B. Gallbladder wall thickening
C. Pericholecystic fluid
D. Gallbladder distention

11. Which of the following is the most common complication of untreated acute cholecystitis?

A. Gallstone ileus
B. Cholecystenteric fistula
C. Gangrenous cholecystitis
D. Emphysematous cholecystitis

12. A 45-year-old female presents with fever, chills, and RUQ abdominal pain for 2 days. Labs show WBC 15, total bilirubin 4, AST 100, ALT 93, and vital signs are remarkable for fever. Which of the following additional symptoms is most concerning for suppurative cholangitis?

A. Confusion
B. Tachycardia
C. Leukopenia
D. Bilious emesis

13. A patient presents to the ED complaining of fever and constant RUQ abdominal pain. Initial vital signs are HR 103 bpm, BP 107/74 mm Hg, So$_2$ 99%, RR 18 breaths/min, and temperature 39.2° C. Physical exam is notable for scleral icterus and RUQ tenderness without rebound or guarding. Notable labs include WBC 14.1, ALT 44, AST 38, alkaline phosphatase 112, total bilirubin 4.6, and lipase 38. What is the best antibiotic regimen?

A. Cefepime and levofloxacin
B. Gentamicin and vancomycin
C. Metronidazole
D. Piperacillin-tazobactam

14. A 46-year-old male presents to the ED with severe RUQ and mid-epigastric pain. The pain is constant and radiates to his back and is associated with nausea and vomiting. Vital signs on presentation are HR 108 bpm, BP 147/74 mm Hg, So$_2$ 100%, RR 14 breaths/min, and temperature 37.8° C. Notable labs include WBC 16, ALT 64, AST 58, alkaline phosphatase 183, total bilirubin 5.6, and lipase 2138. Abdominal ultrasound reveals many small mobile gallstones within the gallbladder and pericholecystic fluid. The gallbladder wall measures 4 cm, and the common bile duct measures 1.4 cm. Which of the following is TRUE regarding pancreatitis?

A. Two-thirds of cases are attributed to alcohol abuse and hypertriglyceridemia
B. An elevated amylase is less specific but more sensitive than an elevated lipase
C. The focus of initial treatment is early aggressive crystalloid resuscitation
D. Early prophylactic antibiotics are associated with a reduction in morbidity and mortality

15. Which of the following medications has a black box warning for an association with acute pancreatitis?

A. Colchicine
B. Valproic acid
C. Zidovudine
D. Amiodarone

16. A 23-year-old male presents to the ED for evaluation of a rapidly enlarging wound to his left shin since having cut his leg 2 weeks prior. Review of symptoms is notable for chronic abdominal pain and bloody diarrhea. Examination of his leg reveals the skin finding in Figure 2.2. Which of the following is the most appropriate treatment strategy?

A. PO antibiotics with gram-positive bacterial coverage
B. IV antibiotics with gram-negative bacterial coverage
C. Local wound care and systemic glucocorticoids
D. Aggressive surgical debridement

17. A 56-year-old man with history of ulcerative colitis presents with several days of bloody diarrhea, severe abdominal pain, and distention. Presenting vital signs are HR 116 bpm, BP 95/68 mm Hg, RR 18 breaths/min, So2 98%, and temperature 39.4° C. An upright abdominal radiograph is obtained (Figure 2.3). Which of the following is the most likely diagnosis?

A. Toxic megacolon
B. Ogilvie's syndrome
C. Neutropenic enterocolitis
D. Sigmoid volvulus

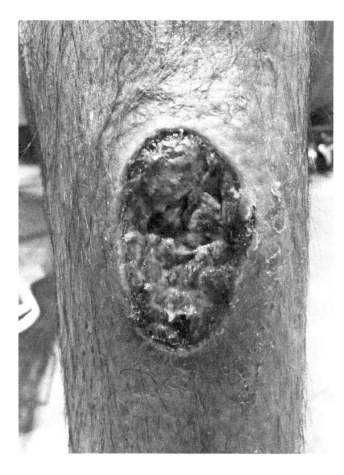

Figure 2.2 Leg wound.

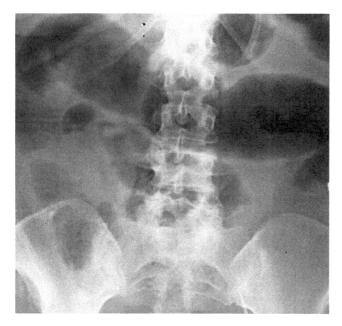

Figure 2.3 Kidneys, ureters, and bladder (KUB) radiograph.

18. A 12-day-old female full term infant with no known medical history is brought into the ED by her mother for repeated vomiting, poor feeding, and increased abdominal distention since birth. The patient passed stool within 48 hours of birth but has passed little stool since then. The patient is afebrile, and her heart rate is 180 bpm. On exam, she appears uncomfortable, and her abdomen is distended. Rectal exam reveals increased tone and absence of stool in the rectal vault. An explosive release of foul-smelling gas and stool occurs after the rectal exam. Which of the following is the most important next step?

A. Start IV antibiotics
B. Emergent surgical intervention
C. Barium enema
D. Observe

19. A 72-year-old male presents from a nursing facility for abdominal distention and decreased oral intake for 2 days. The patient has a prior history of a cerebrovascular accident (CVA) and is nonverbal. On physical exam, the patient's abdomen is significantly distended. but he appears to be in no significant discomfort and his vital signs are within normal limits. An abdominal radiograph demonstrates a large dilated loop of colon with air-fluid levels and an absence of rectal gas. What is the next appropriate step?

A. CT of the abdomen and pelvis
B. Insert nasogastric (NG) tube and admit for observation
C. Discharge with no further workup
D. Emergent surgical consultation

20. A 43-year-old male with no past medical history presents with aching pain on defecation for the past few days. A rectal exam with anoscopy is performed. The external exam and rectal mucosa appear normal, but the patient has significant pain in the lateral rectal wall with palpation. What is the next appropriate step?

A. Perform a bedside incision and drainage (I&D) for suspected perianal abscess
B. Discharge with antibiotics
C. Surgical consultation
D. Discharge with stool softeners

21. A well-appearing 23-year-old female presents with severe pain and swelling over her sacrum. On exam, the patient has a small area of erythema and fluctuance over the natal cleft. What is the appropriate next step?

A. CT of the pelvis
B. Admit for IV antibiotics

C. Discharge with PO antibiotics

D. I&D

22. A 24-year-old male presents with rectal pain and pruritus. He reports unprotected anal intercourse. A rectal exam is performed and finds hyperemic and edematous mucosa and a small amount of purulent fluid. An appropriate treatment plan is which of the following?

A. Supportive care and primary care follow-up

B. Empiric treatment for sexually transmitted infection (STI)

C. Order a CT scan and consult surgery

D. Gram stain and culture purulent fluid and discharge with plan to follow up cultures

23. You are treating a 22-year-old male for proctitis. The patient is HIV positive and on exam is noted to have multiple perianal ulcerations and scant bloody rectal discharge. What is the appropriate treatment?

A. Ceftriaxone 250 mg IM once and doxycycline 100 mg PO twice daily for 7 days

B. Ceftriaxone 250 mg IM once and doxycycline 100 mg PO twice daily for 3 weeks

C. Ceftriaxone 250 mg IM once

D. Doxycycline 100 mg twice daily for 7 days

24. A 7-year-old male presents with rectal pain with defecation ongoing for 2 days. His mother states that he is frequently constipated and often strains with bowel movements. On exam, the patient is noted to have an anal fissure. Most anal fissures occur where?

A. Posterior midline

B. Laterally

C. Anterior midline

D. They occur in all areas equally

25. A 28-year-old female with a history of Crohn's disease presents with malodorous and blood-tinged rectal discharge. Before noticing the discharge the patient states that she had a throbbing pain. However, the pain has since resolved. Vital signs are within normal limits, and labs are unremarkable. On exam, a small opening is appreciated on the anterior anal canal. Which of the following is the most appropriate course of treatment?

A. Emergent surgical consultation

B. Admission for IV antibiotics

C. Bedside I&D

D. Discharge with oral antibiotics and surgical follow-up

26. Which of the following is the most common cause of an anal fistula?

A. Rectal STI

B. Ischiorectal abscesses

C. Malignancy

D. Inflammatory bowel disease

27. A 43-year-old male presents with a bottle in his rectum. Which of the following statements is TRUE?

A. Perianal anesthesia may be performed with 1% lidocaine with epinephrine to facilitate extraction

B. There is no indication for imaging

C. Emergent removal in the ED is indicated if there is any concern for perforation

D. The patient should be admitted for observation even if well-appearing if the bottle is successfully removed in the ED

28. A 47-year-old male with no known medical history presents with extreme rectal pain that started 1 day ago. On exam, the patient's pain is localized to a large thrombosed external hemorrhoid. What is the most appropriate management of this patient?

A. Surgical consultation for excision in the operating room (OR)

B. Discharge with PO antibiotics

C. Discharge with no treatment and referral to surgery

D. Clot excision in the ED

29. Emergent surgical consultation is warranted for internal hemorrhoids in which of the following situations?

A. Grade 4 internal hemorrhoids

B. Grade 3 internal hemorrhoids

C. Always

D. Never, internal hemorrhoids are managed nonoperatively

30. A 67-year-old female with a history of dementia presents from a nursing facility with a rectal prolapse. The patient has thick musculature tissue extending about 6 cm beyond the anal verge with edematous but otherwise well-appearing tissue. Initial attempt at manual reduction with gentle, continuous pressure was unsuccessful. What is the most appropriate next step?

A. Emergent surgical consultation for reduction in the OR

B. Emergent GI consultation for colonoscopy

C. Discharge with close follow-up in surgery clinic

D. Apply a generous amount of granulated sugar and reattempt reduction in 20 minutes

31. A 21-year-old female with no past medical history presents with fatigue, constant RUQ abdominal pain, nausea, vomiting, and jaundice. Her symptoms have progressed over the past week, and during that time she has also noted that her urine has appeared dark colored. Three weeks ago the patient was traveling abroad in Thailand. On exam, she appears jaundiced and is tender to palpation in her RUQ. She is afebrile and her vital signs are within normal limits. Which test is likely to confirm a diagnosis?

A. Viral hepatitis panel
B. Blood smear
C. Abdominal ultrasound
D. CT of the abdomen and pelvis

32. A 55-year-old male with a history of cirrhosis presents with abdominal pain that feels different than normal abdominal distention before paracentesis, which he has done frequently. He is afebrile, and his vital signs are within normal limits. Paracentesis is done, and symptoms improve. Ascitic fluid studies were found to have a negative Gram stain, 270/mL polymorphonuclear leukocytes, and WBC 400/mm³. Fluid cultures are sent. What is the most appropriate next step?

A. Discharge home
B. Wait for ascitic fluid culture
C. Surgical consultation
D. Start IV antibiotics and admit

33. A 63-year-old female with a history of cirrhosis with ascites presented to the ED with abdominal pain. Fluid studies from a paracentesis that was preformed are consistent with spontaneous bacterial peritonitis. Which of the following is the most appropriate antibiotic choices?

A. Vancomycin 1 g IV daily
B. Ceftriaxone 2 g IV daily
C. Azithromycin 500 mg PO daily
D. Metronidazole 500 mg PO every 8 hours

34. A 47-year-old female presents with abdominal pain and distention. She has a known history of alcoholic cirrhosis. She is afebrile, and her vital signs are within normal limits. On exam, she has a distended abdomen with diffuse abdominal tenderness to palpation. She is found to have an international normalized ratio (INR) of 2.7 and a platelet count of 45,000/mm³. You intend to rule out spontaneous bacterial peritonitis. What is the best next step?

A. Give vitamin K before paracentesis
B. Transfuse fresh frozen plasma before paracentesis
C. Transfuse platelets before paracentesis
D. Preform paracentesis

35. A 74-year-male presents with acute onset of abdominal pain several hours before arrival. Pain is described as severe and diffuse and is associated with nausea and an episode of nonbloody loose stool. The patient takes only medications for hypertension and diabetes. Vital signs are temperature 37.7° C, BP 143/85 mm Hg, HR 135 bpm, RR 22 breaths/min, and oxygen saturation 97% on room air. On exam, the patient appears to be in severe pain. His abdomen is soft with mild diffuse tenderness to palpation with no rebound or guarding. Electrocardiogram (EKG) shows atrial fibrillation with no ischemic findings. Labs are unremarkable. The patient continues to have severe pain despite multiple doses of pain medication. Which of the following is the most appropriate next test?

A. RUQ ultrasound
B. Abdominal radiograph
C. Admit for pain control
D. Abdominal CT angiography

36. A 57-year-old male presents with several weeks of malaise, weight loss, and increasing jaundice. Vital signs are within normal limits. He has scleral icterus and appears jaundiced. He has no pain or distention on abdominal examination. Labs include a total bilirubin of 8.1, direct bilirubin 7.2, alkaline phosphatase 240, AST 135, and ALT 123. What is the most likely cause?

A. Pancreatic cancer
B. Cholecystitis
C. Choledocholithiasis
D. Cholangitis

37. A 27-year-old female presents with nausea, vomiting, and upper abdominal pain for a week. Her vital signs are within normal limits. On exam, her abdomen is mildly tender to palpation in the epigastrium and RUQ. Labs include AST 210, ALT 180, bilirubin within normal limits. An abdominal ultrasound is normal. Which of the following is consistent with acute hepatitis B virus (HBV) infection?

A. HBsAb
B. HBcAb
C. HBsAg
D. None of the above will be detected in the acute phase

38. Which of the following is consistent with the presentation of chronic mesenteric ischemia?

    A. 62-year-old female with a history of atrial fibrillation with sudden onset of severe diffuse abdominal pain

    B. 47-year-old female with periodic RUQ pain after meals

    C. 78-year-old male with 6 months of malaise, weight loss, and dark stools

    D. 69-year-old male with a history of peripheral vascular disease with several months of weight loss and recurrent mild diffuse abdominal pain after meals

39. A 59-year-old male presents with concern for weight gain and abdominal distention. On exam, he has a distended abdomen with shifting dullness, gynecomastia, and prominent abdominal veins. Which of the following further pieces of history is the most likely related to the cause of the patient's complaints?

    A. History of alcohol abuse

    B. History of hepatitis A infection

    C. History of taking large daily doses of acetaminophen for chronic back pain

    D. History of travel to South America

40. A 61-year-old male who is currently receiving radiation therapy for prostate cancer presents with 4 days of tenesmus, occasional incontinence of stool, and bloody diarrhea. Vital signs include HR 89 bpm, BP 138/87 mm Hg, and temperature 37.3° C. His abdomen is soft and nontender. On rectal exam he has normal tone and sensation but is diffusely tender, and a small amount of bright red blood is noted. Which of the following is the most appropriate management?

    A. Surgical consultation

    B. Oral steroids

    C. Empiric ceftriaxone and doxycycline

    D. Analgesics and sucralfate

41. A 46-year-old female with a history of alcohol abuse presents with increasing abdominal distention for 2 weeks. She has no other current complaints but notes that she had severe epigastric pain a week prior. She has no known history of cirrhosis or ascites. A bedside ultrasound reveals a moderate amount of ascites, and a paracentesis is performed. Peritoneal fluid is found to have an albumin of 4.7 and serum albumin was 3.7. What is the most likely cause of the patient's ascites?

    A. Cirrhosis

    B. CHF

    C. Pancreatitis

    D. Alcoholic hepatitis

42. A 1-week-old, ex–36 week boy presents with difficulty bottle feeding and bloody stool. His abdomen is distended on exam, and an upright radiograph shows pneumatosis intestinalis. He has an episode of bilious emesis in the ED. His vital signs are temperature 38.5° C, HR 210 bpm, BP 54/32 mm Hg, and RR 62 breaths/min. After starting antibiotics and fluid resuscitation, what is the next step in this patient's management?

    A. Discharge home with follow up in 24 hours with pediatrician

    B. Surgical consult

    C. Admission to telemetry

    D. GI consult for emergent endoscopy

43. A 6-week-old, ex-term baby boy presents with progressively worsening vomiting that is becoming projectile. The patient's mother describes the emesis as curdled milk and states that he seemed very hungry when the vomiting initially started but is not as interested with feeds recently. His exam is unremarkable, and his chemistry shows: Na 134, K 2.8, Cl 87, CO_2 17. You are concerned about a certain diagnosis, and it is confirmed on ultrasound. While waiting for surgery to see the patient, what are important interventions for this patient?

    A. Glucose and electrolyte replacement

    B. Bicarbonate

    C. GI consult for endoscopy

    D. Antibiotics

44. A 3-day-old girl born is brought to the ED after being born at home. She has not had a bowel movement since birth and has been having nonbilious vomiting. On exam, her abdomen is distended, and rectal exam reveals forceful release of meconium with stimulation. Which of the following radiograph findings would be most concerning for this patient?

    A. Double-bubble sign

    B. Pneumatosis

    C. Toxic megacolon

    D. Nonspecific bowel gas pattern

45. A 2-week-old boy presents with bilious emesis for the past 48 hours and has not been feeding well since being discharged from the hospital at day 2 of life. He is fussy, and his vital signs reveal temperature 38.6° C, HR 210 bpm, BP 62/37 mm Hg, RR 40 breaths/min. His abdomen is distended on exam. He had an upper GI contrast study that revealed a corkscrew pattern. What is the next best step in management of this patient?

A. Radiograph
B. Ultrasound
C. CT scan
D. Fluid and antibiotics

46. A precipitous delivery occurs in the ED, and the newborn requires intubation secondary to low Apgar score at 10 minutes. While passing a feeding tube, the nurse notices resistance early on (<10 cm), and the procedure is aborted. Vital signs are otherwise within normal limits, and a radiograph reveals an absence of the gastric bubble but otherwise no acute process. What is the definitive management for this case?

A. GI consult
B. Attempt NG passage with a smaller tube
C. Surgery consult
D. Discharge home

47. A 2-year-old boy presents with intermittent episodes of abdominal pain that are starting to last longer with each episode. The patient's mother states that she has started to notice him bringing his knees to his chest with each bout of pain, and then symptoms resolve after 15 minutes. She has not noticed any other symptoms, and he is otherwise healthy. His vital signs of within normal limits, and he has no tenderness on exam. While talking with his mother, he develops the pain and brings his legs to his chest. Ultrasound shows a "donut" structure. He is sent to interventional radiology for an air enema without improvement of his pathology. What is the next step in management of this patient?

A. Discharge home
B. Admission for observation
C. Surgical consult
D. IV antibiotics

48. What is the most common cause of neonatal jaundice?

A. Sepsis
B. Cephalohematoma
C. Breastfeeding
D. Physiologic

49. A 10-day-old boy is referred to the ED from the pediatric clinic secondary to an elevated bilirubin. He is acting appropriately and has been feeding well, strictly breastfed, but is jaundice on exam. Labs are drawn and reveal a bilirubin total of 21, with most of it being indirect, while the rest of the labs are within normal limits. What is the next appropriate step in management of this patient?

A. Discharge home with follow-up in clinic tomorrow
B. IV hydration
C. Ceftriaxone
D. Phototherapy

50. What is NOT a risk factor for neonatal jaundice?

A. Cephalohematoma
B. Breastfeeding
C. Formula feeding
D. Hemolytic disease

51. A 5-day-old boy presents with odd body movements for the past 12 hours. His mother reports that he will arch his back and neck for minutes and then go flaccid, and he has become harder to arouse over the past couple of hours. On exam, he is jaundice from head to toe, floppy, and not responding to painful stimuli. Most labs are still in process, but bilirubin has come back at 24 mg/dL. What is the best next step?

A. Exchange transfusion
B. Phototherapy
C. Intubation
D. Antibiotics

52. A 3-year-old boy was playing in the kitchen when he started to cry, and when his mother looked over he had a dishwasher detergent pod in his hand that he seemed to have bit into. The mother noticed that he was drooling and seemed to be having trouble swallowing. On presentation to the ED, the patient is still crying and drooling and has an episode of vomiting right when he walks in. His vital signs are HR 115 bpm, RR 18 breaths/min, temperature 37.5° C, and BP 95/70 mm Hg. He doesn't seem to be in respiratory distress at this time and on exam doesn't seem to have any apparent burns to his lips or oral mucosa. What is the next best step?

A. Administer activated charcoal
B. Insert a NG tube for gastric lavage
C. Give pain medication and encourage patient to drink oral fluids to help wash down the ingested material
D. Designate patient as NPO and call GI consult for endoscopy

53. A 16-year-old girl presents after swallowing a sewing needle. She reports that she was holding the needle between her teeth when she accidentally swallowed it. She feels like she has something stuck in her throat, and it hurts to swallow. The patient does not have trouble breathing and has not vomited. On presentation, her vital signs are HR 106 bpm, RR 18 breaths/min,

temperature 37.4° C, and BP 100/70 mm Hg. What is the best next step in management for this patient?

A. Call GI for urgent endoscopy
B. Order a radiograph to determine the location of the needle; no intervention is needed if needle is already in the stomach
C. Do nothing and wait for spontaneous passage
D. Observe with serial radiographs

54. A 60-year-old female presents with diffuse abdominal pain progressively worsening over the past 3 days that is associated with nausea and nonbilious and nonbloody vomiting. She states she had one small bowel movement yesterday. On exam, you notice the abdomen is distended with an old surgical scar to the middle and tender to palpation diffusely. What is the most common cause for this women's presentation?

A. Neoplasm
B. Adhesions
C. Hernia
D. Volvulus

55. A 16-month-old boy is brought in by his mother for abdominal pain since this morning. The mother reports that the patient has been having intermittent episodes when he brings his knees to his chest and cries for about 5 minutes and then feels better until it happens again. He has had three episodes of nonbilious and nonbloody vomiting. On your exam, patient is playful and not in any distress. The abdomen is soft with no tenderness to palpation, rebound tenderness, or guarding. Vital signs are within normal range. What is the best test to help you diagnose and treat the underlying etiology?

A. Abdominal radiograph
B. Abdominal ultrasound
C. Abdominal CT
D. Barium or air enema

56. A 23-month-old boy is brought to the ED by his parents for blood in his stool for the past 2 days. The parents report that they have noticed bright red blood in his diaper for the past 2 days, but the child otherwise seems be doing well and acting his normal self. He has not had any recent fever or vomiting. On exam, the patient is playful and not in any acute distress. The abdomen is soft and nontender to palpation. The diaper contains a small amount of stool with gross blood. What is the most likely diagnosis?

A. Intussusception
B. Anal fissure

C. Meckel's diverticulum
D. Necrotizing enterocolitis

57. A 45-year-old male with past medical history significant for alcohol abuse and cirrhosis presents with abdominal pain, nausea, and vomiting and states that he has noticed a small amount of blood in his vomit. His BP is 98/60 mm Hg, HR 80 bpm, and RR 24 breaths/min. On exam, he has diffuse abdominal tenderness to palpation but no guarding or rebound tenderness. Rectal exam is remarkable for dark tarry stool that is guaiac positive but no frank blood. INR is 3. Which of the following interventions has a mortality benefit in this patient?

A. Proton pump inhibitor
B. Octreotide
C. Ceftriaxone
D. Fresh frozen plasma

58. A 56-year-old male presents with generalized abdominal pain, nausea, vomiting, and a low-grade fever for 1 week and noticed significant bright red blood from his rectum this morning. The patient states that he feels lightheaded. On exam, he appears tired, pale, and diaphoretic; he has an old surgical scar in the mid-abdomen with diffuse abdominal tenderness to palpation but no rebound tenderness or guarding and with gross blood on rectal exam. On further history, he mentions that he had abdominal aortic aneurysm repair 3 years ago. His BP is 83/60 mm Hg, HR 123 bpm, RR 18 breaths/min, oxygen saturation 98% on room air, and temperature 37.8° C (oral). What is the best next step?

A. Abdominal radiograph
B. Emergent endoscopy
C. Call surgeon for emergent laparotomy
D. CT angiography of abdomen and pelvis

59. A 65-year-old male is sent from a nursing facility for abdominal distention and pain associated with nausea. The patient states that he has a history of constipation and has not had a bowel movement for about 2 days now. He denies fever or vomiting. On exam, the abdomen is distended with minimal tenderness diffusely but no rebound tenderness or guarding. An abdominal radiograph is ordered and shows distended loops of bowel with loss of haustral markings. Vital signs are BP 110/80 mm Hg, HR 90 bpm, RR 14 breaths/min, oxygen saturation 96% on room air, and temperature 36.3° C. What is the most likely diagnosis?

A. Small bowel obstruction
B. Cecal volvulus
C. Sigmoid volvulus
D. Mesenteric ischemia

60. Which of the following statements is TRUE in patients with Crohn's disease?

A. Only mucosa and submucosa of the bowel are involved
B. Any part of the GI tract can be involved
C. Bloody diarrhea is common
D. Colonoscopy will show continuous involvement of the bowel

61. A 47-year-old male with past medical history of peptic ulcer disease (PUD) presents for recurrent epigastric pain, nausea, and diarrhea. The patient states that he has tried everything in the past, including H_2 blockers, proton pump inhibitors, and triple therapy with antibiotics and proton pump inhibitors, which seemed to help briefly, but his symptoms tend to recur. He reports losing 15 pounds over the past month. There is a strong family history of PUD. On exam, he appears uncomfortable secondary to pain. The abdomen is soft with epigastric tenderness to palpation but no rebound tenderness or guarding. Vital signs are normal and stable. Which test can best determine the underlying cause of this patient's symptoms?

A. Fasting serum gastrin level
B. Lipase
C. Urease breath test
D. Abdominal radiograph

62. A 42-year-old female with a past medical history significant for hypertension and acid reflux presents with epigastric pain, nausea, and vomiting since earlier this morning. The patient describes the pain as a burning sensation. Pain seems to improve with cold milk but tends to return after eating food. She denies constipation. On presentation, the patient's temperature is 37.5°C, HR 98 bpm, RR 16 breaths/min, and BP 150/ 90 mm Hg. On exam, the patient appears uncomfortable secondary to pain with minimal epigastric tenderness to palpation, has no rebound tenderness or guarding, and is negative for Murphy's sign. What is the most likely diagnosis?

A. Acute coronary syndrome
B. Cholecystitis
C. Gastroesophageal reflux disease (GERD)
D. Small bowel obstruction

63. What is the most common cause of gastritis?

A. Alcohol
B. Nonsteroidal antiinflammatory drugs (NSAIDs)
C. Spicy food
D. *Helicobacter pylori* infection

64. What is the most common cause of large bowel obstruction?

A. Diverticulitis
B. Neoplasm
C. Volvulus
D. Hernia

65. A 50-year-old male is brought in by EMS for multiple bloody bowel movements since this morning. The patient states that he noticed bright red blood in the toilet. He denies abdominal pain but states that he feels lightheaded. On exam, the patient appears tired, and his abdomen is soft with no tenderness to palpation. Vital signs are remarkable for BP 87/60 mm Hg, HR 119 bpm, RR 16 breaths/min, oxygen saturation 96% on room air, and temperature 37° C. What is the next best step after starting resuscitative measures?

A. Consult GI
B. Magnetic resonance imaging (MRI) of the abdomen
C. Angiography
D. Scintigraphy

66. A 14-year-old thin-appearing male presents with abdominal pain that is associated with nausea, vomiting, and anorexia for 8 hours. The patient appears uncomfortable and is lying still on the bed. On presentation, his temperature is 38.4° C, HR 116 bpm, RR 16 breaths/ min, and BP 110/85 mm Hg. The patient states that pain started in the middle of his abdomen and is now mostly in the right lower quadrant. On exam, the patient has tenderness to palpation to the right lower quadrant but no rebound tenderness or guarding. What is the next best step?

A. Abdominal ultrasound
B. Call the surgeon on call for evaluation
C. CT of the abdomen and pelvis with contrast
D. Upright abdominal radiograph

67. A 14-year-old female presents to the ED with right lower quadrant abdominal pain. The pain started 2 days ago and is now worse. She also complains of nausea and vomiting. What is the next best test in her workup?

A. CT of the abdomen and pelvis
B. Ultrasound of the abdomen
C. Pregnancy test
D. Consult surgery

68. A 2-year-old male is brought into the ED after swallowing a button battery. The mother states he was playing with a toy and the battery came out and he

swallowed it before she could get it. What is the initial test you want to help identify the location of the battery?

A. Radiograph
B. Barium swallow
C. Endoscopy
D. CT of the abdomen

69. A 56-year-old male presents to the ED complaining of food stuck in his esophagus. He is leaning forward and cannot swallow his secretions. He states that the food has been lodged for 2 days and he was hoping it would pass on its own so he waited it out at home. The patient has a history of previous food bolus impactions. What is the next best step?

A. Consult GI for endoscopy
B. CT of the chest
C. Chest radiograph
D. Discharge to primary care physician for referral to GI as outpatient

70. A 5-year-old female presents with lower abdominal pain and nausea and vomiting for 1 day. The mother states that the patient is still eating and drinking. Vital signs are temperature 38.5° C, HR 120 bpm, BP 80/60 mm Hg. Her physical exam is unremarkable. What is the next best test to order to make the likely diagnosis?

A. Complete blood count
B. Chemistry 10 panel
C. Urinalysis
D. Ultrasound of the abdomen

71. A 75-year-old male patient presents to the ED with off-and-on abdominal pain for the past day. He has a history of hypertension and coronary artery disease and is a lifelong smoker. He appears pale and ill. Vital signs are BP 80/palp mm Hg, HR 120 bpm, temperature 37.6° C, and RR 20 breaths/min. On exam, the patient has a soft, nondistended abdomen. He is pale and sweaty. Resuscitation is started with IV fluids. What is the best initial imaging for this patient to make the diagnosis?

A. Beside ultrasound
B. CT of the abdomen and pelvis
C. MRI of the abdomen
D. Kidneys, ureters, and bladder (KUB) radiograph

72. A 35-year-old male presents with epigastric abdominal pain with nausea and vomiting. He drank a lot of beer last night at a party, and his pain started this morning. His labs show WBC 17, glucose 300, lipase 230, AST 150, ALT 175, alkaline phosphatase 60, and lactate dehydrogenase 441. What is this patient's estimated mortality based on Ranson's criteria?

A. <3%
B. 10%–15%
C. >40%
D. 100%

73. A male patient presents to the ED with abdominal pain. He has a large abdominal hernia that is easily reducible but causes him discomfort. The patient also has history of cirrhosis and ascites and receives paracentesis biweekly. The family states the patient is Child class C. What is the patient's expected perioperative mortality if the surgeons decide to do an elective hernia repair?

A. 10%
B. 30%
C. 50%
D. 82%

74. A 91-year-old male presents to the ED because his G-tube fell out. He resides in a nursing home. The patient was recently in the hospital for stroke and had a G-tube placed 6 days ago. What is the next step in management for this patient?

A. Replace the G-tube in the ED
B. Consult GI for endoscopic placement of the G tube
C. Discharge back to the facility and have the patient see GI as an outpatient
D. Call surgery

75. A 35-year-old male presents to the ED for profuse diarrhea. He states he was recently on clindamycin for mastoiditis but finished his antibiotics 2 weeks ago. He has had 15 to 20 episodes of diarrhea over the past few days. He states some have blood in them and some do not. What is the next best step in management of this patient?

A. Admission to the hospital and start IV vancomycin
B. Admission to the hospital and start PO vancomycin
C. Admission to the hospital and start PO metronidazole
D. Discharge home with reassurance

76. A 65-year-old well-appearing male is referred to a GI doctor for diarrhea. He has had diarrhea for weeks. The patient denies recent travel, fever, or blood in the stools. An endoscopy is performed and shows pseudomembranous colitis. What is the next best treatment?

A. Start PO metronidazole
B. Admit for IV metronidazole
C. Admit for IV vancomycin
D. Reassurance and supportive measures

1. ANSWER: A

All of the answer choices are recognized precipitants of hepatic encephalopathy, but infection is the most commonly identified precipitant when one is found. Other precipitants include sedative medications, constipation, electrolyte abnormalities, and gastrointestinal (GI) bleeding.

Test-taking tip: This is a "you know it or don't" kind of question. If you don't know it, choose an answer and move on. You can perhaps mark it for review when you are done at the end of the test. Don't, however, let these kinds of questions get you stuck and waste your time.

2. ANSWER: C

Lactulose is a common medication for both the prevention and treatment of hepatic encephalopathy, a common side effect of which is frequent loose bowel movements. Lactulose lowers the colonic pH, increasing the conversion of NH_3 (absorbable) to NH_4^+ (nonabsorbable) and thereby increasing its excretion and reducing plasma concentrations. Oral antibiotics, such as rifaximin, alter gut flora and decrease production of ammonia (choices A and B). Sodium benzoate decreases serum ammonia indirectly by increasing the renal excretion of nitrogen (choice D).

Test-taking tip: This is a "you know it or don't" kind of question. If you don't know it, choose an answer and move on. You can perhaps mark it for review when you are done at the end of the test. Don't, however, let these kinds of questions get you stuck and waste your time.

3. ANSWER: C

The patient in this question is presenting with a pyogenic hepatic abscess, as confirmed by the imaging findings. Etiologies of hepatic abscess include peritonitis, biliary tract disease, and less commonly penetrating hepatic injury. The most common laboratory abnormalities are an elevated white blood cell (WBC) count (most common), hypoalbuminemia, and an elevated alkaline phosphatase level (choice C). Elevations in aspartate aminotransferase (AST), alanine transaminase (ALT), or serum bilirubin are less common than with alkaline phosphatase. (choices A, B, and D).

Test-taking tip: This is a "you know it or don't" kind of question. If you don't know it, choose an answer and move on. You can perhaps mark it for review when you are done at the end of the test. Don't, however, let these kinds of questions get you stuck and waste your time.

4. ANSWER: D

Pyogenic and amebic liver abscesses have similar clinical presentations, but there are certain characteristics that differentiate one from the other. Amebic abscesses are associated with travel to endemic areas of the protozoan *Entamoeba histolytica* (Africa, India, Mexico, and Central and South America). As opposed to pyogenic abscesses, amebic abscesses usually resolve with oral antibiotics and do not require surgical drainage (choices A and C). Amebic abscesses are at higher risk for rupture than pyogenic abscesses (choice D). Aspiration of amebic abscesses reveals an acellular fluid composed mostly of necrotic hepatocytes (trophozoites are not commonly seen), whereas the aspirate of pyogenic abscesses is composed of bacterial and predominantly polymorphonuclear cells (choice B).

Test-taking tip: This is a "you know it or don't" kind of question. If you don't know it, choose an answer and move on. You can perhaps mark it for review when you are done at the end of the test. Don't, however, let these kinds of questions get you stuck and waste your time.

5. ANSWER: D

Hepatocellular carcinoma (HCC) is a primary cancer of the liver that is most commonly seen in patients with chronic liver disease. Patients with liver disease secondary to chronic hepatitis B and C infections are at particular risk for developing HCC. Early HCC is a difficult diagnosis because symptoms are usually limited to symptoms of their underlying disease (choice C). As the cancer progresses one may develop symptoms based on tumor size (pain, palpable mass) or due to invasion. Complications are often associated with extension of the tumor into the hepatic or portal veins (ascites, variceal bleeding) or biliary tree (obstructive jaundice). As with the patient in the question stem, HCC may present as decompensation of previously stable chronic disease. Additionally, patients may exhibit evidence of paraneoplastic syndrome. Hypercalcemia, not hypocalcemia, can be secondary to either bone metastases or paraneoplastic syndrome (choice B). Other manifestations include hypoglycemia, erythrocytosis, and watery diarrhea. Ultrasound will reveal a hypoechoic or hyperechoic, ill-defined mass with coarse internal echoes (choice A). Finally, numerous cutaneous manifestations are associated with HCC, including dermatomyositis, porphyria cutanea tarda, and pemphigus foliaceus (choice D).

Test-taking tip: Complications of chronic diseases are high yield on the exam. It is best to brush up on hepatitis C and its complications.

6. ANSWER: A

The ultrasound reveals a well-defined hyperechoic structure with shadowing contained within the gallbladder. This finding is consistent with cholelithiasis (choice A). Sonographic evidence of cholecystitis includes thickening of the gallbladder wall (>3 mm), pericholecystic fluid, and a positive sonographic Murphy's sign (choices B and C). Choledocholithiasis is suspected when the common bile duct measures more than 6 mm (+1 mm per decade above 60 years of age) (choice D).

Test-taking tip: Brush up on common emergency department (ED) bedside ultrasound findings like right upper quadrant (RUQ) and FAST.

7. ANSWER: C

This patient's presentation is consistent with acute cholecystitis. Although this patient meets systemic inflammatory response syndrome (SIRS) criteria for sepsis and should receive IV antibiotics (choice A), definitive management requires urgent surgical consent for cholecystectomy (choice C). Endoscopic retrograde cholangiopancreatography (ERCP) is not indicated in acute cholelithiasis but is the treatment of choice for choledocholithiasis (choice B). PO challenge with outpatient follow-up is the appropriate treatment of uncomplicated symptomatic cholelithiasis but not of acute cholecystitis (choice D).

Test-taking tip: Brush up on common ED bedside ultrasound findings like RUQ and FAST. The ultrasound showing a thickened wall with a stone is indicative of cholecystitis.

8. ANSWER: B

The patient has choledocholithiasis and possible early gallstone pancreatitis as suggested by the lab abnormalities and ultrasound findings. Magnetic resonance cholangiopancreatography (MRCP) is largely considered the gold standard for diagnosis. In cases in which the diagnosis is already made, one should proceed directly to ERCP for removal of the stone (choice B). Emergent cholecystectomy is the treatment for acute cholecystitis and is not indicated at this time (choice A). Broad-spectrum antibiotics with gram-negative and anaerobic coverage may be warranted, but this alone would not be the most appropriate management (choice C). Hepatobiliary iminodiacetic acid (HIDA) scans are used in the setting of an equivocal ultrasound to confirm acute cholecystitis or biliary obstruction. A HIDA scan is not indicated in this patient (choice B).

Test-taking tip: When thinking about "definitive management" of patients, it is often about treating the suspected underlying cause of their disease, which in this case is removal of the stone that is stuck in the common bile duct by use of ERCP.

9. ANSWER: B

The patient is a presenting with a postoperative bile leak as confirmed by the visualized biloma on ultrasound (choice B). Post-cholecystectomy choledocholithiasis can occur if a gallstone migrates from the gallbladder during cholecystectomy or if there is de novo stone formation within the common bile duct (choice C). MRCP is usually required to make the diagnosis because it is normal for the common bile duct to dilate to 10 mm following gallbladder removal, and therefore ultrasound is less helpful. The patient in this question would likely need MRCP if the ultrasound had not shown a biloma because the clinical presentations are similar. This patient does not have symptoms of an ileus (choice A). Although pneumonia should be on the differential for postoperative fever, it is less likely the etiology of this patient's fever (choice D).

Test-taking tip: Brush up on common complications of common operations like appendicitis and cholecystitis.

10. ANSWER: A

A positive sonographic Murphy's sign in the presence of visualized gallstones is the most sensitive finding for acute cholecystitis. All of the other sonographic findings (gallbladder wall thickening, pericholecystic fluid, etc.) are all commonly found in patients with acute cholecystitis. However, the presence of a sonographic Murphy's sign is the most sensitive for the diagnosis.

Test-taking tip: Brush up on common ED bedside ultrasound findings.

11. ANSWER: C

Gangrenous cholecystitis is the most common complication of acute cholecystitis. In addition to delayed treatment, other risk factors include diabetes and advanced age. The other options, although all known complications of cholecystitis, are less common (choices A, B, and D).

Test-taking tip: Brush up on common complications of common operations like appendicitis and cholecystitis.

12. ANSWER: A

The clinical presentation of jaundice, fever, and RUQ pain is referred to as Charcot's triad and is highly suggestive of cholangitis. The addition of hypotension (shock) and confusion (altered mental status) constitutes Reynold's pentad and is highly suggestive of suppurative cholangitis (choice A). Tachycardia and leukopenia are part of SIRS criteria for sepsis but do not necessarily suggest a diagnosis of suppurative cholangitis (choices B and C). Bilious emesis is not suggestive of suppurative cholangitis (choice D).

Test-taking tip: You can eliminate C and D because low WBC (leukopenia) is not usually associated with infection and bilious emesis is not associated with cholangitis.

13. ANSWER: D

The most common pathogens causing cholecystitis are *Escherichia coli, Klebsiella* species, and *Enterobacter* species. Antibiotic regimens therefore must include both gram-negative and anaerobic coverage. Appropriate antibiotic therapies include the combination of either a second- or third-generation cephalosporin or a fluoroquinolone, plus metronidazole. Another option is solo therapy with piperacillin-tazobactam (choice D). Choices A, B, and C do not provide adequate coverage.

Test-taking tip: This question tests your knowledge of what organisms you need to cover for ascending cholangitis. Brush up on common infectious organisms for common diseases.

14. ANSWER: C

Treatment of acute pancreatitis is focused on aggressive IV crystalloid resuscitation in the first 24 to 48 hours of presentation to prevent hypotension, acute tubular necrosis, and pancreatic hypoperfusion (choice C). Prophylactic antibiotics are not recommended in patients with acute pancreatitis. Fluid resuscitation, not prophylactic antibiotics, is shown to have a morbidity and mortality benefit (choice D). Two thirds of cases of acute pancreatitis are attributed to alcohol abuse and/or gallstones (gallstones being the most common); hypertriglyceridemia accounts for less than 5% of cases (choice A). Other etiologies include infectious, traumatic, hypercalcemia, post-ERCP, medication-induced, and idiopathic. Elevations of lipase are both more sensitive and specific than elevation of amylase (choice B).

Test-taking tip: You can eliminate A because you know gallstones are the most common cause of pancreatitis.

15. ANSWER: B

Valproic acid has black box warnings for hepatotoxicity, major fetal malformations, patients with underlying mitochondrial disease, and acute pancreatitis (choice B). Colchicine does not have any black box warnings or any well-established correlation with pancreatitis (choice A). Zidovudine has black box warnings for hematologic toxicity, myopathy, and lactic acidosis with severe hepatomegaly but not for pancreatitis (choice C). Didanosine, another antiretroviral agent, has a black box warning for pancreatitis. Amiodarone has black box warnings for the development of life-threatening arrhythmias and potentially fatal pulmonary and hepatic toxicities but not for acute pancreatitis (choice D).

Test-taking tip: This is a "you know it or don't" kind of question. If you don't know it, choose an answer and move on. You can perhaps mark it for review when you are done at the end of the test. Don't, however, let these kinds of questions get you stuck and waste your time.

16. ANSWER: C

The above image is an example of pyoderma gangrenosum, an inflammatory-ulcerative disorder of the skin that is characterized by rapid progression of a painful, necrolytic cutaneous ulcer with an irregular, violaceous, and undermined border. Other suggestive features include a history of preceding trauma and a history of underlying autoinflammatory disorders such as inflammatory bowel disease and inflammatory arthritis. First-line therapy typically involves basic local wound care (gentle cleansing and nonadherent dressing) and systemic glucocorticoids (choice C). Because trauma tends to exacerbate these wounds, aggressive surgical debridement is not recommended (choice D). Pyoderma gangrenosum is not infectious and therefore does not require treatment with antibiotics (choices A and B).

Test-taking tip: The key to this question is recognizing that the picture shows pyoderma gangrenosum.

17. ANSWER: A

Toxic megacolon is a potentially lethal complication of inflammatory bowel disease (usually ulcerative colitis) or infectious colitis that is characterized by total or segmental nonobstructive colonic dilation plus systemic toxicity. The transverse or right colon is usually the most dilated, frequently greater than 6 cm with absent or abnormal haustral markings. Ogilvie's syndrome (also known as acute colonic pseudo-obstruction) is characterized by colonic dilation in the absence of an obstructing lesion.

Plain film findings are nonspecific and include diffusely dilated colon with normal haustral markings (choice B). Neutropenic enterocolitis (or typhlitis) is a necrotizing enterocolitis occurring primarily in neutropenic patients. Its presentation may be similar to that of toxic megacolon; however, plain film radiography would reveal a fluid-filled, distended cecum with dilated adjacent small bowel loops, thumbprinting, or localized pneumatosis intestinalis (choice C). A sigmoid volvulus presents with symptoms of bowel obstruction (pain, distention, vomiting, and constipation). Plain film would reveal a large air-filled sigmoid colon extending from the pelvis to the RUQ and the absence of air in the rectum (choice D).

Test-taking tip: To get this answer you need to recognize the very distended loops of bowel on the radiograph as abnormal.

18. ANSWER: A

The question stem notes abdominal distention, increased rectal tone, rectal vault absent of stool, and a large release of foul-smelling stool and gas on exam (squirt sign). These findings are classically described in Hirschsprung's disease. Hirschsprung's disease–associated enterocolitis should be considered in the neonate presenting with abdominal distention or pain, failure to thrive, persistent vomiting, fever, and explosive foul-smelling diarrhea. Mild cases may have less severe symptoms. However, the mainstay of treatment is fluid resuscitation and broad-spectrum IV antibiotics. Emergent surgical intervention may be required in more severe cases. However, many cases may be initially managed nonoperatively, and antibiotics should not be delayed.

Test-taking tip: The key to this question is recognizing classic findings of Hirschsprung's disease and knowing the associated complications of obstructing enterocolitis.

19. ANSWER: D

The differential diagnosis of abdominal distention and/or pain in an elderly patient is huge, but common diagnoses to consider in a non–toxic-appearing patient include:

1. Constipation—always a consideration in elderly and institutionalized patients
2. Small bowel obstruction—often caused by hernias or adhesions
3. Large bowel obstruction—malignancy must be considered, especially in patients older than 60 years

In this case the radiographic findings are consistent with a large bowel obstruction. Complete mechanical obstruction requires surgical intervention in conjunction with fluid resuscitation and preoperative antibiotics.

Test-taking tip: It is important to recognize abnormal imaging findings that require surgical evaluation. Radiographic findings of large bowel obstruction include colonic dilation proximal to the obstruction and collapse distally. Colon measuring more than 6 cm is considered abnormal.

20. ANSWER: C

Differential diagnosis for rectal pain in a middle age male includes:

1. Proctitis—pain would be localized to the prostate on exam and may have other symptoms of anorectal discharge, itching, diarrhea, and abdominal pain
2. Anal fissure—more than 90% occur in the posterior midline and would be visualized on exam
3. Hemorrhoids—external hemorrhoids may be painful with thrombosis; uncomplicated internal hemorrhoids are usually painless, but if they are painful and no thrombosis is visualized, suspect a perirectal abscess or anal fissure
4. Cryptitis—a superficial inflammation of the anal crypts that is treated conservatively with bulk laxatives, high-fiber diet, and sitz baths
5. Perianal abscess—most result from obstruction of an anal gland and abscess forming within the anal crypt; they are superficial and can be seen and/or palpated at the anal verge
6. Perirectal abscess—associated with pain and often purulent discharge; these involve the deeper perirectal spaces and are usually appreciated on the lateral rectal wall or lateral to the anus

Physical examination is key to the diagnosis of anorectal pain. In this question, it is important to recognize that lateral pain or induration is consistent with a perirectal abscess and should be evaluated for surgical drainage. In contrast, perianal abscesses are superficial and should be midline.

Test-taking tip: The exam in the question stem should lead you to the appropriate diagnosis. A patient with internal rectal pain should not be sent home, so you can eliminate B and D because discharge should not happen with this patient.

21. ANSWER: D

The patient in this case has a pilonidal cyst. A pilonidal sinus or cyst is an acquired condition in which a sinus tract forms over the lower sacrum or coccyx at the midline near the natal cleft secondary to a granulomatous reaction due to an ingrown hair. The sinus can become inflamed or infected with abscess formation. Occasionally, these sinus tracts may form draining fistulas that may drain adjacent to the sinus. Treatment is incision and drainage (I&D). Patients may need referral to a surgeon for further excision as these frequently recur. Antibiotics are only necessary if there is surrounding cellulitis.

Testing taking tip: The question is describing a classic appearance and location of a pilonidal cyst; if you remember this, you will know the answer.

22. ANSWER: B

A differential diagnosis for rectal pain in a young person includes perianal and perirectal abscesses, cryptitis, hemorrhoids, anal fissure, and proctitis. The patient in this question is a young, sexually active male. Anal sex is a significant risk factor for proctitis secondary to sexually transmitted infections (STIs). In this case empiric antibiotic treatment would be the most appropriate treatment.

Test-taking tip: It is important to recognize age and risk factors in the question stem to help determine the most likely diagnosis.

23. ANSWER: B

Acute proctitis in males who practice anal receptive intercourse is usually sexually acquired. These patients should be empirically treated with ceftriaxone and doxycycline pending testing for STIs. Gonorrhea and chlamydia are common, and syphilis should always be considered. Men who have sex with men (MSM) who also have proctitis, bloody discharge, and perianal or mucosal ulcerations and who are known to have HIV or chlamydia should be treated to cover for *Lymphogranuloma venereum* with doxycycline for 3 weeks.

Test-taking tip: This question presents a patient who is known to be HIV positive and should lead you to consider alternative treatment choices from standard empiric STI coverage.

24. ANSWER: A

Greater than 90% of anal fissures occur along the posterior midline. They may also be along the anterior midline, but this is more common in women and occurs about 1% of men. Anal fissures are the most common cause of painful rectal bleeding and are frequently seen in patients with constipation and are caused by passing large, hard stool. Treatment includes symptom relief with sitz baths, topical analgesics, and stool-bulking agents. Fissures tend to heal in a few weeks.

Test-taking tip: The location of anal fissures is important to remember because lesions located laterally should increase suspicion for other causes, including assault or abuse, chronic inflammatory conditions, malignancy, and infectious etiologies.

25. ANSWER: D

The differential diagnosis for this case includes perirectal or perianal abscess, anal fissure, and anal fistula. The exam described in the question is consistent with an anal fistula. Patients with inflammatory bowel disease are at risk for developing anal fistulas. Fistulas may also develop from perianal or perirectal abscess. If the fistula tract is open, patients may present with painless and malodorous rectal discharge. They may also have intermittent pain that occurs with inflammation when the fistula tract is obstructed and abscess is formed. This pain may be relieved with rupture of the abscess and obstructed fistula. Patients who are well-appearing are appropriate for discharge with oral antibiotics and follow-up with surgery because surgical excision may be the definitive treatment.

Test-taking tip: The question stem describes a well-appearing, pain-free patient, which should lead you toward less aggressive treatment.

26. ANSWER: B

All of these choices increase the risk for developing an anal fistula. However, ischiorectal abscesses are a relatively common disease process compared with the other choices. When anal glands or crypts are chronically obstructed, polymicrobial abscess may develop. Overtime these abscesses may erode through to the anal canal or skin forming a fistula.

Test-taking tip: Think of eliminating the generally less common answer choices in this question; development of abscess due to obstructed anal crypts is much more common, for example, than colorectal malignancy or inflammatory bowel disease.

27. ANSWER: A

Local infiltration with 1% lidocaine with or without epinephrine may facilitate the exam and extraction of rectal foreign bodies. Viscous lidocaine and conscious sedation may also be used to facilitate the procedure in the ED. Imaging should be used to help identify the shape, number, and location of rectal foreign bodies. Emergent surgical consultation should be done in any case with concerns for bowel perforation and in cases in which the foreign body is unable to be removed in the ED. If the foreign body is successfully removed in the ED and the patient has a normal exam, the patient may be discharged.

Test-taking tip: Know the contraindications to and safe uses of local anesthesia.

28. ANSWER: D

External hemorrhoids can be exquisitely painful when thrombosis is present. Surgical excision in the ED is an appropriate treatment depending on the severity of pain and if the symptoms have been present for less than 48 hours. Clot excision with an elliptical excision may provide significant pain relief. If the pain and thrombosis have been present for more than 48 hours, clot excision may be less beneficial. Clot excision should not be performed in the ED in children, pregnant women, immunocompromised patients, patients with portal hypertension, or patients taking anticoagulation medication or with coagulopathy. It would also be reasonable to discharge this patient with supportive care with sitz baths and a bowel regimen if pain is controlled. Thrombosed external hemorrhoids are usually self-limited with resolution in about 1 week.

Test-taking tip: If you are unsure of the answer to this question, remember to address the patient's symptoms. Excision is the only answer choice that would help alleviate the patient's pain.

29. ANSWER: A

Grade 4 internal hemorrhoids are nonreducible and are at risk for tissue edema and strangulation and incarceration. They require surgical evaluation and treatment. Incarcerated internal hemorrhoids may develop necrosis, significant bleeding, and infection. Surgical consult is also indicated in patients with severe bleeding and intractable pain. Grade 1 to 3 internal hemorrhoids may be managed conservatively with stool softeners, high-fiber diet, and observation (Table 2.1).

Test-taking tip: If you are unsure of the answer, you can narrow down the choices by two because "always" and "never" are not typical answers and are usually wrong.

Table 2.1 GRADES OF INTERNAL HEMORRHOIDS

Grade 1	No extension below the dentate line
Grade 2	Prolapse with straining but spontaneously reduce
Grade 3	Prolapse with straining and require manual reduction
Grade 4	Prolapse and are nonreducible

30. ANSWER: D

Granulated sugar may help reduce tissue edema by osmotic effects, which may allow for reduction of a rectal prolapse. Emergent surgical consultation is warranted if there are concerns about tissue ischemia or gangrene. Surgical consultation should also be obtained if a prolapse is severe, cannot be reduced, or recurs after reduction because these patients may ultimately need operative intervention.

Test-taking tip: The exam in the question stem notes well-appearing and edematous tissue, which should make you think of other options besides immediate surgical consultation.

31. ANSWER: A

Hepatitis A virus (HAV) is transmitted by the fecal-oral route and is commonly transmitted in contaminated water in areas with poor access to safe water sources. HAV has an incubation period of 15 to 30 days, which is followed by nausea, vomiting, abdominal pain, and malaise. Patients may also have dark urine (bilirubinuria) and may later develop light-colored stools and jaundice. There is no chronic component of HAV infection, and life-threatening liver failure is rare.

Test-taking tip: Travel history should lead you to think of specific infections and should help you eliminate the two choices of imaging.

32. ANSWER: D

The differential diagnosis in a cirrhotic patient with abdominal pain is broad because these patients are immunocompromised at baseline. This patient has spontaneous bacterial peritonitis (SBP), which can present with abdominal pain and fever. Symptoms may be also be very subtle or even absent. Ascitic fluid studies with polymorphonuclear leukocytes greater than 250/m:, WBC greater than 1,000/mm³, or bacteria on Gram stain are diagnostic of SBP. Gram stain may be falsely negative in 30% to 40% of cases. If there is any suspicion in the ED or the diagnostic criteria for SBP are met, patients should be admitted and started on IV antibiotics. The incidence of SBP in patients with known ascites approaches 30% annually; recurrence is common, and mortality rates are very high.

Test-taking tip: Commit to memory the diagnostic criteria for SBP.

33. ANSWER: B

The most common organisms causing SBP are Enterobacteriaceae, *Streptococcus pneumoniae,* and enterococci. Recommended antibiotics include cefotaxime, ticarcillin-clavulanic acid, piperacillin-tazobactam, ampicillin-sulbactam, and ceftriaxone. Oral quinolones may be considered in very mild, uncomplicated cases with close follow-up.

Test-taking tip: If you remember the common organisms causing an infection, they can help you narrow down antibiotic choices.

34. ANSWER: D

Patients with alcoholic cirrhosis may require frequent paracentesis both for diagnostic and therapeutic reasons, and as many as three-fourths of these patients will have coagulopathy. Attempting to correct coagulopathy before preforming paracentesis is not routinely advised and should only be done when fibrinolysis and disseminated intravascular coagulation are suspected.

Test-taking tip: Knowing indications and contraindications to common procedures is important and will lead you to the answer of some questions.

35. ANSWER: D

Broad differential diagnoses should be considered in older adult patients with significant abdominal pain. The question stem notes that the patient is in atrial fibrillation, is not on anticoagulation, and has pain out of proportion. This should give you a high suspicion for mesenteric ischemia. Abdominal computed tomography (CT) angiography has a 96% sensitivity for mesenteric ischemia and should not be delayed.

Test-taking tip: You can eliminate RUQ ultrasound and abdominal radiograph because neither is likely to find a cause of severe, diffuse pain.

36. ANSWER: A

Pancreatic cancer must always be considered in patients presenting with painless jaundice. A direct hyperbilirubinemia is consistent with post-hepatic biliary obstruction. However, choledocholithiasis, cholecystitis, and cholangitis will present with RUQ pain. Remember Charcot's triad for cholangitis: RUQ pain, fever, and jaundice; adding hypotension/shock and altered mental status is Reynold's pentad.

Test-taking tip: In this question, all of the answers except pancreatic cancer are typically associated with RUQ pain. Painless jaundice is pancreatic cancer until proved otherwise.

37. ANSWER: C

HBV is transmitted sexually and by blood and has an incubation period of 1 to 3 months. In the acute phase of infection, HBsAg will be positive. HBcAb indicates a prior infection; it appears after HBsAg and will be present for life. HBsAb is present in persons with a history of immunization or prior cleared infection.

Test-taking tip: Choosing "none" is never a good option. Choosing from the other options is a matter of remembering how to interpret hepatitis serology.

38. ANSWER: D

Chronic mesenteric ischemia may present with unintentional weight loss, repeated postprandial pain, and food avoidance (because of recurrent pain with eating). Older adult patients presenting with abdominal pain are at a much higher risk for having serious, surgical pathology than younger patients, and a broad differential should always be considered. Atrial fibrillation and a sudden onset of severe, diffuse abdominal pain should make you think of acute mesenteric ischemia. Consider biliary colic and cholelithiasis in a 47-year-old female with postprandial RUQ pain. Older adult patients with malaise, weight loss, and dark stools may have many disease processes, but malignancy must be considered.

Test-taking tip: Knowing risk factors and common presentations of intraabdominal conditions will help eliminate answer choices.

39. ANSWER: A

The patient described in the question stem has signs of cirrhosis. Abdominal distention and shifting dullness or a fluid wave are findings in patients with large-volume ascites, which is a result of portal hypertension and a decrease in intravascular oncotic pressure. Portal hypertension may also result in prominent epigastric veins and esophageal and rectal varices. Hormonal dysregulation leads to gynecomastia and telangiectasia. The predominate causes of cirrhosis are alcoholism and hepatitis C virus. Parasitic infections, such as schistosomiasis, related to travel in South America are very rare causes of cirrhosis. Chronic or acute acetaminophen ingestion may lead to acute hepatic failure but not cirrhosis.

Test-taking tip: Remembering common conditions and their causes can help you eliminate possible answer choices. The question describes a cirrhotic patient, and alcohol abuse and hepatitis C virus are the most common causes of cirrhosis.

40. ANSWER: D

Radiation colitis or proctitis is common after radiation therapy for cervical or prostate cancer and may present with diarrhea, rectal bleeding, and rectal pain. Symptoms may present months to years after radiation treatment. In many cases a clinical diagnosis can be made, and treatment includes analgesics, sucralfate or steroid enemas, and supportive care. Oral steroids may be used for treatment of ulcerative colitis. Ceftriaxone and doxycycline would be warranted if there were concerns for STIs causing proctitis.

41. ANSWER: C

The patient in this question has a serum albumin ascites gradient (SAAG) of −1 g/dL. An SAAG of less than 1.1 g/dL is consistent with nonportal hypertensive ascites, and pancreatitis is the only answer choice in this question that can cause ascites in the absence of portal hypertension. Pancreatic ascites may present with a history of chronic pancreatitis, a recent episode of acute pancreatitis, or a recent traumatic injury to the pancreas. Portal hypertension leads to an SAAG of more than 1.1 g/dL. Ascites related to cirrhosis, congestive heart failure (CHF), and alcoholic hepatitis are all due to portal hypertension.

Test-taking tip: Cirrhosis, CHF, and alcoholic hepatitis can all cause portal hypertension. If you cannot remember anything about SAAG values, pancreatitis should stand out as a unique answer choice.

42. ANSWER: B

Any child presenting with bilious emesis requires a surgical consult secondary to likely obstructive process requiring close monitoring or emergent surgical intervention. This child specifically has necrotizing enterocolitis (NEC), which is pneumatosis in the intestinal wall due to gas-forming bacteria. While most of these patients do not require surgery, surgery should be involved early in their presentation because of the risk for perforation.

The risk factors for NEC are prematurity and formula-fed neonates. It usually occurs in the first 2 weeks of life. These neonates need to be NPO, be hydrated, have a nasogastric (NG) tube and antibiotics started. Blood in the stool should make you worry about ischemic bowel. Endoscopy is not indicated in this patient, and this patient would benefit from an admission to the intensive care unit.

- Bilious emesis requires a surgery consult
- Blood in stool is concerning for ischemic bowel

Test-taking tip: You can eliminate A because discharge home is not a possibility in this sick baby.

43. ANSWER: A

This patient has pyloric stenosis. Pyloric stenosis is the most common obstructive process in neonates/infants and is more common in boys. It is hypertrophy/hyperplasia of the circular smooth muscle of the pylorus, causing obstruction of the outflow tract of the stomach. These patients have a hypochloremic hypokalemic metabolic acidosis secondary to vomiting and require surgery. Important management for these patients includes replacing electrolytes and giving them a glucose source for nutrition. They do not require antibiotics or GI consult, and bicarbonate has no role in the correction of their acidosis.

- Hypokalemic hypochloremic metabolic acidosis is concerning for pyloric stenosis
- Ultrasound is the imaging modality of choice for pyloric stenosis

Test-taking tip: You can eliminate D because there is no infection that needs antibiotics in pyloric stenosis.

44. ANSWER: B

Pneumatosis is the most concerning radiographic finding for this patient, who likely has Hirschsprung's disease. This is a sign of enterocolitis, which is a surgical emergency and would require close monitoring in the hospital.

The "double-bubble sign" is more often associated with malrotation, which would be associated with bilious emesis. Toxic megacolon is a possibility in Hirschsprung's disease, but pneumatosis is more severe and concerning for ischemic bowel. Hirschsprung's disease is aganglionic megacolon, which is the absence of ganglion in the distal bowel causing chronic contraction of the area and leads to inability to pass stool. Signs of obstruction or enterocolitis or if the child is ill-appearing warrants admission and IV hydration with a surgery consult (Table 2.2).

Table 2.2 PEDIATRIC ABDOMINAL EMERGENCIES

DIAGNOSIS	IMAGING	FINDING
Malrotation with volvulus	Upper gastrointestinal study Upright radiograph	Corkscrew Double-bubble sign
Pyloric stenosis	Ultrasound	Thick pylorus
Necrotizing enterocolitis	Radiograph	Pneumatosis
Intussusception	Ultrasound Air enema	Donut structure Diagnostic and therapeutic

- No passage of meconium in first 48 hours of life is concerning for Hirschsprung's disease.
- Forceful stool with stimulation on exam or history of needing stimulation for bowel movements is concerning for Hirschsprung's disease.

Test-taking tip: You can eliminate D and C because nonspecific gas is not a concerning radiograph and toxic megacolon is not a neonatal finding.

45. ANSWER: D

This patient does require a surgical consult, as does any child presenting with bilious emesis, but should be resuscitated in the ED and started on antibiotics before further interventions secondary to presenting with signs of sepsis.

Ultrasound is not a good imaging modality for this specific patient, with the likely diagnosis being malrotation based on upper GI contrast study. CT scan is also not the best imaging modality at this time, unless you are concerned for perforation or ischemic bowel, which can occur if there is a volvulus wrapping around the superior mesenteric artery. A GI consult would not help with the definitive care of this patient because the patient needs surgical intervention at this time.

Malrotation occurs secondary to incomplete rotation of the bowel at 10 weeks of gestation and usually presents with bilious emesis with abdominal distention. A double-bubble sign may be seen on upright film with contrast, but not always. Risk factors include heterotaxy syndrome, which includes dextrocardia (Table 2.2).

Test-taking tip: This is an action patient. This mindset allows you to eliminate all the imaging (non-action) items.

46. ANSWER: C

Tracheoesophageal fistula and esophageal atresia are difficult to diagnosis in the ED but can be caught when you are trying to pass an NG tube and are unable to get it past 10 cm. With surgical intervention, these patient do well, with a survival rate near 100%.

They are usually started on antibiotics secondary to the risk for aspiration, and those not diagnosed at birth can present with coughing, gagging, cyanosis, vomiting, voluminous oral secretions, and possibly respiratory distress. It is not appropriate to try passing another tube at this time, and discharging a patient home while intubating is not acceptable. GI consult may be made during the patient's hospitalization, but it is not the definitive treatment because this patient will need an operation.

- Inability to pass a feeding tube in neonate/infants past 15 cm is concerning for tracheoesophageal fistula and/or esophageal atresia.

Test-taking tip: Note that the question asks for "definitive management," not the best next step.

47. ANSWER: C

This patient's presentation is concerning for intussusception, which is usually diagnosed and treated with an air enema study. If reduction of the intussusception is not successful with the enema, then surgical intervention is indicated secondary to the risk for necrosis and perforation. While some of these patients can be discharged if their intussusception is successfully reduced and they are observed in the ED for multiple hours after reduction without recurrent symptoms or vital sign derangements, this patient would not be a candidate for discharge because of unsuccessful reduction. The patient has no signs of peritonitis, making antibiotics not helpful in this presentation, and because of the high risk for necrosis, observation is not appropriate. Intussusception is usually idiopathic in children younger than 2 years, but as they get older (>6 years), lymphoma becomes the most common cause. If intussusception is present in an adult, then it is almost always pathologic.

- Intermittent pain with bringing of knees to chest indicates intussusception.
- Intussusception requires reduction emergently.

Test-taking tip: You can eliminate A and B because they are not options in an unreduced intussusception.

48. ANSWER: D

Neonatal jaundice is more prevalent secondary to increased red blood cell (RBC) mass and shorter life span of RBCs. It is more commonly secondary to physiologic processes than pathologic processes. This is because hepatic conjugation and excretion of bilirubin are limiting steps, and neonates also have less binding proteins for bilirubin. Bilirubin typically increases from 1.5 mg/dL to 6.5 mg/dL on day 3 and then gradually declines to less than 1.5 mg/dL by day 10 or 12.

Some of the risk factors for neonatal jaundice are jaundice in the first 24 hours of life, discharged home in high-risk to high-intermediate-risk zone at birth on the bilirubin chart, preterm (<38 weeks), breastfed with excessive weight loss (usually secondary to dehydration and exaggeration of physiologic neonatal jaundice), hemolytic disease, siblings who had neonatal jaundice, cephalohematoma at birth (due to the breakdown of the hematoma), and being of East Asian descent.

Test-taking tip: This is a "you know it or don't" kind of question. If you don't know it, choose an answer and move on. You can perhaps mark it for review when you are done at the end of the test. Don't, however, let these kinds of questions get you stuck and waste your time.

49. ANSWER: D

While risk factors and plotting on the bilirubin chart should be done to risk-stratify these patients, any bilirubin value greater than 20 should prompt phototherapy and require admission.

Phototherapy helps by conjugating indirect bilirubin into direct bilirubin to help with excretion. The goal of phototherapy is to prevent acute bilirubin encephalopathy (ABE) and kernicterus, which have significant morbidity and mortality. This child is well-appearing, with otherwise normal labs, making IV hydration unnecessary along with glucose replacement. In fact, continued breastfeeding during therapy is encouraged. Ceftriaxone can worsen the patient's chances of getting kernicterus, and he is not showing signs of infection at this time.

- Any patient with a bilirubin value greater than 20 should get phototherapy as soon as possible and be admitted.

Test-taking tip: You can eliminate A and C because discharge without intervention is not possible and there is no infection, so antibiotics are not needed.

50. ANSWER: C

Neonatal jaundice is more prevalent secondary to increased RBC mass and shorter life span of RBCs in the neonate, and it is more commonly secondary to physiologic processes than pathologic processes. This is because hepatic conjugation and excretion of bilirubin are limiting steps, and neonates also have less binding proteins for bilirubin. Bilirubin typically increases from 1.5 mg/dL to 6.5 mg/dL on day 3, and then gradually declines to less than 1.5 by day 10 or 12. The risk factors for neonatal jaundice are:

- Jaundice in the first 24 hours of life
- Discharged home in high-risk to high-intermediate-risk zone at birth on the bilirubin chart
- Preterm (<38 weeks)
- Breastfed with excessive weight loss (usually secondary to dehydration and exaggeration of physiologic neonatal jaundice)
- Hemolytic disease
- Siblings who had neonatal jaundice
- Cephalohematoma at birth (due to the breakdown of the hematoma)
- Being of East Asian descent

Test-taking tip: This is a "you know it or don't" kind of question. If you don't know it, choose an answer and move on. You can perhaps mark it for review when you are done at the end of the test. Don't, however, let these kinds of questions get you stuck and waste your time.

51. ANSWER: C

Just like with any patient, ABCs are the first part of an emergency medicine physician's algorithm. This neonate is not responding to stimuli and is floppy, making the chance for aspiration high. This child needs intubation and resuscitation at this time. The underlying cause of this patient's altered mental status is likely ABE (kernicterus is defined after a week of life, while ABE is in the first week of life) and would require exchange transfusion along with phototherapy, but not before his airway is secured. The child is likely dehydrated and possibly septic, but securing his airway is the priority. The alternating between the arching of the back and flaccid tone is called retrocollis-opisthotonos and, along with jaundice in the neonate, is pathognomonic for ABE and kernicterus. The signs of symptoms of ABE and kernicterus are:

- *Early*: poor suck, decreased urine output, fussy, hypotonia, lethargy

- *Intermediate:* high-pitched cry, irritable, increased tone with arching of neck and trunk alternating with hypotonia (retrocollis-opisthotonos), fever
- *Severe:* pronounced retrocollis-opisthotonos, semicoma/seizure, bicycling movement

Test-taking tip: This is an action patient. Any patient who is critical needs fast intervention, so look for the answer that is fast and effective. This mindset allows you to eliminate answers A, B, and D because those are not action answers.

52. ANSWER: D

Many household items have caustic potential; these include detergent, dishwasher soap or pods, drain cleaners, stove cleaners, and bleach. Obtain a history to determine the type of agent, amount, and time of ingestion. Patients may present with mouth pain, throat pain, drooling, stridor, hoarseness, respiratory distress, vomiting, or abdominal pain. In a patient with respiratory distress, consider early intubation because laryngeal edema may progress and require surgical airway later.

Caustic materials are classified into two categories—acidic or alkaline—because they cause different types of injuries. Acidic ingestion leads to coagulation necrosis, whereas alkaline ingestion leads to liquefaction necrosis resulting in deep and progressive mucosal burns. Liquefaction necrosis is worse than coagulation necrosis. Management is mostly supportive, and if the patient is stable, institute NPO and call the on-call GI specialist for endoscopy, which is the gold standard for evaluating the severity and location of injury to the GI tract. Endoscopy should be done as early as possible and at least within 24 to 48 hours after ingestion. Avoid administering activated charcoal (choice A) because it does not bind well with most of the caustic material and impedes visualization during endoscopy. Avoid inserting an NG tube (choice B) until after endoscopy. You can give the patient pain medication to help with discomfort, but avoid oral fluids until after evaluation by endoscopy (choice C). In addition, avoid inducing vomiting or attempting pH neutralization.

Test-taking tip: You can eliminate A and C because after the mouth or esophagus is burned, nothing should be put in the mouth before GI consult performing an endoscopy.

53. ANSWER: A

The patient swallowed a sharp object, which is an indication for urgent endoscopy despite the patient being asymptomatic or the location of the object in the GI tract. Because the risk for intestinal perforation from ingested sharp objects is high, the American Society for Gastrointestinal Endoscopy Guidelines recommend removal of sharp objects while they are in the stomach or duodenum. Even though 80% to 90% of foreign bodies pass spontaneously once they reach the stomach, the risk for perforation with sharp objects is too high (15%–35%) to not intervene. Circumstances that warrant urgent endoscopy for esophageal foreign bodies are presence of sharp or elongated objects, button batteries, multiple foreign bodies, evidence of perforation, a coin at the level of the cricopharyngeus muscle in a child, airway compromise, and presence of foreign body for more than 24 hours.

Test-taking tip: You can eliminate C and D because not doing an intervention on a sharp, long object is not an option.

54. ANSWER: B

The patient in this case most likely has a small bowel obstruction. Bowel obstruction should be on the differential for anyone presenting with abdominal pain and vomiting, especially if they have had abdominal surgery in the past. Abdominal pain is usually the presenting sign, followed by vomiting, constipation, and then distention. Some patients will continue to pass flatus and have bowel movements after obstruction has occurred because they still have feces and gas distal to the obstruction. Patients with partial obstruction will often have diarrhea. Small bowel obstruction is more common than large bowel obstruction, and the most common cause of small bowel obstruction is fibrous adhesions and scar tissue after an abdominal surgery. The second most common cause of small bowel obstruction is hernia. Neoplasm is the most common cause of large bowel obstruction, followed by volvulus and diverticulitis.

Test-taking tip: This is a "you know it or don't" kind of question. If you don't know it, choose an answer and move on. You can perhaps mark it for review when you are done at the end of the test. Don't, however, let these kinds of questions get you stuck and waste your time.

55. ANSWER: D

Intussusception most often occurs when a proximal portion of intestine telescopes into the distal, adjacent portion. Its typical presentation involves intermittent episodes of abdominal pain that lasts a few seconds to minutes, and parents may describe their child holding their knees to their chest and crying inconsolably, followed by an asymptomatic interval. Most patients present with colicky abdominal pain and vomiting only. The classic triad of paroxysmal abdominal pain, vomiting, and bloody stools (or currant-jelly stool) is only seen in 25% to 65% of patients.

The gold standard test for diagnosing and treating intussusception is barium or air enema. Successful reduction rates using air or barium enema range between 80% and 90%. Air enema is favored over barium enema given the high risk for chemical peritonitis with barium if perforation were to occur. Ultrasound has high sensitivity (98%–100%) and specificity (88%–100%) and is used by many hospitals now as the initial diagnostic test. However, it is not the correct answer choice because it is only diagnostic and not therapeutic and is dependent on a radiologist's experience. Abdominal radiograph is not correct because abdominal radiographs are often normal or equivocal, particularly during the early course of disease, and thus they require a follow-up ultrasound or enema study in cases highly suspicious for intussusception. Abdominal CT can accurately diagnose intussusception but is usually the last imaging test ordered given the risk of high radiation.

Test-taking tip: Be aware of the question asking for the "best test" to diagnose and treat. Many tests can diagnose, but only enema can treat.

56. ANSWER: C

Meckel's diverticulum is a true diverticulum (i.e., it involves all three layers of small intestine) and contains ectopic gastric tissue that can ulcerate and cause painless rectal bleeding. Meckel's diverticulum tends to follow the "rule of 2s": it is present in 2% of population, presents at 2 years of age, is located 2 feet from the ileocecal valve, and is 2 inches long. It is diagnosed using a technetium-99m pertechnetate scan, and treatment usually involves resuscitation followed by surgical resection.

Intussusception can present with bloody stool, classically known as currant-jelly stool, but that is a rare and late finding of the disease and usually presents with paroxysmal abdominal pain and vomiting. Meckel's diverticulum can form a lead point for intussusception. Anal fissure is one of the common causes of rectal bleeding, but bleeding is often light, and it is associated with constipation and diarrhea. NEC is mainly seen in premature neonates and usually presents with bilious vomiting, abdominal distention, and constipation, followed by diarrhea and gross blood per rectum.

Test-taking tip: For painless rectal bleeding around 2 years of age, think of Meckel's diverticulum.

57. ANSWER: C

GI bleeds due to variceal bleeding have a very high mortality rate. Of the choices listed. only ceftriaxone has been shown to have mortality benefit because up to 20% of patients with cirrhosis have an infection at the time of admission and half of the patients with cirrhosis go on to develop an infection during their hospitalization. In addition, antibiotic administration has also been shown to decrease rebleeding events and length of hospitalization.

Proton pump inhibitor use is controversial because it has shown no mortality benefit, decrease in rebleeding events, or decrease in the need for transfusion compared with placebo but is still part of the upper GI variceal bleed protocols at most hospitals, and most gastroenterologists recommend it. Octreotide is a synthetic analog of somatostatin and reduces portal hypertension by reducing splanchnic blood flow and also reduces acid production, but it does not have a mortality benefit. It does help prevent rebleeding events in both variceal and nonvariceal upper GI bleeds. Most patients with cirrhosis also have coagulopathy with elevated international normalized ratio (INR), and thus fresh frozen plasma is recommended if the INR is greater than 1.5, but this has not been shown to have a mortality benefit.

Test-taking tip: Of all the medications that are given to cirrhotic patients with an upper GI bleed, antibiotics (usually third-generation cephalosporin, i.e., ceftriaxone) are the only ones shown to have a mortality benefit.

58. ANSWER: C

Aortoenteric fistula is a rare complication of aortic graft placement but is associated with a high mortality rate of 50% even with operative management. Many patients will present with nonspecific abdominal pain, back pain, nausea, vomiting, and GI bleeding in the form of hematemesis or hematochezia or even melena. Patients with underlying graft infection, such as this case, may even have low-grade fever before signs of GI bleed, which results from infection leading to secondary aortoenteric fistula formation. For unstable patients, one should not wait for diagnostic studies such as abdominal radiograph or abdominal CT and should contact the surgeon immediately for emergent laparotomy because these patients can deteriorate quickly and the definitive treatment is surgical intervention.

Patients who are stable can undergo CT angiography or endoscopy for further evaluation and to rule out any other causes of GI bleeding. CT angiography is the fastest and least invasive diagnostic modality, but its sensitivity for diagnosing aortoenteric fistula is between 30% to 80%.

Test-taking tip: Always consider aortoenteric fistula when a patient with history of aortic graft presents with new onset of GI bleed.

59. ANSWER: C

Sigmoid volvulus is most commonly seen in older adults (>60 years) and is usually associated with constipation, inactivity, and neurologic or psychiatric conditions. Diagnosis is usually made with abdominal radiographs that show markedly distended loops of bowel with loss of haustral markings and a characteristic "bent inner tube" appearance.

If abdominal radiographs are inconclusive, a contrast enema can be used and will often show a characteristic "bird's beak" sign. Abdominal CT can also be used. Sigmoid volvulus can be treated with endoscopic reduction such as flexible sigmoidoscopy, but the recurrence rate is approximately 60%, and many patients will require definitive surgical management.

Small bowel obstruction usually presents with abdominal distention, pain, nausea, vomiting, and obstipation. Small intestines can be differentiated from large bowel on abdominal radiograph by valvulae conniventes—mucosal folds that cross the full width of the bowel. Cecal volvulus is less common than sigmoid volvulus and is usually present in middle-aged patients (30s–50s) and is frequently seen in marathon runners. Cecal volvulus usually presents with abdominal pain/distention, nausea, vomiting, and obstipation. Abdominal radiograph usually shows a characteristic "coffee bean" appearance. Management is surgical decompression and resection. Mesenteric ischemia has many subtypes, but patients often experience pain out of proportion to their examination and may have different radiograph findings such as bowel thickening or pneumatosis intestinalis—air in the bowel wall due to necrosis.

Sigmoid volvulus is more common than cecal volvulus, is usually seen in older adult (>60 years) patients, and is associated with inactivity, constipation, and neurologic and psychiatric conditions. Cecal volvulus is more common in younger patients (30s–50s) and is associated with marathon runners.

Test-taking tip: This is a "you know it or don't" kind of question. If you don't know it, choose an answer and move on. You can perhaps mark it for review when you are done at the end of the test. Don't, however, let these kinds of questions get you stuck and waste your time.

60. ANSWER: B

Any part of the GI tract can be involved in Crohn's disease. Inflammatory bowel disease (IBD) is an autoimmune disease characterized by chronic inflammation of the GI tract. Crohn's and ulcerative colitis have many similarities and some differences. Patients with Crohn's usually present with cramping abdominal pain, chronic diarrhea that is nonbloody, fever, rectal fistula, perianal abscess, and occult blood. Crohn's can involve any part of the GI tract (from mouth to anus), involves all three layers of the bowel, and on colonoscopy is noted to have "skip lesions"—normal areas of bowel between areas with lesions. Patients with ulcerative colitis usually present with cramping abdominal pain, chronic diarrhea that is bloody, and fever. Ulcerative colitis is a disease of the colon and always involves the rectum but involves only the superficial layers of the bowel (mucosa and submucosa), and continuous bowel involvement is noted on colonoscopy.

Test-taking tip: This is a "you know it or don't" kind of question. If you don't know it, choose an answer and move on. You can perhaps mark it for review when you are done at the end of the test. Don't, however, let these kinds of questions get you stuck and waste your time.

61. ANSWER: A

This patient's presentation of recurrent peptic ulcer disease (PUD) and associated weight loss is concerning for an underlying etiology such as Zollinger-Ellison syndrome (ZES). ZES is caused by secretion of gastrin by duodenal or pancreatic neuroendocrine tumors. The most common presenting symptoms are abdominal pain and chronic diarrhea, but some patients also have symptoms of gastroesophageal reflux disease (GERD), weight loss, and GI bleeding. Chronic diarrhea is secondary to acid secretion and the high acidic environment that impairs pancreatic digestive enzymes, interferes with emulsification, and results in maldigestion. Fasting serum gastrin level and gastric pH should be measured in patients with high suspicion for ZES.

A serum gastrin level greater than 10 times the upper limit of normal and gastric pH below 2 is diagnostic of ZES. Lipase is usually measured in patients with suspicion for acute or chronic pancreatitis and is a not a specific test for ZES. Urease breath test is used to diagnose *Helicobacter pylori* infection, which can cause PUD but is not associated with chronic diarrhea and significant weight loss, as seen in this patient. *H. pylori* would be appropriate testing to do during the initial workup of PUD. Abdominal radiograph is not indicated in ZES workup, and CT of the abdomen and pelvis and endoscopic ultrasound are more beneficial in ZES because they can help identify tumors and lesions.

The rate of gastric acid secretion exceeds the neutralizing capacity of pancreatic bicarbonate secretion, resulting in an abnormally low pH of intestinal contents. The low pH inactivates pancreatic digestive enzymes, interfering with the emulsification of fat by bile acids, and damages intestinal epithelial cells and villi. Maldigestion and malabsorption both result in steatorrhea.

Test-taking tip: ZES should be considered in patients with recurrent PUD and chronic diarrhea. Serum gastrin level greater than 10 times the upper normal limit of gastrin and gastric pH of less than 2 are diagnostic of ZES.

move on. You can perhaps mark it for review when you are done at the end of the test. Don't, however, let these kinds of questions get you stuck and waste your time.

62. ANSWER: C

This patient's presentation of burning epigastric pain associated with nausea and vomiting, which tends to occur after eating food, correlates with GERD. GERD is caused by reflux of stomach contents and tends to present with burning epigastric pain that occurs after eating food and resolves spontaneously and sometimes is associated with regurgitation of stomach content. Acute coronary syndrome (ACS) is less likely given that other than hypertension, the patient does not have risk factors for ACS. Patients with a history of ACS or high risk for ACS who present with epigastric pain with nausea and vomiting may need additional ACS workup. Cholecystitis is less likely owing to no RUQ tenderness and negative Murphy's sign. Patients with cholecystitis tend to present with RUQ pain with nausea and vomiting that tend to occur after a large fatty meal. Small bowel obstruction is less likely because the patient reports no change in bowel movement and no other history is noted, such as past surgeries that increases her risk for small bowel obstruction.

Test-taking tip: Common things are common. If a patient with history of acid reflux presents with typical acid reflux presentation of epigastric burning pain with nausea and vomiting, it is more likely secondary to GERD than any other etiology.

63. ANSWER: D

Gastritis is inflammation of the lining of the stomach and is usually asymptomatic but can present with epigastric pain, nausea, and vomiting. It is most commonly caused by the bacteria *H. pylori*. *H. pylori* infection can be diagnosed with noninvasive means such as urea breath test or stool antigen testing or using invasive means such as endoscopic biopsy. *H. pylori* can be treated with triple therapy of (1) proton pump inhibitor, (2) amoxicillin (1 g twice daily), and (3) clarithromycin (500 mg twice daily) for a total of 14 days.

Gastritis can also be caused by GI irritants such as nonsteroidal antiinflammatory drugs (NSAIDs), alcohol, and iron supplements, but this is less common than *H. pylori* and is most commonly known as reactive gastritis. There has been no evidence to suggest that eating habits such as spicy foods cause gastritis.

Test-taking tip: This is a "you know it or don't" kind of question. If you don't know it, choose an answer and

64. ANSWER: B

Large bowel obstruction is most commonly caused by neoplasm (~60%), followed by diverticulitis. These two together account for about 90% all cases of large bowel obstruction. Other less common causes include volvulus (sigmoid more than cecal), ischemic colitis, and fecal impaction. Hernias are an uncommon cause of large bowel obstruction. Large bowel obstruction tends to present with diffuse or poorly localized abdominal pain and distention. Nausea and vomiting are less common compared with small bowel obstruction. Most cases can be diagnosed with plan film, which will show dilated loops of large bowel, but this is often followed up with CT because it not only can help diagnose obstruction but in many cases can identify the underlying cause.

Test-taking tip: Neoplasm is the most common cause of large bowel obstruction, followed by diverticulitis. Adhesions are the most common cause of small bowel obstruction.

65. ANSWER: A

In patients with lower GI bleed who are hemodynamically unstable, the first step should be to resuscitate, and the second step should be to consult GI for endoscopy and colonoscopy. Upper endoscopy should be done before colonoscopy because colonoscopy is only done when the patient is stable. Angiography involves injecting dye directly into the mesenteric arteries to evaluate for extravasation and will be the next step if the patient is found to have no upper GI bleed source on endoscopy but continues to have a significant amount of lower GI bleeding and is still hemodynamically unstable. Angiography can help determine the site of bleeding and also allows therapeutic interventions such as embolization. Scintigraphy involves injecting a radiotracer into the blood and capturing images to detect extravasation and is indicated when unable to determine the source of a GI bleed with endoscopy and colonoscopy. It can help localize the site of a small bleed with a rate as low as 0.1 mL/min and is sometimes used to determine whether the patient would benefit from angiography or surgical intervention.

Test-taking tip: This is an unstable GI bleed and needs an action as the correct answer. The only action presented is to consult GI.

66. ANSWER: A

For adolescents, presentation of appendicitis is very similar to that in adults, with symptoms such as periumbilical pain that migrates to the right lower quadrant, nausea, anorexia, and vomiting that starts after abdominal pain. Ultrasound is the first choice of imaging in the pediatric population, and if positive it prevents radiation exposure. Ultrasound has been found to be 90% sensitive and 95% specific for diagnosing appendicitis but can be limited because of the patient's body habitus and sonographer's experience.

Ultrasound findings consistent with appendicitis are a tender, noncompressible structure, without peristalsis that is more than 6 mm in diameter. If the appendix is not visualized, it still may not be necessary to obtain CT of the abdomen and pelvis to rule out appendicitis because the negative predictive value for ultrasound when appendix is not visualized is 85% to 95%. CT of the abdomen and pelvis is the most accurate study for appendicitis; however, for the pediatric population, it is recommended to start with ultrasound to reduce radiation exposure. Abdominal radiographs have limited value in appendicitis and are usually only used to rule out other causes of abdominal pain, such as bowel obstruction or severe constipation, rather than to look for a rare "fecalith" plugging the opening of the appendix.

Test-taking tip: For pediatric patients, ultrasound is preferred over CT of the abdomen and pelvis for evaluation of appendicitis given the high radiation exposure associated with CT.

67. ANSWER: C

A young female with abdominal pain is pregnant until proved otherwise. The differential diagnosis in this patients includes appendicitis, ovarian torsion, and ectopic pregnancy.

The best test to evaluate for appendicitis would be an abdominal ultrasound. However, if the pregnancy test is positive, ectopic pregnancy will rise to the top of your differential.

Test-taking tip: Always rule out pregnancy in a young female with abdominal pain.

68. ANSWER: A

Abdominal radiographs are the initial diagnostic modality of choice to reveal the location of the battery. If the radiograph is negative and your suspicion is high, consider a barium swallow or GI consult for endoscopy. In this case, your suspicion is very high because the mother witnessed the event. Button batteries in the esophagus are very serious, so urgent GI consult for endoscopy is the definitive treatment. Button batteries can be corrosive and if in the esophagus can have high mortality because the tissue on both sides of the battery actives the electrical circuit and the patient gets liquefactive necrosis.

Test-taking tip: Note that the question stem asks for best initial test (not definitive treatment).

69. ANSWER: A

Endoscopy is indicated if impaction present for more than 24 hours or the patient is unable to swallow secretions or is in distress.

There is a high incidence of underlying pathology in the esophagus (e.g., cancer, scarring) in adults who present with food bolus impaction. Medication that may help promote spontaneous passage is glucagon.

This is not an outpatient disease. The food bolus needs to be taken care of before discharge of the patient.

Test-taking tip: The question is asking for the next best step. Given the food bolus has been present for more than 24 hours, GI consult is the best course of action.

70. ANSWER: C

Urinalysis is the test of choice in a febrile young child with lower abdominal pain. Bag specimens are unsuitable for the diagnosis and need to be a clean catch or in-and-out urine. Dipstick urinalysis is only 83% sensitive. The gold standard is urine culture, which should be sent on all pediatric patients if the urinalysis is positive, the patient is febrile, or the patient is a child with previous urinary tract infection.

Treatment should be antibiotics and follow-up with the pediatrician. Admission is only indicated for toxic patients who present with dehydration, vomiting, or other symptoms. This patient appears healthy and can be discharged home with outpatient antibiotics.

Test-taking tip: Note that the question is asking for the next best test.

71. ANSWER: A

This patient's presentation is very concerning for ruptured abdominal aortic aneurysm (AAA). Bedside ultrasound is convenient and fast. It is very accurate, and its sensitivity approaches 100% in the trained provider. A CT scan of the abdomen is the test of choice because it shows if the AAA has ruptured and gives the extent of the disease. However, if the patient has unstable vital signs, then CT should not be done. Kidneys, ureters, and bladder radiograph (KUB) is a rapid screen and may reveal an aortic calcification. However, it is low yield because 20% of aortas with calcifications do not have an AAA. Magnetic resonance imaging is accurate but very time-consuming.

Treatment is operative management, and surgery should be consulted. Risks for AAA include use of tobacco, age greater than 65 years, male sex, and hypertension. This patient has all of these risk factors.

Test-taking tip: The question is asking for the initial imaging of choice in this unstable patient. You need to recognize that he likely has an AAA to get the right answer.

72. ANSWER: B

This patient has three signs on Ranson's criteria so has a predicted mortality of 10% to 15%.

Ranson's criteria is a scoring system for pancreatitis to gauge the severity and outcome and what the predicted mortality for the patient will be based on lab values on admission.

You get one point for each of the following:

Age >55 years
WBC >16,000
Lactate dehydrogenase >350
AST >250
Glucose >200

Mortality rates based on points are as follows:

<3 points: 0%–3%
3–4 points: 11%–15%
5–6 points: 40%
>7 points: 100%

Test-taking tip: Brush up on common scoring systems like Ranson's criteria before the exam.

73. ANSWER: D

This question is asking about the Child-Pugh Liver Disease Classification score. This score helps look at perioperative mortality given the patients underlying liver disease (Table 2.3).

Table 2.3 CHILD-PUGH LIVER DISEASE CLASSIFICATION

POINTS	1	2	3
Bilirubin	<2 mg/dL	2–3 mg/dL	>3 mg/dL
Albumin	>3.5 g/dL	2.8–3.5 g/dL	<2.8 g/dL
International normalized ratio	<1.7	1.71–2.2	>2.2
Ascites	None	Medication controlled	Yes
Encephalopathy	None	Medication controlled	Yes

PERIOPERATIVE mortality: class A, 5–6 points (10%); class B, 7–9 points (30%); class C, 10–15 points (82%).

Test-taking tip: Review common scoring systems like the Child-Pugh score before the exam.

74. ANSWER: B

This G-tube was only placed 6 days ago. A mature fistula needs to form for the ED to be able to try to replace the tube. It usually takes at least 1 week for a mature track to form. It is most common for G-tube dislodgment to happen in the first 2 weeks after placement. If you try to replace a G-tube and a mature track is not present, a false track can easily be created.

If a G-tube is replaced in the ED, *always* confirm placement with a Gastrografin radiograph.

Test-taking tip: Know the common complications with G-tubes because they are common to present to the ED.

75. ANSWER: C

Clostridium difficile is an anaerobic, gram-positive, spore-forming bacillus. Antibiotic use is a common risk factor, especially if antibiotics are used within the prior 2 to 10 weeks. It is the leading cause of antibiotic-associated diarrhea/colitis and infectious diarrhea in the health care setting.

Treatment for mild to moderate disease is PO metronidazole.

Test-taking tip: You can eliminate D because discharge home with that much diarrhea is not possible.

76. ANSWER: A

Pseudomembranous colitis is pathognomonic for *C. difficile* infection.

C. difficile is an anaerobic, gram-positive, spore-forming bacillus. Antibiotic use is a common risk factor, especially if antibiotics are used within the prior 2 to 10 weeks. It is the leading cause of antibiotic-associated diarrhea/colitis and infectious diarrhea in the health care setting.

Test-taking tip: You can eliminate B and C because admission is not needed when the patient appears healthy and PO medication is preferred to treat *C. difficile*.

3.

CARDIOVASCULAR EMERGENCIES

Kurt Brueggeman, Seth Eidemiller, Michael Kukurza, Leann Manis, and James McCue

1. A 46-year-old female with a past medical history of asthma presents to the emergency department (ED) from her primary doctor's office for new-onset hypertension. Her blood pressure (BP) is now 170/100 mm Hg. The patient denies any complaints, including chest pain, shortness of breath, headache, or visual changes. What is the best next step in this patient's management?

A. Refer to her primary care for further evaluation and treatment
B. Start a nicardipine drip for a goal BP <140/90 mm Hg
C. Start the patient on oral metoprolol
D. Obtain screening labs to look for end-organ damage

2. A 25-year-old male presents after being brought to the ED by friends for altered mental status. He is noted to be tachycardic, hypertensive, diaphoretic, and combative. His initial BP is 200/110 mm Hg. His pupils are 8 mm bilaterally. He has no evidence of trauma. What is the next best step in this patient's management?

A. Emergent head computed tomography (CT)
B. Start an esmolol drip
C. Give IV lorazepam (Ativan) as needed
D. Start a nicardipine drip

3. A 25-year-old male with a past medical history of nonischemic cardiomyopathy presents to the ED with shortness of breath and chest pain. He is noted to have a BP of 200/100 mm Hg with a heart rate (HR) of 95 bpm. He is tachypneic with a respiratory rate (RR) of 30 breaths/min with an increased work of breathing. He has crackles in his lung bases and 3+ pitting edema to his thighs bilaterally. What is the best next step in the management of this patient?

A. Give a 2-liter normal saline (NS) bolus
B. Obtain a chest radiograph, complete blood count (CBC), chemistry 10 panel, troponin, and brain natriuretic peptide (BNP)

C. Start biphasic positive airway pressure (BiPAP) and a nitroglycerin drip
D. Give IV furosemide (Lasix)

4. A 1-year-old otherwise healthy male presents to the ED after he collapsed. His mother reports that this happened after his older sister stole his teddy bear. He was crying before it happened. His mother notes that he turned very red. He collapsed to the ground but quickly regained consciousness. He had no jerking. He was acting normally immediately when he woke up. In the ED he has normal vital signs, is acting age appropriately, and has a normal exam. What is next best step in management?

A. Electrocardiogram (EKG)
B. Electroencephalogram (EEG)
C. Transthoracic echocardiogram
D. Discharge home with primary care follow-up

5. Which of the following patients with syncope can be safely discharged home from the ED without any workup?

A. An 18-year-old male presents with exertional syncope after playing basketball
B. A 39-year-old female presents with syncope after giving blood
C. A 75-year-old female presents with syncope after having a bowel movement
D. A 30-year-old male presents with syncope and a history of a harsh systolic murmur

6. A 25-year-old Lao male presents to the ED after an unprovoked syncopal event 3 hours before arrival. He has no complaints now. Labs are unremarkable, including CBC, comprehensive metabolic panel (CMP), and troponin. His EKG is shown in Figure 3.1. What is the next step in management?

A. Admit for percutaneous coronary intervention (PCI)
B. Admit for automated implantable cardiac device (AICD)

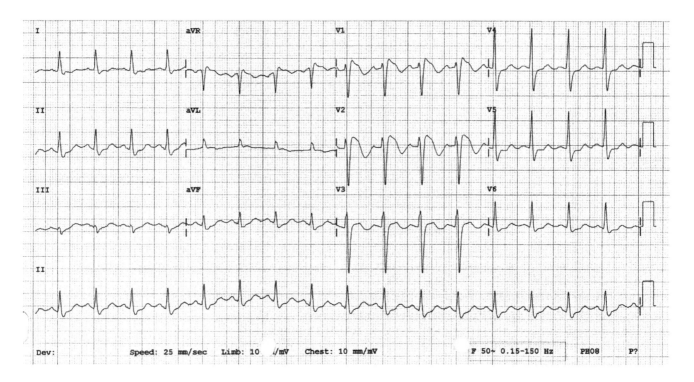

Figure 3.1 Electrocardiogram.

C. Admit for serial troponins

D. Discharge with home with Holter monitor

7. A 75-year-old female presents after a syncopal event, witnessed by her husband. She is currently alert but confused. Her husband reports that she was cooking and collapsed to the ground. Her BP is 75/palp mm Hg. Her initial EKG is shown in Figure 3.2. What is the next best step in the management of this patient?

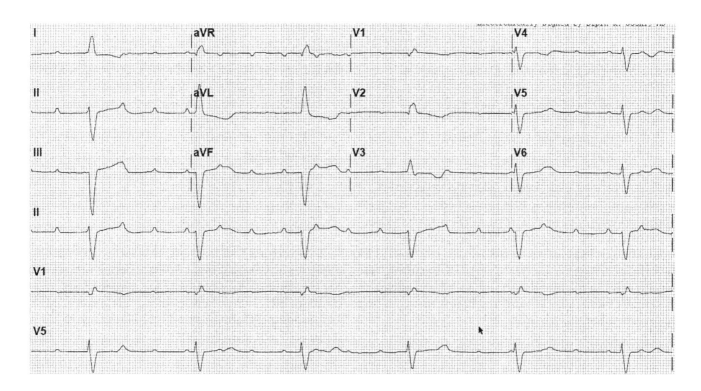

Figure 3.2 Electrocardiogram.

A. Cardiology consult for AICD
B. 0.5 mg IV atropine
C. Transcutaneous pacing
D. Transvenous pacing

8. A 25-year-old female presents with right calf swelling for 3 days after being discharged from the hospital after her first cesarean delivery. She has pitting edema of the right leg with tenderness to palpation of the calf. There is mild erythema of the calf. What is the best test to order for this patient to make the correct diagnosis?

A. D-dimer
B. Deep venous thrombosis (DVT) ultrasound of the right lower leg
C. Radiograph of the right lower leg
D. CT venography

9. A 35-year-old female presents with left calf swelling. She is currently undergoing treatment for thyroid cancer. She noticed her leg was swollen about a week ago, and it has been getting worse. She has pitting edema of the left lower extremity as well. Her DVT ultrasound is negative. What is the best next step in the management of this patient?

A. Order a D-dimer
B. Empirically treat at DVT
C. Repeat the ultrasound in 1 week
D. Discharge home with primary care follow-up

10. A thrombus in which vein does not necessarily require anticoagulation?

A. Popliteal vein
B. Superficial femoral vein
C. Axillary vein
D. Cephalic vein

11. A 65-year-old male with a past medical history of chronic obstructive pulmonary disease (COPD) presents with abrupt onset of dyspnea. Emergency medical services (EMS) started him on continuous positive airway pressure (CPAP). On arrival, the patient is diaphoretic, hypotensive at 70/40 mm Hg, tachycardic at 125 bpm, with an oxygen saturation of 85% on CPAP. Lungs are clear bilaterally. His left calf is swollen with pitting edema. His right calf is normal. What is the next best step in the management of this patient?

A. Obtain a CT angiogram of the chest
B. Start albuterol-ipratropium through his CPAP
C. Administer full-dose tissue plasminogen activator (tPA)
D. Administer half-dose streptokinase

12. Which anticoagulant is appropriate to start for a new diagnosis of pulmonary embolism (PE) in a pregnant patient?

A. Enoxaparin
B. Rivaroxaban
C. Warfarin
D. Clopidogrel

13. Which of the following are *not* indications for an inferior vena cava (IVC) filter placement in the setting of venous thromboembolism?

A. Trauma
B. Malignancy
C. Prophylaxis
D. Large clot burden

14. In a markedly hypertensive patient who presents with confusion for which the suspect cause is hypertensive emergency, what is the goal reduction of mean arterial pressure (MAP) and diastolic BP in the first hour?

A. 5%
B. 10%
C. 25%
D. 50%

15. An 85-year-old female presents with acute onset of pain and discoloration in her leg. On exam, her leg is a dark discoloration (Figure 3.3) with no palpable distal pulse. What is the next best step in the management of this patient?

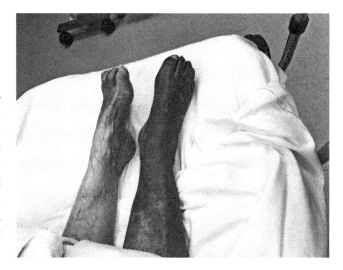

Figure 3.3 Leg.

A. Antibiotics
B. DVT ultrasound

C. Vascular consult

D. CT angiogram

16. A 55-year-old male with history of uncontrolled hypertension presents with tearing chest pain radiating to the back, BP 200/100 mm Hg, and HR 100 bpm. Which medication should be used to lower this patient's BP acutely?

A. Nifedipine

B. Hydralazine

C. Esmolol

D. Nitroprusside

17. A 24-year-old female presents with right lower quadrant (RLQ) abdominal pain and syncope. CBC shows mild anemia but no leukocytosis. Chemistry panel is unremarkable. Vital signs show tachycardia and mild hypertension. Which other test would best help to make the correct diagnosis?

A. Liver function tests (LFTs) and lipase

B. Pregnancy test

C. Urinalysis

D. EKG

18. A 40-year-old male presents after being found in his enclosed garage after he was working on his 1960s Chevy truck with the motor running. His wife heard him collapse. He awoke with a headache. He arrived at the hospital with normal vital signs, but he has a worsening headache and nausea. What is the next best step in the management of this patient?

A. CT of the head

B. EKG

C. 15 L of oxygen

D. Arterial blood gas (ABG) test

19. A 26-year-old male presents after a syncopal event after he started treatment for pneumonia. He regained consciousness almost immediately. His EKG is seen in Figure 3.4. Which drug likely precipitated this rhythm?

A. Azithromycin

B. Levofloxacin

C. Amoxicillin–clavulanic acid

D. Doxycycline

20. Which of the following is not part of Wells' criteria for DVT risk stratification?

A. Unilateral pitting edema

B. Recent immobilization of the lower extremities

C. Collateral superficial veins

D. Exogenous estrogen use

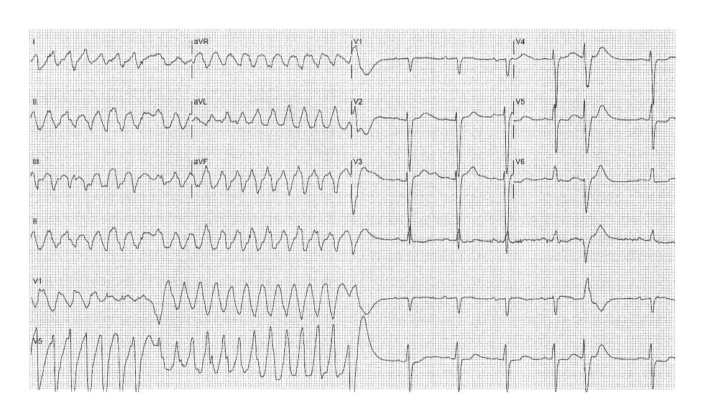

Figure 3.4 Electrocardiogram.

21. Which patient is a candidate for thrombolysis in the setting of an acute PE?

   A. A patient with a saddle PE with normal vital signs
   B. A patient found to have a PE on CT scan that presented after a major motor vehicle collision and is tachycardic and normotensive
   C. A patient with normal vital signs who has evidence of right ventricular dysfunction on bedside echocardiogram
   D. A patient with a subsegmental PE who is tachycardic and hypotensive

22. A 76-year-old male presents with a chest pain and a BP of 200/110 mm Hg. The patient states he takes clonidine, lisinopril, hydrochlorothiazide (HCTZ), and amlodipine for his BP, metformin and insulin for his diabetes, and atorvastatin for his cholesterol. He says he ran out of a medication yesterday but doesn't know which one. Which medication most likely precipitated his hypertension by not taking it?

   A. Lisinopril
   B. HCTZ
   C. Amlodipine
   D. Clonidine

23. What is the pathophysiology of Brugada's syndrome?

   A. Sodium channelopathy
   B. Potassium channelopathy
   C. Sodium-potassium adenosine triphosphatase (ATPase) dysfunction
   D. Calcium channelopathy

24. A 73-year-old male with a known history of congestive heart failure (CHF) presents to the ED with shortness of breath that began 2 hours ago on awakening. He denies recent fevers, vomiting, or unilateral leg swelling. Initial vital signs show temperature 37° C, HR 110 bpm, RR 22 breaths/min, BP 120/76 mm Hg, and oxygen saturation 93%. Physical exam demonstrates regular rate and rhythm of the heart, rales at lung bases bilaterally, an abdomen that is soft and nontender, and 1+ pitting edema in the bilateral lower extremities. The patient has two large-bore IV lines placed, O_2 is started by nasal cannula, and the patient is placed on a cardiac monitor demonstrating no ST changes. On reassessment, the SpO_2 increases to 98%. What is the next best step in this patient?

   A. Begin IV furosemide (Lasix)
   B. Give sublingual nitroglycerin
   C. Place the patient on BiPAP
   D. Obtain a chest radiograph

25. Which of the following interventions has been shown to decrease morbidity and mortality in acute decompensated heart failure (ADHF)?

   A. Inotropes
   B. Furosemide (Lasix)
   C. Nitroglycerin
   D. Noninvasive positive pressure

26. Which of the following is not part of the physiology regarding using BiPAP in acute decompensated heart patients?

   A. Recruitment of atelectatic alveoli
   B. Increasing intrathoracic pressure
   C. Decreasing pulmonary compliance
   D. Decreasing work of breathing

27. An 83-year-old female is brought to the ED by EMS. The EMS personnel report the patient became increasingly short of breath throughout the day and her family called EMS when the patient became confused. The family told EMS the patient had been out of medications for a week. Oxygen saturation in the ambulance was 83%, and the patient was given sublingual nitro and placed on BiPAP en route. In the ED, the patient remains confused on BiPAP after 30 minutes, and her oxygen saturation has improved to 86%. A brief physical exam demonstrates 3+ pitting edema bilaterally in the lower extremities, diffuse rales in the lungs bilaterally, and tachycardia to 120 bpm but with a regular rhythm. What is the next best step in the management of this patient?

   A. Prepare for endotracheal Intubation
   B. IV nitroglycerin
   C. Obtain a chest radiograph and EKG
   D. Intensive care unit (ICU) consult

28. Which of the following is the most common etiology of pericarditis?

   A. Malignancy
   B. Idiopathic
   C. Post–myocardial infarction (MI)
   D. Infectious

29. A 72-year-old female comes to the ED with recurrent chest pain. The patient states that the pain feels exactly like the pain she had 2 weeks ago in the ED when she was evaluated and subsequently admitted for an ST elevation anterior MI. She states the pain is central, constant, and radiates to both shoulders. Vital signs are temperature 37.2° C, HR 89 bpm, RR 16 breaths/min, BP 130/90 mm Hg, and SpO_2 98% on room air.

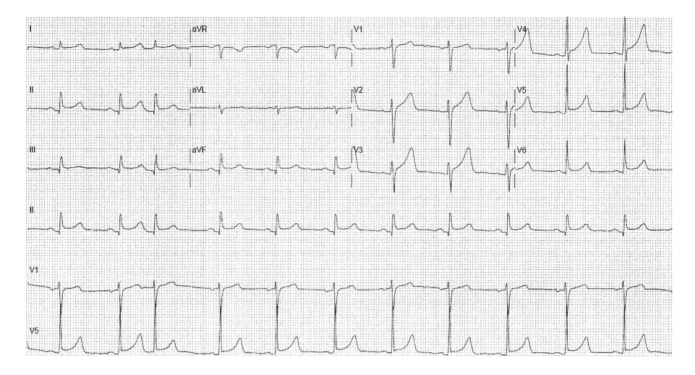

Figure 3.5 Electrocardiogram.

Her physical exam is unremarkable. Her initial workup demonstrates a normal chest radiograph, and her labs are significant for troponin 0.03, WBC 12.6, normal BNP. Her EKG is shown in Figure 3.5. Which of the following therapies is most appropriate for this patient?

A. Anticoagulation with heparin
B. Coronary arteriography
C. Aspirin and close follow-up
D. Sublingual nitroglycerin

30. A 30-year-old previously healthy male presents to the ED with chest pain. The patient initially seems rather anxious. He tells you the pain began suddenly, is substernal, radiates to his left shoulder, and worsens with movement, and he notes associated nausea. The patient states he had flu-like symptoms a week prior. He denies recent travel, unilateral leg swelling, or recent surgeries. Vital signs are temperature 37.1° C, HR 99 bpm, RR 18 breaths/min, BP 118/76 mm Hg, and SpO₂ 98% on room air. Labs are significant for WBC of 12.4, and his troponin is elevated at 0.12. An EKG is obtained and is shown in Figure 3.6. Which of the following is the most likely diagnosis?

A. Pericarditis
B. MI
C. Anxiety attack
D. PE

31. A 65-year-old female present to the ED with epigastric abdominal pain for 2 months that has worsened over the past week and states, "I just got tired of the pain, so I decided to see a doctor." Vital signs show temperature 36.9° C, HR 48 bpm, RR 14 breaths/min, BP 140/90 mm Hg, and oxygen saturation 98% on room air. Physical exam demonstrates an obese female with no jugular venous distention (JVD), normal heart sounds, lungs that are clear to auscultation, 1+ distal radial and dorsalis pedis pulses, and no peripheral edema. Labs show normal lipase and LFTs. Abdominal CT scan is normal. EKG is normal sinus rhythm (NSR), and chest radiograph demonstrates enlarged cardiac silhouette. A bedside echo is performed that shows a large pericardial effusion without evidence of tamponade. Which of the following labs would be most helpful in the diagnosis of this patient?

A. Thyroid-stimulating hormone and free thyroxine
B. BNP
C. Procalcitonin
D. Erythrocyte sedimentation rate (ESR) and C-reactive protein (CRP)

32. A 42-year-old homeless male comes to the ED complaining of a right anterior chest wall laceration after an altercation. He denies heart palpitations, sob, or chest pains. He does admit to fevers, a cough, and night sweats. He was recently released from the county jail.

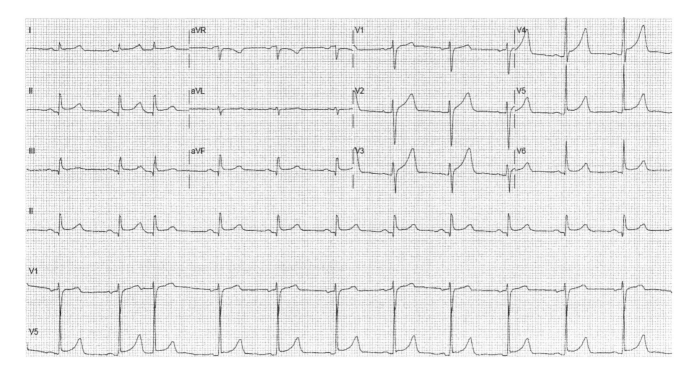

Figure 3.6 Electrocardiogram.

Vital signs show temperature 38.6° C, HR 78 bpm, RR 14 breaths/min, BP 143/92 mm Hg, and oxygen saturation 96% on room air. Chest radiograph demonstrates an enlarged cardiac silhouette and an infiltrate in the right upper lobe. Bedside ultrasound demonstrates a small pericardial effusion with no right ventricular collapse during diastole and a normal IVC with respiratory variation. Which of the following is the most appropriate step in the management of this patient?

A. Urgent pericardiocentesis
B. Administer ASA and colchicine
C. Obtain a blood smear
D. Isolation and antibiotic therapy

33. A 54-year-old female with stage IV breast cancer, undergoing radiation and chemotherapy, is brought to the ED by ambulance due to chest pain. Initial impressions show a pale, diaphoretic patient who is able to speak in full sentences. She describes the pain as substernal, sharp, and constant. There is no change with position. Vital signs show temperature 37.2° C HR 130 bpm, RR 20 breaths/min, BP 82/58 mm Hg, and oxygen saturation 94% on room air. Physical exam demonstrates a friction rub. JVD is absent. Bedside ultrasound shows a pericardial effusion with right ventricular collapse during diastole and IVC dilation without respiratory variation. What is the next best step in the care of this patient?

A. Prepare for endotracheal intubation
B. Give high-dose IM ketorolac
C. 2 L NS followed by 2 units of packed red blood cells
D. Prepare for pericardiocentesis

34. A 73-year-old female presents to the ED by ambulance for an episode of syncope that occurred this morning while the patient was rising from bed. She denies recent fevers, chills, chest pains, or dyspnea. She tells you she had heart surgery about 6 months ago to "fix a murmur" and has been on warfarin since. Physical exam demonstrates an aortic regurgitation murmur, lungs clear to auscultation, and abdomen soft and nontender. Vital signs include temperature 36.9° C, HR 103 bpm, RR 16 breaths/min, BP 120/80 mm Hg, and oxygen saturation 98% on room air. Chest radiograph is unchanged from previous, and an EKG shows sinus rhythm with no acute changes. A bedside ultrasound shows a mass seen on the aortic valve. Labs are pertinent for a prothrombin time (PT)/international normalized ratio (INR) that is subtherapeutic. What is the next best step in the management of this patient?

A. Begin anticoagulation with heparin
B. Initiate antibiotic therapy with vancomycin and gentamicin
C. Outpatient referral to cardiology for transesophageal echocardiography
D. Surgical thrombectomy

35. A 69-year-old male is brought in by ambulance to the ED after being found down at his nursing home. Vital signs show temperature 37°C, HR 128 bpm, RR 18 breaths/min, BP 85/53 mm Hg, and SpO₂ 97% on room air. Physical exam demonstrates a pale-appearing patient with 1+ distal pulses and a widened pulse pressure. A diastolic murmur is heard at the left sternal border, lungs are clear to auscultation, and the abdomen is soft and nontender. The EMS personnel report that the wife mentioned the patient has diabetes and high BP and had a heart valve replacement 1 year ago. Two large-bore IV lines are established, a 2-L bolus of NS is given without improvement, and the patient is placed on oxygen delivered by nasal cannula. What is the next best step in the management of this patient?

A. Initiate a dobutamine drip
B. Urgent surgical consult for valve replacement
C. Initiate a norepinephrine drip
D. Antibiotics and continued fluid boluses

36. A 75-year-old female with a past medical history of type 1 diabetes, hypertension, hyperlipidemia, and previous heart valve replacement comes to the ED for 1 week of fevers and general body aches. The patient denies cough, chills, vomiting, shortness of breath, dysuria, urinary frequency, or abdominal pain. She denies a history of IV drug use, recent dental work, or history of sexually transmitted disease. Physical exam demonstrates a regular HR and rhythm without murmurs, lungs clear to auscultation, a soft and nontender abdomen with no costovertebral angle tenderness. There are small, red, flat, nontender lesions on the palms and purple-brown lesions under the nail beds. Vital signs include temperature 39° C, HR 85 bpm, RR 16 breaths/min, BP 140/93 mm Hg, and SpO₂ 99% on room air. Chest radiograph reveals a 4-mm nodule noted in the left upper lobe. Labs are significant for WBC 12.1, an elevated CRP, and a urinalysis demonstrating few bacteria with positive leukocyte esterase. Which of the following is the most likely diagnosis?

A. Secondary syphilis
B. Infective endocarditis
C. Pyelonephritis
D. Viral upper respiratory illness

37. Which of the following is the most significant risk factor for thoracic aortic dissections?

A. Diabetes
B. Hyperlipidemia
C. Hypertension
D. Coronary artery disease (CAD)

38. A 61-year-old male presents to the ED with central chest pain that began abruptly 2 hours prior while on a walk. He describes the pain as severe and constant but denies radiation. Vital signs show temperature 37.2° C, HR 120 bpm, RR 16 breaths/min, BP 160/100 mm Hg, and SpO₂ 98% on room air. Physical exam demonstrates the heart is tachycardic without murmurs, rubs, or gallops, lungs are clear to auscultation, and abdomen is soft and nontender. Pulses are 1+ in the right dorsalis pedis and 3+ in the left dorsalis pedis. An EKG demonstrates NSR with nonspecific ST changes and no previous EKG available for comparison. The chest radiograph is shown in Figure 3.7. What is the most appropriate next step in the management of this patient?

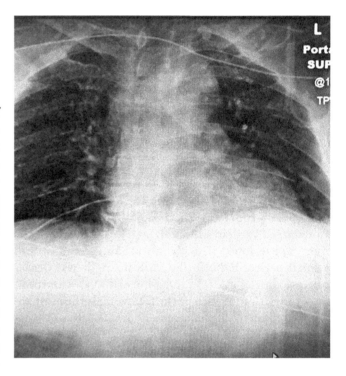

Figure 3.7 Chest radiograph.

A. Activate the catheterization lab
B. Order a CT aorta angiogram
C. Order a CT PE study
D. Begin a nitroglycerin drip for BP control

39. A 71-year-old female presents to the ED with central chest pain radiating to the back that began abruptly 3 hours before arrival. Initial vital signs show temperature 37° C, HR 120 bpm, RR 16 breaths/min, BP 180/120 mm Hg, and SpO₂ 96% on room air. CT of the aorta is ordered and shows a descending thoracic aortic dissection beginning after the left subclavian artery. What is the next most appropriate step in the management of this patient?

A. Contact vascular surgery for immediate surgical intervention

B. Begin esmolol IV drip followed by nitroprusside IV

C. Begin nitroprusside IV followed by esmolol

D. Begin oral metoprolol followed by oral morphine

40. A 62-year-old male presents to the ED with bilateral leg weakness that caused him to fall this morning. The patient states he was walking around the mall when he suddenly developed shortness of breath and chest pains, and then felt as if his legs would not function correctly. He denies any facial asymmetry or slurred speech. He admits to a history of smoking, hypertension, hyperlipidemia, and diabetes. He continues to endorse chest pressures and leg weakness. Vital signs in the ED show temperature 37.2° C, HR 115 bpm, RR 22 breaths/min, BP 190/115 mm Hg, and SpO$_2$ 97% on room air. Physical exam demonstrates an anxious-appearing male who is diaphoretic. Cardiac exam shows tachycardia with regular rhythm and no murmurs, rubs, or gallops. Lungs are clear to auscultation, and he has 5/5 strength in bilateral upper extremities and 3/5 strength in bilateral lower extremities. Cranial nerves II to XII are intact. There is no facial droop or slurred speech. Which of the following is the most likely diagnosis?

A. Cauda equina syndrome

B. MI

C. Stroke

D. Aortic dissection

41. A 45-year-old male presents to the ED with left groin pain that has been worsening for the past 12 hours. The patient states that he was recently discharged from the hospital after undergoing a femoral-femoral bypass for severe atherosclerosis of his left femoral artery. Today, the patient states the pain is constant, worse with movement, and throbbing, and he complains of tingling in his left lower leg. Physical exam demonstrates a warm leg with full range of motion in the knee and ankle, but the patient is unable to cooperate with hip ranging because of pain. A well-healing surgical scar is present over the left groin. Bedside ultrasound demonstrates a pulsatile mass. Vital signs are normal. Which of the following is the next best step in management of this patient?

A. Heparinization

B. Esmolol and nitroprusside

C. Urgent vascular surgery consult

D. Pain control with outpatient follow-up with surgery

42. An obese 62-year-old male arrives by EMS with complaints of right arm bleeding. The patient denies any recent trauma to the site. He admits to recent chills and cold symptoms. He states he called EMS because his right arm began oozing yesterday at the site of his dialysis fistula and he could not control the bleeding with pressure, and it continued to bleed more heavily overnight. He notes now that he is feeling lightheaded, admits to some shortness of breath, but denies chest or abdominal pain. Initial vital signs are temperature 39.2° C, HR 123 bpm, RR 22 breaths/min, BP 87/60 mm Hg, and SpO$_2$ 97% on room air. Brief physical exam demonstrates a bandage on the right arm soaked in bright red blood. Heart is tachycardic but regular rhythm. Lungs are clear to auscultation bilaterally, and the abdomen is soft and nontender. What is the next best step in the management of this patient?

A. Begin empiric treatment for *Staphylococcus* with IV antibiotics

B. Place two large-bore IV lines and bolus 2 L of NS

C. Obtain Duplex ultrasound of the right arm

D. Obtain EKG and chest radiograph

43. A 73-year-old male is brought in by EMS in extremis. EMS reports that the patient's family called after they found him in bed with abdominal pain. The patient became unconscious en route. The family of the patient report a history of smoking, hyperlipidemia, diabetes, and hypertension. A point-of-care glucose is 85, vital signs are temperature 36° C, HR 135 bpm, BP 82/54 mm Hg, RR 20 breaths/min, and SpO$_2$ 97% on room air. Two large-bore IV lines are placed, 2 L of crystalloid is hung, oxygen by nasal cannula is placed, and the patient is attached to the cardiac monitor. Brief physical exam demonstrates cool extremities, a soft abdomen with an epigastric mass, and 1+ distal radial and dorsalis pedis pulses. Which of the following is the next best step in management of this patient?

A. Bedside ultrasound

B. CT scan

C. Magnetic resonance imaging (MRI)

D. Start IV vasopressors

44. A 62-year-old male presents to the ED with periumbilical abdominal pain. The patient reports the pain began 3 days ago, is dull and constant, has been worsening, and is nonradiating. Physical exam is unremarkable. Vital signs are normal. Labs including LFTs, lipase, CBC, and chemistry panel are unremarkable. A urinalysis shows rare bacteria and 2+ leukocyte esterase with no nitrites, three squamous cells, and no WBCs. Bedside ultrasound demonstrates a 5-cm dilation of the infrarenal aorta with no free fluid in the abdomen. Which of the following is the next best step in management?

A. Urgent vascular consult

B. Discharge home on nitrofurantoin

C. Discharge home with outpatient vascular surgery follow-up

D. Reassurance, discharge home, and close follow-up with primary care physician

45. A 54-year-old male with CHF, CAD, COPD, and Marfan's syndrome presents to the ED with abdominal pain. He states the pain has been worsening for the past 3 days, is constant, and radiates to his low back, and he admits to generally feeling weak. He denies any fevers, chills, IV drug use, diarrhea, hematuria, hematochezia, or dysuria. The abdomen is soft and nontender with no rebound. Which of the following is the most likely diagnosis in this patient?

    A. Mesenteric ischemia
    B. Diverticulitis
    C. Abdominal aortic aneurysm (AAA)
    D. Perforated viscus

46. A 72-year-old female presents to the ED complaining of left foot pain. She states the pain began this morning around 8 AM while lying in bed watching TV and has continued to the point she can no longer walk. She states the pain gets better when she hangs her leg over the side of the bed but also notes that she has had leg and foot discomfort for "years" but that this feels worse than usual. She states that she bumped her leg into the dresser last night while walking to the bathroom in the dark. After waking today, she now notes a pins-and-needles sensation in her leg. Chart review shows the patient has diabetes mellitus, hypertension, and hyperlipidemia and has smoked a pack a day of cigarettes for 30 years. What is the next best step in the management of this patient?

    A. Obtain a three-view radiograph of the left foot and leg
    B. Perform ankle-brachial indexes (ABIs)
    C. Get an MRI of the left lower extremity
    D. Send the patient home with directions to rest, apply ice, use compression stockings, and elevate the affected area

47. A 52-year-old male presents to the ED with left arm pain. He tells you the pain began 2 hours ago, is felt mostly over his forearm and wrist, and is "aching" and that he cannot move his fingers very well anymore. He tells you that his medical history includes CHF, COPD, and atrial fibrillation for which he is not on anticoagulation. Exam demonstrates a cool extremity with 1+ radial pulse in the left arm. What is the next best step in the management of this patient?

    A. Give an aspirin and begin heparinization
    B. Order a CT angiography study of the left arm
    C. Consult vascular surgery
    D. Consult interventional radiology

48. A 53-year-old African American female who has been treated with prednisone in the past and is now on azathioprine for sarcoidosis presents after a syncopal episode. She has been experiencing increased dyspnea, fatigue, and dizziness for the past year. Vital signs are notable RR of 22 breaths/min and Sao_2 91%. Her hemoglobin is 9.3, and her EKG is shown in Figure 3.8. What is the most likely underlying etiology for her syncope?

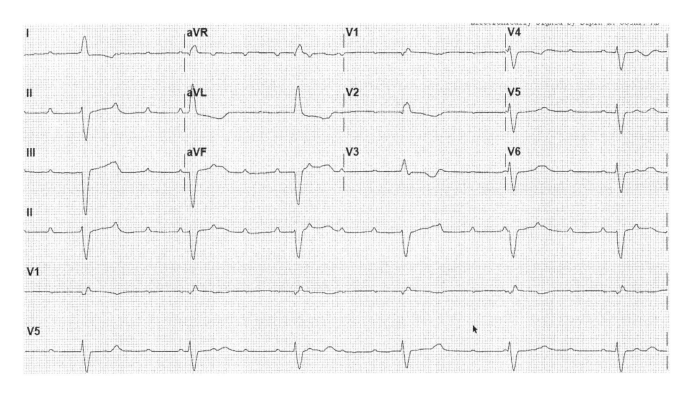

Figure 3.8 Electrocardiogram.

A. Hypoxia from interstitial lung disease
B. Anemia from azathioprine
C. Cardiac sarcoidosis
D. Increased vagal tone

49. A 43-year-old homeless male is brought in by ambulance after experiencing sharp chest pain earlier in the day. His pain has since resolved. The patient is unclear about any prior cardiac or medical history. He does state that he smoked methamphetamine with a friend this morning. Vital signs are BP 157/93 mm Hg, HR 108 bpm, and Sao$_2$ 96%. An EKG is obtained by EMS on arrival to the ED and is shown in Figure 3.9. What is the next best step in the management of this patient?

A. Drug abuse counseling
B. Catheterization lab activation
C. Potassium administration
D. Cardiac stress testing

50. A 23-year-old female college student was brought in by ambulance after a witnessed seizure while in class. Medical records list a prior seizure when she was 3 years old following a febrile illness and a hospitalization for depression at 18 years old. Initial vital signs include HR 127 bpm, BP 83/52 mm Hg, and Sao$_2$ 98% on room air. Her EKG is shown in Figure

3.10. What is the most likely cause of this patient's presentation?

A. Drug overdose
B. Inherited sodium channelopathy
C. Sequelae related to primary seizure disorder
D. Sinus tachycardia

51. A 35-year-old female with a past medical history of amenorrhea presents to the ED. She reports that her legs "didn't want to work" this morning but that she only decided to come to the hospital when she began vomiting. She additionally describes ongoing skin pigmentation changes with severe muscle aches recently. Triage vital signs are notable for HR 43 bpm. The patient's EKG is shown in Figure 3.11. What is the most likely cause of her presentation?

A. Thyroid disease
B. Electrolyte disturbances
C. Propranolol
D. Hypothermia

52. A 63-year-old male presents with chest pain radiating to his jaw and right arm. His past medical history includes hypertension, diabetes, and obesity. He is pale and diaphoretic. His initial EKG is shown in Figure 3.12. What is the most likely cause of this presentation?

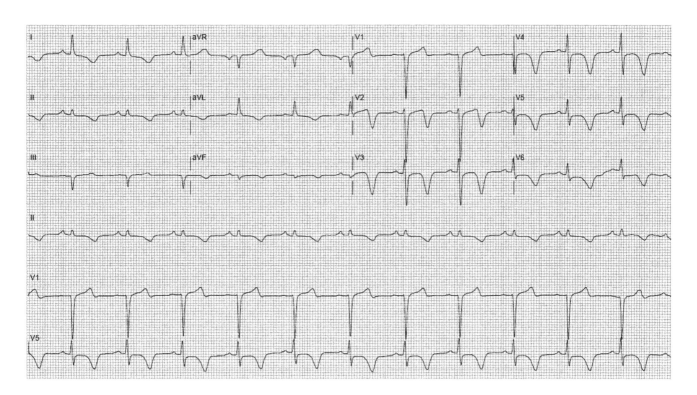

Figure 3.9 Electrocardiogram.

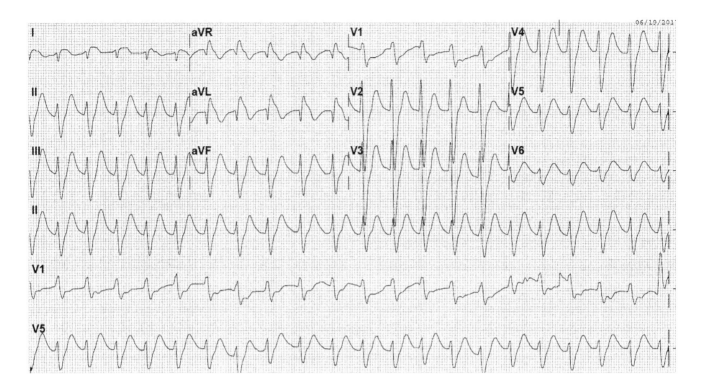

Figure 3.10 Electrocardiogram.

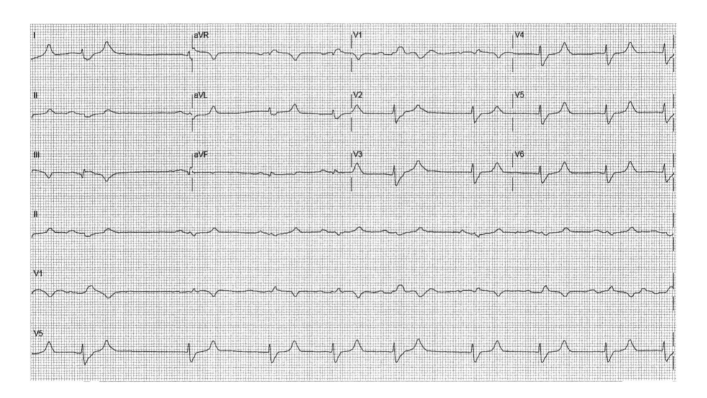

Figure 3.11 Electrocardiogram.

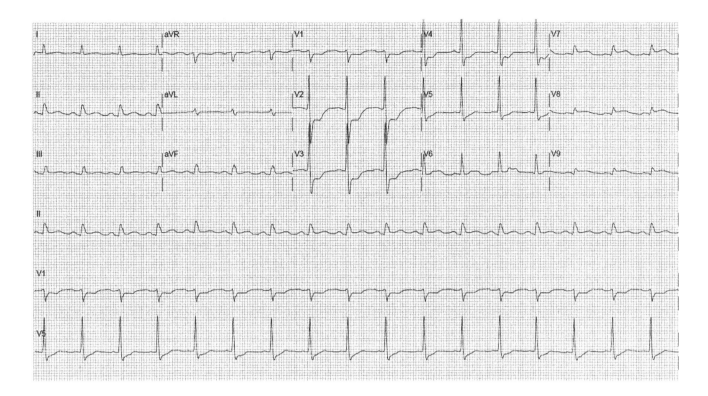

Figure 3.12 Electrocardiogram.

A. Posterior infarction
B. Inferior infarction
C. Lateral infarction
D. Septal infarction

53. A 67-year-old male presents to the ED with request for medication refills and multiple vague complaints. The patient has a history of CHF, hypertension, and COPD. As part of his ED workup, the EKG shown in Figure 3.13

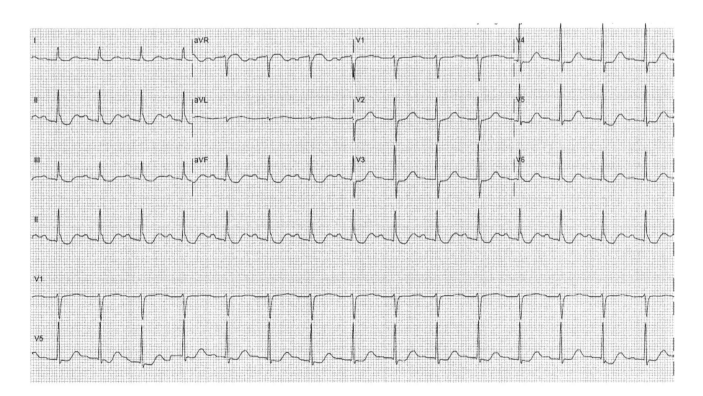

Figure 3.13 Electrocardiogram.

is obtained. What is the most likely cause of the EKG changes shown?

  A. Non–ST elevation myocardial infarction (NSTEMI)
  B. Hyperkalemia
  C. Sick sinus syndrome
  D. Medication effect

54. You get a radio report that EMS is bringing in patient from the field with an EKG concerning for MI. On arrival, the patient is 67-year-old female with known history of CAD, hypertension, and COPD. She is pale and diaphoretic. Her chest pain began earlier that morning and has improved after EMS administration of aspirin and sublingual nitroglycerin. Her vital signs include HR 114 bpm, BP 103/72 mm Hg, and Sao$_2$ 94% on 4 L by nasal cannula. Her EKG is shown in Figure 3.14. What is the most likely location of her lesion?

  A. Left anterior descending (LAD) artery
  B. Left dominant circumflex artery
  C. Right circumflex artery
  D. Left main coronary artery (LMCA)

55. A 19-year-old female is brought in by her boyfriend after she began experiencing palpitations. Her past medical history is unremarkable, and there is no family history of cardiac problems. She denies chest pain. Her palpitations began after inhalation of cocaine while at a concert. Vital signs are notable for tachycardia. Her EKG is shown in Figure 3.15. What is the next best step in the management of this patient?

  A. IV lorazepam (Ativan)
  B. 1 L bolus NS
  C. Adenosine 6 mg IV
  D. Observation

56. A 43-year-old male presents to the ED with chest pain. His past medical history includes a recent diagnosis of hyperlipidemia for which he was placed on a statin. The patient denies prior cardiac history in himself or in his family. His initial EKG is shown in Figure 3.16. What is the next best step in the management of this patient?

  A. Catheterization lab activation
  B. Aspirin and sublingual nitroglycerin
  C. Insulin and D50
  D. Repeat EKG in 20 minutes

57. A 37-year-old female who is well known to hospital staff because of a history of schizophrenia and prior history of suicide attempts is found down in the hospital

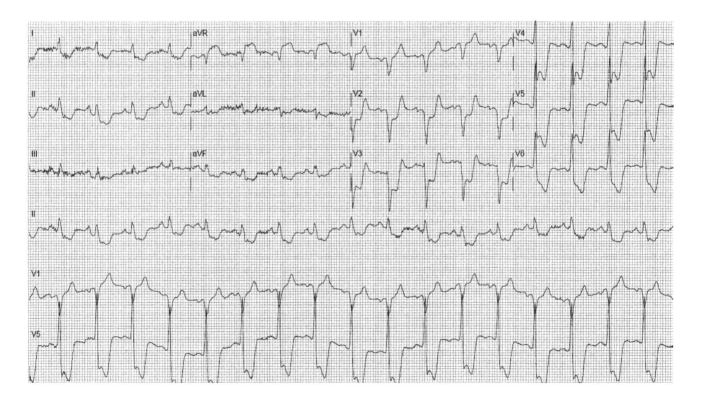

Figure 3.14 Electrocardiogram.

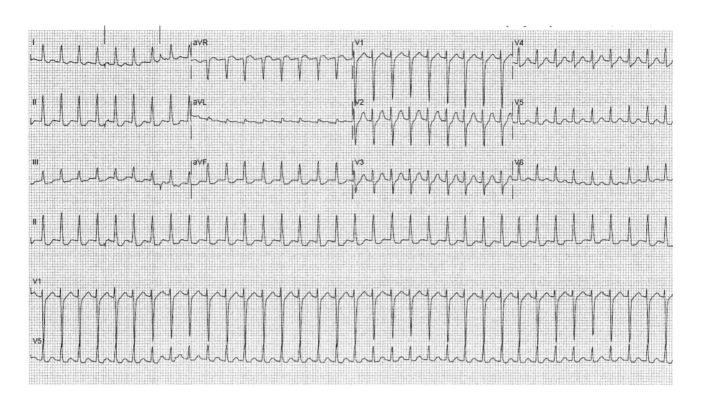

Figure 3.15 Electrocardiogram.

bathroom. Her vital signs include BP 70/palp mm Hg, HR 205 bpm, Sao$_2$ 97%, and RR 24 breaths/min. Her EKG is shown in Figure 3.17. What is the patient at immediate risk for?

A. Respiratory failure
B. Anoxic brain injury
C. Ventricular fibrillation
D. Ischemic stroke

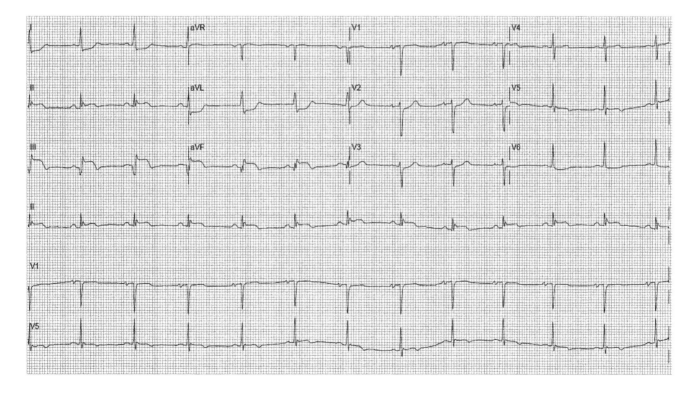

Figure 3.16 Electrocardiogram.

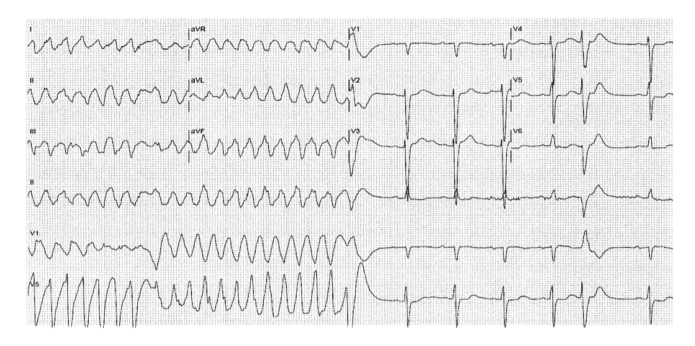

Figure 3.17 Electrocardiogram.

58. What is the most effective way to treat ventricular fibrillation?

A. Electrical defibrillation
B. Cardiopulmonary resuscitation (CPR)
C. Amiodarone
D. Epinephrine

59. An 83-year-old female is brought in by ambulance from her skilled nursing facility after she is noted to be hypoxic. Per the EMS report, initial vital signs were BP 163/94 mm Hg, HR 142 bpm, Sao$_2$ 87% on 4 L NC, and RR 30 breaths/min. The patient has an extensive smoking history and COPD. EMS put her on a non-rebreather mask and gave her a duo-neb treatment. Sao$_2$ improved to 92%. An EKG is obtained, which is shown in Figure 3.18. What rhythm is shown on her EKG?

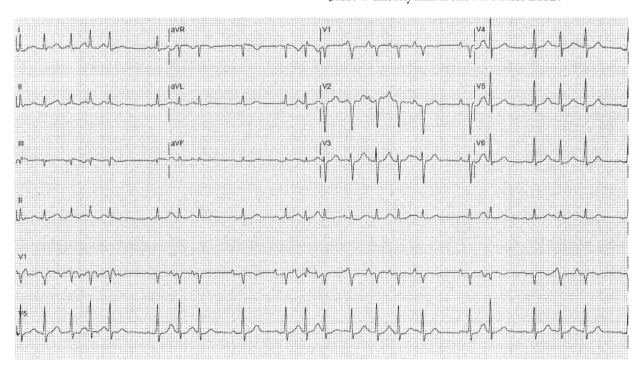

Figure 3.18 Electrocardiogram.

A. Atrial flutter
B. Atrial fibrillation
C. Premature atrial contractions
D. Multifocal atrial tachycardia (MAT)

60. A 43-year-old Mexican male presents with increased dizziness and heart palpitations. He has been having palpitations for several months but ignored them. He is coming in now because they are getting worse, and his dizziness has started affecting his job as a landscaper. He immigrated to the United States 7 years ago. His EKG is shown in Figure 3.19. What feature is shown on his EKG?

A. Premature atrial contractions
B. Complete heart block
C. Mobitz type II
D. Sick sinus syndrome

61. EMS found a 53-year-old female after they were called by her dialysis nurse when she didn't show up for treatment and failed to answer her phone. They found her lethargic and lying on the floor. On arrival to the ED, a stat EKG is obtained, which is shown in Figure 3.20. What are the findings on this EKG most consistent with?

A. β-Blocker overdose
B. Hyperkalemia

C. Hypothermia
D. Increased intracranial pressure

62. A 73-year-old male presents to the ED with the complaint that he is "feeling worse than normal." He is being actively treated for lung cancer at the VA hospital. When asked for further details, he specifies that he has had an upset stomach with increased nausea and vomiting for a few days. He is also more constipated and tired than normal. His EKG is shown in Figure 3.21. What is your interpretation of the EKG?

A. No abnormalities
B. Changes due to electrolyte imbalance
C. Ischemic changes
D. Cardiac arrhythmia

63. A 67-year-old male with COPD and chronic atrial fibrillation presents after experiencing palpitations and dizziness. An initial EKG shows that he is in atrial fibrillation with rapid ventricular rate (RVR) and HR 138 bpm, BP 156/98 mm Hg, RR 22 breaths/min, and Sao$_2$ 94% on 2 L NC. He is rate-controlled with diltiazem. Later in the shift, while he is waiting to be admitted, his nurse informs you that his monitors are showing 3-second pauses. He is awake and intermittently dizzy. His new EKG is shown in Figure 3.22. What is the most likely cause of these new findings?

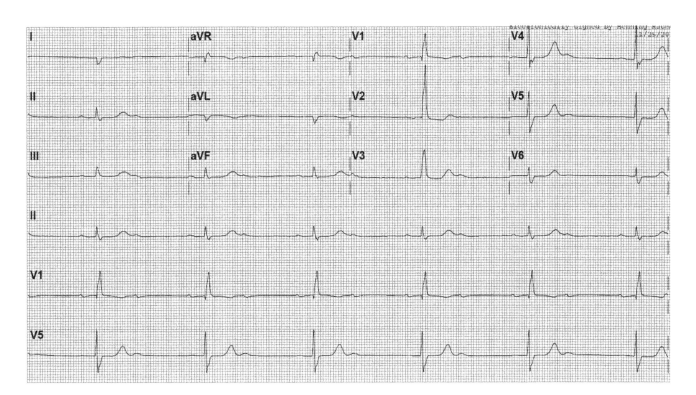

Figure 3.19 Electrocardiogram.

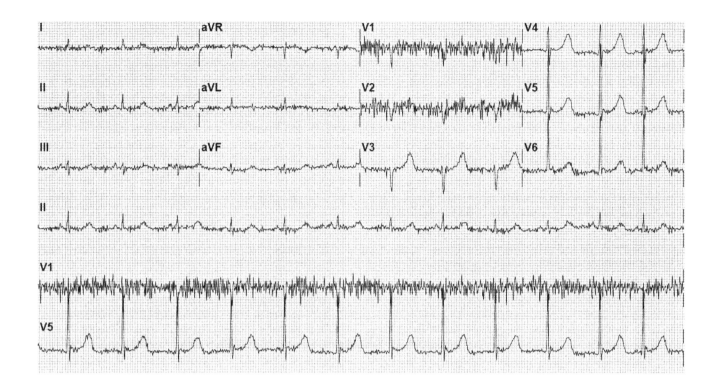

Figure 3.20 Electrocardiogram.

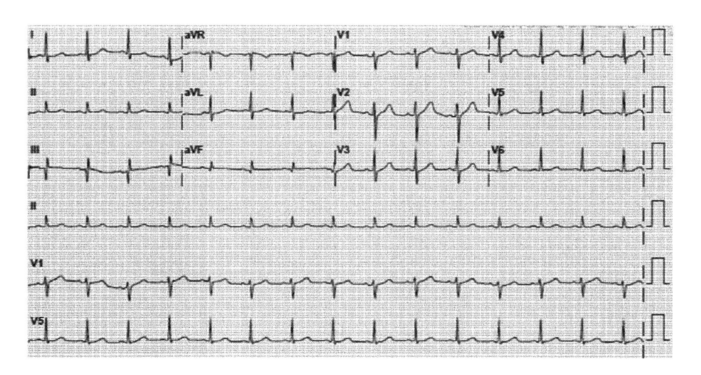

Figure 3.21 Electrocardiogram.

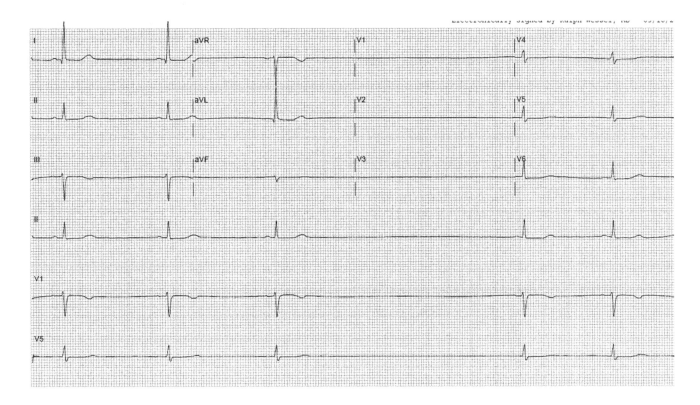

Figure 3.22 Electrocardiogram.

A. High vagal tone
B. Second-degree type I block
C. Sick sinus syndrome
D. Ischemia

64. A 57-year-old female presents with the complaint of persistent tachycardia. She was working in her garden that morning when she suddenly felt palpitations. They did not resolve after rest, so she called her primary care doctor who advised to go to the ED. She has experienced this before, but it has always gotten better with rest. She has no past medical history. HR is 163 bpm and regular. BP is 147/88 mm Hg. Her EKG is shown in Figure 3.23. What is your interpretation of this EKG?

A. NSTEMI
B. Atrioventricular node reentry tachycardia (AVNRT)
C. Accelerated junctional escape rhythm
D. Sinus tachycardia

65. An 83-year-old male presents to the ED with complaints of dizziness and palpitations. His past medical history is notable for MI 3 weeks ago. HR is 164 bpm, and BP is 123/72 mm Hg. He is talking coherently and worried that he is having another heart attack. His EKG is shown in Figure 3.24. What is the next most appropriate step in the management of this patient?

A. Cardioversion
B. Catheterization lab activation
C. Sotalol
D. Procainamide

66. An 83-year-old female with a past medical history of hypertension presents to the ED complaining of fatigue and dyspnea. An EKG is obtained at triage and is shown in Figure 3.25. What is the best interpretation of this EKG?

A. Atrial flutter
B. Sinus tachycardia
C. Atrial fibrillation
D. Premature atrial contractions

67. A 15-year-old female collapses at school following an argument with another girl. After she does not regain consciousness, CPR is initiated quickly, an automated external defibrillator is applied, and a shock is delivered. After the shock, she regains consciousness. School officials tell EMS on arrival that she had recently had two syncopal events during physical education class. The mother provides additional information when she arrives to the hospital that one of patient's

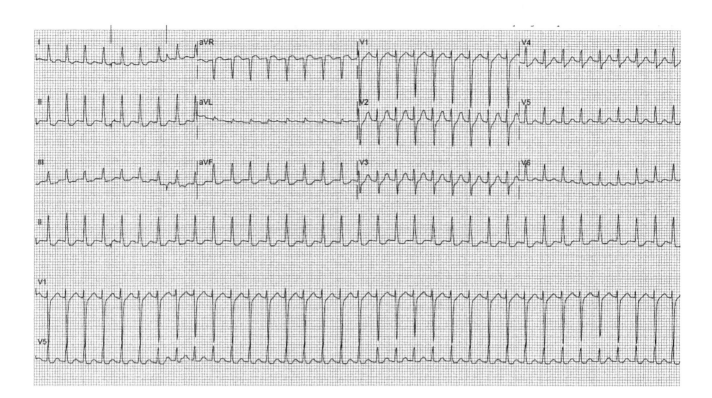

Figure 3.23 Electrocardiogram.

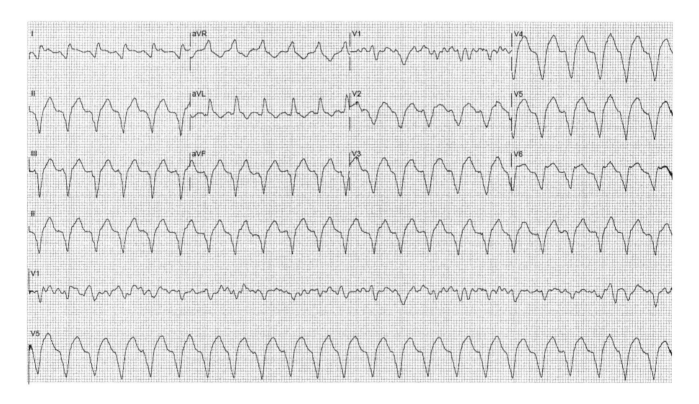

Figure 3.24 Electrocardiogram.

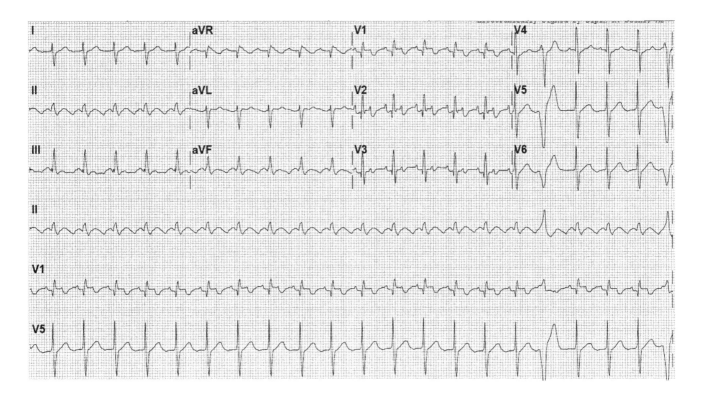

Figure 3.25 Electrocardiogram.

paternal uncles died in his early 20s. Her initial EKG is obtained immediately on arrival to the ED and is shown in Figure 3.26. What is the most likely cause of her collapse?

A. Antidromic Wolff-Parkinson-White (WPW) syndrome
B. Prolonged QT syndrome
C. Sympathomimetic drug use
D. Hypertrophic obstructive cardiomyopathy (HOCM)

68. A 32-year-old male was recently participating in a 50-mile mountain bike race when he began experiencing palpitations. He was able to get to the next aid station where paramedics assessed him and transported him to the closest ED. On arrival, the EKG shown in Figure 3.27 is obtained. There is no prior history of family cardiac problems, and he denies any past medical history. Other than the palpitations, he was asymptomatic during the event. A repeat EKG an hour later is normal. What is the most likely disorder explaining this patient's symptoms and EKG?

A. Brugada's syndrome
B. WPW syndrome
C. Right ventricular outflow tract (RVOT) tachycardia
D. Prolonged QT syndrome

69. In cases of wide complex tachycardia, which of the following is most specific for determining whether the rhythm is ventricular tachycardia (VT) or supraventricular tachycardia (SVT) with aberrancy?

A. HR >150 bpm
B. Age >50 years
C. Prior cardiac history
D. The lack of a RS complex in any precordial leads

70. A 36-year-old female is brought in by ambulance after being found acting weirdly at her home by her son. Current vital signs are HR 37 bpm and BP 80/53 mm Hg. Her initial EKG is shown in Figure 3.28. The patient admits to taking some of her father's pills, but she doesn't know what they are. The only thing she knows is that her father has high BP and takes multiple medications for it. What is the next most appropriate step in the management of this patient?

A. Administer IV atropine
B. Administer IV calcium gluconate
C. Administer IV sodium bicarbonate
D. Administer IV glucagon

71. A 56-year-old male was sent by his primary care physician to the ED with shortness of breath for 3 weeks. He has a history of diabetes, hypertension, and

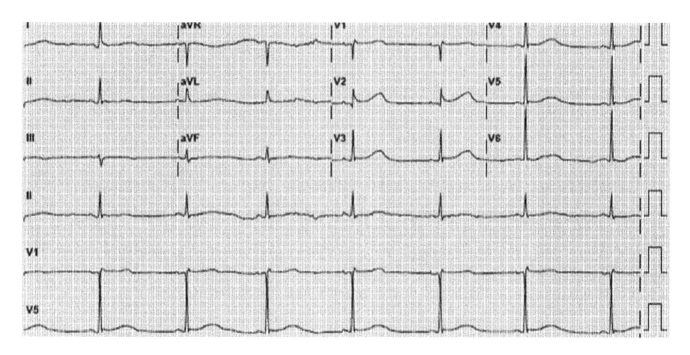

Figure 3.26 Electrocardiogram.

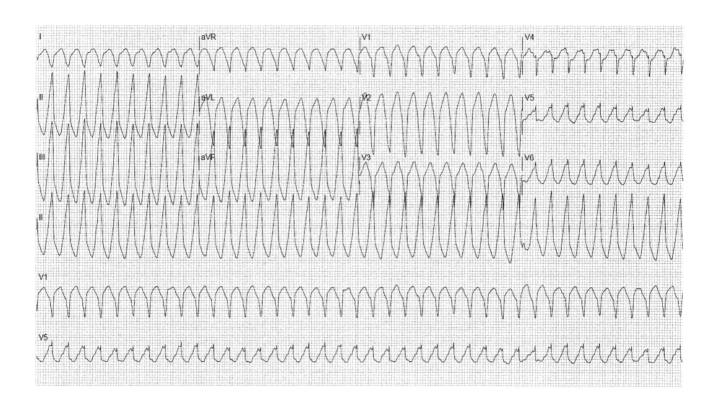

Figure 3.27 Electrocardiogram.

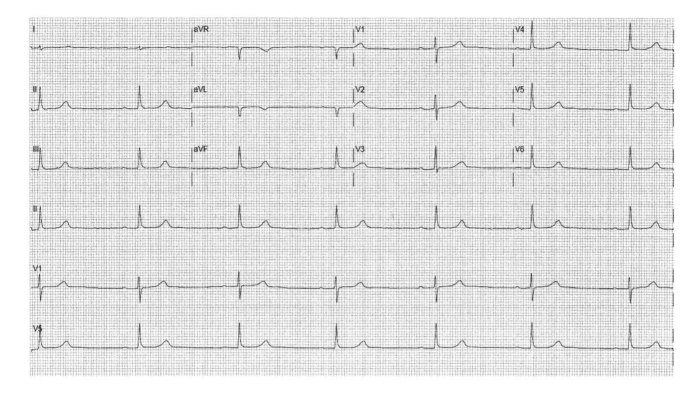

Figure 3.28 Electrocardiogram.

smoking. His dyspnea began when he was building a fence around his property. He had some chest pain initially with the dyspnea that resolved after some rest. He denies chest pain since that moment and any currently. His dyspnea is constant and worse with exertion. His EKG is shown in Figure 3.29. What is the most likely diagnosis?

A. Left ventricular aneurysm
B. ST elevation myocardial infarction (STEMI)

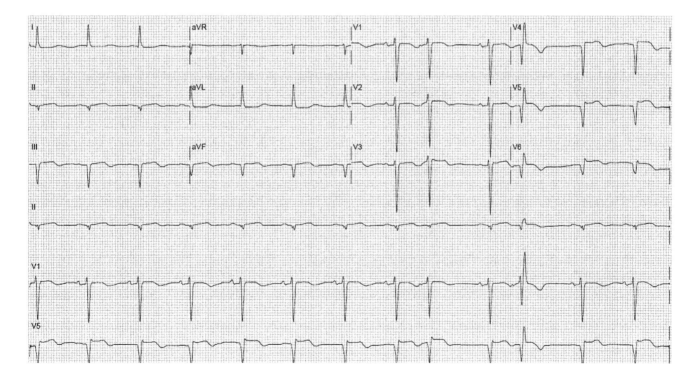

Figure 3.29 Electrocardiogram.

C. Wellens' syndrome
D. PE

72. A 42-year-old male experienced a syncopal episode while eating dinner in a restaurant with his family. The patient regained consciousness shortly afterward when EMS arrived. He denied any prodrome or prior history of syncope. There is no family history of cardiac disease. He does report fever with a productive cough for 4 days and is currently experiencing palpitations. He had a physical with his primary doctor a few weeks ago that included a normal EKG. His current EKG is shown in Figure 3.30. What is the most likely diagnosis?

A. PE
B. Brugada's syndrome
C. Aortic stenosis
D. Wellens' syndrome

73. An 83-year-old female is brought to the ED after her family found her to be suddenly confused and vomiting. She is on multiple medications for heart failure and has an extensive past medical history including hypothyroidism, diabetes, end-stage renal disease (ESRD), COPD, and atrial fibrillation. She was recently seen and diagnosed with gastroenteritis by her primary doctor. Her EKG on presentation to the ED is show in Figure 3.31. What is the most likely cause of this presentation?

A. Inferior STEMI
B. New left bundle branch block
C. Myxedemic coma
D. Medication toxicity

74. A previously healthy 6-year-old male presents with increased work of breathing that has progressively worsened over the past day. He has also had a fever during this time and had a recent respiratory illness 2 weeks ago. On exam, he is tachycardic with rales on lung exam, but he is normotensive and afebrile. His EKG shows sinus tachycardia, and his radiograph shows pulmonary edema. What is the most appropriate disposition for this patient?

A. Home with close follow-up
B. Emergent surgery for valve repair
C. Admission to telemetry
D. Observation in the ED for 6 hours

75. A 25-year-old male presents with altered mental status and increased work of breathing. He is not able to provide a history, but exam reveals track marks to bilateral antecubital fossa, heart murmur, and temperature of 39.1° C. He is intubated because of depressed mental status and inability to handle his secretions. What is the next best step in the management of this patient?

A. Emergent surgical consultation
B. Aggressive fluid resuscitation

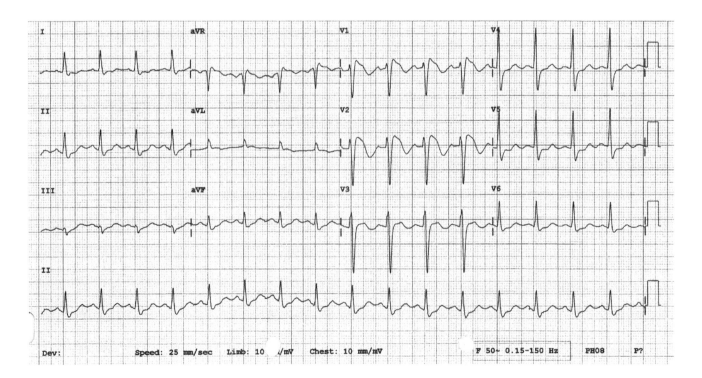

Figure 3.30 Electrocardiogram.

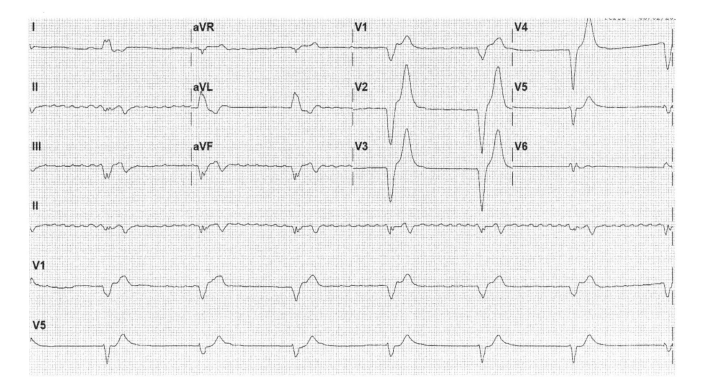

Figure 3.31 Electrocardiogram.

C. Emergent echocardiogram

D. Administer broad-spectrum antibiotics

76. A 22-year-old male presents to the ED with palpitations, and on the monitor, he has a narrow complex tachycardia without obviously discernible P waves. He is normotensive without any other complaints. Vagal maneuvers are not successful with cardioversion, and the patient is given adenosine. After administration, the patient decompensates into ventricular fibrillation. What was the likely underlying rhythm?

A. Atrial fibrillation with WPW syndrome

B. Sinus tachycardia

C. SVT

D. Atrial flutter with 2:1 block

77. A 9-year-old girl presents with palpitations. She has no other complaints and is normotensive. She is found to be in a narrow complex tachycardia at 280 bpm. What is the next best step in management of this patient?

A. Adenosine

B. Carotid massage

C. Vagal maneuvers

D. IV fluid bolus

78. A 45-year-old man with a history of stents presents with shortness of breath and chest pain. He is hypotensive and found to have a regular narrow complex tachycardia at a rate of 210 bpm. What is the next best step in management of this patient?

A. Synchronized cardioversion

B. Adenosine

C. Vagal maneuvers

D. Carotid massage

79. A 12-year-old female presents after passing out while at cross-country practice without any prodromal symptoms. She has no complaints in the ED, and her vital signs are normal for her age group. Her EKG is shown in Figure 3.32. What is the most likely underlying diagnosis?

A. Prolonged QT syndrome

B. First-degree AV block

C. WPW syndrome

D. Hypertrophic obstructive cardiomyopathy (HOCM)

80. A 62-year-old male presents with acute-onset shortness of breath an hour before arrival. He was recently released from the hospital after suffering an MI that required stenting. His oxygen saturation is in the 80s. On exam, there are rales in all lung fields, and he has a holosystolic murmur that radiates to the left axilla. What is the definitive treatment that this patient needs?

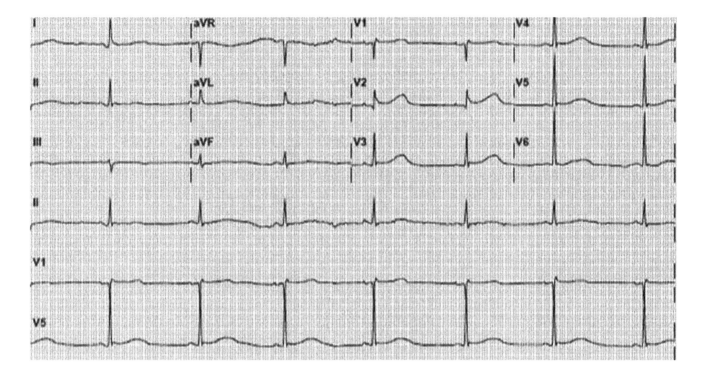

Figure 3.32 Electrocardiogram.

A. Admission for observation
B. Emergent surgical intervention
C. Broad-spectrum IV antibiotics
D. Aggressive fluid resuscitation

81. A 72-year-old male presents with tearing back pain that started suddenly 2 hours before arrival. He has numbness in his left lower extremity and has markedly different BPs when comparing his right and left arms. While being worked up for an aortic dissection, he develops sudden onset of shortness of breath and on exam has bilateral rales with a high-pitched blowing decrescendo diastolic murmur over his left upper sternal border. What valvular dysfunction is likely present?

A. Aortic regurgitation
B. Pulmonary regurgitation
C. Mitral regurgitation
D. Mitral stenosis

82. A 74-year-old male with a history of CHF presents with worsening shortness of breath, bilateral lower extremity swelling, and dyspnea on exertion. His vital signs are within normal limits, and his exam reveals bibasilar rales and crescendo-decrescendo systolic murmur that radiates to the carotids. What agent should be avoided in this patient for the treatment of his heart failure?

A. Digoxin
B. Lisinopril
C. Nitrates
D. Statins

83. A 44-year-old female with a history of lupus presents with worsening dyspnea on exertion and shortness of breath over the past 2 to 3 weeks, with bilateral lower extremity edema. Her vital signs are within normal limits, and her exam reveals bibasilar wheezing with a loud opening snap and a diastolic rumble heart murmur. What is the most likely valvular dysfunction?

A. Mitral stenosis
B. Pulmonary stenosis
C. Tricuspid regurgitation
D. Pulmonary regurgitation

84. A 26-year-old man with a history of IV drug use presents with malaise and fevers for the past month. His vital signs reveal a temperature of 38.4° C, HR 106 bpm, BP 96/57 mm Hg, and RR 24 breaths/min. He is diaphoretic, his lungs are clear, and heart exam reveals a holosystolic murmur over the left upper sternal border. What is the likely organism causing this patient's infection?

A. *Staphylococcus aureus*
B. *Streptococcus viridans*

C. Coagulase-negative staphylococcus
D. *Enterococcus* species

85. A 14-year-old female presents after developing palpitations while playing basketball. She is more than 6 feet tall, and her arms appear disproportionately long for her height. She has no other complaints, and her vital signs are within normal limits. Her exam is normal except for a mid-systolic click over the apex of her heart. Her workup is negative, and her symptoms have resolved. What is the most appropriate disposition for this patient?

A. Follow-up with a cardiologist as an outpatient
B. Admission to a telemetry floor
C. Urgent surgical intervention
D. Admission to the pediatric ICU

86. A 2-week-old male infant who was born at home presents with difficulty feeding over the past few days. His vital signs are within normal limits, and his exam reveals a holosystolic murmur with a thrill over the left sternal border. He is also hypotonic. While working up the patient for sepsis, what else should be ruled out emergently in the ED?

A. Hypothyroidism
B. Hyponatremia
C. Intracranial hemorrhage
D. Hypoglycemia

87. A 3-year-old male is brought into the ED because his parents are concerned that he is turning blue and having difficulty getting around without developing shortness of breath. They state this has happened in the past, and he had required surgery at that time. He is cyanotic on exam, and his oxygen saturation is between 65% and 70% on room air. His exam reveals a sternotomy scar and diffuse cyanosis. What is the definitive treatment for this child?

A. Supplemental oxygen
B. Broad-spectrum antibiotics
C. Urgent cardiac surgery
D. Discharge home with cardiology follow-up

88. A 2-year-old male presents with congestion and fever for the past 3 days. He is still eating well and acting like himself, and many other kids are sick with similar symptoms at his group child care. His vital signs are within normal limits, and his exam is unremarkable except for a vibratory murmur best heard over the left sternal border while the child is lying flat. A radiograph

reveals no acute process. What is the best disposition for this patient?

A. Home with general pediatric follow-up
B. Emergent surgical evaluation
C. Admission for IV antibiotics
D. Admission to the telemetry floor

89. A 2-month-old female presents with discoloration to the bottom half of her body that has progressively worsened over the past few days. She is otherwise eating well, making six to eight wet diapers a day, and acting herself. Her vital signs are within normal limits, and her exam reveals cyanosis to her lower extremities compared with her upper extremities. If her underlying condition were to progress further, what is a potential finding on chest radiograph?

A. Bilateral infiltrates
B. Rib notching
C. Deep sulcus sign
D. Pleural effusion

90. A 16-year-old boy presents with difficulty breathing and almost passing out while he was running a track event. He has a history of being a "blue baby" but had a pulmonary valve replacement early in life and has been okay since. His vital signs are within normal limits at rest, and his exam reveals a holosystolic murmur along the left sternal border. What diagnostic study will best determine this patient's diagnosis?

A. Chest CT
B. Treadmill testing
C. Chest radiograph
D. Echocardiogram

91. A 24-year-old woman has a precipitous delivery in the ED, and 10 minutes after delivery the baby is still cyanotic. The baby continues to have an oxygen saturation that is in the low 80s despite blow by oxygenation. His pulse is still greater than 60 bpm, and he has a decent cry. What is the most appropriate disposition for this patient?

A. Admission to the neonatal ICU
B. Admission to the newborn nursery on high-flow oxygen
C. Transfer to the operating room for emergent surgery
D. None of the above

92. A 2-month-old male presents because of intermittent discoloration around his lips and nails after

crying and feeding. It has progressively worsened over the past few days, and he has been more restless during this time. He has a crying episode during your exam, when he develops bluish coloration around his lips and nails, which improves with flexing of his knees and hips. What diagnostic test is most likely to make the correct diagnosis for this patient?

A. Chest radiograph
B. Chest CT
C. Echocardiogram
D. Pulmonary function testing

93. A 65-year-old male with a history of diabetes mellitus, CAD, hypertension, and CHF presents to the ED stating that his AICD has shocked him three times in the past 2 hours. He denies chest pain or shortness of breath but states he now feels weak and tired. He has been placed on a monitor, which shows a normal sinus rhythm with a rate of 68 bpm. What is the next most appropriate step in the management of this patient?

A. Discharge home with referral to his cardiologist within 1 week
B. Admit to a telemetry floor for cardiac monitoring
C. Administer IV amiodarone
D. Have the patient's AICD interrogated in the ED

94. A 73-year-old female is brought into the ED by EMS after collapsing at home. She is noted to have an AICD. For EMS providers, she has a pulse and agonal respirations. They establish an IV line and assist respirations with bag-valve-mask ventilation. On arrival to the ED, she loses pulses and her AICD is noted to be firing. You place her on a monitor, and she is in ventricular fibrillation. What is true about the initial management of this patient?

A. Do not perform chest compressions because the person performing compressions may be shocked
B. Do not attempt to externally defibrillate because the patient's AICD is already firing
C. Perform cardiac life support as you would in any pulseless patient
D. Arrange for immediate interrogation of the AICD

1. ANSWER: A

This is a case of asymptomatic hypertension. The patient has had two readings of elevated BP, one at her primary doctor's office and one in the ED. Per American College of Emergency Physicians clinical policy, it is reasonable to discharge the patient with no screening labs or intervention.

It would be appropriate to start medication or screen patients with poor follow-up, however in this case, she came from her primary care provider's office. Dropping the BP acutely is potentially harmful for the patient and should not attempt to be achieved during an ED visit.

Test-taking tip: In a well-appearing, asymptomatic patient with follow-up, less being done is sometimes better, even on standardized tests.

2. ANSWER: C

This patient is likely suffering from acute sympathomimetic crisis secondary to stimulant drug use, such as methamphetamine or cocaine. The treatment of choice for both these drugs is lorazepam (Ativan) or midazolam (Versed) as needed until the patient calms down and is less combative.

A head CT can be done after the patient is stable. CT is needed if the patient has any focal neurologic chances or does not metabolize appropriately.

Esmolol is relatively contraindicated in this case. If the patient used cocaine, there would be a theoretical unopposed β-blockade leading to worsening of the hypertension.

Nicardipine is a second-line treatment if Ativan fails to achieve results related to controlling the BP.

Test-taking tip: This is an action patient, so any answer that is not an acute intervention can be excluded. Remember, that with anything toxicology-related in the setting of an agitated patient, benzodiazepines are usually the answer as first line therapy.

3. ANSWER: C

This patient appears to have an acute decompensation of his CHF with respiratory distress. This patient has clinical signs and symptoms of volume overload. Given his clinical findings, the first line of treatment for a patient in respiratory distress from volume overload with hypertension is respiratory support with BiPAP and a nitroglycerin drip. A nitroglycerin drip causes an acute decrease in the afterload, easing the strain of the heart. BiPAP in this setting has been shown to reduce the time to resolution of dyspnea and reduce need for intubation. It has become the mainstay of acute CHF exacerbations with respiratory distress.

Giving a bolus to this person would worsen his fluid overload and is contraindicated in this patient. Labs and a chest radiograph will need to be done to rule out other causes but should be done after intervention has been started because this patient has acute respiratory distress that needs to be addressed.

Although furosemide (Lasix) will need to be given, patients with CHF can have decreased renal perfusion and acute kidney injury (AKI). It would be prudent to delay Lasix administration until renal function is assessed.

Test-taking tip: This is an action patient, so any answer that is not an acute intervention can be excluded. Some of the answers may be appropriate at some time during the patient's care, but when the question states "next best," focus on the answer that will treat the patient's immediate life threat.

4. ANSWER: D

This patient had a syncopal event following a breath-holding spell. This typically occurs in children 6 to 18 months old after an emotional inciting event. They may have myoclonic jerks that could simulate a small seizure but typically have no postictal period. If the syncope event was unexplained, an EKG or transthoracic echocardiogram would be warranted to assess for structural cardiac abnormalities. An EEG would be warranted if there were signs/symptoms of a seizure. For breath-holding spells, there is no intervention. The patient should be referred to their primary care physician for follow-up.

Test-taking tip: Children who are healthy tend not to require much intervention in the ED.

5. ANSWER: B

The only patient who can be sent home from these brief scenarios is choice B because this is likely vasovagal syncope after giving blood.

Choices A, C, and D all need further workup. The 18-year-old male at least needs an EKG to rule out hypertrophic cardiomyopathy. The 75-year-old female will likely be able to go home but is at higher risk and warrants further workup. The 30-year-old male with a harsh murmur may have aortic stenosis and is at high risk for cardiac arrhythmias. He also requires further workup. Although no one set of clinical decision rules is perfect, high-risk patients have a history of cardiac disease and are prone to arrhythmias.

Test-taking tip: It frequently helps to eliminate outliers—the older and younger patient in this case. Then choose between the remaining two. In this case, one has a medical problem and the other was situational.

6. ANSWER: B

This is a case of Brugada's syndrome. Brugada's is sodium channelopathy that leads to sudden cardiac death in young patients; it is typically due to a ventricular dysrhythmias like ventricular fibrillation. It is frequently found in people of Asian descent. The typical EKG of type 1 Brugada's syndrome is a coved ST elevation in V_1 to V_3 with a T wave inversion in V_1 to V_3. This should prompt admission for an AICD because it is the only treatment shown to improve mortality.

The patient is unlikely to have acute coronary syndrome because he is asymptomatic and has no other evidence of an ischemic etiology of his syncope. Discharging with a Holter monitor would detect any arrhythmia that precipitated his syncope but would not treat the potentially fatal arrhythmia. Discharging home with no intervention would be inappropriate for a patient with an abnormal EKG.

Test-taking tip: This question is dependent on you recognizing the classic pattern of Brugada's syndrome on the EKG and knowing that this syndrome can lead to fatal arrhythmias. Brush up on classic EKG findings (Brugada's, Wellens', Winter's, etc.) before the test.

7. ANSWER: C

This syncopal episode is due to the patients' complete heart block and hypotension. Because she is altered and hypotensive, she will need overdrive pacing. The quickest way to do that is to transcutaneous pace the patient.

Transvenous pacing may need to happen if the cardiologist is unable to place a permanent pacemaker in a timely manner or if the transcutaneous pacing fails to capture. Although some bradyarrhythmias respond to atropine, complete heart block rarely does, making transcutaneous pacing the most appropriate initial management of this unstable patient.

Test-taking tip: This is an action patient. Any patient who is critical needs fast intervention, so look for the answer that is fast and effective. This mindset allows you to eliminate choices A and C.

8. ANSWER: B

This patient is high risk per the Wells' criteria for DVT. This patient has major surgery (cesarean delivery), tenderness along the deep venous system, calf swelling, and edema giving her a score of 3. The next best step is to order an ultrasound to evaluate for a DVT.

Because the clinical probability is high, the D-dimer will not change the decision management. A radiograph will not evaluate the venous system, and there is no history of trauma, limiting the usefulness of this diagnostic test. Venography is not the first line for diagnosing a DVT and exposes the patient to radiation, which may not be needed if the ultrasound is positive.

WELLS' SCORE AND PROBABILITY

One point for each: active cancer; paralysis, paresis, recent immobilization of lower extremities; localized tenderness along the deep venous system; entire leg swollen; calf swelling >3 cm larger than asymptomatic side; unilateral pitting edema; collateral superficial veins; previous history of DVT

Negative two points for alterative diagnosis is as likely or more likely than a DVT.

Score higher than two suggests high probability.

Score less than two suggests low probability.

Test-taking tip: Brush up on clinical decision rules and scores (Wells', PECARN, etc.) because they are useful in clinical practice and on standardized tests.

9. ANSWER: A

The patient has a high probability of DVT, and if the ultrasound is negative, the next step is to obtain a D-dimer. If the D-dimer is negative, then DVT is ruled out. If the D-dimer is positive, then the ultrasound will need to be repeated in 1 week. Empirically treating at this point is not necessary because the DVT has not been formally ruled in. Completely ruling out a DVT at this point and discharging the patient home would be dangerous and could potentially lead to a PE if she had a DVT missed on ultrasound.

Test-taking tip: Brush up on come clinical treatment pathways, such as for DVT and PE, before the test.

10. ANSWER: D

Only thrombosis of the deep venous system requires anticoagulation. Of the veins listed, the cephalic is the only superficial vein. The deep veins of the arm include the subclavian, axillary, brachial, paired radial, paired ulnar, and interosseous veins. The deep veins of the leg include the popliteal, superficial femoral, common femoral, and calf veins (anterior tibia, peroneal, and posterior tibial).

Test-taking tip: This is a "you know it or don't" kind of question. If you don't know it, choose an answer and move on. You can perhaps mark it for review when you are done at the end of the test. Don't, however, let these kinds of questions get you stuck and waste your time.

11. ANSWER: C

This patient's presentation is consistent with a PE, and he meets criteria for a massive PE. For massive PE, the treatment is full-dose tPA, streptokinase, or urokinase.

Half-dose thrombolytics can be considered in a person with a submassive PE, but this patient's presentation is not consistent with a submassive PE. This patient is not stable enough for a CT scan now, and it would be dangerous to send him. The patient has no evidence of COPD exacerbation currently because his lungs have no wheezing.

Test-taking tip: This patient is unstable, suggesting the need for immediate action. Going to the CT scan with an unstable patient is always a bad idea, helping you to eliminate this answer. The fact that he has no wheezing helps to eliminate the use of nebulized treatments through CPAP, leaving you two choices.

12. ANSWER: A

The patient requires anticoagulation that is safe for her and her fetus. Enoxaparin is recommended by the American College of Obstetricians and Gynecologists for treatment of PE; it is safe for the fetus because it does not cross the placenta.

Warfarin is a known teratogen and is contraindicated in pregnancy. Warfarin can cause neurocognitive developmental abnormalities.

Clopidogrel is not indicated for PE but is a cardiac antiplatelet medication used in CAD and CVA patients.

Rivaroxaban has not been formally studied in pregnancy, but a small case study suggests it may be deemed safe in the future.

Test-taking tip: This is a "you know it or don't" kind of question. If you don't know it, choose an answer and move on. You can perhaps mark it for review when you are done at the end of the test. Don't, however, let these kinds of questions get you stuck and waste your time.

13. ANSWER: C

IVC filters are generally placed when anticoagulation fails, there is a reason to discontinue anticoagulation, or the risk for recurrence is high. In the setting of venous thromboembolism in trauma, there is a high risk for both bleeding (from the injuries) and clot formation (from the hypercoagulable state in trauma). There is high risk for recurrence in malignancy and in patients with a large clot burden.

Prophylaxis as a reason for IVC placement is not recommended by the 2012 American College of Chest Physicians guidelines because there is no evidence an IVC filter is better than pharmacologic prophylaxis.

Test-taking tip: Three of the answers suggest high-risk disease states that might benefit from an invasive procedure. Prophylaxis does not, making it a good guess for the correct answer.

14. ANSWER: C

In a patient with hypertensive emergency as suggested by the confusion, the goal reduction in MAP is 25% over the first hour or a goal reduction of the diastolic BP to 100 or 110 mm Hg. These patients have lost their ability to autoregulate their cerebral perfusion, but they also have a tolerance to hypertension. Lowering the MAP to a normal range can cause a drop in cerebral perfusion, leading to ischemia. Lowering the BP insignificantly will not reverse the cerebral dysfunction.

Test-taking tip: Avoid picking the extreme answers, when it comes to answers with numbers in them, because they are not usually correct.

15. ANSWER: C

This patient has a pulseless leg that results from a large arterial occlusion that causes limb cyanosis and diffuse pain. This is a vascular emergency. A vascular surgeon should be consulted immediately.

This patient is unlikely to have diffuse cellulitis of her leg. Imaging would delay definitive management of this patient.

Test-taking tip: Blue is bad. If there is threat to a limb, call the specialist.

16. ANSWER: C

This patient presents with hypertension and symptoms concerning for aortic dissection. This is a hypertensive emergency. The best medication to lower BP initially is esmolol because it reduces the shearing force on the aorta by reducing the change in BP with each heartbeat. The target BP is 100 to 120 mm Hg with a goal HR around 60 bpm.

If esmolol doesn't adequately reduce the BP, nitroprusside can be added. Nitroprusside should not be started first because it can raise the HR and increase shearing forces.

Nifedipine is not indicated because it has minimal inotropic effect and may even result in reflex sympathomimetic stimulation. Hydralazine is also not indicated in aortic dissection, nor does it lend to titratable dosing.

Test-taking tip: In critically ill patients, you want to use medications that have quick onset of action but also can be discontinued/reversed quickly. Nifedipine and hydralazine do not meet these two criteria for medications in the critically ill patient, allowing you to eliminate them.

17. ANSWER: B

In a woman of childbearing age with abdominal pain and syncope, a ruptured ectopic is extremely high on the differential and must be ruled out first. The test that would likely give you the diagnosis first is a pregnancy test.

Although she may have hepatobiliary disease, it is unlikely that this would cause syncope. Pyelonephritis would more likely have flank pain and a leukocytosis, but again does not usually cause syncope.

An EKG is probably indicated in this patient but will not answer the diagnostic dilemma.

Test-taking tip: Syncope and abdominal pain in women of childbearing age equals ectopic pregnancy until ruled out.

18. ANSWER: C

Given the clinical scenario, this patient is presumed to have carbon monoxide poisoning as demonstrated by the headache, syncope, and nausea. The treatment is high-flow oxygen by non-rebreather mask first before any studies are done. A head CT, EKG, and ABG test can all be done after starting high-flow oxygen.

Test-taking tip: When thinking about "next best steps" in management of patients, it is often about treating the suspected underlying cause of the disease with an agent that works quickly. Administering oxygen in this patient meets this criterion. All the other actions are tests to further clarify the correct diagnosis.

19. ANSWER: A

Azithromycin likely precipitated this patient's syncope. It is commonly used for pneumonia in young patients and can prolong a QTc. QTc prolongation can lead to torsades, which is what is shown on the EKG and what led to his syncope. The other choices do not commonly prolong a QTc interval.

Test-taking tip: This is a "you know it or don't" kind of question. If you don't know it, choose an answer and move on. You can perhaps mark it for review when you are done at the end of the test. Don't, however, let these kinds of questions get you stuck and waste your time.

20. ANSWER: D

WELLS' SCORE AND PROBABILITY

One point for each: active cancer; paralysis, paresis, recent immobilization of lower extremities; localized tenderness along the deep venous system; entire leg swollen; calf swelling >3 cm larger than asymptomatic side; unilateral pitting edema; collateral superficial veins; previous history of DVT

Negative two points for alterative diagnosis is as likely or more likely than a DVT.

Score higher than two suggests high probability

Score less than two suggests low probability.

Wells' score stratifies the risk for DVT. Exogenous use of estrogen is not part of the Wells' criteria; however, it is part of the Pulmonary Embolism Rule-out Criteria (PERC) rules.

Test-taking tip: Three of the answers involve the leg (the location of the DVT). Choosing the outlier in this case may help you select the correct answer.

21. ANSWER: D

This patient described in D is the only patient of the group with hemodynamic compromise. Currently, the only strong recommendation for thrombolytics is in the setting of a massive PE, as defined by hemodynamic compromise.

The patient described in choice C likely has a submassive PE and warrants very close monitoring.

The patient in B may have many reasons to be tachycardic, and thrombolytics are contraindicated within 3 weeks of major trauma or surgery.

Although the patient described in A has a saddle PE, that patient is hemodynamically stable, and the risk for bleeding does not outweigh the benefit of thrombolytics.

Test-taking tip: Find the patient who meets the action. Thrombolytics in the setting of PE are a heroic attempt to save a life. Find the unstable patient who needs the treatment, and you will select the correct answer.

22. ANSWER: D

Clonidine is known to cause rebound hypertension because there is overactivity of the sympathetic system (the α-agonism is absent). The other medications don't generally cause a rebound hypertension like clonidine.

Test-taking tip: This is a "you know it or don't" kind of question. If you don't know it, choose an answer and move on. You can perhaps mark it for review when you are done at the end of the test. Don't, however, let these kinds of questions get you stuck and waste your time.

23. ANSWER: A

Brugada's syndrome is a dysfunction in the sodium channel that is inherited in an autosomal dominant manner. It is unclear why there is a male predominance. It is proposed that there is increased transmural dispersion of ventricular repolarization, leading to a predisposition to dysrhythmias; however, it is poorly understood.

Potassium channelopathies have been associated with prolonged QT syndrome. Calcium channelopathies can lead to a wide variety of dysrhythmias and have been associated with short QT syndrome. Sodium-potassium ATPase dysfunction does not give any specific arrhythmia but will present like digoxin overdose with variable dysrhythmias.

Test-taking tip: This is a "you know it or don't" kind of question. If you don't know it, choose an answer and move on. You can perhaps mark it for review when you are done at the end of the test. Don't, however, let these kinds of questions get you stuck and waste your time.

24. ANSWER: B

This patient with a known history of CHF and presents with signs and symptoms of a mild to moderate CHF exacerbation. The key to this question is that the patient has a decent oxygen saturation and is normotensive. In these cases, sublingual nitroglycerin is the initial therapy of choice because nitroglycerin lowers preload and after load, which improves pulmonary congestion. Nitroglycerin would be contraindicated if the patient were hypotensive.

Most patients with CHF exacerbations should be started on supplemental oxygen; however, this patient with a mild CHF exacerbation may not need BiPAP because he has responded to oxygen by nasal cannula.

A chest radiograph is seldom useful in evaluating for pulmonary edema in the acute phase because there may be no radiographic evidence initially.

IV furosemide (Lasix) is not an initial therapy of choice because of its prolonged onset of physical diuresis. Moreover, many acute decompensated heart failure patients have low renal blood flow due to vasoconstriction and thus a relative inability to diurese effectively.

Test-taking tip: When thinking about "next best steps" in management of patients, it is often about treating the suspected underlying cause of the disease with an agent that works quickly. This allows you to eliminate choices A and D, leaving you two choices.

25. ANSWER: D

Several studies have shown that noninvasive positive pressure ventilation decreases both morbidity and mortality in ADHF patients. This has resulted in increased use of noninvasive ventilation for any patients not responding to initial oxygen therapy by nasal cannula. None of the other answers have been shown to decrease morbidity and mortality.

Test-taking tip: This is a "you know it or don't" kind of question. If you don't know it, choose an answer and move on. You can perhaps mark it for review when you are done at the end of the test. Don't, however, let these kinds of questions get you stuck and waste your time.

26. ANSWER: C

This question asks you to know how BiPAP helps in heart failure, but even if you do not know the answer off the top of your head, it can be reasoned out by thinking through the effects of noninvasive positive pressure ventilation.

Noninvasive ventilation has been shown to decrease the need for endotracheal intubation in ADHF patients by increasing intrathoracic pressure due to the positive pressure. This increasing intrathoracic pressure helps to recruit atelectatic alveoli by essentially forcing open more alveoli. This helps to change the ventilation and perfusion within the lung, causing fluid to shift back into the capillaries and thereby decreasing the work of breathing. It also works to increase pulmonary compliance, not decrease compliance.

Test-taking tip: Decreased compliance is a bad thing when it comes to lungs, making it different from the rest of the answers.

27. ANSWER: A

This patient has continued confusion and hypoxia with coarse rales bilaterally despite being on noninvasive ventilation, which all point toward the patient being unstable. Any of the other answers would delay the next critical step of immediate endotracheal intubation and should only be considered after intubation is successfully performed.

Test-taking tip: When thinking about "next best steps" in management of patients, it is often about treating the suspected underlying cause of the disease with an agent or action that works quickly. This allows you to eliminate choices C and D, leaving you two choices.

28. ANSWER: B

In the majority of pericarditis cases the etiology is unknown. While many are thought to be viral in origin, only a relatively small number have proved to be due to infection.

Malignancy and MI also cause pericarditis, but these etiologies are much less common. Post-MI pericarditis can be early in onset (within a few days) or late in onset (called Dressler's syndrome).

Test-taking tip: This is a "you know it or don't" kind of question. If you don't know it, choose an answer and move on. You can perhaps mark it for review when you are done at the end of the test. Don't, however, let these kinds of questions get you stuck and waste your time.

29. ANSWER: C

This patient had a recent STEMI 2 weeks prior and is now presenting with chest pain that is described as the same as her last STEMI. While this is always a concerning story to hear from patients, the EKG is more suggestive of pericarditis rather than acute ischemia.

Determination of pericarditis versus recurrent MI is imperative to avoid potentially giving anticoagulation or performing coronary arteriography erroneously because both of these can have serious complications and side effects.

Given the timing of the recurrence of chest pain, the negative troponin, and the EKG findings, this is most likely post-MI pericarditis, also known as Dressler's syndrome. Of note, a mild troponin elevation and leukocytosis can also be present in Dressler's syndrome.

Sublingual nitro is not warranted, and while it may have few negative side effects in this patient, pericarditis is the most likely diagnosis, and thus the best therapy is high-dose aspirin or nonsteroidal antiinflammatory drugs (NSAIDs).

Test-taking tip: Part of choosing the correct answer is in interpreting the EKG correctly, but even if you are not able to do so, three of the answers treat coronary ischemia. Only choice C stands out as different.

30. ANSWER: A

Pericarditis can present similarly to both MI and PE. In this patient, PE is unlikely because by PERC he would be low risk (<2% chance of having a PE).

While there is an elevation in troponin level, both MI and pericarditis can cause troponin elevations. However, the EKG shows ST elevations in noncontiguous leads, which argues against MI and for pericarditis.

Test-taking tip: Recent viral syndrome in a young, otherwise healthy patient should make you think pericarditis or myocarditis.

31. ANSWER: A

This patient has an incidental finding of a large pericardial effusion but no tamponade physiology, warranting further investigation into the cause.

Hypothyroidism can often present with myxedema in the pericardial sac and can be quite large but rarely causes tamponade. Thyroid labs can diagnose hypothyroidism, and the myxedema responds to thyroid replacement.

None of the other labs would be helpful in determining a possible etiology for incidental large pericardial effusion. BNP is used to diagnose and determine whether heart failure is worsening or improving. ESR and CRP are inflammatory markers that may suggest inflammation or infection but are not specific to help diagnose the causes of a pericardial effusion. Procalcitonin can aid in the diagnosis and risk stratification of bacterial sepsis but is not helpful in the diagnosis of pericardial effusion.

Test-taking tip: This is a "you know it or don't" kind of question. If you don't know it, choose an answer and move on. You can perhaps mark it for review when you are done at the end of the test. Don't, however, let these kinds of questions get you stuck and waste your time.

32. ANSWER: D

This patient presents after an altercation and has an incidental finding of a pericardial effusion. No evidence of tamponade is shown on his ultrasound, but he does have a history and radiographic findings concerning for tuberculosis. Patients with tuberculosis are at increased risk for developing a pericardial effusion. Thus, this effusion is most likely chronic and does not to be emergently drained by pericardiocentesis.

The best treatment for this patient is isolation and antibiotic treatment with rifampin, isoniazid, pyrazinamide, and ethambutol.

High-dose aspirin and colchicine are used to treat pericarditis, which this patient does not have evidence of.

Labs may be helpful, but blood smears would not be applicable here because it is unlikely this patient needs a leukemia/lymphoma workup.

Test-taking tip: When thinking about "next best steps" in management of patients, it is often about treating the suspected underlying cause of the disease with an agent or action that works quickly. The patient does not have tamponade, so urgent pericardiocentesis is not indicated, and a blood smear will not help in the acute management of this patient, leaving you two answers to choose from.

33. ANSWER: D

This patient is undergoing chemotherapy and radiation for metastatic breast cancer and is at increased risk for pericarditis. While Beck's triad for pericardial tamponade is not present, there are signs of tamponade, including hypotension and right atrial collapse on ultrasound. The next step is to perform a pericardiocentesis to remove fluid from the pericardial sac and improve cardiac output.

Although this patient is critically ill, she is speaking in full sentences and is not tachypneic or hypoxic. Thus, intubation is not the best next step in her care.

High-dose NSAIDs, like ketorolac, can be used in the treatment of pericarditis, but this case is not consistent with the presentation of this disease process.

Although this patient is hypotensive and in shock, it is due to pericardial tamponade not hemorrhage; thus volume repletion, including blood, is not immediately indicated.

Test-taking tip: This patient is in shock and has pericardial tamponade, for which the only emergent appropriate treatment is pericardiocentesis.

34. ANSWER: D

This patient most likely had a previous valve replacement surgery and now presents with an aortic regurgitation murmur. Thrombosis is a common complication of valve replacements, and while murmurs in older adults are unreliable diagnostic indicators, the bedside ultrasound confirms an aortic valve thrombosis.

This patient is unlikely to have infective endocarditis given lack of fevers, normal vital signs, and few risk factors, so antibiotic therapy is not warranted for empiric treatment.

In this case, surgical thrombectomy or fibrinolysis is the treatment option of choice for prosthetic valve thrombosis. Anticoagulation has no place currently because there is a thrombosis that needs to be specifically managed to avoid further complications such as emboli causing stroke or peripheral arterial emboli.

An outpatient referral for a transesophageal echocardiography in this patient is not appropriate because the thrombosis needs to be managed urgently and not as an outpatient.

Test-taking tip: Choices B and C are easy to eliminate, given the scenario in the question, leaving you two choices.

35. ANSWER: A

This patient with a previous heart valve replacement is now presenting with signs of cardiogenic shock. This is most likely due to a recent valvular dysfunction, but the emergent issue is the shock from aortic regurgitation. Thus, surgical consult may be needed but not before addressing the shock.

There is no evidence of septic shock in this patient, so antibiotics and fluid boluses may not fix the problem. Patients with valve dysfunction may often be refractory to fluids and require vasopressors to maintain cardiac output and distal organ perfusion.

The pressor of choice when regurgitation is suspected (as the patient has a diastolic murmur and a widened pulse pressure) is Dobutamine or low dose dopamine rather than a potent alpha vasoconstrictor like Norepinephrine, as Norepinephrine may worsen valvular regurgitation and cardiogenic shock.

Test-taking tip: This is a "you know it or don't" kind of question. If you don't know it, choose an answer and move on. You can perhaps mark it for review when you are done at the end of the test. Don't, however, let these kinds of questions get you stuck and waste your time.

36. ANSWER: B

This patient presents to the ED with fever of unknown etiology for more than a week. Given the history of a valve replacement, presence of Janeway lesions (red nontender lesions on the palms), and splinter hemorrhages, this patient most likely has an infective endocarditis and will require further intervention and workup including antibiotics and a TTE.

While infective endocarditis can be very difficult to definitively diagnose in the ED by Duke's Criteria, ED providers need to have a high index of suspicion in patients with risk factors (including IV drug use, prosthetic valves with recent dental work, or patients who regularly use injection medications, such as those with type 1 diabetes).

Secondary syphilis can also present with painless lesions of the palms and soles, but this patient has no history of sexually transmitted infections and secondary syphilis typically has a diffuse maculopapular rash also present.

Pyelonephritis is unlikely in this patient because there are no casts in the urine and no costovertebral angle tenderness. A viral upper respiratory illness is also unlikely given the lack of associated symptoms.

Test-taking tip: Fever in a patient with a history of valve replacement and hand lesions should make you think endocarditis.

37. ANSWER: C

Uncontrolled hypertension is the number one predisposing risk factor in thoracic aortic dissection. Other risk factors include known atherosclerosis or aortic aneurysm, bicuspid aortic valve, congenital aortic coarctation, and collagen vascular diseases such as Marfan's syndrome.

Test-taking tip: This is a "you know it or don't" kind of question. If you don't know it, choose an answer and move on. You can perhaps mark it for review when you are done at the end of the test. Don't, however, let these kinds of questions get you stuck and waste your time.

38. ANSWER: B

This patient is presenting with sudden onset of chest pain associated with tachycardia, hypertension, and different pulses in the lower extremities. His chest radiograph shows a widened mediastinum. This clinical picture is strongly suggestive of aortic dissection, and the confirmatory test is CT of the aorta with contrast.

This helps to determine whether a dissection is present and where the dissection is located to help further guide appropriate management. In this patient, there is enough of a suspicion for dissection that an argument could be made for beginning management before confirmatory testing; however, the correct management includes esmolol IV first, then nitroprusside IV for BP control. Nitroglycerin alone is not an appropriate therapy in this setting.

Test-taking tip: Nontraumatic chest pain with a widened mediastinum equals thoracic aneurysm or

dissection until proved otherwise. This allows you to eliminate A and C as possible answers.

39. ANSWER: B

This patient has a confirmed aortic dissection. Dissection can be classified by the Stanford classification as either type A (involving the ascending aorta) or type B (beginning after the left subclavian artery).

Type A dissections are considered true surgical emergencies; however, this patient has a type B dissection and can be reasonably managed with medications.

Oral medications are never to be used in an acute dissection. The correct order of medicines is esmolol IV followed by nitroprusside to give β-blockade of the heart and then provide BP relief. Giving nitroprusside first may result in rebound tachycardia, potentially worsening the dissection.

Test-taking tip: Brush up on classifications, such as the Stanford classification for aortic dissection, that help you decide how to manage patients.

40. ANSWER: D

This patient presents with a variety of signs and symptoms that could be attributed to many things. However, the combination of neurologic symptoms and chest pain should raise concern for an aortic dissection. The patient also has risk factors for dissection including hypertension, hyperlipidemia, and smoking.

A stroke is unlikely in this patient given the bilateral lower extremity distribution without any arm weakness.

Cauda equina can cause lower extremity weakness; however, there is no mention of saddle anesthesia or urinary retention, and there are no red flags such as fevers, back pains, IV drug use, or immunosuppression.

An MI can cause chest pains and vital sign abnormalities, but the combination of hypertension, bilateral lower extremity weakness, and dissection risk factors makes aortic dissection the most likely diagnosis.

Test-taking tip: Neurologic symptoms and chest pain equal aortic dissection until proved otherwise.

41. ANSWER: C

This patient most likely has a pseudoaneurysm in his left femoral artery. Pseudoaneurysms form most commonly at graft sites and occur when there is disruption of the suture line at an anastomosis.

This patient underwent a recent femoral-femoral bypass for an occluded femoral artery and now returns with severe pain and a pulsatile mass. Pseudoaneurysms are managed surgically and should be addressed emergently because they can rupture, causing hemorrhage or limb ischemia.

Heparinization is not indicated in this patient and may worsen his condition if the pseudoaneurysm ruptures. Esmolol and nitroprusside are medications to control BP in the setting of aortic dissection. Although pain control is indicated, this condition cannot be managed as an outpatient because of the high likelihood of complications.

Test-taking tip: Pulsatile masses are never good, allowing you to eliminate choice D, and the patient has a normal BP, allowing you to eliminate choice B and leaving you two options.

42. ANSWER: B

This patient has a right arm dialysis fistula with continued heavy bleeding. Dialysis fistulas are at an increased risk for pseudoaneurysm because of the recurrent perforation by dialysis needles. If a pseudoaneurysm grows it can erode into the overlying skin, risking serious infection, or it can cause heavy bleeding.

While there are very few clues for pseudoaneurysm in this patient, a high index of suspicion should be kept in any dialysis patient for hemorrhage or infection. A noncomplicated pseudoaneurysm should be dealt with surgically; however, this patient presents hypotensive, tachycardic, and lightheaded.

The care of this patient should follow the essential steps of ABCs, so the correct first step would be to place two large-bore IV lines and begin fluid resuscitation.

Test-taking tip: When thinking about "next best steps" in management of patients, it is often about treating the suspected underlying cause of the disease with an agent or action that works quickly. This patient is in hemorrhagic shock, which points to the correct answer of B.

43. ANSWER: A

Bedside ultrasound to assess for free fluid in the abdomen and pelvis is the imaging modality of choice in this patient presenting with signs and symptoms of shock. While the abdomen is soft on exam, older adult patients often do not develop guarding and rigidity in the presence of free fluid.

This patient has an epigastric mass with AAA risk factors including smoking, diabetes, hyperlipidemia, and hypertension. Many patients with AAA have no known history, so a high index of suspicion is required. When AAA is suspected and a patient is unstable, immediate evaluation

for free fluid from rupture should be obtained. An ultrasound can identify free fluid rapidly and is a great modality for determining the presence of AAA at the bedside.

CT scan is the imaging modality of choice to detect rupture in stable patients, but this patient is too unstable to be sent for CT or MRI.

Vasopressors may be required but no reassessment of pressures has taken place yet, and aggressive fluid resuscitation should be done first. Thus, beginning with a bedside ultrasound is best. Of note, ultrasound alone cannot be used to rule out a nonruptured aneurysm, so do not be reassured by a negative FAST exam.

Test-taking tip: The patient is in extremis, making advanced imaging such as CT or MRI not appropriate, leaving you two answers to choose from.

44. ANSWER: A

This patient has a 5-cm abdominal aortic dilation in the setting of abdominal pain. Infrarenal dilations greater than 3 cm are diagnostic of an aneurysm. The risk for rupture of an aneurysm varies with the size of an aneurysm: 3- to 5.4-cm aneurysms are at low risk for rupture, and 5.5- to 6-9 cm are at moderate risk with a 9.4% to 10.2% risk for rupture within 1 year. Aneurysms 7 cm or larger have a 32.5% risk for rupture in 1 year.

This patient's pain is most likely due to his AAA. Symptomatic AAAs are presumed ruptured until proved otherwise. This patient should have a CT scan to evaluate for rupture and a prompt surgical consultation, even in the setting of hemodynamic stability, because these patients can quickly decompensate.

Test-taking tip: Three of the answers involve discharge; choose the answer that is the outlier (vascular consult).

45. ANSWER: C

Marfan's syndrome is a connective tissue disorder that is a significant risk factor for AAA because these patients have blood vessel walls that are weak and can stretch. This patient has vague symptoms, including general weakness and abdominal pain that radiates to the low back. This should make the provider have a high suspicion for AAA in this patient.

The physical exam does not specifically mention a pulsatile mass, but the physical exam for AAA is highly unreliable and should not be relied on to rule in or out an aneurysm.

While mesenteric ischemia is a possibility, the story is atypical because mesenteric ischemia usually has an acute presentation of mid-abdominal pain that is out of proportion to the physical exam.

Diverticulitis is less likely because this patient has no fever, bowel changes, hematochezia, or history of diverticulosis. A perforated viscus is also less likely given the lack of trauma or history of ulcers in the setting of a soft, nonsurgical-appearing abdomen.

Test-taking tip: Marfan's syndrome with chest or abdominal pain equals aortic aneurysm or dissection until proven otherwise.

46. ANSWER: B

This patient is most likely having a critical ischemic event because of her chronic peripheral arterial disease. This is evidenced by her medical history risk factors, pain that gets worse with lying down and better with dependent blood flow (i.e., hanging a leg over the bed), and leg pain that has been ongoing for years but that has acutely worsened.

When evaluating for limb ischemia, keep in mind the six Ps: pain, paresthesias, poikilothermia, paralysis, pulselessness, and pallor. In this case, the patient is exhibiting pain out of proportion (unable to bear weight) and paresthesias. Given the suspicion for an acute ischemic event, this should be further evaluated.

The quickest and best evaluation modality for an arterial thromboembolism is an ABI. A radiograph may be beneficial to evaluate for fractures, but given the critical time period for discovering acute limb ischemia, it is not the best option. Likewise, an MRI could potentially be beneficial, but MRIs are expensive and slower than getting an ABI, which is quick and easy.

Test-taking tip: The patient has no history of significant trauma, allowing you to eliminate A as the correct answer, and you do not send patients who can't walk home, allowing you to eliminate answer D, leaving you two options as answers.

47. ANSWER: A

This patient has obvious signs of an acute ischemic event, most likely embolic in nature given the history of being non-anticoagulated with atrial fibrillation. When evaluating for limb ischemia, keep in mind the 6 Ps: pain, paresthesias, poikilothermia, paralysis, pulselessness, and pallor.

This patient has several signs, including pain, paralysis, paresthesias, and poikilothermia, as well as decreased pulses. With obvious hard signs that are concerning, immediate anticoagulation should be started by giving an aspirin and treating with weight-based heparin.

While vascular surgery or interventional radiology are definitive treatment options, the textbook answer for all thromboembolic patients is to first begin heparinization.

A CT angiography study would be helpful when there is need for further investigation about occlusion, but in this patient with obvious signs, a CT will only further delay treatment and intervention.

Test-taking tip: When thinking about "next best steps" in management of patients, it is often about treating the suspected underlying cause of the disease with an agent or action that works quickly. Answer A is the only one that accomplishes this goal.

48. ANSWER: C

This patient's past medical history of steroid-resistant sarcoidosis is a clue to her current symptoms. Her hypoxia is notable and is a known secondary effect of sarcoidosis, but hypoxia in and of itself does not cause syncope.

Her hemoglobin of 9.3 is low and may be contributing to her chronic symptoms but would also be an unlikely cause of syncope.

Increased vagal tone can cause atrioventricular (AV) blocks, but a complete block from it is unlikely, particularly in the presence of a disease with AV block as a known complication.

This question is about recognizing the EKG findings and linking them to a known disease process. Her sarcoidosis has likely progressed to the point that granulomas are influencing the cardiac conduction system. This patient has a type III or complete heart block as seen in the EKG by isolated P waves. The other answer choices are also possibilities but less likely with the given information.

Test-taking tip: Correctly interpreting the EKG as complete heart block is key to selecting the correct answer because anemia, hypoxia, and increased vagal tone do not cause this.

49. ANSWER: B

In this scenario, there are two important clues to the correct diagnosis, including recent methamphetamine use and the EKG findings. Methamphetamine is well known to cause cardiac vasospasms, which could have caused the chest pain but does not account for the EKG findings.

Wellens' syndrome is a recognized STEMI equivalent that presents with deeply inverted or biphasic T waves in V_2–V_3 with possible involvement of all precordial EKG leads. This EKG pattern is suspicious enough for high-grade LAD stenosis that it warrants immediate catheterization lab activation.

Patients can present with waxing and waning chest pain and EKGs that demonstrate the pattern shown or clear signs of anterolateral STEMI depending on whether they are experiencing active ischemia.

Cardiac stress testing is highly discouraged in these patients. Hypokalemia presents with U waves in the precordial leads.

Test-taking tip: This question is dependent on you recognizing the classic pattern of Wellens' syndrome on the EKG and knowing that this syndrome is a STEMI equivalent. Brush up on classic EKG findings (Brugada's, Wellens', and Winter's syndromes, etc.) before the test.

50. ANSWER: A

The key clinical findings in this question are new seizure with tachycardia and hypotension. Tricyclic antidepressants (TCAs) are well known to produce this triad of symptoms.

TCA overdose can mimic or expose underlying, undiagnosed Brugada's syndrome on EKG, but the EKG findings must be taken in the context of the clinical picture. Notice the wide QRS and terminal R wave in aVR on the EKG in Figure 3.10. Both of these EKG findings signify a significant TCA toxicity. Treatment for wide QRS is sodium bicarbonate.

Test-taking tip: Even if you can't correctly interpret the EKG findings as being related to a TCA overdose, this patient is in extremis, allowing you to eliminate answers C and D as being causes of her presentation.

51. ANSWER: B

This patient is presenting with several complaints suggesting a multisystem disease. Vomiting, leg weakness, and EKG changes are concerning for electrolyte disturbances, specifically hyperkalemia. Thyroid disease is a possibility in this scenario, but the EKG allows for differentiation between the two given the information provided.

Notice on EKG the wide complex bradycardia. This patient has Addison's disease, which is known to cause hyperkalemia. Thyroid disease can have a similar presentation and causes a narrow complex bradycardia. Hypothermia and propranolol can also cause bradycardia but typically also produce narrow complex QRS patterns.

Test-taking tip: The key to choosing the correct answer is recognizing that, of the choices, only hyperkalemia causes a wide complex bradycardia.

52. ANSWER: A

This clinical picture is concerning for an MI given the patient's presentation, and this is reflected in the answer choices. The question involves the distribution of the infarction. The EKG shows only depression in the precordial leads. Isolated posterior infarct must be on the differential with these EKG findings.

This could also be subendocardial ischemia, but that it is not an answer choice. Because the two diseases have very different treatment needs, it is important to distinguish between the two. An EKG with posterior lead placement can help significantly with this decision. Also consider the patient's overall clinical picture and risk factors for each of these diseases. The other choices would present with ST elevation in the appropriate leads.

Test-taking tip: Choosing the correct answer for this question is completely dependent on correctly interpreting the EKG. Brush up on the different STEMI patterns before the test.

53. ANSWER D

There is not much information given in this question stem, so it is important to focus on where most of the information is given, which is the EKG. This EKG demonstrates the digitalis effect. This series of EKG findings indicates only that the patient is on digitalis and has no correlation to toxicity. These findings commonly involve T wave changes that include shortening of the QT interval and flattening and inversion of the T wave. The most famous finding of the digitalis effect is described as a "hockey stick" or "Dali's moustache" pattern that refers to ST depression with an additional scooped appearance that is seen in the precordial leads.

Test-taking tip: This is a "you know it or don't" kind of question. If you don't know it, choose an answer and move on. You can perhaps mark it for review when you are done at the end of the test. Don't, however, let these kinds of questions get you stuck and waste your time.

54. ANSWER: D

The patterns on this EKG indicate a large blockage given the number of leads with changes in them. It is important to recognize that this indicates increased disease in comparison to more common obstructive patterns.

The differential for aVR ST elevation includes LMCA and LAD occlusion, three-vessel disease, and diffuse ischemia. LAD is the only other choice in the answers that this EKG could belong to but recognizing the large ST elevation present in aVR compared to V1 indicates that this is likely a LMCA lesion.

Test-taking tip: Choosing the correct answer for this question is completely dependent on correctly interpreting the EKG. Brush up on the different STEMI patterns before the test.

55. ANSWER: C

The differential diagnosis for a regular, narrow complex SVT includes sinus tachycardia, atrial flutter with a block, AVNRT, WPW syndrome with orthodromic AV reentry, and atrial tachycardia.

This EKG shows a high rate of tachycardia with a narrow complex. There are no discernable P waves. The next best step would be to use adenosine to narrow the differential diagnosis.

Test-taking tip: A regular, narrow complex tachycardia without discernable P waves is paroxysmal SVT until proved otherwise.

56. ANSWER: A

This EKG shows a large inferior STEMI with ST elevation prominent in the inferior leads (II, III, aVF) and reciprocal depression in leads I and aVL. This signifies occlusion of the right coronary artery.

Aspirin and nitroglycerin are adjuncts to treating coronary ischemia, but they are not the best next step in the care of this patient, who needs reperfusion. Insulin and D50 would be treatment for hyperkalemia, but this story and the EKG are not consistent with this diagnosis. This patient needs prompt reperfusion, and thus waiting for a repeat EKG is not wise.

Test-taking tip: This question is dependent on you recognizing the classic pattern of inferior STEMI on EKG. Brush up on classic EKG findings (Brugada's, Wellens', Winter's syndromes, etc.) before the test.

57. ANSWER: C

This patient is in torsades de pointes. This question requires recognition of that and knowing that it is likely, from the prolonged QT interval, to be due to an overdose of antipsychotics.

Antipsychotics are believed to cause QT prolongation by preventing or slowing outward potassium flow during repolarization. The altered membrane potential may then provoke an inward depolarizing current, causing increased action potential duration simultaneously with an early afterdepolarization. This creates a unidirectional block and reentry circuit, which can further degenerate into ventricular fibrillation.

This patient's presentation is not most consistent with ischemic stroke, and although she may be at risk for anoxic brain injury or respiratory failure if she is not appropriately resuscitated, it is ventricular fibrillation that she is at immediate risk for developing.

Test-taking tip: The key to this question is "immediate risk." The patient may be at risk from other sequelae, but the immediate risk is ventricular fibrillation.

58. ANSWER: A

According to the American Heart Association (AHA), electrical defibrillation is the most effective way to treat ventricular fibrillation. Survival rates decrease considerably as time to defibrillation increases. Effective CPR is important in all patients who are pulseless and apneic but is not the best treatment for ventricular fibrillation.

Test-taking tip: Ventricular fibrillation equals electricity. All the other treatments are also helpful, but the key to this question is "most effective."

59. ANSWER: D

This EKG shows an irregular rhythm with multiple shapes for P waves. This is a description of MAT.

MAT is closely linked to COPD, particularly COPD exacerbations. COPD has been linked to the other answer choices as well, but the EKG demonstrates MAT. Several factors likely combine to produce arrhythmias as a natural sequela of COPD. These include pulmonary hypertension, chronic inflammation, hypoxia, atrial stretch, and others.

Atrial flutter and atrial fibrillation can be confused with MAT, but neither has P waves with multiple shapes. Atrial flutter may have flutter waves, and usually with atrial fibrillation you will not see P waves.

Test-taking tip: Chronic respiratory problems should make you think of MAT.

60. ANSWER: C

It is important to develop a system for reading EKGs in order not to miss any findings. This EKG shows second-degree type II heart block, also known as Mobitz II. This type of heart block is usually related to physical damage to the His-Purkinje system, which allows for consistent transmission of electrical stimuli until the entire conduction is blocked, as opposed to the variable block caused by decreased AV conduction of Mobitz I. Given this patient's age and his origin, it would be worthwhile to include Chagas' disease in the differential.

In complete heart block, the P waves have not been associated with the QRS complexes. Sick sinus syndrome may present with many different EKG findings, from sinus bradycardia to atrial fibrillation.

Test-taking tip: This question is dependent on you recognizing the classic pattern of Mobitz II second-degree AV block on the EKG. Brush up on classic EKG findings (Brugada's syndrome, Wellens' syndrome, Mobitz I and II, etc.) before the test.

61. ANSWER: C

The differential for this case is large. Little information is provided in the question stem, except the fact that the patient undergoes dialysis, leaving the answer to be obtained from correct interpretation of the EKG.

The EKG shows bradycardia with PR, QRS, and QT prolongation. These changes are common in β-blocker overdose, hyperkalemia, and hypothermia. The only difference is the presence of J (Osborn) waves. J waves have been found in other medical conditions and even incidentally. However, they are still considered to be highly sensitive and specific for hypothermia.

Test-taking tip: The key to this question is spotting the J wave and realizing that the artifact on the EKG is due to shivering, a response to the hypothermia.

62. ANSWER: B

This question is about EKG interpretation and recognizing abnormal findings. This patient is exhibiting symptoms of hypercalcemia, which is a recognized occurrence in cancer patients. This EKG shows a shortened QT interval that is common in hypercalcemia. Shortened QT intervals can degenerate into VT or fibrillation. Short QT is defined as QT < 370 msec.

Test-taking tip: There are no finding consistent with ischemic changes or arrhythmia on this EKG, making these answers easy to eliminate.

63. ANSWER: C

This EKG shows alternating tachycardia and bradycardia. Of the choices listed, this is most likely tachy-brady syndrome, which is a subset of sick sinus syndrome. The patient's age, symptoms, and history of atrial fibrillation are contributing factors to this diagnosis.

Patients with high vagal tone are generally younger and asymptomatic. The P waves here are regularly spaced, making second-degree type I block less likely. There are no ST-T elevations or depressions, making ischemia less likely.

Test-taking tip: Alternating tachycardia and bradycardia should make you think sick sinus syndrome.

64. ANSWER: B

Answering this question depends entirely on EKG reading skills because the information in the stem could be valid for any arrhythmia.

The pseudo R wave in the precordial leads is actually a P wave. In AV nodal reentrant tachycardia (AVNRT), the reentry pathway is within the AV node itself, which causes P waves to be found after the QRS. Pseudo R waves can be found in atrioventricular reentry tachycardia (AVRT), but they are much more likely to be in AVNRT.

ST depression is commonly found in AVNRT, but it should resolve after adenosine treatment. If it does not, then an NSTEMI should be considered.

In an accelerated junctional escape rhythm, the P waves would be inverted. In sinus tachycardia, the P waves would have normal morphology and be in front of the QRS complexes.

Test-taking tip: This question is dependent on you recognizing the classic pattern of AVNRT on the EKG. Brush up on classic EKG findings (Brugada's syndrome, Wellens' syndrome, AVNRT, etc.) before the test.

65. ANSWER: D

Although this patient is clinically stable, his EKG shows monomorphic ventricular tachycardia (VT).

Cardioversion is the most successful treatment method for VT. However, the AHA currently recommends treatment of stable patients first with procainamide, amiodarone, or sotalol.

Procainamide has demonstrated efficacy over amiodarone and sotalol, earning it a class IIa recommendation from the AHA, while amiodarone and sotalol are class IIb, making procainamide the first-line drug of choice.

Test-taking tip: Brush up on your advance cardiac life support (ACLS) algorithms because they are frequently sources for questions on standardized emergency medicine tests.

66. ANSWER: A

EKG reading abilities are key to this question. The first clue is the rate. HR of 130 to 170 bpm should trigger suspicion for atrial flutter with a 2:1 conduction block. It is caused by a reentrant atrial circuit, and progression through the AV node determines the ventricular rate. Leads II, III, and aVF are best for viewing flutter waves.

Atrial fibrillation is often confused for a flutter and vice versa. However, once you look for them, the flutter waves are present. The QRS waves are also too regular for atrial fibrillation, although this could occur with a superimposed block.

With sinus tachycardia, you should see a P wave in front of every QRS complex.

Test-taking tip: With regularly irregular rhythms, look for flutter waves to distinguish between atrial fibrillation and flutter.

67. ANSWER: B

The differential for syncope is lengthy, but with EKGs, there are five main arrhythmias to be concerned about: WPW, HOCM, Brugada's, prolonged QT, and AV blocks.

Prolonged QT syndrome is a common cause of death in the young. It is a cardiac arrhythmia typically presenting with syncope or cardiac arrest after emotional or physically strenuous events. This disease is a physical ramification of several genetic disorders relating to sodium or potassium channel function allowing for R-on-T occurrence during tachycardia that degrades into torsades de pointes, VT, or ventricular fibrillation.

WPW syndrome and HOCM belong in the differential, but the EKG lacks findings characteristic for these disorders. Sympathomimetic drug use does not affect the QT interval.

Test-taking tip: Remember the five main arrhythmias associated with syncope and look for them on the EKG.

68. ANSWER: C

This EKG shows a wide complex tachycardia with an inferior axis deviation and left bundle branch block morphology consistent with RVOT tachycardia. RVOT is a form of idiopathic VT that is not usually associated with underlying structural heart disease. It generally arises from the outflow tract of the right ventricle or possibly from the tricuspid annulus.

In Brugada's syndrome, the arrhythmia leads to a polymorphic VT that presents with syncope and sudden death.

WPW and long QT syndromes are possibilities but are less likely with an EKG that returns to normal.

Test-taking tip: This question is dependent on you recognizing the classic pattern of RVOT on the EKG. Brush up on classic EKG findings (Brugada's syndrome, Wellens' syndrome, RVOT, etc.) before the test.

69. ANSWER: D

For this question, it is important to recognize that SVT and VT are readily confused, which is why it is recommended to treat for VT regardless. However, EKG differentiators do exist. SVT with aberrancy is a result of abnormal conduction occurring with SVT. When the aberrancy is a bundle branch block, then SVT mimics VT. Brugada and colleagues developed a four-step algorithm to help differentiate between the two. The first criterion is the lack of an RS complex in any of the precordial leads. It has a specificity of 1.0 for VT, although its sensitivity is rather low.

Test-taking tip: This is a "you know it or don't" kind of question. If you don't know it, choose an answer and move on. You can perhaps mark it for review when you are done at the end of the test. Don't, however, let these kinds of questions get you stuck and waste your time.

70. ANSWER: D

This question stem provides important information in the patient's vital signs and in the mechanism of a likely overdose of hypertensive medications. The EKG shows bradycardia and a first-degree AV block. This information makes it most likely that she ingested β-blockers and/or calcium channel blockers.

The immediate treatment for this is glucagon because it bypasses adrenergic receptors and stimulates cyclic adenosine monophosphate. which counterattacks the β-blockade.

This question involves compiling multiple pieces of information to reach the most likely scenario. None of the other medications listed will have the same clinic effects as glucagon.

Test-taking tip: In the setting of overdose and antihypertensives, always think β-blocker or calcium channel blocker, and glucagon is first-line therapy.

71. ANSWER: A

This question provides a clue in the 3 weeks of dyspnea that occurred with chest pain initially. The EKG provides further information in the diffuse ST elevation combined with pronounced Q waves and a lack of reciprocal ST depression. Left ventricular aneurysm occurs at least 2 weeks after an MI. Residual ST segment elevation can be found in EKGs because of the aneurysm.

It is doubtful that the patient would still be alive if he was having ongoing symptoms from a STEMI or PE for 3 weeks.

Test-taking tip: With this question, the guidance toward the correct answer is in the history provided in the question stem, not necessarily in the EKG findings.

72. ANSWER: B

With syncope and abnormal EKG findings, there are five key etiologies to be concerned about: AV blocks, prolonged QT syndromes, WPW syndrome, and hypertrophic obstructive cardiomyopathy.

Multiple other diseases cause syncope that have high mortality associated with them, such as PE and aortic stenosis, but EKG findings from these etiologies are much more subtle.

This patient had a normal EKG during a routine checkup a few weeks ago, but that does not preclude Brugada's syndrome because some variants allow sodium channels to function normally until other factors are added to them. Fever is a well-recognized symptom to unmask Brugada's syndrome.

Test-taking tip: Remember the five main arrhythmias associated with syncope and look for them on the EKG.

73. ANSWER: D

The differential diagnosis for this patient is extensive. The EKG shows cardiac involvement and provides several clues to the correct diagnosis.

The changes in the EKG are more extensive than what could be commonly explained by an inferior STEMI or a new left bundle branch block.

Myxedemic coma is generally linked to bradycardia, low QRS voltage, and diffuses T wave inversions. It can also be linked to AV blocks and QT prolongation.

Medication toxicity should be high on the differential for anyone on multiple medications, and the fact that the patient has heart failure, ESRD, and recent gastroenteritis increases the risk of this.

EKG changes from digoxin toxicity are diverse given its mechanism of action and include rate changes of tachycardia or bradycardia, AV blocks, premature ventricular contractions, bundle branch blocks, and T wave inversions. It can also produce ST changes of either depression or elevation.

Test-taking tip: This is a "you know it or don't" kind of question. If you don't know it, choose an answer and move on. You can perhaps mark it for review when you are done at the end of the test. Don't, however, let these kinds of questions get you stuck and waste your time.

74. ANSWER: C

This child is presenting with heart failure, which is likely secondary to myocarditis. Myocarditis is the most common cause of heart failure in the pediatric population, and most cases are secondary to a viral illness and have associated viral prodromes. It is the cause of sudden cardiac death in 15% to 20% of individuals younger than 40 years. Other causes include drugs, autoimmune diseases, and peripartum cardiomyopathy. Many of these cases are asymptomatic.

These patients require admission to the telemetry floor to monitor for possible dysrhythmias. There is no mention of a heart murmur, making valvular pathology less likely Observation would not be the best disposition for this patient because these patients are at risk for dysrhythmias, including VT and ventricular fibrillation. It is not appropriate to discharge this patient because the presentation is consistent with heart failure.

Test-taking tip: It is easy to eliminate answers A and D because new-onset heart failure in any age group requires admission for further workup and management.

75. ANSWER: D

This patient is septic from an unknown source but with a presentation concerning for endocarditis. Early antibiotics are an important part of the management in early sepsis.

While fluid resuscitation is also crucial, antibiotics early have shown to have a better outcome than fluid resuscitation alone.

It is premature to get surgery involved in the patient's care at this time without a confirmed diagnosis, and antibiotics should not be delayed for an echocardiogram.

There should be a high index of suspicion for endocarditis for this patient based on the fever and murmur with an exam concerning for IV drug use. The depressed mental status may be secondary to the patient being septic, but it is possible that the patient is having a stroke secondary to septic emboli. Antibiotic coverage for methicillin-resistant *Staphylococcus aureus* (MRSA) should be included based on the high probability of the patient having an IV drug use history.

Test-taking tip: Fever in a patient with a history if IV drug use should make you think endocarditis until proved otherwise, and in these patients, antibiotics should be administered early.

76. ANSWER: A

Atrial fibrillation with WPW syndrome is likely to be the cause of this patient's decompensation into ventricular fibrillation. Adenosine causes AV nodal blockade, but in WPW syndrome the accessory pathway feeds into the AV node. Without it being able to conduct through the AV node after the administration of adenosine, this puts the patient at an increased risk for ventricular fibrillation due to continuous signals entering the accessory pathway.

The patient would then require electrical unsynchronized cardioversion for the ventricular fibrillation. In a patient who requires cardioversion and has a known history of WPW syndrome, procainamide is the most suitable agent.

The other listed rhythms are all supraventricular rhythms without reentrant pathways, making the likelihood of decompensation into a ventricular dysrhythmia less likely.

Test-taking tip: Decompensation to ventricular fibrillation after administration of adenosine should make you think WPW syndrome.

77. ANSWER: C

When a patient is in SVT, it is recommended to attempt the following, in the order listed, as long as the patient is hemodynamically stable (systolic BP >90 mm Hg, no chest pain, no altered mental status, and not short of breath):

- **Vagal maneuvers**
  - Bearing down
  - Trying to blow a plunger out of a syringe
  - Ice to the face (most appropriate in children)
- **Carotid massage**
  - Be careful in older patients because of the possibility of dislodging a plaque and causing a stroke
- **Cardioversion**
  - Chemical
  - Electrical

If a patient is hemodynamically unstable, then electrical cardioversion is the method of choice using synchronized cardioversion.

Fluids could be beneficial with these patients, but while IV access is being established, there is little harm in trying vagal maneuvers and potentially carotid massage.

Test-taking tip: All these answers are potentially correct, but in a stable patient, there is time to start with the least invasive, which helps you eliminate A and D.

78. ANSWER: A

When a patient is in SVT, it is recommended to attempt the following as long as the patient is hemodynamically stable (systolic BP >90 mm Hg, no chest pain, no altered mental status, and not short of breath):

- *Vagal maneuvers*
  - Bearing down
  - Trying to blow a plunger out of a syringe
  - Ice to the face (most appropriate in children)
- *Carotid massage*
  - Be careful in older patients because of the possibility of dislodging a plaque and causing a stroke
- *Cardioversion*
  - Chemical
  - Electrical

If a patient is hemodynamically unstable, like the patient presented in this question, then electrical cardioversion is the method of choice using synchronized cardioversion. Using synchronized cardioversion prevents an R-on-T phenomenon, which puts the patient at risk for decompensation into a ventricular dysrhythmia.

Test-taking tip: In unstable patients with a tachyarrhythmia, electricity is almost always the correct answer.

79. ANSWER: A

Based on the patient's history and EKG, there is a high concern for prolonged QT syndrome. While definitions for a prolonged QT can vary, it is considered >460 milliseconds for men and >480 milliseconds for woman, making anything >500 milliseconds for any sex abnormal. There are many causes of QT prolongation, with medications being the highest culprit, but in the pediatric population congenital prolonged QT syndrome must be considered.

The PR interval is not greater than 200 milliseconds, making first-degree AV block unlikely. There are no delta waves, there are P waves, and there are no signs of left ventricular hypertrophy (LVH), making the other diagnoses unlikely.

These patients do not require admission to the hospital unless they are unstable, have another reason for admission, or are unable to get adequate follow-up as an outpatient. If they are able to follow up with their primary care physician and/or a cardiologist in a reasonable time period, then discharge home can be done with the instructions of no sports or exertional activities until they are cleared by their general pediatrician or a cardiologist.

Avoiding QT prolonging agents is also recommended. If there is concern for electrolyte abnormalities (i.e., malnutrition or eating disorders), then electrolytes should be evaluated.

Test-taking tip: Remember the five main arrhythmias associated with syncope and look for them on the EKG.

80. ANSWER: B

Ruptured papillary muscle after an MI is one of the potential sequelae that occurs approximately 5 to 7 days after the event. When this occurs, the symptoms are sudden in onset, and mitral regurgitation is one of the possible murmurs present (Table 3.1). Pulmonary edema is one of the potential hallmarks of valvular rupture and when present requires emergent repair.

When it comes to the other possible answers for this patient, IV antibiotics and fluids are not going to treat the underlying disorder, and admission to observation is not appropriate for this patient's management. IV fluids could actually worse his condition because he has pulmonary edema.

Test-taking tip: Brush up on the delayed complications of MI, including papillary muscle rupture, tamponade, aneurysm of the ventricle, and others.

81. ANSWER: A

This patient has a presentation concerning for his aortic dissection down into his heart and causing dysfunction of the aortic valve, leading to aortic regurgitation. Please see Table 3.1 for reference.

Test-taking tip: If you are thinking aortic dissection, think about involvement of the aortic valve.

82. ANSWER: C

While rare, it is always concerning when a patient with aortic stenosis presents with fluid overload. The mainstay of treatment for heart failure is to decrease afterload and preload to help the heart pump more efficiently. Unfortunately, in aortic stenosis, these patient are dependent on a narrow gradient across that aortic valve to keep it functioning properly. Administration of nitrates and afterload reducers affects that gradient and puts the patient at risk for further complications, including death.

Digoxin is appropriate in patient with aortic stenosis and heart failure. They can also be gently diuresed if needed. If antibiotics are required, there are no contraindications with regard to the diagnosis of aortic stenosis.

Test-taking tip: Brush up on the classic findings of important cardiac murmurs before the test.

83. ANSWER: A

When a patient presents with new-onset pulmonary edema, the goal should be to figure out why the patient has gone into heart failure. Based on this patient's exam and history, it is concerning that she has worsening mitral stenosis, which can be caused by rheumatologic disorders (including lupus), rheumatic fever, tumors, and congenital defects. While all left-sided heart murmurs can potential cause pulmonary edema, that patient's murmur is most consistent with mitral stenosis. Please see Table 3.1 for reference.

Test-taking tip: Brush up on the classic findings of important cardiac murmurs before the test.

Table 3.1 HEART MURMURS

- **Mitral stenosis:** loud opening snap with a diastolic rumble over the apex of the heart
- **Mitral regurgitation:** holosystolic murmur radiating to the left axilla
- **Aortic stenosis:** crescendo-decrescendo systolic murmur that radiates to the carotids
- **Aortic regurgitation:** high-pitched blowing decrescendo diastolic murmur over the left upper sternal border
- **Pulmonary stenosis:** crescendo-decrescendo ejection murmur best heard over the left upper sternal border that does not radiate
- **Pulmonary regurgitation:** holosystolic murmur over the left upper sternal border
- **Tricuspid stenosis:** uncommon, often inaudible, may produce soft opening snap and a mid-diastolic rumble over the left lower sternal border
- **Tricuspid regurgitation:** frequently not heard, but holosystolic murmur best heard over the left lower border
- **VSD:** holosystolic murmur over the left sternal border with a palpable thrill
- **Mitral valve prolapse:** mid-systolic click over the apex of the heart

84. ANSWER: A

This patient's presentation is highly concerning for endocarditis, and in patients with a history of IV drug use, it is most likely secondary to *S. aureus,* specifically MRSA.

While the other pathogens are also possible, *S. aureus* is the most common in this patient population.

Test-taking tip: Think *S. aureus* with fever in IV drug use patients.

85. ANSWER: A

This patient's body habitus is most likely secondary to an underlying collagen disorder, specifically Marfan's syndrome. These patient are at a higher risk for developing mitral valve prolapse. While there are other causes for mitral valve prolapse, including lupus and polycystic kidney disease, collagen disorders are the most common associated genetic disorders. Marfan's syndrome is more common in women than men and usually is diagnosed at about 10 to 16 year of age. Palpitations are the most common presenting symptoms.

As long as the patient is hemodynamically stable and the rest of the workup is unremarkable, discharge home with outpatient follow-up with a cardiologist is appropriate. The patient should be instructed to refrain from exertional activities and sports until an evaluation is complete.

Test-taking tip: Sometimes less is better in patients who are clinically stable, even on standardized examinations.

86. ANSWER: D

This question is about the basic approach to the resuscitation of an altered patient, which always includes ruling out hypoglycemia as a cause. It is one of the quickest tests to be performed and resolved in the ED, and one that can be easily reversed. While the other answers are also possible, evaluating for hypoglycemia can be done the fastest.

This patient likely has a ventricular septal defect (VSD) and with the hypotonia has a higher concern for Down syndrome. Down syndrome patients are at an increased risk for tetralogy of Fallot, and the most common heart murmurs in these patients are associated with VSD.

Test-taking tip: Altered equals point-of-care glucose during the initial resuscitation.

87. ANSWER: C

Children with hypoplastic left heart syndrome are very intimidating when they present to the ED. They are born with only one functional ventricle, which indiscriminately pumps blood to both the pulmonary and systemic systems. Over the first 3 years of their life, they require three surgeries to correct this malformation, with the first being in the first week of life, the second at about 6 months of life, and the third occurring at about 2 to 3 years of age.

These patients usually declare themselves for the next surgery by presenting with worsening oxygen saturation and worsening cyanosis. It is not uncommon for these children to have baseline oxygen saturation in the mid-80s, and when it drops below that baseline, surgical evaluation is indicated.

The patient in this question likely is a hypoplastic heart patient who is ready for the third part of his surgical repair. He warrants a surgical consultation with admission to the ICU.

Supplemental oxygen may be helpful for him but is not the definitive treatment he needs. It is not appropriate to discharge this patient home without surgical consultation, and antibiotics are not the definitive treatment for this surgical problem.

Test-taking tip: The key to this question is "definitive treatment," and of the potential answers, only cardiac surgery fits this description.

88. ANSWER: A

It is very common for pediatric patients to have murmurs, and most of them are benign. This patient likely has a Still's murmur, which is classified by a musical/vibratory murmur that is accentuated with lying flat. It is most common between the ages of 2 and 5 years, can be intermittent, and usually does not require follow-up with cardiology.

If a patient has a murmur before 1 year of age, it may be beneficial to suggest a referral to cardiology, but it is not necessary when the patient is stable from a cardiac standpoint. This patient was incidentally found to have this murmur while presenting with a respiratory complaint, likely secondary to a viral illness, and it is appropriate to discharge this patient home with primary care follow-up because he is hemodynamically stable.

This patient does not require surgical intervention or IV antibiotics. Admission to telemetry would also not be beneficial for this child.

Test-taking tip: Sometimes less is better in patients who are clinically stable, even on standardized examinations.

89. ANSWER: B

This patient's exam is most concerning for coarctation of the aorta because of the normal skin color of the upper extremities with cyanosis of the lower extremities. This is a result of the decreased blood flow due to the narrowing at the distal end of the aortic arch. Coarctation can be missed at birth because the defect is ductal dependent. Once the patent ductus arteriosus closes, symptoms can present, as in this patient. If the diagnosis goes undetected, then rib notching can occur, which is a late sign of this disease process.

Deep sulcus sign is associated with pneumothorax, which is an unlikely sequela of this disease process. These patients are not at increased risk for pneumonia, making bilateral infiltrates less likely. Pleural effusions are also unlikely because fluid overload is not usually associated with coarctation.

Test-taking tip: Brush up on presentations of common congenital heart conditions because they are frequently covered on standardized emergency medicine tests.

90. ANSWER: D

Patients with a history of tetralogy of Fallot have the classic presentation of:

- Pulmonary stenosis
- Right ventricular hypertrophy
- Overriding aorta
- VSD

It is not uncommon for these patients to undergo a surgical intervention, whether it is VSD closure or pulmonary valve replacement. Patients who undergo a pulmonary valve replacement are at risk for developing pulmonary regurgitation due to the increased leaking/stretching of the valve as they grow. This would require revision/replacement if they develop symptoms.

This patient had a near syncopal event with exertion, and based on his history, should be evaluated with an echocardiogram and a cardiology consult owing to possible valve failure.

CT is not the best study for the evaluation of murmurs, and a chest radiograph will likely be unremarkable. Treadmill testing is also not helpful with the evaluation of a murmur.

Test-taking tip: When you think congenital heart disease, think echocardiogram as the usual diagnostic test.

91. ANSWER: A

There are myriad reasons that a child may become cyanotic, ranging from congenital defects to toxicologic emergencies like methemoglobinemia. These patients require testing,

including an echocardiogram, and may requiring intubation if they are listless or not responding to noninvasive ventilation.

This patient warrants an admission to the neonatal ICU because of the hypoxia and potential for further decompensation. The newborn nursery is not an appropriate level of care. The cause of this infant's cyanosis has not yet been identified, and thus surgery is not yet indicated.

Test-taking tip: Blue is bad; send the patient to the ICU.

92. ANSWER: C

This patient's presentation is concerning for a tet spell, which is classic for a patient with Tetralogy of Fallot. What happens is the patient becomes agitated, cries, or is feeding and has a sudden decreased in oxygen because of shunting from the VSD. The child may then attempt to bear down or need to have flexion of the hips and knees to help with increasing the peripheral vascular resistance and decrease the shunting that occurs across that VSD.

Tetralogy of Fallot patients have the classic presentation of:

- Pulmonary stenosis
- Right ventricular hypertrophy
- Overriding aorta
- VSD

While it is difficult to make this diagnosis in the ED, an echocardiogram is the best test to make this diagnosis. None of the other tests listed will help in making this diagnosis.

Test-taking tip: When you think congenital heart disease, think echocardiogram as the usual diagnostic test.

93. ANSWER: D

For stable, asymptomatic patients who have experienced multiple shocks from their AICD, an important first step after placing them on a monitor is to have their AICD interrogated to determine whether the shocks were given appropriately, because of a cardiac arrhythmia, or because of malfunction.

Patients who received only a single shock and had no cardiac-related symptoms do not need immediate AICD interrogation and can be discharged home with follow-up with their cardiologist within 1 week.

Three or more appropriate shocks within 24 hours are concerning. These patient require further workup, including evaluation for electrolyte abnormalities, acute coronary syndrome, and medication side effects. These patients may require treatment with antiarrhythmics and need to be admitted to the hospital for further workup and monitoring.

Test-taking tip: All of these answers may be appropriate at some point in the care of this patient; however, the "next most appropriate" step is to figure out whether the AICD is functioning correctly.

94. ANSWER: C

All patients who are pulseless and not breathing should receive cardiac life support in the same manner, including chest compressions, external defibrillation, and appropriate administration of ACLS medications.

There is no danger to performing chest compressions on a patient whose AICD is delivering shocks. The person providing chest compressions may feel a tingling sensation that can be unpleasant, but this can be ameliorated by wearing gloves.

If a patient's AICD is firing and the patient is still pulseless, it suggests that the AICD is not working, and external defibrillation is indicated. There is some risk for damage to the AICD with external defibrillation. This risk can be decreased by not putting the defibrillator pads directly over or too close to the AICD.

If the patient has return of spontaneous circulation and is stabilized, the AICD will require interrogation to assess function, but this is not of immediate concern in the initial resuscitation of a pulseless patient with an AICD in place.

Test-taking tip: All pulseless and apneic patient need ABCs and ACLS.

4.

CUTANEOUS DISORDERS

Fred Wu

1. A 36-year-old male presents with a rash for 3 days after starting phenytoin. The rash is pictured in Figure 4.1. He is also complaining of sores in his mouth. The rash is not pruritic but burns and is blistering. He reports chills at home and a mild cough. Vital signs include temperature 39.2° C (102.6° F), heart rate (HR) 124 bpm, blood pressure (BP) 94/70 mm Hg, and pulse oximetry 93% on room air. What is the most appropriate treatment for this patient?

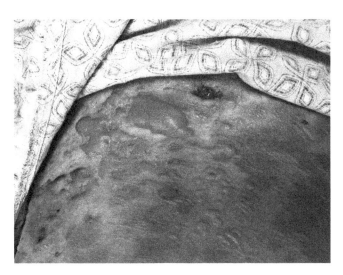

Figure 4.1 Rash.

A. Discharge home as viral exanthem
B. Admission for IV steroids
C. Discharge home with oral steroids
D. Admission for possible sepsis, fluid resuscitation, and antibiotics

2. A 2-year-old male presents with a rash for 2 days. The rash is pictured in Figure 4.2. The mother reports decreased oral intake and irritability. There is no cough, nasal congestion, vomiting, or diarrhea. The rash does not involve the mucous membranes, but the mother

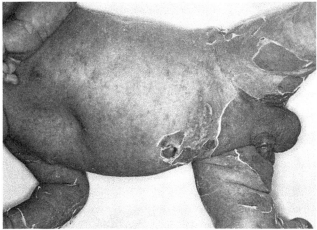

Figure 4.2 Rash.
(Reprinted from Habif TP. Clinical Dermatology. 6th ed. 2016. With permission from Elsevier.)

states that he looks "sunburned," especially in the groin region. Immunizations are up to date. Vital signs include temperature 6° F 38.5° C (101.3° F), HR 144 bpm, respiratory rate (RR) 30 breaths/min, and pulse oximetry 98% on room air. What is the most likely diagnosis?

A. Scarlet fever
B. Staphylococcal scalded skin syndrome
C. Toxic epidermal necrolysis
D. Bullous impetigo

3. A 19-year-old female presents with a rash on her right wrist for 5 days. The rash is pictured in Figure 4.3. She reports wearing a new bracelet that her boyfriend gave her. The rash is associated with intense itching, and she thinks it may be infected. There is no history of fever, vomiting, diarrhea, or other constitutional symptoms. What is the most likely diagnosis?

A. Herpes zoster
B. Impetigo

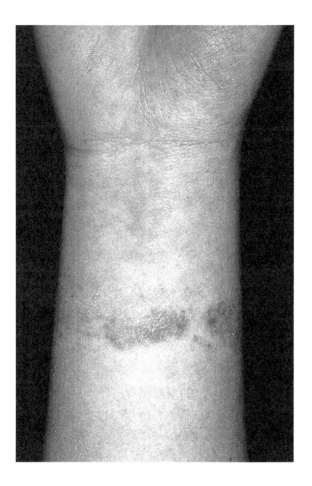

Figure 4.3 Rash.
(Reprinted from Habif TP. Clinical Dermatology. 6th ed. 2016. With permission from Elsevier.)

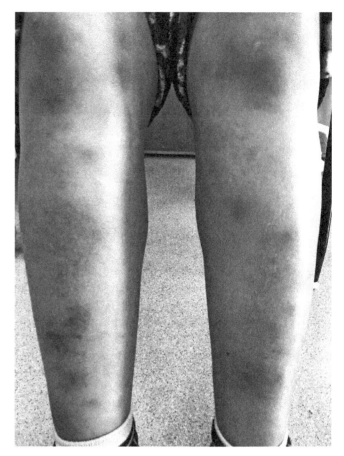

Figure 4.4 Rash.

C. Contact dermatitis
D. Psoriasis

4. A 32-year-old male presents with a painful rash on both lower legs for 1 week. The rash is pictured in Figure 4.4. He reports a tactile fever at home. He denies any new contacts to foods or medications. The patient has no past medical problems. His social history reveals that he is a migrant farm worker currently working in the central valley of California. What is the most likely diagnosis?

A. Erythema nodosum
B. Erythema induratum
C. Cold panniculitis
D. Multiple abscesses

5. A 36-year-old male presents to the emergency department (ED) complaining of a rash for 4 days. The rash is pictured is pictured in Figure 4.5. It is widespread, but he shows you his palms and states the lesions are identical elsewhere. He reports fatigue over the past week but no fever. He also denies taking any medications.

When you examine his mouth, you notice a few scattered ulcerations. His vital signs are within normal limits. What is the most likely diagnosis?

A. Erythema multiforme
B. Syphilis

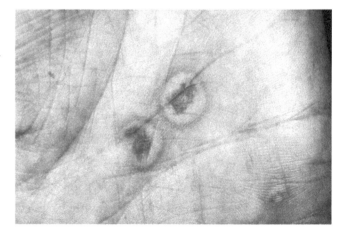

Figure 4.5 Rash.
(Reprinted from Burge S et al. Oxford Handbook of Medical Dermatology. 2nd ed. 2016. With permission from Oxford University Press.)

C. Pityriasis rosea
D. Urticaria

6. A 16-year-old female presents to the ED with a rash on her arms and legs for 3 days. The rash is pictured in Figure 4.6. She reports hiking in the foothills last weekend. There is no history of fever or vomiting. She is not on any medications. Her vital signs are within normal limits. She only complains that the "itching is killing me!" What is the most likely diagnosis?

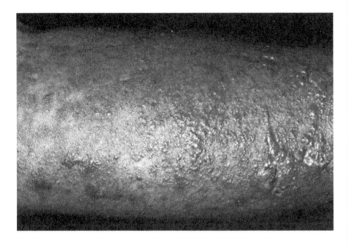

Figure 4.6 Rash.
(Reprinted from Habif TP. Clinical Dermatology. 6th ed. 2016. With permission from Elsevier)

A. Herpes zoster
B. Rhus dermatitis
C. Scabies
D. Urticaria

7. A 68-year-old male presents with a rash on his abdomen for 2 days. On examination you notice the rash shown in Figure 4.7 on the right side of his abdomen. His past medical history includes hypertension, which is controlled with lisinopril. His vital signs are within normal limits. There is no history of fever. What is the most likely diagnosis?

A. Varicella
B. Molluscum contagiosum (MC)
C. Hand-foot-and-mouth disease
D. Herpes zoster

8. A mother brings her 2-year-old son to the ED for evaluation of a rash for 4 days. She states that it started as a blister on his knee that popped and is now shiny and scaly, as pictured in Figure 4.8. There is no fever or vomiting, but the mother reports diarrhea. He is feeding normally. Vital signs are within normal limits. What is the most likely diagnosis?

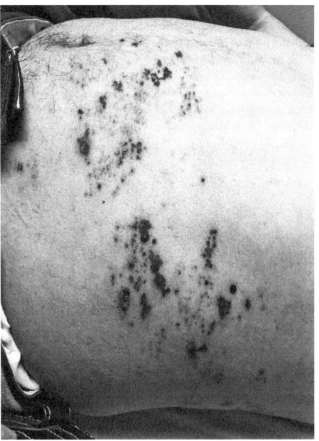

Figure 4.7 Rash.

A. Classic impetigo
B. Atopic dermatitis
C. Bullous impetigo
D. Bullous pemphigoid

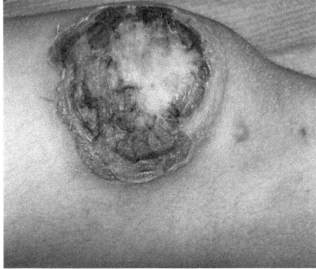

Figure 4.8 Rash.
(Reprinted from Burge S et al. Oxford Handbook of Medical Dermatology. 2nd ed. 2016. With permission from Oxford University Press.)

9. A 2-year-old female is brought in to the ED by her parents with a rash for 2 weeks. The parents state she is itching uncontrollably to the point at which she is crying with discomfort. She is scratching her neck, hands, and feet. The rash on her foot is pictured in Figure 4.9. There has been no change in her diet. The parents report no fever and no new soaps, lotions, or detergents. What is the most likely diagnosis?

A. Classic impetigo
B. Scabies
C. Atopic dermatitis
D. Pityriasis rosea

10. A 19-year-old female presents to the ED because of a rash on her neck for 1 month. The rash is pictured in Figure 4.10. She has minimal discomfort, and there is no fever. There is no history of new exposures to soaps, medicines, lotions, or shampoos. What is the most likely diagnosis?

A. Molluscum contagiosum (MC)
B. Varicella
C. Atopic dermatitis
D. Herpes zoster

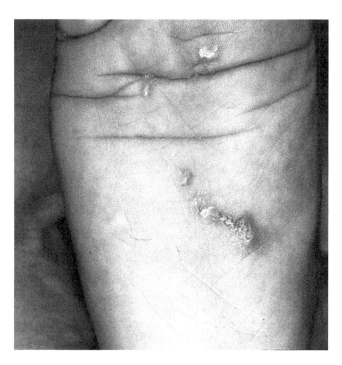

Figure 4.9 Rash.
(Reprinted from Burge S et al. Oxford Handbook of Medical Dermatology. 2nd ed. 2016. With permission from Oxford University Press.)

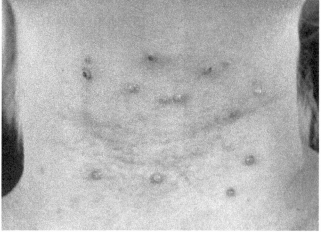

Figure 4.10 Rash.
(Reprinted from Lewis-Jones S. OSH Paediatric Dermatology. 2010. With permission from Oxford University Press.)

ANSWERS

1. ANSWER: D

The above case is classic for Stevens-Johnson syndrome (SJS), a severe variant of erythema multiforme (EM). SJS is commonly caused by medications (e.g., nonsteroidal antiinflammatory drugs [NSAIDs], antibiotics, anticonvulsants) or infections (e.g., *Mycoplasma pneumoniae*, herpes simplex). Physical exam findings include rash with mucous membrane and eye involvement. The rash may present as target lesions, erythematous macules, purpura, and blisters or bullae. Blistering typically involves less than 10% of total body surface area (TBSA), whereas toxic epidermal necrolysis involves greater than 30% TBSA. Mucous membrane involvement may present with erosions to the genitalia, mouth, and pharynx. Ocular findings include conjunctivitis.

Treatment is supportive and includes IV fluids, pain control, and treating underlying infections. Use of steroids is controversial and currently not recommended. Gram-negative pneumonia has been implicated as a frequent cause of sepsis. Burn center admission may be needed because there are similarities in treatment.

Patients with suspected SJS should never be discharged home because the disease can rapidly progress and there is significant associated morbidity and mortality.

Test-taking tip: The patient presented is unstable based on his vital signs, easily eliminating the two answers that involve discharge home.

2. ANSWER: B

Staphylococcal scalded skin syndrome (SSSS) is a childhood disease, usually affecting children younger than 6 years. The responsible agent is *Staphylococcus aureus,* which releases an exotoxin that causes generalized intradermal exfoliation. It presents with diffuse erythema that can resemble a "sunburn" and is prominent in the intertriginous areas (axilla, groin) and near the eyes and mouth. Bullae can exhibit Nikolsky's sign, where slight rubbing of the skin results in exfoliation of the outermost layer. Mucous membranes are not affected. There may be a concurrent skin infection, but sometimes no source is identified.

Treatment is similar to that for burn patients and includes fluid resuscitation, analgesia, and avoiding excess heat loss. Antibiotic choice should be effective against penicillinase-resistant *S. aureus* (e.g., cefazolin, nafcillin, dicloxacillin, cephalexin). Children who appear toxic with widespread skin involvement and/or dehydration should be admitted.

The rash associated with scarlet fever is erythematous, covers most of the body, and classically feels like sandpaper when touched. Scarlet fever predominantly occurs in children aged 1 to 10 years.

The rash associated with toxic epidermal necrolysis (TEN) is characterized by widespread erythema, necrosis, and bullous detachment of the epidermis and mucous membranes resulting in exfoliation. TEN is commonly drug induced but can be caused by infection, malignancy, and other factors. TEN is more common in adults.

Bullous impetigo tends to affect the face, extremities, axillae, trunk, and perianal region of neonates, but older children and adults can also be affected.

Test-taking tip: Knowing the distribution of common rashes and the age groups in which they typically occur can help you reach the correct answer.

3. ANSWER: C

Contact dermatitis is an inflammatory, hypersensitivity reaction. It can be caused by an irritant, such as soaps, chemicals, or urine, or can be due to an allergic reaction to plants, metals, leather, or topical medications. The presentation includes skin erythema, edema, papules, vesicles, crusting, and pruritus at the site of contact.

Treatment includes removing the offending agent, cool compresses, antipruritic medications, and topical/oral steroids depending on the severity.

Herpes zoster is a painful rash that follows a unilateral dermatomal distribution in immunocompetent individuals.

Impetigo is a bacterial infection that usually presents with honey-colored crusting on the face and extremities. It is most common in the pediatric population.

Psoriasis presents with scaly, well-delineated lesions that mostly affect the extensor surfaces and scalp.

Test-taking tip: Knowing the distribution of common rashes and the age groups in which they typically occur can help you reach the correct answer.

4. ANSWER: A

Erythema nodosum is a common skin disorder caused by an immune-mediated response. It is often a sign of an underlying disease process, but etiologies include medications (oral contraceptives, sulfonamides), HIV, malignancy, infections (streptococcal, coccidioidomycosis, *Mycobacterium tuberculosis,* syphilis), and systemic diseases (sarcoidosis, inflammatory bowel disease). The clinical presentation includes tender subcutaneous, erythematous nodules on the extensor surface of the lower legs. It can also present on the hands, thighs, and arms. The nodules are symmetrically distributed and vary in size from 1 to 10 cm. Patients may also have fever, hilar adenopathy, arthralgias, and leukocytosis. Treatment is based on the underlying etiology.

Erythema induratum is panniculitis on the back of the calves.

Cold panniculitis occurs after exposure to cold and usually occurs in the pediatric population.

Abscesses can occur anywhere on the skin but do not usually present in a symmetric fashion in the previously mentioned geographical locations.

Test-taking tip: This is a "you know it or don't" kind of question. If you don't know it, choose an answer and move on. You can perhaps mark it for review when you are done with the test. Don't, however, let these kinds of questions get you stuck and waste your time.

5. ANSWER: A

EM is a hypersensitivity reaction most commonly caused by herpes simplex virus (HSV). Other causes include malignancy, *Mycoplasma* infections, idiopathic, and medications (phenytoin, antibiotics, NSAIDS). EM can be divided into minor and major, with the latter referring to severe disease (TEN and SJS). A nonspecific prodrome of fever and fatigue may precede the rash. The rash presents as red macules and papules that evolve into distinctive "target" lesions with central clearing and can be present in various stages. The rash can be found on the extremities, trunk, hands, feet, palms, and soles. Treatment is targeted at removing or treating the underlying cause.

A rash associated with syphilis usually occurs with secondary syphilis and can involve the palms of the hands and soles of the feet as well as other body parts. The rash is usually not pruritic but can be associated with mild flu-like symptoms.

Pityriasis rosea is a common skin rash that typically begins with a single red and slightly scaly lesion. This is followed by a generalized body rash of many small patches of pink or red flaky lesions. These lesions typically spread across the chest first, following the ribs in a classic "Christmas tree" distribution. This rash is benign and usually resolves without treatment.

Urticaria appears as raised, well circumscribed areas of erythema and edema that are very pruritic. Urticaria is usually a benign, self-limited skin disease but can be a clinical manifestation of a serious allergic reaction.

Test-taking tip: There are a limited number of rashes that show up on the palms of the hands, including EM, Coxsackie virus, Rocky Mountain spotted fever, syphilis, and measles. Knowing these can help you choose the right answer if the rash involves the palms.

6. ANSWER: B

Rhus dermatitis refers to the rash caused by poison ivy, poison oak, and poison sumac. Contact with the plant's oleoresin (urushiol) results in the rash. The rash presents with erythema, edema, vesicles, pruritus, and sometimes bullae. The characteristic linear lesions are a result of the plant being drawn across the skin or from scratching and spreading the urushiol. The blister fluid is not infective and cannot spread the rash. Wet compresses and antihistamines may help with symptomatic relief. Topical steroids may also help with mild symptoms. Moderate to severe symptoms may benefit from systemic corticosteroids (2–3 weeks with gradual taper), but be aware that premature termination of corticosteroids may result in a rebound of symptoms.

Herpes zoster is a painful rash that follows a dermatomal pattern.

Scabies is a pruritic rash that frequently involves the interdigital areas and the elbows and wrist. The lesions appear as tracks or burrows.

Urticaria appears as raised, well-circumscribed areas of erythema and edema that are very pruritic. Urticaria is usually a benign, self-limited skin disease but can be a clinical manifestation of a serious allergic reaction.

Test-taking tip: Spend some time looking at pictures of common rashes. The visual cue and the history of recent hiking should direct you to the correct answer.

7. ANSWER: D

Herpes zoster (shingles) is caused by the varicella-zoster virus, which lies dormant in the dorsal root ganglia after initial infection as chickenpox. When the rash remerges, it usually presents as grouped vesicles on an erythematous base, which then scab and crust over. The rash usually follows one dermatome and rarely crosses the midline. The most common nerve distributions are T2 to L2. If lesions are on the face, be aware of ocular involvement and Ramsay Hunt syndrome. There may be a prodrome of pain and paresthesias to the skin before the rash appears. Postherpetic neuralgia may persist after rash resolution. Treatment is with antivirals (acyclovir, valacyclovir, or famciclovir) and should be started within 72 hours of rash onset.

Varicella (chickenpox) is a primary infection with the varicella-zoster virus and presents as a diffuse vesicular rash associated with fever. It typically occurs in younger individuals.

MC is a nonvesicular, flesh-colored papule, sometimes with central umbilication.

Hand-foot-and-mouth disease is caused by Coxsackie virus and typically presents as painful ulcerations to the palms, soles, and mouth. It is most common in the pediatric population.

Test-taking tip: Knowing the distribution of common rashes and the age groups in which they typically occur can help you reach the correct answer.

8. ANSWER: C

Bullous impetigo is caused by *S. aureus,* specifically by its exotoxin, which causes epidermal cleavage. Unlike classic impetigo, *Streptococcus* is not a causative organism. It is mostly seen in children but can occur in adults. Bullous impetigo usually presents with a large bullae that has ruptured, leaving an erythematous, shiny base with scaling/peeling edges. Some areas may develop a honey-colored or dark brown crust. There may be drainage of serum. Any surface of the body can be involved, although it usually presents on the face. Associated systemic symptoms may include diarrhea, fever, and weakness. The diagnosis is made by clinical exam, but culturing the bullous fluid may be considered. Small lesions may be treated with topical therapy, but because bullous impetigo lesions are larger and more widespread, systemic therapy is usually recommended. Options for antimicrobial therapy include macrolides, β-lactamase–resistant penicillins or cephalosporins.

Classic impetigo is caused by *Staphylococcus* or *Streptococcus* and does not involve bullae or systemic symptoms. It also typically involves the face but can affect any skin surface.

Atopic dermatitis is an inflammation of the skin that results in itchy, red, swollen and cracked skin. It usually begins in childhood but can persist into adulthood. In infants it presents most typically on the face, but in older children it tends to occur at the elbow and knee flexor surfaces.

Bullous pemphigoid classically presents with tense, fluid-filled bullae. It is a rarer skin condition and is most common in older adults.

Test-taking tip: Knowing the distribution of common rashes and the age groups in which they typically occur can help you reach the correct answer.

9. ANSWER: B

Scabies is a reaction to the saliva, eggs, and excrement of the mite *Sarcoptes scabiei* variant *hominis.* Mites mate on the skin surface, and the female mite burrows into the epidermis to lay eggs. Scabies produces intense pruritus, usually nocturnal, and rash. The rash is classically found in the web spaces of fingers, groin, feet, elbows, wrists, breasts, and axillary folds. The head and neck are infrequently affected in adults but more commonly affected in children. The rash can present as linear burrows, finger-web crusting, blisters, pustules, excoriations, and papules. At the end of linear papules or burrows, there is usually a vesicle with a black dot, which represents the mite. Permethrin cream is the treatment of choice, with an optional retreatment 1 to 2 weeks after the initial treatment. Patients should be advised that itching may persist up to 4 weeks after successful treatment. Oral antihistamines may also help with pruritic symptoms. All bedding and clothes will need to be washed and dried on hot cycle to exterminate remaining mites.

Classic impetigo is caused by *Staphylococcus* or *Streptococcus* and does not involve bullae or systemic symptoms. It also typically involves the face but can affect any skin surface.

Atopic dermatitis is an inflammation of the skin that results in itchy, red, swollen and cracked skin. It usually begins in childhood but can persist into adulthood. In infants it presents most typically on the face, but in older children it tends to occur at the elbow and knee flexor surfaces.

Pityriasis rosea is a common skin rash that typically begins with a single red and slightly scaly lesion. This is followed by a generalized body rash of many small patches of pink or red flaky lesions. These lesions typically spread across the chest first, following the ribs in a classic "Christmas tree" distribution. This rash is benign and usually resolves without treatment.

Test-taking tip: This picture is classic for scabies; spend some time reviewing pictures of classic rashes.

10. ANSWER: A

Molluscum contagiosum (MC) is a common, benign infection caused by a poxvirus. In children it is usually spread skin to skin, while in adults it is usually by sexual contact. The lesions may be large and numerous if co-infected with HIV. MC presents with firm, spherical papules that may be flesh colored, white, or light yellow. Some may present with an umbilicated center. The lesions may self-resolve after a few months but may last up to 5 years. Treatment is usually in the primary care setting and may include curettage, cryotherapy, podophyllin, or trichloroacetic acid. Lesions can become superinfected.

Varicella (chicken pox) is a primary infection with the varicella-zoster virus and presents as a diffuse vesicular rash associated with fever. It typically occurs in younger individuals.

Atopic dermatitis is an inflammation of the skin that results in itchy, red, swollen and cracked skin. It usually begins in childhood but can persist into adulthood. In infants it presents most typically on the face, but in older children it tends to occur at the elbow and knee flexor surfaces.

Herpes zoster (shingles) is caused by the varicella-zoster virus, which lies dormant in the dorsal root ganglia after initial infection as chickenpox. When the rash re-emerges, it usually presents as grouped vesicles on an erythematous base, which then scab and crust over. The rash usually follows one dermatome and rarely crosses the midline. The most common nerve distributions are T2 to L2.

Test-taking tip: Knowing the distribution of common rashes and the age groups in which they typically occur can help you reach the correct answer.

5.

ENDOCRINE, METABOLIC, AND NUTRITIONAL EMERGENCIES

Lily Hitchner

1. A 72-year-old male presents with altered mental status. Labs reveal a serum sodium level of 118. While you are assessing his fluid status to determine the next step, he begins seizing. What do you administer now?

A. 50 mL of D5W
B. 100 mL of hypertonic 3% NaCl
C. 500 mL of 2% NaCl
D. 1,000 mL of 0.9% NaCl

2. A 70-year-old male presents to the emergency department (ED) with heart rate (HR) 130 bpm, blood pressure (BP) 90/60 mm Hg, dry lips, generalized weakness, and diarrhea for 3 days. Serum sodium is measured at 155, and urine sodium is less than 20 mEq/L. Based on his clinical history presentation, what is the initial treatment of choice?

A. Fluid restriction
B. Fluid resuscitation with 3% NaCl
C. Fluid resuscitation with isotonic or hypotonic NaCl solutions
D. Trial of desmopressin

3. A patient presents with a glucose of 700 and serum sodium of 130. What is the corrected serum sodium?

A. 125
B. 136
C. 140
D. 152

4. A 12-year-old male presents to the ED saying that he can barely move. His arms and legs feel weak. He denies difficulty breathing or swallowing. On exam, he is non-toxic appearing, his proximal muscles are affected more than distal muscles, and his reflexes are slow. He recalls a similar episode last month that lasted for several hours. He denies any symptoms in between the attacks. His father reports having similar attacks. What is the most likely diagnosis?

A. Hypokalemic periodic paralysis
B. Myasthenia gravis
C. Renal tubular acidosis
D. Transverse myelitis

5. A 60-year-old female with end-stage renal disease (ESRD) on M/W/F dialysis presents with generalized weakness and this electrocardiogram (EKG) (Figure 5.1). What is the definitive treatment for this patient?

A. Calcium chloride administration
B. Cardiac catheterization
C. Fluid resuscitation
D. Hemodialysis

6. This EKG is from a post-thyroidectomy patient with hypocalcemia. What is the most characteristic EKG finding (present in the EKG in Figure 5.2) present in hypocalcemia?

A. Deep S waves in lateral leads
B. Prominent T waves
C. QRS widening
D. QTc prolongation

7. A 73-year-old female with breast cancer metastatic to bone presents with abdominal pain and confusion. Her calcium level is 14.2 mg/dL. Which option should you avoid in the treatment of hypercalcemia?

A. Bisphosphonates
B. Calcitonin
C. Normal saline
D. Thiazide diuretics

Electronically signed by ... ... MD 10/29/2...

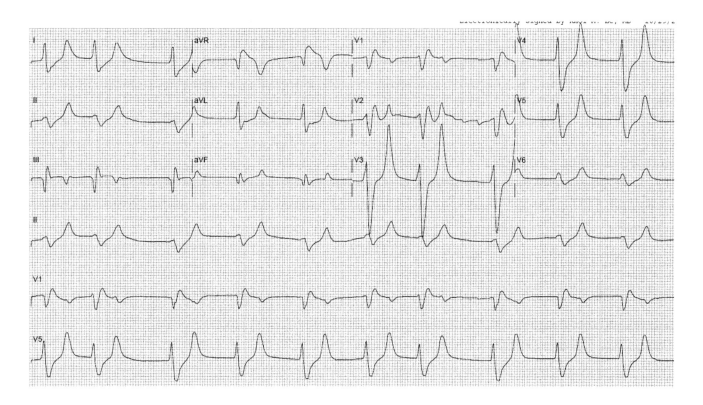

Figure 5.1 Electrocardiogram

... ...

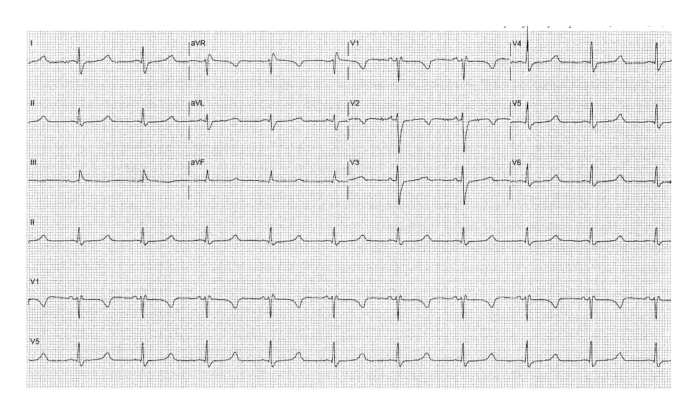

Figure 5.2 Electrocardiogram

8. A malnourished chronic alcoholic patient presents with shock-resistant ventricular fibrillation arrest. What medication should be included in your resuscitation?

A. IV calcium
B. IV magnesium
C. IV lidocaine
D. IV procainamide

9. A 32-year-old male with history of alcohol abuse and frequent ED visits for alcohol-induced gastritis presents to the ED with generalized weakness, bilateral upper extremity paresthesias, anorexia, nausea and vomiting, and diarrhea. His phosphorus level returns as less than 1 mg/dL. What is your initial treatment?

A. IV calcium therapy
B. IV phosphate therapy
C. Oral phosphate therapy
D. Skim milk

10. A 30-year-old female presents with shallow rapid respirations, nausea and vomiting, urinary frequency, and elevated blood glucose. Initial arterial blood gas (ABG) test shows pH 7.06, Pco_2 12, and bicarbonate 4. What type of acid-base disorder is this?

A. Combined metabolic and respiratory acidosis
B. Metabolic acidosis with compensatory respiratory alkalosis
C. Metabolic alkalosis with compensatory respiratory acidosis
D. Respiratory acidosis with metabolic alkalosis

11. A 21-year-old male with type 1 diabetes presents to the ED with a blood glucose of 400 after running out of his insulin 4 days ago. His chemistry panel shows sodium 140, potassium 4.0, chloride 109, HCO_2 8, creatinine 0.9. What is his anion gap?

A. 7
B. 14
C. 23
D. 27

12. A 61-year-old male with type 2 diabetes is brought in by his family because he "is acting drunk," diaphoretic, and complaining of frequent urination. The patient was started on a steroid burst for gout 5 days ago. The patient is ill-appearing on arrival with HR 137 bpm, diaphoresis, and respiratory rate (RR) 22 breaths/min. Initial ED labs reveal a white blood cell (WBC) count 17.1, sodium 135, potassium 4.3, chloride 103, anion gap 14, CO_2 18,

glucose 850, osmolality 340, and β-hydroxybutyrate 5.3. What is the most likely diagnosis?

A. Alcoholic ketoacidosis
B. Diabetic ketoacidosis (DKA)
C. Hyperglycemic hyperosmolar nonketotic state
D. Lactic acidosis

13. A 50-year-old male presents to the ED complaining of generalized abdominal pain, weakness, nausea, and vomiting. He is well known to the ED for alcohol abuse and says he has been trying to stop drinking lately. Labs reveal an anion gap metabolic acidosis with serum ketones and a glucose of 80. What is the initial treatment for this patient?

A. Bicarbonate drip
B. Fluid resuscitation with D5 normal saline (NS)
C. Fluid resuscitation with NS
D. Insulin drip

14. What is your differential for a wide anion gap metabolic acidosis?

A. Gastrointestinal (GI) losses, renal tubular acidosis, acetazolamide
B. Organophosphates, opioids, muscle relaxants
C. Uremia, ketoacidosis, lactic acidosis, toxic ingestions
D. Vomiting, diuretics, antacid use, Cushing's syndrome

15. A 45-year-old female with known hyperthyroidism presents to the ED with agitated delirium the day after an orthopedic surgery. Her triage vital signs are HR 140 bpm, RR 24 breaths/min, BP 85/60 mm Hg, oxygen saturation 98%, and temperature 40.6° C (105° F). Her thyroid-stimulating hormone (TSH) level is low and thyroxine (T_4) is high. What treatments, and in which order, should you give?

A. Iodine → propranolol → propylthiouracil (PTU)/ methimazole
B. Iodine → PTU/methimazole → propranolol
C. Propranolol → iodine → PTU/methimazole
D. Propranolol → PTU/methimazole → iodine

16. A 42-year-old female presents with altered mental status. Initial vital signs are HR 42 bpm, BP 85/42 mm Hg, RR 8 breaths/min, and temperature 34° C. A quick physical exam reveals a Glasgow Coma Scale score of 12, periorbital edema, extremity edema, delayed tendon reflexes, and dry skin. A family member arrives and tells you that the patient is taking a medication to help her thyroid but ran out several months ago. What is your

initial ED management beyond supportive care and airway management?

    A. Do nothing until the TSH returns
    B. Either IV or PO hydrocortisone alone
    C. IV thyroxine plus IV hydrocortisone
    D. PO thyroxine plus PO hydrocortisone

17. A 5-year-old male presents to the ED for generalized weakness, lethargy, and vomiting for 4 days. One week before the start of the illness, the patient was treated with a steroid burst for an asthma exacerbation. The patient is afebrile, has a normal HR, and borderline low BP. You check a blood glucose almost immediately on arrival, and it is 45. Additional labs show sodium 115 and potassium 6.3. What diagnosis is most likely in this patient?

    A. Acute adrenal insufficiency
    B. DKA
    C. Myxedema coma
    D. Surreptitious insulin use

18. You are managing a critical patient with shock due to presumed urosepsis. Despite maximal efforts at resuscitation with fluid and vasopressors, the patient remains hypotensive. What additional therapy should be considered for refractory septic shock?

    A. High-dose insulin drip
    B. Hydrocortisone

    C. Lipid emulsion therapy
    D. Streptokinase

19. A 2-week-old female neonate presents with poor feeding and excessive sleepiness. The baby was born at 39 weeks' gestational age with no complications. The neonate is afebrile and lethargic and has decreased skin turgor. On genitourinary exam, you note fused labia and an enlarged clitoris. What laboratory values do you expect to find?

    A. Hyperglycemia, normal sodium, and normal potassium levels
    B. Hypoglycemia, normal sodium, and normal potassium levels
    C. Normoglycemia, hypernatremia, and hypokalemia
    D. Normoglycemia, hyponatremia, and hyperkalemia

20. A 2-week-old female neonate presents with poor feeding and excessive sleepiness. The baby was born at 39 weeks' gestational age with no complications. The neonate is afebrile and lethargic and has decreased skin turgor. On genitourinary exam, you note fused labia and an enlarged clitoris. What is your initial treatment?

    A. IV fluid bolus alone
    B. IV fluid bolus, hydrocortisone
    C. IV fluid bolus, glucose and insulin
    D. Observation

ANSWERS

1. ANSWER: B

Hypertonic (3%) saline is indicated in patients with significant altered mental status/coma or in patients who are actively seizing and hyponatremia is the presumed cause. The goal of hypertonic saline administration is to stop the progression of mental status changes due to cerebral edema and/or to stop seizure activity. An increase in serum sodium by 4 to 6 mEq/L is usually sufficient. This can be achieved by administering 100 mL of 3% NaCl every 10 minutes up to 300 mL or termination of seizure activity. After this is achieved, the goal is to increase serum sodium by 8 to 10 mEq/L over 24 hours. In patients with chronic hyponatremia, it is critical to avoid rapid correction of serum sodium at the risk of causing central pontine myelinolysis. As a general rule of thumb, serum sodium should not be corrected to greater than 0.5 mEq/L/hr in these patients.

Test-taking tip: Skimming the answers before reading a long question stem can often save you time while reading to determine what is pertinent to answer the question.

2. ANSWER: C

This patient has hypovolemic hypernatremia. He shows signs of dehydration, including tachycardia, hypotension, and dry mucous membranes. The history of diarrhea for 3 days points to extrarenal fluid loss from GI losses. Other causes include excessive sweating, vomiting, and GI drainage tubes. In these patients, free water is lost to a greater extent than sodium. The young and the old are particularly prone to hypovolemic hypernatremia because they either do not have access to free water, are unable to sense thirst, or respond to thirst abnormally. The key to treating these patients is fluid resuscitation. It is reasonable to start with 0.9% NS to treat hypotension, then proceed with a hypotonic solution such as 0.45% NS. Desmopressin is not indicated in this case because the patient is hypovolemic and does not meet criteria for diabetes insipidus.

Test-taking tip: This question stem is pointing to the fact that the patient is in hypovolemic shock. Although sometimes important in your workup of hypernatremia, don't get too hung up on the significance of the urine sodium level, use clinical skills to evaluate fluid status, and correct the vital sign abnormalities first!

3. ANSWER: C

Low sodium laboratory measurements occur with hyperglycemia because of the movement of free water. The accumulation of extracellular glucose causes water to move out of the cell, causing hypertonic hypernatremia, which is not physiologically significant. This is a phenomenon that ED physicians need to be aware of in order to properly evaluate the sodium and fluid status in these patients. The formula to calculate this is:

Corrected Na = Na + 0.016 × (glucose − 100)

Pseudohyponatremia occurs in patients whose plasma has abnormally elevated levels of lipid or protein. Despite that the concentration of sodium in serum water is normal, the concentration of sodium in serum is low. This occurs in patients with hyperlipidemia or multiple myeloma or patients in who have received IV immunoglobulin.

Test-taking tip: This is a "you know it or don't" kind of question. If you don't know it, choose an answer and move on. You can perhaps mark it for review when you are done at the end of the test. Don't, however, let these kinds of questions get you stuck and waste your time.

4. ANSWER: A

Hypokalemic periodic paralysis is a rare genetic cause of episodic painless muscle weakness caused by a defect in skeletal muscle ion channels. Attacks are of sudden onset, often hours after strenuous exercise, stress, or heavy meals. Bulbar muscles are generally spared, and patients have no respiratory compromise. Between attacks, patients have little to no muscle weakness. Potassium levels during the attack are low, but they normalize between attacks. A broader differential should be considered if this is the first attack, but given this is a repeat attack and there is a familiar component, the answer is hypokalemic periodic paralysis.

Test-taking tip: Don't be distracted by the reasonable differential diagnoses; go for the most likely cause.

5. ANSWER: D

This EKG shows symmetric peaked T waves, wide QRS, and flattened P waves, which are pathognomonic for hyperkalemia. There is not a reliable correlation between serum potassium levels and EKG changes, but the EKG changes generally occur stepwise and as follows: symmetric T wave peaking, P wave flattening, QRS widening, and sinusoidal pattern.

Several strategies are commonly employed in the ED for patients with hyperkalemia. These include cardiac membrane stabilization with calcium salts; moving potassium into cells with insulin, glucose, albuterol, and sodium bicarbonate; and removing potassium from the body with dialysis. Treatment must also be aimed at the underlying cause of the hyperkalemia, such as diuretic use, Bactrim use, digoxin toxicity, or an addisonian crisis. In patients who are on dialysis who present with hyperkalemia, hemodialysis is the most effective way to excrete potassium from the body and is the definitive treatment for these patients.

Test-taking tip: If you skim through the question and answers first, you can save time on this one. You don't need to pour time and energy over this EKG. The question asks for the "definitive treatment" (dialysis), not the initial treatment (calcium).

6. ANSWER: D

Hypocalcemia most commonly causes QT prolongation. The QTc in the EKG is 579. This places the patient at risk for torsades de pointes, although patients are at greater risk for this fatal dysrhythmia with hypokalemia or hypomagnesemia. Atrial fibrillation has been reported in cases of hypocalcemia, but dysrhythmias are rare. T waves are usually not affected.

Test-taking tip: Remember that as a general rule of thumb, the QT segment should be less than half the RR.

7. ANSWER: D

Patients with symptomatic or severe hypercalcemia require emergent treatment to lower serum calcium levels. Several treatment modalities exist, including forced diuresis, inhibiting further bone resorption, and decreasing gut absorption of calcium. Volume expansion and forced diuresis are achieved with isotonic solutions such as NS. Calcitonin decreases bone resorption and increases renal excretion of calcium. Bisphosphonates also decrease bone resorption but don't reach peak effect for several days. Thiazide diuretics should be avoided, along with volume depletion, high calcium diet, and prolonged inactivity, because these can worsen hypercalcemia. Thiazide diuretics increase the reabsorption of calcium in the distal tubule.

Test-taking tip: In many hospital systems you would be calling your specialist or admitting physician before initiating these therapies, but they will still be tested.

8. ANSWER: B

Advanced cardiac life support (ACLS) guidelines recommend considering IV magnesium in patients with cardiac arrest due to torsades de points and in patients with suspected magnesium deficiency with ventricular fibrillation or ventricular tachycardia arrest. Hypomagnesium deficiency should be suspected in patients with increased GI

losses due to diarrhea, medications, alcohol, or malnutrition; in those with redistribution due to refeeding syndrome; in those receiving treatment for DKA or pancreatitis; or in certain cases of TPN use, diabetes, and hyperthyroidism. Magnesium should be given as 2 g IV over 30 to 60 seconds.

Test-taking tip: If you don't have your ACLS algorithms memorized completely, the question stem here helps you out by having the patient be a malnourished alcoholic. If you are at a loss, look for these clues.

9. ANSWER: B

Hypophosphatemia is rare because of the abundance of phosphorus in foods and its easy digestion. It is caused by decreased GI absorption, increased renal excretion, and/or cellular shifts. Severe symptoms usually present when the phosphorus level is less than 1 mg/dL. When cells are starved of phosphorus, they are unable to produce adenosine triphosphate, resulting in cellular dysfunction and lack of oxygen. This manifests clinically as weakness, tremors, paresthesias, anorexia, and decreased deep tendon reflexes. Patients can also present in heart failure. Treatment involves repletion with either oral or IV phosphate, and disposition will be determined by severity of symptoms. IV therapy is required when the patient is unable to tolerate oral replacement or in patients with severe symptomatic hypophosphatemia (generally considered <1 mg/mL).

Test-taking tip: Make sure to use reference values if you are unsure of the significance of lab values.

10. ANSWER: B

Interpreting ABG values is a stepwise process. Firstly, determine whether the patient is acidotic (pH < 7.35) or alkalotic (pH > 7.45). Second, look at the $Paco_2$ to evaluate the respiratory component. A normal range is between 35 and 45 mm Hg. Here the pH is acidotic and the $Paco_2$ is less than 35 mm Hg, which indicates a compensatory respiratory alkalosis because a primary acid-base disorder would have caused alkalosis. Next, look at the bicarbonate level for the metabolic component. A normal HCO_3^- is 22 to 26 mmol/L. In our scenario, the patient is acidotic and the bicarbonate level is 4, indicating a primary metabolic acidosis.

This patient is in DKA, an acute life-threatening complication of diabetes. Of note, ABG tests are not always necessary because venous blood gasses can provide sufficient information. Arterial pH is approximately 0.03 higher than venous pH.

Test-taking tip: Remember to use the reference value page when needed.

11. ANSWER: C

A high anion gap is caused by elevation in unmeasured anions. Unmeasured anions can be caused by lactic acid, ketones, uremia, salicylates, methanol, and ethylene glycol. In this scenario, the patient is likely in DKA and has elevated ketones.

The formula to calculate this is:

$$AG = Na - (Cl + HCO_2)$$

Test-taking tip: Recall that a normal anion gap is 8 to 16. The question stem implies that the patient has an elevated anion gap, so that narrows your possible answers to two.

12. ANSWER: C

This patient is in a hyperglycemic hyperosmolar nonketotic state (hyperglycemic hyperosmolar syndrome, or HHS). HHS is typically a complication of type 2 diabetes and is less common than DKA. This condition is characterized by hyperglycemia, high serum osmolality, mild ketosis, and altered mental status. A minority of patients will present with coma. Because of the osmotic diuresis of glucose caused by hyperglycemia, these patients will be severely dehydrated and have dry mucosa, tachycardia, dizziness, and generalized weakness. Bedside ultrasound will show a collapsible inferior vena cava. The illness is generally precipitated by medical illness, including myocardial infarction (MI), infection, and pancreatitis, and can also be caused by medications, such as steroids and second-generation antipsychotics.

Test-taking tip: Although type 2 diabetic patients can go into DKA, it is less likely, especially if they are older and have a relative, rather than absolute, deficiency of insulin.

13. ANSWER: B

This patient is presenting with alcoholic ketoacidosis. This acid-base disorder is often seen in chronic alcoholics who have a cessation or reduction in alcohol use. These patients have depleted glycogen stores leading to ketoacidosis, nausea, vomiting, and vague abdominal pain. Methanol and ethylene glycol can also produce an anion gap acidosis, but they do not produce ketones.

The mainstay of treatment is fluid resuscitation and glucose therapy. Glucose is critical to trigger the body to produce insulin that will stop lipolysis and ketone formation. D5 NS should be given until the patient can tolerate PO intake.

NS alone is not sufficient to reverse the ketone production. Bicarbonate therapy is not indicated unless pH is less than 7.0 and if the patient's bicarbonate level does not respond to fluid and glucose. Insulin therapy is not indicated and can be deleterious given relative depletion of glycogen stores in these patients.

Test-taking tip: You can use process of elimination on a question like this if you don't know the answer off the top of your head. Insulin is dangerous with a glucose of 80, and bicarbonate administration seems unlikely if the question stem doesn't give you a pH. Now you are left with two answers, giving you a 50/50 chance of choosing the correct answer.

14. ANSWER: C

Anion gap refers to the unmeasured anion concentration in serum. The formula to calculate the anion gap is:

$$AG = Na - (Cl + HCO_2)$$

A normal anion gap is considered 8 to 16 mEq/L. The presence of an anion gap warrants consideration of what unmeasured anions are present in the blood and is generally considered in the context of metabolic acidosis. MUDPILES is a classic mnemonic to help with the differential:

M = Methanol
U = Uremia
D = DKA
P = Propylene glycol
I = Isoniazid
L = Lactic acidosis
E = Ethylene glycol
S = Salicylates

This list is certainly not exhaustive.

A normal anion gap is cause by bicarbonate loss. This can be due to GI losses, renal tubular acidosis, and carbonic anhydrase inhibitors. GI losses can include diarrhea and fistulas causing drainage of pancreatic secretions or bile. Metabolic alkalosis is caused by excess base or increased acid loss through GI or renal loss. Medications that cause decreased or shallow respirations, such as organophosphates, opioids, and muscle relaxants, can lead to CO_2 retention and a respiratory acidosis.

Test-taking tip: In certain cases, formulating your answer before looking at the options is helpful. In this question, you may be tempted to err, but you can keep your wits about you if you don't get bogged down in the options and have your answer in mind before looking.

15. ANSWER: D

This patient is presenting with thyroid storm. Thyroid storm is a life-threatening presentation of hyperthyroidism with a high mortality rate. Patients present with thyrotoxicosis along with altered mental status and significant vital sign abnormalities. Temperature higher than 40° C (104° F) and tachycardia are common findings. Hypotension, arrhythmia, and death and cardiac arrest can also occur. The diagnosis of thyroid storm is based on the vital sign abnormalities, central nervous system involvement, and lab evidence of hyperthyroidism. Thyroid storm is often triggered by an acute stressor in a patient with underlying thyroid disease, such as infection, trauma, surgery, amiodarone, pregnancy, and iodine contrast load.

The treatment of thyroid storm involves a stepwise approach. Acute stabilization and resuscitation are critical, including assessing the airway, fluid repletion, and rapid cooling. β-Blockers are used to treat the peripheral actions of thyroid hormones and block the peripheral β-receptors. Propranolol specifically has the added benefit of blocking the peripheral conversion of T_4 to its more active form, triiodothyronine (T_3). A thionamide, such as PTU or methimazole, stops the synthesis of new thyroid hormone, stops the release of stored hormone, and prevents the conversion of T_4 to T_3. One hour after the first dose of PTU or methimazole is given, administer iodine. Iodine halts the release of thyroid hormone and reduces the organification of thyroglobulin. It is critical to give this after the administration of a thionamide; otherwise, iodine will be used for new hormone synthesis. Corticosteroids may also be given to decrease the peripheral conversion of thyroid hormone.

In addition to the previous treatments, it is critical to search for the underlying and precipitating cause of thyroid storm. Investigations and subsequent treatments for sepsis, MI, cerebrovascular accident (CVA), congestive heart failure (CHF), and pulmonary embolism (PE) must be undertaken, depending on the clinical picture.

Test-taking tip: This is a "you know it or don't" kind of question. If you don't know it, choose an answer and move on. You can perhaps mark it for review when you are done at the end of the test. Don't, however, let these kinds of questions get you stuck and waste your time.

16. ANSWER: C

Myxedema coma or myxedema crisis is a rare and extreme form of hypothyroidism with multiorgan dysfunction and high mortality rates. These patients present with altered mental status, bradycardia, hypotension, respiratory depression, and hypothermia. Many stressors can cause a crisis, including sepsis, acute coronary syndrome/MI, CHF, trauma, CVA, electrolyte abnormalities, and medication noncompliance.

The diagnosis of myxedema coma is a clinical diagnosis. Treatment should not be delayed while awaiting results of TSH, T_3, T_4, and cortisol levels. These should be drawn before the initiation of treatment, however, to confirm the diagnosis and evaluate the response to therapy.

ED treatment includes evaluation and management of the ABCs. Intubation, vasopressors, patient warming, and intensive care are often required for these patients. Further treatment includes thyroid hormone replacement and steroids for increased metabolic stress. Either IV T_4 or IV T_3 may be used. IV T_4 is preferred in patients with or at risk for cardiac disease because of the risk for infarction or dysrhythmias with IV T_3. Initial ED treatment should be IV instead or PO owing to reduced GI motility and absorption. Furthermore, the ED provider must identify and treat underlying precipitators of disease.

Test-taking tip: Some test takers prefer to read the answers before reading the question stem. This question is an example of when this may save some time by not focusing on the diagnosis because the stem gives it away.

17. ANSWER: A

This patient has an altered mental status, low BP, hypoglycemia, hypernatremia, and hyperkalemia. These electrolyte abnormalities and clinical presentation are concerning for acute adrenal insufficiency. Glucocorticoid deficiency can manifest with nausea, vomiting, hypoglycemia, hypotension, and shock. Mineralocorticoid deficiency can lead to intravascular volume depletion, hypernatremia, hyperkalemia, and acidosis. Adrenal insufficiency can be both congenital and acquired. Congenital adrenal hyperplasia (CAH) refers to primary adrenal insufficiency of newborns. Most newborn screening programs will test for CAH, but it is possible that these infants present to the ED before the results of the screening test. The most common cause of adrenal insufficiency occurs later in childhood, adolescents, and adults after exposure to steroid use. Patients who are treated with steroids for chronic medical issues can be predisposed to acute adrenal insufficiency when these steroids are discontinued and the patient is exposed to a physiologic stressor.

ED management of acute adrenal insufficiency includes addressing ABCs, treating shock, correcting hypoglycemia, treating hyperkalemia, giving stress dose steroids, and searching for precipitating causes of the event. Before administering steroids, laboratory investigations for specific endocrine hormones should be drawn, if possible.

Test-taking tip: If you don't immediately recognize the electrolyte abnormalities in the question, look for other clues. You will often find other clues in a question stem that can lead you to the right answer. In this case, the patient recently completed a course of steroids.

18. ANSWER: B

In some cases of severe sepsis, the body cannot mount a sufficient hypothalamic-pituitary axis or adrenal response, leading to cardiovascular compromise and overwhelming systemic inflammation. Several studies and meta-analyses have shown that glucocorticoids have a mortality benefit for patients with pressor-dependent shock. Although the data are somewhat controversial, the general consensus is to administer low-dose hydrocortisone to patients with refractory septic shock. Hydrocortisone is preferred over other glucocorticoids because it provides both glucocorticoid and mineralocorticoid affects.

Lipid emulsion therapy is used for local anesthetic toxicity and in overdoses of β-blockers, tricyclic antidepressants, and calcium channel blockers. High-dose insulin can be used in certain cases of calcium channel and β-blocker overdose. Streptokinase is a thrombolytic used in suspected ST elevation MI, PE, and arterial thromboembolism.

Test-taking tip: Don't get caught up in the controversial literature on this one; if persistent shock, give steroids.

19. ANSWER: D

This patient is presenting with findings consistent with congenital adrenal hyperplasia (CAH). The salt-wasting form of CAH presents early in life with poor feeding, lethargy, vomiting, and poor weight gain. Physical exam may reveal hyperpigmentation, fused labia and an enlarged clitoris in females, and normal or a small phallus in males. These patients may present before the parents know the results of the newborn screening tests.

Rapid point-of-care glucose is important for infants with these presenting symptoms because inborn errors of metabolism and sepsis are in your differential. However, hypoglycemia is rare unless the neonate is presenting late with significant vomiting and poor intake. The typical laboratory abnormalities for patients with salt-wasting CAH is hyponatremia and hyperkalemia. It is important to obtain blood hormone levels and an EKG if hyperkalemia is found.

Test-taking tip: Use the process of elimination for this question if you are unsure of the answer. You may not be able to narrow it down to one, but you can increase your odds of choosing the right answer.

20. ANSWER: B

This neonate is presenting with salt-wasting congenital adrenal hyperplasia (CAH). In addition to fluid resuscitation with 10 to 20 mL/kg NS, steroid replacement should be administered emergently. The dose is 25 mg of hydrocortisone IV or IO in neonates. The hyponatremia should resolve with hydrocortisone and NS. Hyperkalemia can be observed unless there are EKG changes and should resolve with hydrocortisone and fluid resuscitation alone. If EKG changes or arrhythmias accompany hyperkalemia, treat with IV calcium with or without sodium bicarbonate. Insulin and glucose should be avoided in neonates and infants because of the risk for significant hypoglycemia.

Test-taking tip: This question asks about the initial treatment of a neonate who is afebrile and lethargic. The clues in the question stem should give you the diagnosis of CAH. If not, you can likely guess that it is some type of endocrine abnormality, which could lead you to eliminate A and D as answer choices.

6.

ENVIRONMENTAL EMERGENCIES

Michael A. Darracq

1. A 27-year-old female scuba diver with no past medical history completes a dive to 60 feet for 30 minutes. Immediately on reaching the surface, she experiences a seizure and is confused and postictal with a return to normal in 20 minutes. Which of the following is the most appropriate treatment?

A. Oxygen administration by nasal cannula
B. Hyperbaric oxygen therapy
C. Transport to nearest hospital for electrocardiogram (EKG), head computed tomography (CT) scan, and admission for new-onset seizures
D. Encourage the patient to hyperventilate

2. A 24-year-old male presents to the emergency department (ED) with the complaint of eye and face discomfort after scuba diving with his wife while on their honeymoon. On exam you see significant scleral redness and a non-blanching rash around his eyes. He was using appropriate scuba dive gear. His face is shown in Figure 6.1. What is your diagnosis?

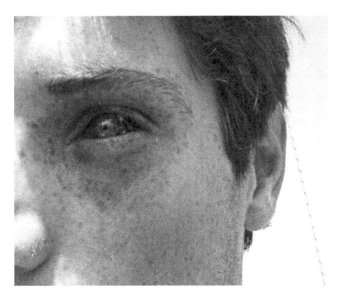

Figure 6.1 Eye.

A. Facial barotrauma
B. Barodontalgia
C. Ocular trauma
D. Middle ear barotrauma

3. A 45-year-old male scuba diver does not follow the recommendation of his dive master and is bitten by the marine animal pictured in Figure 6.2. What clinical effects can be expected following this bite?

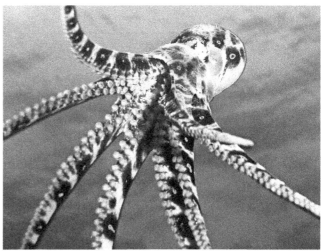

Figure 6.2 Octopus.

A. Extreme pain
B. Paralysis, including respiratory paralysis
C. Intractable nausea, vomiting, and diarrhea
D. Bleeding

4. You and your friend are body surfing off the coast of San Diego. Immediately on entering the water, your friend lets out a yell and states as he begins crying that he has severe pain in his left leg. You both exit the water where you see a single wound with bleeding present as shown in Figure 6.3. Several bystanders gather around and recommend various treatments. Which of the following treatments is most appropriate?

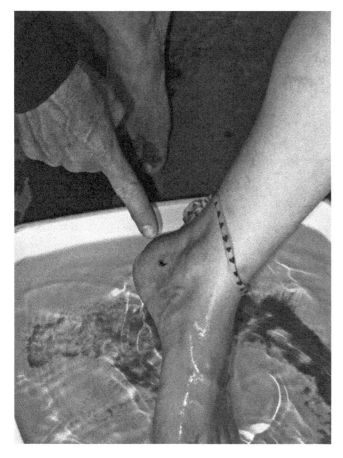

Figure 6.3 Foot.

A. Hot water immersion
B. Cold water immersion
C. Vinegar
D. Salt water rinses

5. A 42-year-old male who appears intoxicated presents to the ED with a swollen, ecchymotic, and tense left ankle. The swelling extends to the knee. He denies any numbness, weakness, or paresthesias but has considerable pain at the ankle. He states that a snake bit him

after he found it on his property and was trying to remove it with a stick. The snake that bit him is pictured in Figure 6.4. Which of the following is the most appropriate ED therapy?

A. Elevation and antibiotics
B. Incision and suction to remove venom
C. Placement of a tourniquet to prevent venom spread
D. Administer antivenom

6. A 45-year-old female truck driver is brought to the ED by emergency medical services EMS after being bitten by a snake on the left hand. She states that she found a snake near her truck, killed it by cutting it in half, and then attempted to pick it up. The snake "doubled back" and bit her. She describes that snake as having a triangular head and a rattle on its tail. This occurred 30 minutes ago. Physical examination reveals fang marks, but she has no pain, swelling, ecchymosis, blebs, or systemic symptoms. Her blood pressure and heart rate are normal, as are her laboratory findings. What is the most appropriate therapy?

A. Administration of antivenom
B. Immediate fasciotomy
C. Prophylactic oral antibiotics
D. Observation for 6 to 8 hours

7. A 23-year-old male presents to your rural Florida ED after being bitten by a snake on the forearm while removing brush from his property. He took a picture of the snake, that shows a snake with red and yellow bands touching, which is seen in Figure 6.5. He initially had no pain or other symptoms, but 1 hour later he develops tingling and fasciculations in the same arm, and he subsequently started to experience profound fatigue, double vision, and difficulty with swallowing.

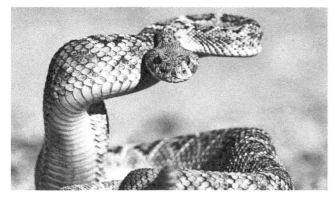

Figure 6.4 Snake.

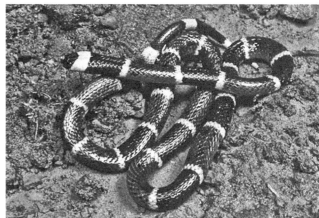

Figure 6.5 Snake.

On arrival to the ED, the patient is awake, alert, and oriented with normal vital signs. Physical examination reveals dysarthria, disconjugate gaze, and two small puncture marks to the forearm. What is the most likely snake responsible for this presentation?

A. Eastern diamondback *(Crotalus adamanteus)*
B. Eastern coral snake *(Micrurus fulvius)*
C. Indian cobra *(Naja naja)*
D. King snake *(Lampropeltis getula)*

8. A 45-year-old female presents to your rural Louisiana ED after being bitten on the hand by a small red, black, and yellow snake while foraging in the woods. She initially had no symptoms but then developed tingling in the involved arm, followed by double vision and difficulty with swallowing. On arrival to the ED, she is awake, alert, and anxious. Physical examination reveals ptosis, dysarthria, and two small puncture marks to the hand. She has progressive shortness of breath with shallow breathing and stridulous breath sounds. What is the most appropriate treatment for this snake envenomation?

A. Administration of antivenom and supportive care
B. Immediate fasciotomy
C. Prophylactic antibiotics
D. Neurology consultation

9. A 6-year old female presents to the ED after playing in the yard and experiencing severe immediate pain on her left ankle. Physical examination reveals two puncture marks, oozing, ecchymosis, and edema extending to the midcalf. You appropriately suspect a rattlesnake bite. What is the most appropriate initial dose of antivenom?

A. Two to three vials of Crotalidae Fab Antivenom
B. Four to six vials of Crotalidae Fab Antivenom
C. There is no indication for antivenom in this patient
D. The treatment for lower extremity edema, ecchymosis, and oozing following rattlesnake envenomation is always fasciotomy

10. A 4-year-old girl experiences immediate pain after putting on her shoe. The spider with a red hourglass on his abdomen is pictured in Figure 6.6 is seen by her father after he shakes out the shoe. Which of the following is the most appropriate initial treatment?

A. Morphine IV
B. Calcium IV
C. Antivenom IV
D. Isotonic fluids IV

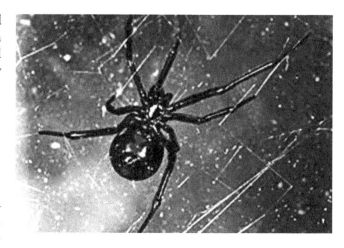

Figure 6.6 Spider.

11. A 37-year-old female in Kansas reports to the ED following a spider bite with a necrotic wound. The offending spider is shown in Figure 6.7. Which of the following is the component of the venom that is responsible for necrosis?

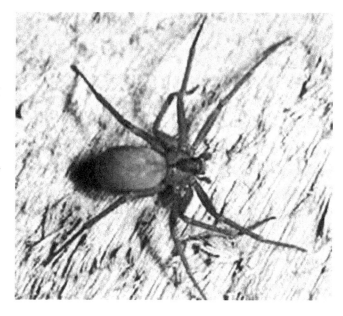

Figure 6.7 Spider.

A. Calcium
B. Substance P
C. Latrotoxin
D. Sphingomyelinase

12. A 6-year-old girl is brought to your ED after being pulled from her backyard swimming pool after falling in. She has a depressed level of consciousness. Which of

the following is true regarding resuscitation following drowning?

A. Prophylactic antibiotics should be routinely administered
B. Regurgitation of stomach contents is rare
C. Traditional ABCs is the recommended approach to cardiopulmonary resuscitation (CPR)
D. Ventricular fibrillation is the predominant cardiac arrest rhythm

13. Which of the following correctly describes how acetazolamide (Diamox) can prevent and treat acute mountain sickness (AMS)?

A. Acts as osmotic diuretic
B. Causes a metabolic acidosis
C. Decreases respiratory rate
D. Increases hypoxia

14. Which of the following is true regarding drowning?

A. Cervical spine injury is common among drowning incidents of all causes
B. It is a leading cause of death among children 5 to 14 years of age in the United States
C. Resuscitation should include active efforts to expel water from the airway
D. Any patient who required resuscitation should be taken to an ED

15. A 3-year-old female who lives in Arizona presents to the ED for finger pain. Her vital signs are blood pressure (BP) 90/palp mm Hg, pulse 176 bpm, respiratory rate (RR) 36 breaths/min, temperature 38.1°C (100.6°F), and SpO$_2$ 97% on room air. She is restless and ataxic and has excessive oral secretions, jerking muscular movements, and rapid, wandering eye movements. No abnormality is seen on her hand. Which envenomation is most consistent with this presentation?

A. Black widow spider
B. Bark scorpion
C. Brown recluse spider
D. Rattlesnake

16. You are climbing Aconcagua (22,841 feet) in South America. One of the individuals in your climbing party begins to act strangely, and you suspect high-altitude cerebral edema (HACE). Which of the following is the definitive treatment for this condition?

A. Acetazolamide
B. Gamow bag
C. Nifedipine
D. Descent to a lower altitude

17. You are practicing in a brown recluse endemic area. A 23-year-old male presents after being bitten by a brown recluse. He has normal vital signs, minimal discomfort, and only mild erythema at bite site. Which of the following is the most appropriate management?

A. Discharge home with primary care follow-up and return precautions
B. Admission for immediate hyperbaric oxygen
C. Administration of antivenom
D. Incision and drainage of the bite location

18. A 23-year-old electrician presents to the ED after sustaining an electric shock while working in a customer's bedroom. He denies any loss of consciousness or other symptoms. Physical examination and EKG are normal. Which of the following is the most appropriate management?

A. Admission with telemetry
B. Discharge home with primary care follow-up and return precautions
C. Order complete blood count (CBC), creatine kinase (CK), and coagulation studies before determining disposition
D. Observe for 6 hours before discharging to home

19. A 4-year-old boy presents with crying after his mother found him biting an electrical cord plugged into the outlet. He has a deep laceration to his lower lip that bled but stopped after 15 minutes of direct pressure. Which of the following is most appropriate management?

A. Discharge home with outpatient plastic surgery follow-up and return precautions
B. Admission with serial EKGs and telemetry
C. Observe for 6 hours before discharge to home to ensure no deterioration
D. Laboratory studies including CBC and creatine phosphokinase (CPK) and admission

20. A 55-year-old male walks into your ED, confused and disheveled. His vital signs are BP 145/90 mm Hg, heart rate (HR) 135 bpm, RR 22 breaths/min, and temperature 36.7° C. His back looks like the image in Figure 6.8. What happened to this individual?

A. Sustained a scald burn due to hot liquid
B. Was exposed to toxicodendron diversilobum (poison oak)
C. Was struck by lightning
D. Sustained a chemical burn caused by concrete mix

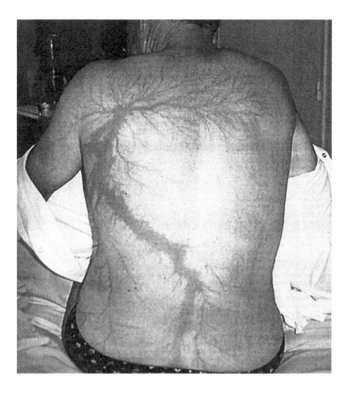

Figure 6.8 Back.

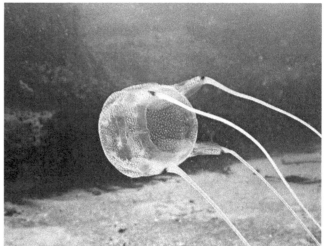

Figure 6.9 Jellyfish.

A. Administer antivenom
B. Immerse the affected area in hot water
C. Immerse the affected area in cold water
D. Wash the affected area with vinegar

21. You come on a scene with several members of a Boy Scout troop who have been struck by lightning. There are 15 people who are down with various degrees of injury. Which of the following individuals should be treated first?

A. Patient who states he is paralyzed from the waist down
B. Patient with confusion and severe left ear pain
C. Patient who is pulseless and not breathing
D. Patient who is bleeding from an open distal radius fracture

22. Immediate death resulting from envenomation by the animal pictured in Figure 6.9 is most typically caused by which disease process?

A. Anaphylaxis
B. Respiratory arrest
C. Disseminated intravascular coagulation
D. Sepsis

23. A 16 year old female swimmer comes to the ED following a trip to the beach in Southern California. She complains of pain on her right thigh. Direct examination reveals multiple linear marks, and the patient tells you that she thinks she was stung by a jellyfish. Which of the following is the most appropriate treatment for this patient?

24. You are climbing Mt. Kilimanjaro and are not feeling well. You are concerned that you might have AMS. Which of the following symptoms is necessary to make the diagnosis of AMS?

A. Headache
B. Nausea
C. Vomiting
D. Sleep disturbance

25. A 36-year-old male presents to your ED with complaints of extreme fatigue associated with severe shoulder and elbow pain bilaterally. He just returned from Jamaica where he went scuba diving on several occasions during the past 24 hours before presentation. His vital signs are normal, and his physical exam is unremarkable except that he is unwilling to actively range his shoulders or elbows and will not let you passively range them. What is the most appropriate definitive treatment for this condition?

A. IV hydration and analgesia
B. Discharge home with ibuprofen and primary care follow-up
C. Arrange for hyperbaric oxygen therapy
D. Immediately heparinize the patient and arrange for emergent CT pulmonary angiogram

26. A 65-year-old male presents to the ED in the middle of January after being found down outside on a lawn. He presents altered and cold to touch. He is wet and

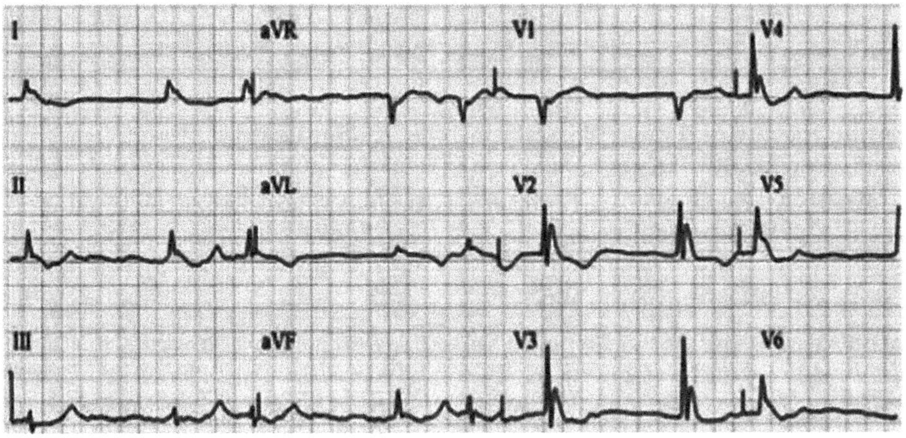

Figure 6.10 Electrocardiogram.

the temperature outside is 2.2° C (36° F). You obtain an EKG, which is shown in Figure 6.10. At what core temperature would you expect to see these EKG findings?

A. 37° C (98.6° F)
B. 35.6° C (96° F)
C. 33.3° C (92° F)
D. 30° C (86° F)

27. Which of the following distinguishes classic heat stroke from exertional heat stroke?

A. Presence of sweating
B. Altered mental status
C. Nausea and vomiting
D. Body temperature

28. A 35-year-old male presents to the ED confused, without sweating and with alteration in mental status. He is a roofer in Las Vegas and is presenting during the summer months. You diagnose a heat illness and begin to cool him. Your nurse asks you what the goal temperature of cooling is. What do you tell him?

A. 37° C
B. 40° C
C. 36° C
D. 39° C

29. You are taking care of a 12-year-old female who sustained a single bee sting to the left forearm. It is mildly red and swollen. The patient's mother asks you about "Africanized honeybees" and how dangerous they really are. She wants to know how many bee stings are really necessary to kill someone. What is the median lethal dose (LD_{50}) of simultaneous bee stings?

A. 25–50 stings
B. 100–200 stings
C. 200–500 stings
D. 500–1000 stings

1. ANSWER: B

This patient experienced a neurologic sign and symptom immediately on reaching the surface. This is extremely concerning for air gas embolism (AGE). The appropriate treatment for AGE is immediate hyperbaric oxygen therapy. Hyperbaric oxygen therapy theoretically crushes the oxygen bubbles that are thought to be occluding blood flow to the brain and allows restoration of normal blood flow.

Normobaric oxygen administration, such as that administered by nasal cannula, is not sufficient to treat AGE. Administration of 100% oxygen by non-rebreather can improve outcomes and should be provided until definitive treatment can be arranged.

Transport to the nearest hospital may delay definitive treatment with hyperbaric oxygen. The patient should be transported to a facility that has hyperbaric oxygen. Divers Alert Network (DAN) has an emergency hotline to locate the nearest facility with hyperbaric oxygen therapy available.

Hyperventilation is not recommended in this situation.

Test-taking tip: Tests questions may have two answers that are very similar to one another and two answers that are not like the others. As a general rule, one of the two similar answer choices is going to be the right answer.

2. ANSWER: A

This individual is demonstrating subconjunctival hemorrhage and petechial rash around his eye. This is classic for mask squeeze. As a diver descends, pressure increases on the diver and on the mask. This reduces the volume of air that exists between the patient's face and the mask. If the diver doesn't exhale a little bit of air through the nose into the mask, a "vacuum" effect can suck the mask onto the diver's face. This results in increased capillary leak and petechial and subconjunctival hemorrhages.

Barodontalgia is dental pain due to air trapped beneath a poorly filled dental cavity that expands on ascent. It is relatively benign and self-limited.

Ocular trauma can occur while diving, but the presentation does not suggest trauma, and the patient was wearing scuba dive gear that includes a mask, which should be protective of direct trauma.

Middle ear barotrauma is the most common complaint of scuba divers. It occurs on descent. Divers typically perform maneuvers in an attempt to maintain equal pressures across the tympanic membrane. If they are unable to maintain equal pressures, it leads to ear pain and at times associated tinnitus and even vertigo.

Test-taking tip: In questions with visual stimuli, often the correct answer can be reached looking at the stem alone with the image simply confirming what is described in the stem.

3. ANSWER: B

The blue-ringed octopus bit this diver. While the bite is not particularly painful and only results when the octopus feels threatened, this is a potentially lethal marine envenomation.

The blue-ringed octopus injects tetrodotoxin (TTX), which acts to block sodium channels throughout the body. Sodium channels are important to many bodily functions, including nerve conduction and respiratory function. Paralysis, including respiratory paralysis, is a common effect following envenomation.

Pain, nausea, vomiting, diarrhea, and bleeding are not expected following envenomation by the blue-ringed octopus.

Test-taking tip: Toxicology involves only a handful of mechanisms. If in doubt, sodium channel blockade is a great choice to guess because it is so common with both pharmaceutical and natural toxins.

4. ANSWER: A

Your friend has been stung by a stingray. The stingray is a member of the shark family. Stingrays frequently bury themselves in the sand of shallow water, where they can be inadvertently stepped on. A person who is stung usually experiences immediate pain and typically has a single wound that may be either a puncture wound or a jagged laceration. A spine of the stingray may still be present in the wound.

The best treatment for a stingray sting is to soak the wound in hot water for 30 to 90 minutes. During the hot water soak, the wound should be explored and debrided of any visible pieces of sting that may continue to envenom the patient.

If hot water for immersion is not immediately available, the wound can be irrigated with nonheated water or saline until heated water becomes available. The use of salt water rinses or vinegar is not indicated.

Test-taking tip: There are two answers that are opposite to each other (hot water versus cold water), suggesting that one of these is the correct answer.

5. ANSWER: D

This patient has been bitten by a western diamondback rattlesnake *(Crotalus atrox)*. The most common signs of envenomation by a rattlesnake are immediate burning pain at the bite site with surrounding edema that gradually spreads proximally.

The only proven therapy is antivenom. ED care of a poisonous snakebite must focus on supportive care and rapid treatment with the appropriate antivenom.

Many therapies for snakebite envenomation have been suggested in the past, but most have been found to be ineffective if not actually dangerous. Incision of bite wounds should be avoided because of lack of proven efficacy and potential danger to underlying structures and infection. Tourniquets should also not be placed because they can increase tissue damage in this situation. The use of suction devices has also not been shown to be beneficial.

Test-taking tip: Make sure to read questions thoroughly, paying particular attention to keywords like "appropriate," "best," or "most." Many answers may be correct, but only one is "most" correct or "best."

6. ANSWER: D

This patient was most likely bitten by a rattlesnake, but there are currently has no signs of envenomation. One-fourth of bites by poisonous snakes result in no envenomation (grade 0 envenomation or a "dry bite"). Therefore, she does not require immediate administration of antivenom. Patients with a suspected bite by a venomous snake who have no immediate signs or symptoms should be observed for 6 to 8 hours. If there is no progression of local or systemic symptoms, they can safely be discharged home.

Immediate fasciotomy is not indicated because the patient has no signs of increased compartment pressure.

Despite an abundance of oral flora cultured from the mouths of rattlesnakes, their venom is actually antibacterial, and therefore antibiotics are not indicated.

Test-taking tip: Study up on the indications and contraindications for administering antivenom for poisonous envenomations.

7. ANSWER: B

This patient has been bitten by an eastern coral snake *(Micrurus fulvius)*. Their bites are usually associated with limited pain or swelling. Their venom contains compounds that block neuromuscular transmission at the acetylcholine receptor sites. Common signs and symptoms include ptosis, paresthesias, fasciculations, slurred speech, drowsiness, dysphagia, nausea, and proximal motor weakness. Death is usually due to respiratory failure.

The eastern coral snake is found in North Carolina, South Carolina, Florida, Louisiana, Mississippi, Georgia,

and Texas. Coral snakes can be readily identified by their color pattern. At first glance, they resemble one of several varieties of king snake found in the southern United States. The coral snake can be differentiated from the king snake by two characteristics: the nose of the coral snake is black, and the red and yellow bands are adjacent on the coral snake but separated by a black band on the king snake. The popular rhyme is as follows: Red next to yellow, kill a fellow. Red next to black, venom lack.

The eastern diamondback *(Crotalus adamanteus)* is a pit viper found in the southeastern United States. Its venom causes more local effects, such as pain and swelling, rather than neurologic effects. It is generally brownish in color with a series of dark brown to black diamonds.

The Indian cobra is not found in the United States except at zoos and as exotic pets and is not red, yellow, and black in color.

The king snake is a member of the Colubridae family of snakes and is red, black, and yellow. King snakes do not cause serious envenomations such as that described in the clinical vignette.

Test-taking tip: You should be able to eliminate the Indian cobra based on geography and the king snake based on its lack of toxicity, leaving two possible answers.

8. ANSWER: A

All victims of bites by the eastern coral snake *(Micrurus fulvius)* should be given antivenom even before any symptoms develop. The toxicity of this venom has a rapid onset, and once symptoms develop, it may be too late to reverse the effects. The recommended dose is three to five vials in 300 to 500 mL of normal saline. Antivenom should be given based on the clinical response. Patients should also be treated supportively with close observation and mechanical ventilation as indicated.

Coral snakes do not cause swelling and do not cause compartment syndrome, so fasciotomy is not indicated.

Antibiotics are not needed prophylactically in snake bites, only if signs and symptoms of infection develop.

Although this patient has neurologic symptoms, you know the cause and the treatment, so neurology consult is not indicated.

Test-taking tip: Study up on the indications and contraindications for administering antivenom for poisonous envenomations.

9. ANSWER: B

Dosage of antivenom is based on a typical envenomation rather than age or weight, so dose is the same for children and adults. The patient meets criteria for administration of antivenom that includes progression of swelling proximal to the bite site (moderate envenomation, grade II)

The recommended initial dose of CroFab is four to six vials. Dosage requirements are dependent on the individual patient response. The use of the recommended adult dosages in the pediatric population appears to be safe. The initial dose should not be reduced in pediatric patients because, despite their smaller size, the volume of venom to be neutralized is not reduced.

Fasciotomy is rarely indicated in the treatment of rattlesnake envenomation and is associated with considerable morbidity.

Test-taking tip: You can eliminate choice D because it contains the word "always," and the patient has signs and symptoms suggesting some treatment is necessary thus eliminating choice C.

10. ANSWER: A

The patient has been bitten by a black widow spider *(Latrodectus mactans)*. In the image, one can see a distinct red hourglass on the abdomen of the offending spider. Pain is the most immediate and most important symptom of black widow bites. Parenteral analgesics such as morphine are recommended first-line treatment, as are benzodiazepines if the patient has significant muscle cramps.

Calcium used to be recommended but no longer is because it showed no efficacy.

Antivenom is controversial because deaths have been reported following use of antivenom, and deaths from black widow bites alone are extremely rare. Antivenom should not be the first-line of therapy, except in patients with severe symptoms such as seizures, respiratory failure, or uncontrolled hypertension.

IV fluids alone are not going to treat the pain or other symptoms related to a black widow spider bite.

Test-taking tip: There are only two spiders of interest medically in North America. The black widow *(Latrodectus)* bite causes immediate pain, while the brown recluse spider bite does not cause immediate pain.

11. ANSWER: D

The spider picture is the brown recluse *(Loxosceles reclusa)*. It has a limited geographical distribution (most typically midwestern states like Kansas). The main component of the venom that causes complications, including necrosis, is sphingomyelinase.

Latrotoxin is the component of black widow venom that causes symptoms including the pain and cramping.

Substance P, which is involved in pain transmission in the central nervous system, and calcium are not in venom.

Test-taking tip: Knowing the major component of animal venoms is important and also commonly tested on board examinations

12. ANSWER: C

Traditional ABCs is the recommended method for resuscitation following drowning. Because death due to drowning is a hypoxic driven event, this is a situation in which compression-only CPR may not be as effective as CPR with assisted ventilations.

Antibiotics should not be routinely administered. Aspiration of water on chest radiographs is often misdiagnosed as pneumonia, but true pneumonia develops infrequently, and indiscriminate administration of antibiotics can lead to resistant and aggressive organisms.

Regurgitation is very common following drowning.

Asystole is the most common cardiac arrest rhythm following drowning, not ventricular fibrillation.

Test-taking tip: Words such as "routinely," "always," and "never" should help you to eliminate incorrect answers.

13. ANSWER: B

Acute mountain sickness (AMS) is a syndrome of high-altitude ascent characterized by headache in combination with one or more symptoms of gastrointestinal disturbance (i.e., anorexia, nausea, vomiting), dizziness, fatigue, or sleep disturbance. Hypoxia is thought to be the causative mechanism.

Acetazolamide (Diamox) induces a nongap metabolic acidosis. To maintain serum pH, the body must decrease P_{CO_2} through increased respiration; this in turn raises serum P_{O_2}.

Acetazolamide is not an osmotic diuretic.

Acetazolamide increases respiratory rate and thus decreases hypoxia.

Test-taking tip: Knowing the pathophysiology of the disease or the mechanism of drug action will help answer questions like this.

14. ANSWER: D

Resuscitative efforts needed on scene predict the potential for delayed symptoms, thus all victims of drowning who require resuscitation in the prehospital setting should be transported to an ED.

Injuries to the spine from drowning are rare (<0.5% of persons who drowned) and usually associated with someone diving into a shallow body of water.

Unintentional injuries (accidents) are the most common cause of death in the United States for persons 5 to 14 years of age. Drowning is the second leading cause of death among children 1 to 4 years of age.

Active expelling of water actually delays initiation of ventilation and increases the risk for vomiting and increase in rate of mortality.

Test-taking tip: Epidemiology is fair game for board examinations, so study up on some of the basics related to common disease processes.

15. ANSWER: B

The bark scorpion is the most venomous scorpion in North America and inhabits the deserts of the southwest, especially Arizona. Their venom is predominantly excitatory and acts to cause pain, paralysis, paresthesias, and muscular jerking. Fatalities are rare but can be seen in small children, older adults, and adults with compromised immune systems. An antivenom is available.

Black widow venom causes predominantly pain and muscle spasms.

Brown recluse spider venom causes dermatonecrosis, which is delayed in onset.

Rattlesnake venom is a local tissue toxin causing hemolysis, bleeding, and tissue breakdown.

Test-taking tip: Cranial nerve dysfunction is a hallmark of bark scorpion venom. Brush up on the primary presenting symptoms of envenomations.

16. ANSWER: D

The only definitive treatment for all altitude-related illnesses is descent. Descents of as little as 3,000 feet may improve symptoms; however, descent should be continued until symptoms resolve.

All of the other modalities have been used in the treatment or prevention of altitude-related illness.

Acetazolamide is used both in the prevention and treatment of altitude illness. For prevention, it can be started 24 hours before ascent to prevent AMS. It can be used in the treatment of high-altitude pulmonary edema (HAPE) if descent is not possible.

A Gamow bag is a portable hyperbaric chamber that can be used for the treatment of HACE or HAPE. These chambers generate 103 mm Hg (2 psi) above ambient pressure, simulating a descent of 4,000 to 5,000 feet.

Nifedipine is the first-line medication for the treatment of HAPE if descent is not possible.

Test-taking tip: Descent is always the preferred treatment for severe forms of high-altitude illness, so this will usually be the correct answer in these scenarios unless descent is not possible.

17. ANSWER: A

Brown recluse spider bites may result in delayed tissue necrosis and hyperbaric oxygen, and several other therapies have been described. Unfortunately, none of these therapies has been proved beneficial.

Generally, the recommendation is to wait for tissue edges to demarcate before skin grafting. There is no way to predict which wounds will develop tissue necrosis, and incision and drainage may add unnecessary trauma to the tissues.

There is no commercial available antivenom for brown recluse spider bites.

The appropriate treatment is discharge to home with follow-up and return precautions.

Test-taking tip: Knowing which envenomations have an antidote or antivenom and which do not will help in questions like this.

18. ANSWER: B

The most appropriate management is discharge to home with follow-up. Household current is low voltage and is not associated with serious injury if there are no immediate injuries present.

Exposure to higher voltage (>600 V), as can be seen in industrial settings, is associated with delayed injuries in the absence of immediate presenting complications. These patients should have laboratory studies, telemetry, and serial examinations looking for delayed complications such as compartment syndrome or rhabdomyolysis.

Test-taking tip: Knowing that low-voltage injuries, such as those sustained in household accidents, rarely cause internal injury lets you eliminate choices A and C.

19. ANSWER: A

This patient has a cosmetic lesion at this point that is best served by outpatient plastic surgery. Appropriate return precautions should be given for recurrent bleeding because the patient is at risk for labial artery bleeding. A period of observation in the ED is not indicated because these recurrent bleeds are often delayed.

Admission with serial EKGs and telemetry is not going to change this outcome, and delayed injuries from household current exposures are unlikely. Laboratory studies are similarly not advised.

Test-taking tip: Knowing that low-voltage injuries, such as those sustained in household accidents, rarely cause internal injury lets you eliminate choices B and D.

20. ANSWER: C

This is a classic visual diagnosis and represents a Lichtenberg figure. Lichtenberg figures are associated with lightning strikes and fade over time. The most likely cause is the rupture of capillaries beneath the skin caused by the electrical discharge.

Scald burns due to hot liquid tend to be spotty in nature and in adults tend to be on the anterior aspect of the body because of kitchen accidents and car radiator explosions.

Chemical burns due to cement would most likely occur in industrial workers who work with cement. Some of the worst burns occur when cement gets into boots, gloves, or clothing. Dry cement is less caustic than wet cement because when cement reacts with water, it produces a highly alkaline calcium hydroxide.

A rash due to poison oak occurs in people allergic to the oil urushiol, which is released from the poison oak when damaged. It causes a rash that is erythematous and pruritic and can progress to form large blisters that ooze. Poison oak rash is most likely to appear around the wrists, ankles, and neck.

Test-taking tip: Visual diagnoses are classic board questions, especially when related to dermatologic questions. Spend some time looking at pictures related to common visual diagnoses.

21. ANSWER: C

Lightning strikes require "reverse" triage. Typically, a patient without breathing or a pulse in a multiple or mass casualty situation, using conventional triage rules, would be considered "black" or deceased, and no attempts at resuscitation would be started.

With lightning strikes, cardiac arrest is often precipitated by primary respiratory arrest and associated asystole. Cardiac function often returns before respiratory function, and thus these patients need immediate CPR with ventilator support (not compressions only CPR) to improve survival.

Tympanic membrane rupture with associated hearing loss and apparent confusion is common in lightning strikes but not life-threatening.

Neurologic symptoms, including paralysis, can occur after a lightning strike but are not usually life-threatening and frequently resolve with time.

Direct trauma can also occur with lightning strikes, and bleeding should be controlled as soon as possible, but the patient who is not breathing and without a pulse takes precedent in this scenario.

Test-taking tip: Knowing exceptions to the rules, such as in this question, can be important in test-taking situations.

22. ANSWER: B

This is a box jellyfish *(Chironex fleckeri),* which is among the most dangerous of jellyfish envenomations. Deaths are typically the result of respiratory arrest.

Disseminated intravascular coagulation and sepsis do not typically cause immediate death, and anaphylaxis would be extremely rare because it would require previous exposure to the components of box jellyfish venom.

Test-taking tip: Choices C and D can be easily eliminated because they do not cause "immediate" death.

23. ANSWER: B

Jellyfish envenomations may occur during beach trips. Multiple linear marks are common and represent the multiple tentacles that make contact with the patient.

Numerous studies have suggested that hot water is the most appropriate treatment for jellyfish envenomation. Vinegar has been suggested as treatment when box jellyfish or *Physalia* species envenomations are known to be the cause. In this case, the cause of the envenomation is not known.

There is not antivenom available for all jellyfish envenomations (only for the box jellyfish and only in Australia).

Test-taking tip: Hot water is a good guess for treatment of most marine envenomations.

24. ANSWER: A

Acute mountain sickness (AMS) may occur during ascents of relatively low-altitude elevations. Headache is the only symptom listed that is necessary to make the diagnosis of AMS. The Lake Louise Scoring System requires an increase in elevation over the preceding 4 days, headache, and at least one other symptom from the following categories: gastrointestinal, fatigue or weakness, dizziness or lightheadedness, and difficulty sleeping.

Test-taking tip: Scoring systems are often a tested element on board examinations and are good to brush up on.

25. ANSWER: C

This patient is suffering from decompression sickness (DCS), commonly referred to as "the bends," which occurs when dissolved gases (mainly nitrogen) come out of solution in bubbles. These bubbles can affect any part of the body but most commonly affect the nervous and musculoskeletal systems. Symptoms usually occur within 48 hours of diving.

Hyperbaric oxygen treatment is the definitive therapy for DCS. During decompression, the hyperbaric chamber gets pressurized to simulated depths of 30 to 60 feet, allowing the gas bubbles to dissolve back into solution.

IV hydration and analgesia may help with musculoskeletal symptoms but will not reverse the pathology of this disease process.

Discharging home is not appropriate because this process is very painful and is readily treatable.

This patient is not at high risk for a pulmonary embolism, especially given that he has normal vital signs and no respiratory symptoms.

Test-taking tip: As descent is usually the correct answer in the setting of high-altitude illness, hyperbaric therapy is usually the correct answer in patients with serious symptoms related to scuba diving.

26. ANSWER: D

The finding on EKG is an extra deflection at the end of the QRS complex. This is called a J wave or Osborn wave and is a finding associated with hypothermia. At a temperature of 30° C (86° F), 80% of patients will have an Osborn wave present.

Test-taking tip: You can easily eliminate A and B because they are normal or near-normal body temperatures, and J waves are a rare finding on more severe hypothermia.

27. ANSWER: A

Heat illnesses such as heat stroke result from impairments in the body's ability to self-regulate temperature. Heat stroke represents the most severe impairment in this ability.

Classic heat stroke typically affects very young children, older adults, or debilitated people and is characterized by altered mental status and the absence of sweating.

Exertional heat stroke victims, who are usually fit athletes or outdoor workers, are usually still sweating.

In both classic and exertional heat stroke, the body temperature is usually 40.° C (105° F) or higher and the patient is altered.

Nausea and vomiting are not common findings in heat stroke.

Test-taking tip: Having a clear idea of how diseases and syndromes are different is important in the setting of standardized medical tests.

28. ANSWER: D

The most important element of the treatment of heat stroke patients is rapid cooling. Patients presenting to the ED with heat stroke have a high mortality rate, up to 63%. Evaporative cooling is the most commonly recommended method in the ED because it is effective and does not interfere with other resuscitative efforts. Immersion in ice water is also effective but can be difficult to accomplish and hinders other treatment.

The end point of cooling is a temperature of 38.5° to 39° C to avoid overcooling and the development of hypothermia.

Test-taking tip: With numerical answers, if you don't know, guessing that the answer is somewhere in the middle is usually reasonable.

29. ANSWER: D

Fatalities may occur when a large amount of bee venom is absorbed following a massive envenomation such as that which occurs with "Africanized honeybees." These bees are much more aggressive than standard honeybees, and these bees often swarm a victim. The LD_{50} for honeybee stings is estimated between 500 and 1,200 stings, and death results from multiorgan failure.

Test-taking tip: Many questions on board examinations will offer answer choices that represent general ranges. It is a good idea to have a general sense of relative frequencies, doses, and so forth rather than absolute numbers.

7.

DENTAL, HEAD, EYE, EAR, NOSE, AND THROAT EMERGENCIES

Rene Ramirez and John Ramos

1. A mother presents to the emergency department (ED) with her 4-year-old son who has burning eye pain that started immediately after rubbing a commercial grade degreasing soap on his face and eyes 1 hour ago. There was no pain relief after his mother washed his face and eyes with tap water at home. He is in severe distress, crying, and refusing to open his eyes. A piece of litmus paper is applied to each eye that shows a dark blue stain (pH >7.5) (Figure 7.1). Which of the following is the next best step?

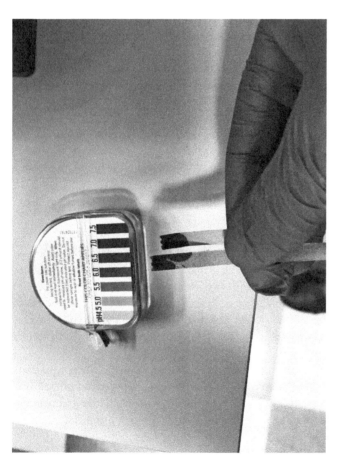

Figure 7.1 Litmus paper.

A. Apply proparacaine and fluorescein stain to visualize corneal abrasions
B. Irrigate eyes with normal saline, reassess pH at 5 and 30 minutes, apply fluorescein stain to visualize potential corneal injury
C. Irrigate eyes to achieve a pH less than 7 and discharge home with outpatient follow-up
D. Apply proparacaine and discharge home

2. A 65-year-old female with hypertension, diabetes, and chronic kidney disease presents with a worsening rash for 3 days (Figure 7.2). The patient notes that before the rash appeared, she felt burning and tingling on the left side of her face. She denies any changes in sensation. Visual acuity is 20/20 in the right, left, and both eyes. Which of the following statements regarding management is true?

A. Discharge orders should include oral acyclovir and prednisone, with ophthalmology follow-up
B. If slit lamp examination is positive for punctate lesions, consult ophthalmology, and administer IV acyclovir
C. Administer acyclovir because this patient displays Hutchinson's sign
D. If slit lamp examination is positive for dendritic lesions, consult ophthalmology and administer acyclovir, corticosteroids, and diazepam intravenously

3. A 60-year-old male presents to the ED with gradually worsening left-sided blurred vision and "spots" over the past 3 days. Patient denies eye pain. Left pupil is reactive to direct and consensual light. An ultrasound of the left eye is completed (Figure 7.3). Which of the following statements is most relevant to educating the patient about his condition?

A. Ocular massage is a treatment option to restore retinal artery blood flow

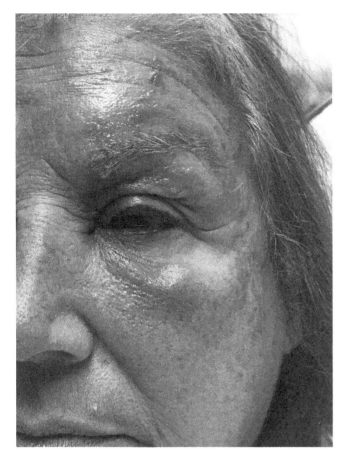

Figure 7.2 Face.

B. High-dose IV methylprednisolone is a sight-saving treatment
C. Compared with macula-off retinal detachment, macula-on retinal detachment has a worse prognosis for vision restoration
D. Compared with macula-on retinal detachment, macula-off retinal detachment has a worse prognosis for vision restoration

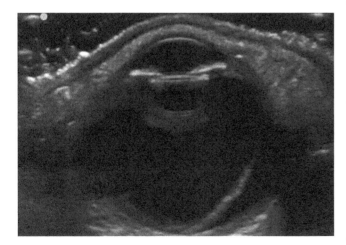

Figure 7.3 Ultrasound of eye.

4. A 31-year-old female presents with a 1-day history of worsening left-sided eye pain, vision loss, and photophobia. She is not tachycardic or febrile. Visual acuity is 20/25 on the right and 20/100 on the left. Tonometry is 16 mm Hg on the right and 17 mm Hg on the left. Pupils are reactive to direct and consensual light, but shining a light in the patient's right eye intensifies the patient's pain. Which of the following is the most likely diagnosis?

    A. Iritis
    B. Acute angle closure glaucoma
    C. Central retinal artery occlusion
    D. Optic neuritis

5. A 32-year-old male presents 8 hours after a physical assault with blunt facial trauma. He complains of right-sided pain and blurry vision, which has acutely worsened in the past 2 hours. On physical exam he has decreased visual acuity at near and far distances. Which of the following findings warrants emergent ophthalmology consultation?

    A. Ocular ultrasound shows lens subluxation
    B. Increased intraocular pressure (IOP)
    C. Subconjunctival hemorrhage
    D. Corneal abrasion

6. A 74-year-old female with a past medical history including atrial fibrillation, diabetes, and glaucoma presents with painless, left-sided vision loss. "Thirty minutes ago I was just watching TV and all of a sudden it was like the room was turning black in one eye." The patient takes all of her home medications as prescribed. "I went to the optometrist 3 years ago, I thought everything was fine." The patients vital signs are heart rate (HR) 92 bpm, blood pressure (BP) 130/83 mm Hg, respiratory rate (RR) 16 breaths/min, and temperature 36.9° C. On physical examination, the patient has intact light perception, and visual acuity is 20/25 on the right and 20/100 on the left. "Something's wrong, I was able to dial 9-1-1 on the phone 15 minutes ago." You recognize the time-sensitive nature of this sight-threatening emergency, initiate treatment to reduce IOP, and consult ophthalmology after you visualize which of the following fundoscopic findings?

    A. Visualization obscured by cloudy vitreous
    B. Optic disc pallor, cherry-red macula
    C. Blood and thunder fundus
    D. Retinal hemorrhages

7. A 35-year-old female with a history of cluster headaches presents to the ED with worsening right-sided head and eye pain along with blurred and decreased vision from her right eye and photophobia for 3 hours. The patient's

heart rate is 120 bpm and temperature is 37° C. While you are interviewing the patient, she refuses to open her right eye. At home, her headache symptoms are typically relieved with oxygen 2 L/min by nasal cannula. "The headache feels the same, but it never lasts for this long and my eye never hurts." After treating the patient's pain, her HR is 92 bpm and you start a physical exam. The patient still has difficulty opening the eye because of pain with light. In her right eye, you observe minimal diffuse conjunctival redness and a constricted pupil. What information would increase your suspicion for uveitis?

A. Patient's age is less than 50 years and erythrocyte sedimentation rate is elevated
B. Right-sided IOP more than 20 mm Hg with a hazy cornea
C. Ciliary injection, constricted pupil
D. Patient is 1 week postpartum and was diagnosed with preeclampsia

8. A 33-year-old female with no past medical history presents with sudden onset of pain and blurred vision in her right eye. Her son accidentally broke a light bulb above their heads with a broom while cleaning but she did not feel glass get into her eye. She has decreased

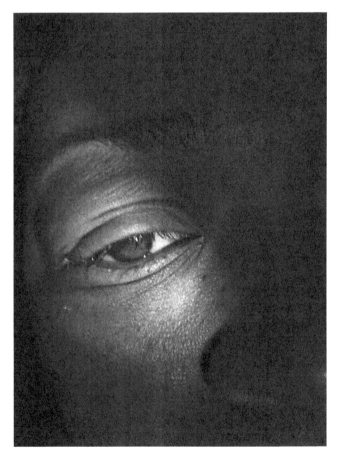

Figure 7.4 Eye.

vision in her right eye and normal vision in her left eye. Pain is relieved with topical proparacaine, and an exam with fluorescein is done that shows fluorescein uptake across the bottom half of the iris (Figure 7.4). Which of the following is the correct diagnosis?

A. Penetrating intraocular foreign body
B. Hyphema
C. Corneal ulceration
D. Corneal abrasion

9. You are working in triage when a 53-year-old male is brought in by emergency medical services (EMS) with right-sided eye pain, temporal headache, and vision loss. His symptoms started 2 hours ago and have progressively worsened. His medical history is significant for polymyalgia rheumatica, and he wears corrective lenses. Vital signs are unremarkable. Physical exam of the orbit is unremarkable for redness or swelling. The patient has marked visual field deficits (20/40 left eye, 20/100 right eye), with worsening light perception in the right eye. Given the history and physical exam findings, which of the following treatments is most likely indicated?

A. Surgical intervention for drainage
B. Oral prednisone
C. IV lasix
D. IV acetazolamide

10. A 30-year-old male presents to the ED with sudden onset of bilateral eye pain that started 30 minutes ago while he was welding. The patient admits to welding without protective eyewear. Administering proparacaine causes complete relief of the patient's symptoms, and visual acuity is 20/20 with testing of the right, left, and bilateral eyes. You apply fluorescein to both eyes and perform a slit lamp examination. Which of the following is the most likely finding?

A. Focal punctate abrasion
B. Diffuse punctate abrasions
C. Linear corneal laceration
D. Diffuse dendritic lesions

11. A 70-year-old male presents to the ED by ambulance after a physical altercation with blunt-force impact to the left orbit. He complains of pain and complete vision loss in the left eye. On exam, you see the eye as presented in Figure 7.5. Which of the following is indicated for the management of this patient's condition?

A. Fluorescein staining and slit lamp examination
B. Tonometry
C. IV administration of morphine
D. Topical administration of proparacaine

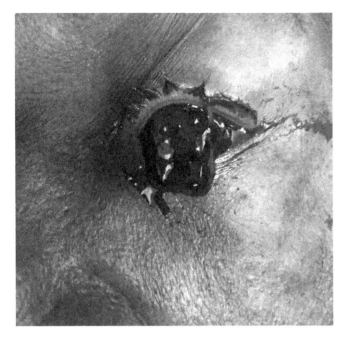

Figure 7.5 Eye.

12. A 20-year-old female with a history of uncontrolled diabetes presents with right-sided eye pain for 1 day. Additional symptoms include sinus pain and congestion for the past 2 weeks. She was diagnosed with bacterial sinusitis at an urgent care 2 days ago. She has been compliant with levofloxacin for the past 2 days. On external examination of her right eye, it is swollen and red (Figure 7.6). Which of the following physical exam findings would increase your suspicion for orbital cellulitis and *not* periorbital cellulitis?

    A. IOP more than 20 mm Hg in both eyes by tonometry
    B. IOP less than 20 mm Hg in the right eye by tonometry
    C. Conjunctival injection in the right eye
    D. Pain with right eye movement

13. A 32-year-old male presents with right-sided eye pain and redness for 3 days. The patient states the pain started after he got a bug bite near his eye. Physical exam is remarkable for conjunctival injection and mild erythema of the periorbital soft tissue. There is no pain with extraocular movements, and visual acuity testing is 20/25 right, 20/20 left, and 20/25 bilaterally. Slit lamp examination is unremarkable. Which of the following is the most likely diagnosis and treatment?

    A. Periorbital cellulitis, outpatient treatment with clindamycin
    B. Periorbital cellulitis, administer IV antibiotics

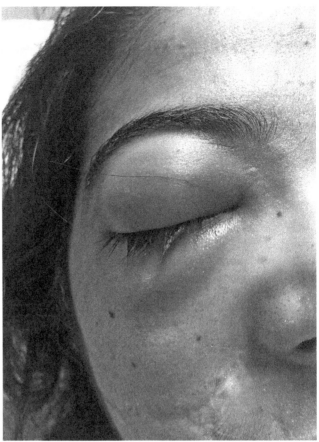

Figure 7.6 Eye.

    C. Orbital cellulitis, administer IV antibiotics
    D. Order computed tomography (CT) scan of the orbits

14. A 52-year-old male presents to the ED 1 day after being struck in the face with fists during an altercation. He complains of pain and tearing in his right eye. On physical examination, the patient has periorbital ecchymosis. The eye has an injected sclera, negative fluorescein uptake, and normal pupils. When checking his pupils with a pen light, he has pain when you shine the light into the affected eye and pain when you shine the light into the good eye. What is his most likely diagnosis?

    A. Iritis
    B. Optic neuritis
    C. Blepharitis
    D. Acute angle closure glaucoma

15. A-34-year old female presents to the ED with bilateral, watery eye discharge for 2 days. She has had a sore throat and cough for the past 2 days, which she says are the same symptoms her entire family is experiencing. This morning she woke with her eyes matted shut. She is afebrile and not tachycardic. Physical exam is

remarkable for mild conjunctival injection bilaterally, and visual acuity is normal. Which of the following is the most likely diagnosis?

A. Allergic conjunctivitis
B. Bacterial conjunctivitis
C. Viral conjunctivitis
D. Orbital cellulitis

16. A 19-year-old male presents to the ED with left-sided eye redness and discharge. His symptoms started 2 days ago, but he denies any recent illnesses. The patient is afebrile and not tachycardic. Physical exam is remarkable for conjunctival injection in the left eye with some mucopurulent discharge noted. Visual acuity exam is 20/30 for both eyes, and the patient is not currently wearing his corrective contact lenses. Which of the following is the best next step in managing this patient's condition?

A. Collect a sample of discharge for polymerase chain reaction amplification
B. Collect a sample for viral culture
C. Treat empirically with ofloxacin drops
D. Treat empirically with polymyxin B/trimethoprim eye drops

17. A 58-year-old female with diabetes mellitus presents with worsening left-sided eye pain and blurry vision that started 3 hours. The patient's vital signs are HR 80 bpm, BP 156/80 mm Hg, RR 18 breaths/min, and temperature 37.6° C. On physical examination you observe a steamy cornea in the left eye. Tonometry reveals IOPs of 30 on the left and 18 on the right. What is the next appropriate step for definitive management?

A. Immediate ophthalmology consult
B. Treatment with pilocarpine 2% eye drops to improve aqueous humor outflow
C. Treatment with timolol 0.5% eye drops to inhibit aqueous humor production
D. Treatment with IV mannitol to reduce aqueous humor volume

18. A 27-year-old female presents to the ED with severe vision loss and eye pain in her right eye. She first noticed some right-sided vision loss (described as blurred vision) and pain with eye movement 2 weeks ago and was diagnosed with conjunctivitis at an urgent care facility. She states she has never had pain this bad before, although she had a similar episode of eye pain and vision loss 1 year ago that resolved in 3 to 4 weeks. Her vital signs are unremarkable. A full neurologic exam is remarkable for decreased visual acuity in the right eye compared with the left, and you also note that the

patient's pupils constrict less when you swing a light from the left eye to the right. Which of the following is the most likely underlying medical condition?

A. Temporal arteritis
B. Orbital cellulitis
C. Retinal detachment
D. Multiple sclerosis

19. A 52-year-old male presents with a painless bump on his right eye lid. Weeks ago, the patient was diagnosed with a hordeolum on his right eyelid. Physical examination of the right eye reveals a 0.5-cm, firm, nontender lesion on the inferior eyelid margin. Pupils are 5 mm and equally reactive to light. Extraocular movements are intact and do not illicit pain. Which of the following is the most likely diagnosis?

A. Hordeolum
B. Chalazion
C. Blepharitis
D. Periorbital cellulitis

20. A 34-year-old female presents with unilateral eye pain without associated visual deficits. Symptoms started 2 days ago and have progressively worsened despite compressions with a warm washcloth at home. Physical examination of the left eye reveals a small red, swollen lesion on the external aspect of the inferior eye lid (Figure 7.7). The lesion is extremely tender to palpation. The patient is not tachycardic or febrile. Which of the following is appropriate in the management of this patient's condition?

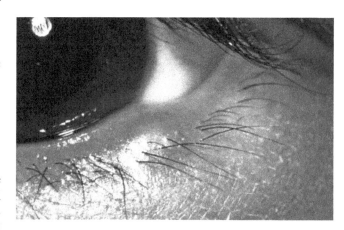

Figure 7.7 Eyelid.

A. Continue warm compresses
B. Daily treatment with baby shampoo
C. Incision and drainage
D. IV antibiotics and hospital admission

21. A 4-year-old female presents with multiple puncture wounds to her forehead after being attacked by her family's dog. There are multiple small puncture wounds to the left side of the patient's forehead and orbit, with no observable puncture wounds to the eye. Of note, there is a laceration through the medial area of the left lower eyelid. Although the patient is no longer crying or in distress, you notice tearing at the left eye. Surgical consultation is necessary because:

A. All eyelid lacerations require surgical consultation
B. Physical exam findings are consistent with damage to the lacrimal glands
C. Physical exam findings are consistent with globe rupture
D. Physical exam is concerning for compromise of the gray line

22. A 45-year-old male with a past medical history of diabetes and hypertension presents to the ED with ear pain. He states that for the past week his ear has gotten gotten painful with redness and swolling, as seen in the photo (Figure 7.8). What is the best treatment for this patient?

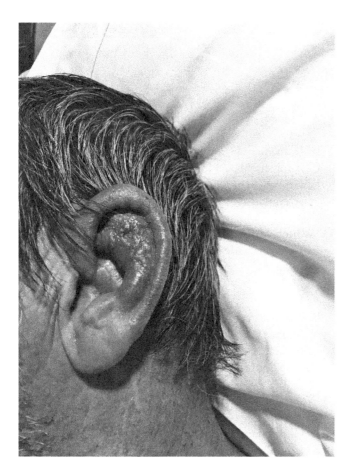

Figure 7.8 Ear.

A. Ciprofloxacin and admit
B. Incision and drainage and discharge home
C. Warm compresses, conservative treatment, and discharge home
D. Unasyn/vancomycin and admit

23. A mother presents because she is concerned about her 1-week-old male infant. In the past day the mother noticed redness, swelling, and drainage in her infant's left eye. The mother received no prenatal care and delivered outside of the hospital by water birth at home. She denies any history of recent trauma. The infant weighs 3.2 kg and has a HR of 130 bpm and temperature of 37.6° C. The infant cries but is consolable and not toxic appearing. Physical examination of the left eye reveals red and swollen eyelids with colorless discharge. Which of the following is the most appropriate treatment for the infant?

A. Erythromycin ointment
B. Erythromycin oral suspension
C. Intramuscular ceftriaxone
D. Silver nitrate

24. A 14-year-old girl who is vacationing with her family and has made extensive use of the resort's swimming pool presents with 2 days of progressive moderate pain and swelling to her right ear canal with moderate white discharge. The discharge is removed with a curette, revealing a small perforation of the tympanic membrane. The best choice of antibiotic to prescribe is:

A. Cortisporin
B. Acetic acid with hydrocortisone
C. Ofloxacin Otic
D. Cipro HC Otic

25. Flora that are known to naturally reside within healthy ears of patients include each of the following *except*:

A. *Staphylococcus epidermidis*
B. *Corynebacterium* species
C. *Pseudomonas aeruginosa*
D. *Haemophilus influenzae*

26. Of the following choices, which bacteria is the most common cause of acute otitis media (AOM) in adults?

A. *Streptococcus pneumoniae*
B. Group A β-hemolytic *Streptococcus*
C. *Staphylococcus aureus*
D. *Moraxella catarrhalis*

27. An 8-year-old male presents with a 2-day history of progressive left ear pain, rhinorrhea, cough,

subjective fever, injected sclera, and conjunctival exudate. Otoscopy reveals an injected tympanic membrane with an effusion. The most common causative organism in children to account for these symptoms is:

A. Nontypeable *H. influenzae*
B. *S. pneumoniae*
C. *Chlamydia trachomatis*
D. *M. catarrhalis*

28. A 14-year-old male presents to the ED complaining of mild pain and swelling to his left ear after sustaining a roundhouse kick during a martial arts tournament. Physical exam reveals bruising and swelling about 2 cm in diameter to the upper pinna of his left ear consistent with a hematoma. What is the next best choice in management of this patient?

A. Scalpel or needle incision and drainage
B. Pressure dressing to the ear
C. Ibuprofen and reassurance
D. IV antibiotics and admission

29. A 4-year-old male presents to the ED after placing a popcorn kernel in his left ear. Which of the following is *false* regarding aural foreign bodies?

A. Irrigation has been established as an effective mechanism for foreign body removal
B. Irrigation can induce swelling of organic foreign bodies
C. Popcorn kernels can swell sufficiently to lodge tight in an ear canal of patients younger than 1 year
D. Kidney beans can swell up to 1,268% of their dry size in water

30. Which of the following is known to be a cause of sudden hearing loss?

A. Barotrauma
B. Pregnancy
C. Salicylates
D. All of the above

31. A 65-year-old hypertensive male taking rivaroxaban (Xarelto) for atrial fibrillation presents to the ED for a nose bleed. It has been steady for more than 30 minutes, and the patient ends up requiring the placement of bilateral posterior packing. What is the next appropriate step?

A. Admission to the hospital for close observation
B. Admission to the hospital and IV antibiotics
C. Discharge home with oral antibiotics
D. Observe the patient in the ED for 4 hours and, if stable, discharge home

32. A 22-year-old male presents to the ED after being assaulted with fists. A CT scan is obtained secondary to head and facial trauma with epistaxis (Figure 7.9). Exam with a nasal speculum reveals a purple/bluish mass. Which of the following is true with this finding?

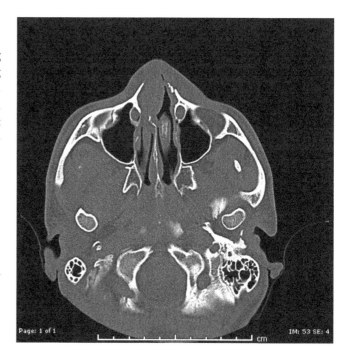

Figure 7.9 Face computed tomography.

A. Immediate incision and drainage (I&D) is warranted
B. Immediate IV antibiotics are warranted
C. Apply nasal packing to the right nares
D. Urgent ear, nose, and throat (ENT) specialist referral

33. Which of the following is the most appropriate diagnostic test to rule out the diagnosis of cavernous sinus thrombosis?

A. D-dimer
B. Noncontrast CT
C. Magnetic resonance imaging (MRI)/magnetic resonance venography (MRV)
D) Ultrasound

34. Which of the following are causes of sialadenitis?

A. Chronic juvenile recurrent parotitis (CJRP)
B. Immunoglobulin G4-RS (IgG4-RS)
C. Cat-scratch disease
D. All of the above

35. A 65-year-old female presents to the ED with a complaint of throat pain after accidentally swallowing an earring mistaking it for her morning medications. In which clinical phase are complications most likely to occur in the setting of aspiration and ingestion of foreign bodies?

A. Initial stage
B. Second stage
C. Third stage
D. Fourth stage

36. A 65-year-old female presents to the ED with a complaint of throat pain after accidentally swallowing an earring mistaking it for her morning medications. She is calm and is speaking full sentences. The earring is seen on a radiograph (Figure 7.10). Which additional option of visualization might one consider for removal of this foreign body?

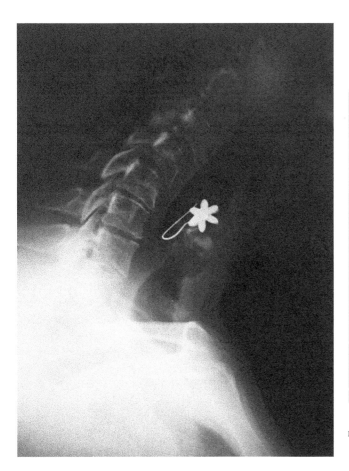

Figure 7.10 Soft tissue neck radiograph.

A. Flexible bronchoscopy
B. Video-assisted Laryngoscopy
C. Tongue blade
D. Rigid bronchoscopy

37. A 4-year-old unvaccinated child is brought in by EMS with abrupt onset of stridor, dysphagia, fever, and sore throat. The patient is observed sitting in a tripod position with increased work of breathing. He is holding his head forward in a "sniffing position." Which of the following findings on radiography would help you confirm your diagnosis?

A. Thumb sign
B. Narrowed vallecula
C. Increased opacity of the larynx
D. All of the above

38. A 3-year-old female presents to the ED at 0300 with her mother complaining of a loud barking cough. She is well-appearing and generally asymptomatic at rest. She has a fever. Her chest radiograph is shown in Figure 7.11. The most common cause of this condition is:

A. Diphtheria
B. Parainfluenza
C. Influenza
D. Respiratory syncytial virus (RSV)

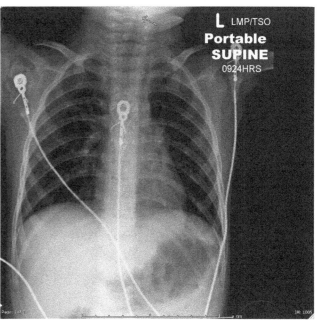

Figure 7.11 Chest radiograph.

39. The treatment of choice for a 3-year-old child with croup is:

A. Solumedrol
B. Dexamethasone
C. Prednisone
D. Azithromycin

40. Which of the following is the most common cause of Ludwig's angina?

A. Otitis media
B. Peritonsillar abscess
C. Submandibular sialadenitis
D. Dental disease

41. A 33-year-old male presents with fever, sore throat, and odynophagia with intermittent gagging sensation. Physical exam reveals pharyngitis and an enlarged, edematous uvula with an accentuated gag reflex (Figure 7.12). The most common bacterial etiology associated with this finding is:

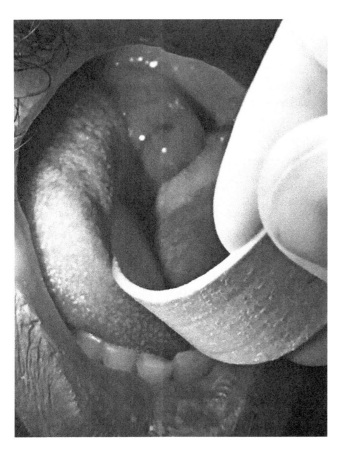

Figure 7.12 Posterior pharynx.

A. *H. influenzae* type b
B. Group A *Streptococcus*
C. *S. pneumoniae*
D. *Fusobacterium nucleatum*

42. A 33-year-old male presents with fever, sore throat, and odynophagia with intermittent gagging sensation. Physical exam reveals pharyngitis with a very red post pharynx and an enlarged, edematous uvula with an

accentuated gag reflex. What is the best treatment for this patient?

A. Antibiotics
B. Aggressive airway management including uvular amputation or decompression
C. Lateral neck radiograph
D. Antihistamines and steroids

43. A 35-year-old male presents with a muffled voice, trismus, fever, and sore throat. Physical exam reveals right-sided peritonsillar swelling. Bedside intraoral ultrasound shows an abscess cavity approximately 1.5 cm in depth from the surface. While setting up for I&D of the abscess you recall the internal carotid artery's depth from the tonsil is:

A. 1.5 cm
B. 2 cm
C. 2.5 cm
D. 3 cm

44. A 4-year-old male presents to the ED complaining of progressive neck pain for 2 weeks with a change in his voice. Physical exam reveals trismus, fever, and a muffled voice. The child will not look up. Which of these prevertebral measurements would make you mostly suspect a retropharyngeal abscess based off of a soft tissue neck radiograph?

A. 7.5 mm at C2
B. 7.5 mm at C6
C. 17 cm at C6
D. 17.5 cm at C6

45. You decide that the patient's soft tissue radiograph is unremarkable measuring 7 mm at C2 and 17 cm at C6. The patient appears stable, with improvement of pain after analgesia and improved temperature after antipyretics. The next imaging modality of choice would be:

A. Repeat soft tissue neck radiograph
B. Neck CT with IV contrast
C. Neck CT without contrast
D. Neck MRI

46. A 17-year-old male is punched at school and has an avulsed tooth. Which of the following is the best choice of storage medium for the avulsed tooth while the patient travels from school to the ED?

A. Saline
B. Hank's Balanced Salt Solution (HBSS)
C. Milk
D. Saliva

47. A 55-year-old diabetic male comes in to the ED with 2 days of mouth pain and foul-smelling breath. He is afebrile and well-appearing. The physical exam of the patients' mouth shows gum bleeding and ulcerations (Figure 7.13). What is the recommended treatment for this condition?

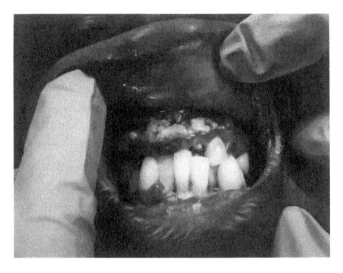

Figure 7.13 Mouth.

A. Urgent dental consult
B. IV antibiotics and admission
C. Chlorhexidine rinse
D. Magic mouthwash

48. A 65-year male is sent in to the ED by his primary care doctor for diabetic ketoacidosis. He is seen in your high-acuity area and appears ill. He is breathing rapidly, his labs show a pH of 7.1, sugar >500, and ketones in the urine. IV fluids and an insulin drip are started. On physical exam, you notice a well-developed male with dry mucous membranes and Kussmaul breathing. On examination of the eye, you notice a proptotic right eye that is immobile, and the pupil is fixed in size. On further questioning, the patient states his eye started like this 1 day ago and his vision has been blurry with only light/dark perception for 1 day. CT scan of the head and orbits is normal. What is the most likely causative organism for this patient's eye infection?

A. Streptococcal infection
B. Methicillin-resistant *S. aureus* (MRSA)
C. Mucor
D. Candidal infection

ANSWERS

1. ANSWER: B

The question addresses the management of ocular chemical exposure. The severity of a chemical burn is dependent on the chemical involved, exposure duration, and depth of penetration. Severity of the burn is also dependent on the strength of the chemical involved because commercial-strength products are often less concentrated than industrial-strength products. Acidic chemicals (toilet bowl cleaner, grout cleaner, rust remover, glass etching agents, car battery fluid) cause coagulation necrosis, which can result in corneal scarring. Alkaline chemicals (ammonia, bleach, fertilizers, hair dyes, dishwasher detergent) cause liquefication necrosis and are often more severe than acidic burns because of saponification of cellular phospholipid membranes. Depending on strength and exposure length of the offending agent, prolonged management may be necessary. Management involves irrigating the ocular membranes to achieve a neutral pH between 7 and 7.3 with water or isotonic saline. It should be noted that exposures to dry lime (calcium oxide), elemental metals, and phenol (carbolic acid) require different management and should not be immediately irrigated. When irrigating, complete eyelid retraction is essential, and this is best achieved with a polymethylmethacrylate scleral lens. Proparacaine may be necessary for symptomatic relief before irrigation. Although the patient in this question has a normal ocular pH (between 7 and 7.5), irrigation and pain management are warranted because the patient is symptomatic without intervention.

Test-taking tip: The key to this question is that the patient is still having severe eye pain. With any chemical exposure to the eyes, copious amounts of irrigation are needed until the pH is normal. You can exclude A and D right away because irrigation is not part of the answer choice.

2. ANSWER: B

Herpes zoster ophthalmicus is a serious sight-threatening condition. At least 50% of patients with dermatomal involvement of the frontal trigeminal nerve branch will have ocular involvement. Nearly two-thirds of patients will have physical exam findings diagnostic of herpes zoster ophthalmicus, including punctate or dendritic lesions on slit lamp examination. Hutchinson's sign (vesicular lesions on the nose) indicates involvement of the nasociliary nerve, which innervates the globe. This patient does not display Hutchison's sign. In immunocompromised patients, rapid detection and treatment with IV acyclovir is crucial. Additional treatment with corticosteroids and diazepam is recommended for Ramsay Hunt syndrome, which may present with vertigo and vesicular lesions in the ear canal and auricle.

Test-taking tip: This question is asking for the management of herpes ophthalmicus. All answer choices include acyclovir. You can narrow the answers down to two (B and D) because with a positive slit lamp examination with dendritic lesions, admission is needed for IV acyclovir and an ophthalmology consult.

3. ANSWER: D

This particular case represents an ophthalmologic emergency with a sight-threatening condition. The following list addresses the differential diagnoses for a patient with painless monocular vision loss:

1. **Retinal detachment:** gradual-onset unilateral blurred vision, painless, associated with spots in vision occurring after light perception decreases. Ocular ultrasound will show a detached retina as seen in Figure 7.3. This is the most likely cause of the patient's symptoms. Macula-off retinal detachment is associated with a worse prognosis for return of vision after surgical intervention.
2. **Central retinal artery occlusion**: retinal ischemia leads to unilateral painless vision loss. Patients may present with an afferent pupillary light defect on physical examination (i.e., no pupillary constriction with direct and consensual light in the affected eye). Retinal infarction usually causes irreparable damage if blood flow is not restored within 90 minutes.
3. **Complete or incomplete lens dislocation (subluxation)**: occurs with trauma or with underlying connective tissue disorders. Lens subluxation can lead to glaucoma or uveitis.

Test-taking tip: The image shown in Figure 7.3 is an ultrasound of the eye with a flap showing a retinal detachment. If you recognize this image, you can immediately narrow your answers down to C and D.

4. ANSWER: A

This question addresses the differential diagnosis for sudden onset of painful vision loss and an abnormal pupil exam. The information essential to make a diagnosis is worsening of the patient's symptoms with consensual light in the unaffected eye. Pain in the effected eye with consensual light in the unaffected eye is highly suggestive for iritis. Anatomically, the uvea includes the iris, ciliary body, and choroid, so uveitis is the general diagnosis for inflammation of the anterior segment of the uveal tract.

Managing inflammation in uveitis/iritis consists of a long-acting cycloplegic agent (to reduce pupillary sphincter action and further irritation) and 24-hour follow-up with ophthalmology.

Test-taking tip: Classically, the pupillary exam in acute angle closure glaucoma is described as fixed and mid-position in the affected eye with a steamy cornea, so with normal eye pressures you can exclude B. Physical exam findings in the question do not describe the afferent pupillary defect found in patients with optic neuritis or central retinal artery occlusion (C and D).

5. ANSWER: B

Lens dislocation or subluxation most commonly occurs following traumatic injury to the orbit, and symptoms include vision loss and pain in the injured eye. While lens dislocation requires ophthalmologic referral for surgical repair, emergent ophthalmologic consultation is necessary when IOP is elevated, which can progress to optic neuropathy. Anterior subluxation of the lens can cause pupillary block, an obstruction in aqueous humor flow, and subsequently increased IOP.

Test-taking tip: The question is asking about conditions that need *emergent* ophthalmology consult. You can eliminate C and D right away because those are both pretty benign conditions.

6. ANSWER: B

This particular case assesses fundoscopic examination finding recognition in an ophthalmologic emergency with a sight-threatening condition. In painless monocular vision loss, the differential diagnoses include retinal detachment, central retinal artery occlusion, and lens dislocation. The patient's symptoms are sudden in onset without any reported history of trauma. Additionally, the patient has underlying medical conditions that increase the risk for retinal artery occlusion.

Central retinal artery occlusion is a sight-threatening emergency, which can result in permanent monocular blindness if treatment is not started within 90 minutes. Treatment options focus on restoring blood flow to the retina and include ocular massage and reducing IOP.

Fundoscopic examination can be helpful in distinguishing retinal artery occlusion (optic disc pallor, cherry-red macula) from retinal vein occlusion (dilated and tortuous veins, retinal and macular edema). Retinal hemorrhages may also be associated with retinal vein

occlusion; however, they can also be associated with giant cell arteritis, hypertension, or diabetes. Cloudy vitreous or vitreous exudate is classically associated with uveitis, which typically presents as painful vision loss.

Test-taking tip: This is a "you know it or don't" kind of question. If you don't know it, choose an answer and move on. You can perhaps mark it for review when you are done at the end of the test. Don't, however, let these kinds of questions get you stuck and waste your time.

7. ANSWER: C

This question addresses the differential diagnosis for sudden onset of painful vision loss and selecting history or physical examination findings consistent with uveitis. Anatomically, the uvea is the iris, ciliary body, and choroid. Inflammation of these structures is referred to as uveitis. Physical exam findings associated with uveitis include ciliary injection, pupillary constriction, and normal ocular pressure. On slit lamp examination, you will see flare ("smoke in a projector beam"); this is the protein in the fluid. Choice A refers to temporal arteritis, which is more common in patients 50 years or older but can present with painful monocular vision loss and an elevated erythrocyte sedimentation rate. Choice B, increased IOP, is associated with acute angle closure glaucoma. Choice D refers to risk factors associated with cerebral venous sinus thrombosis, which can present with neurologic deficits and headache.

Test-taking tip: This is asking about painful monocular vision loss with a normal IOP. You can eliminate B and D easily and narrow down the choices because choice B shows high IOP and choice D (preeclampsia) has no association with the eye.

8. ANSWER: D

This question is concerning for sudden onset of eye pain and loss of vision and a potential ocular foreign body. It is critical to recognize globe rupture and penetrating foreign bodies because these require emergent ophthalmologic consultation, and further medical interventions may worsen ocular damage. An initial physical examination should include visualization for signs of trauma in the orbit and eye. Extruding aqueous humor (Seidel's test), prolapsed internal ocular structures, afferent pupillary defect, and tenting at the site of puncture are findings that, if visualized, raise the suspicion for a globe rupture, and further interventions that increase IOP should be avoided (including topical medication administration, eyelid inversion, and tonometry). This patient, however, has a physical exam more consistent with a corneal abrasion. There is a generous amount of fluorescein uptake, likely indicating damage caused by the chemical contents that line the surface of many household light bulbs.

Test-taking tip: You can eliminate B because you cannot easily visualize a hyphema with fluorescein. You can also eliminate A because there is no mention of an irregular pupil.

9. ANSWER: B

The differential diagnoses for painful monocular vision loss should include acute glaucoma, iritis, uveitis, periorbital or orbital cellulitis, and temporal arteritis. Giant cell arteritis is an inflammatory condition of medium-sized arteries. Temporal headache, eye pain, and vision loss can be manifesting symptoms when the temporal artery is involved. The condition is more common in individuals 50 years or older and in individuals with a past medical history of polymyalgia rheumatica. The definitive diagnosis is made with temporal artery biopsy, but laboratory abnormalities may include elevated erythrocyte sedimentation rate and anemia (normal laboratory values do not exclude temporal arteritis). Corticosteroids are indicated in the treatment of temporal arteritis. Acetazolamide would be indicated if the patient had acute angle closure glaucoma.

Test-taking tip: There are certain conditions that predispose to other conditions. When you hear of polymyalgia rheumatica with an eye complaint, think temporal arteritis.

10. ANSWER: B

The question addresses slit lamp examination findings for a patient with recent high-intensity light exposure. Welding without protective eyewear is a risk factor for actinic keratitis (snow blindness, flash burn, welder's arch burn), a condition caused by ultraviolet damage to the conjunctiva. Chronic ultraviolet exposure can lead to actinic keratitis, particularly in individuals who spend prolonged periods in sunlight without protective eyewear. Slit lamp examination of actinic keratitis usually shows diffuse punctate abrasions, although this finding may not present until 6 to 12 hours after the initial exposure. This particular patient may routinely weld without protective eyewear, and slit lamp findings are present from previous ultraviolet exposure. Focal punctate abrasions are more consistent with corneal abrasion. Dendritic lesions are more consistent with herpes zoster.

Test-taking tip: This is a "you know it or don't" kind of question. If you don't know it, choose an answer and move on. You can perhaps mark it for review when you are done

at the end of the test. Don't, however, let these kinds of questions get you stuck and waste your time.

11. ANSWER: C

It is critical to recognize ocular globe rupture because this condition requires emergent ophthalmologic consultation and further medical interventions may worsen ocular damage. High-velocity projectiles, blunt ocular impact, and penetrating trauma are commonly associated with open globe injuries. An initial physical examination should include visualization for signs of trauma at the orbit and eye. Extruding aqueous humor (Seidel's test), prolapsed internal ocular structures, afferent pupillary defect, and tenting at site of puncture are findings that, if visualized, raise the suspicion for a globe rupture. With patients for whom you have a high suspicion, any interventions that increase IOP should be avoided (including topical medication administration, eyelid inversion, and tonometry). Treatment should focus on treating pain through nonocular administration routes, tetanus, antibiotic prophylaxis, and emergent ophthalmology consultation.

Test-taking tip: You can eliminate answers A, C, and D because they all can increase IOP, and if you suspect a globe rupture, these tests can make the rupture worse.

12. ANSWER: D

Periorbital cellulitis and orbital cellulitis are infections of the preseptal and septal soft tissues, respectively. They are typically caused by *S. aureus, S. pneumoniae, H. influenzae,* and anaerobes. Most commonly, periorbital cellulitis and orbital cellulitis are preceded by local skin trauma or sinus infections. It can be difficult to distinguish between the diseases because they both present with severe eye pain, warmth, redness, and swelling. Identifying anatomic location of the infection is essential for diagnosis and management. Periorbital cellulitis does not extend past the orbital septum.

Orbital cellulitis, an infection posterior to the orbital septum, can cause a variety of symptoms and physical exam findings, including unilateral proptosis and/or increased IOP, visual acuity defects (secondary to increased pressure on the optic nerve), pain with eye movement, and unilaterally decreased sensation of the face (secondary to involvement of the ophthalmic and maxillary branches of the trigeminal nerve). While early periorbital cellulitis can be managed with outpatient antibiotics, it is recommended that patients with periorbital cellulitis and orbital cellulitis be admitted for IV antibiotics.

Test-taking tip: This is a "you know it or don't" kind of question. If you don't know it, choose an answer and move on. You can perhaps mark it for review when you are done at the end of the test. Don't, however, let these kinds of questions get you stuck and waste your time.

13. ANSWER: A

This question refers to the recognition and management of periorbital cellulitis. Periorbital cellulitis is a soft tissue infection anterior to the orbital septum. Orbital cellulitis, an infection posterior to the orbital septum, can cause a variety of symptoms and physical exam findings, none of which are consistent with this patient's presentation. This patient may be treated in the outpatient setting with PO antibiotics and strict return precautions. If the patient presented with any symptoms concerning for orbital cellulitis, it would be prudent to consider hospital admission, IV antibiotics, and advanced imaging of the orbit and/or sinuses. Advanced imaging can help to distinguish the extent of the infection (preseptal vs. septal) and the need for ophthalmology consultation.

Test-taking tip: You can eliminate C and D and narrow your choices because this is *not* orbital cellulitis. The hint of no pain with extraocular movements is key to the diagnosis.

14. ANSWER: A

Traumatic iritis occurs after blunt trauma to the eye. Iritis can also occur in patients with autoimmune diseases, especially diseases related to HLA-B27. The diagnosis is made with the clinical symptoms of unilateral eye pain with a painful red eye. There is usually blurry vision present with direct and consensual photophobia.

IOP can be normal or low. If IOPs are high (>20) you need to consider the diagnosis of glaucoma. On slit lamp examination, you can see flare. Flare is protein in the fluid that looks like "smoke in a projector beam."

Treatment is ophthalmology consult and usually steroid drops.

Test-taking tip: Consensual photophobia is the key to the diagnosis of Iritis.

15. ANSWER: C

The goal of this question is to distinguish the symptoms and physical exam findings of viral conjunctivitis from bacterial and allergic conjunctivitis. Red flags for bacterial conjunctivitis include mucopurulent discharge in addition to pruritis and redness. Drainage from viral and bacterial conjunctivitis can cause crusting or sticking of the eyelids.

Viral and allergic conjunctivitis can both present with bilateral colorless or watery discharge and can be preceded by upper respiratory symptoms. This patient presents with ocular symptoms preceded by an upper respiratory infection (URI). Her symptoms are most likely viral in etiology because she does not present with any history of seasonal allergies, has no mucopurulent discharge, and does not complain of eye pain or pruritus.

Test-taking tip: The hint of bilateral eye involvement preceded by a URI should help you choose C.

16. ANSWER: C

The goals of this question are to distinguish the symptoms and physical exam findings of bacterial conjunctivitis from allergic and viral conjunctivitis and to identify appropriate management considering the patient's use of contact lenses. Red flags for bacterial conjunctivitis include mucopurulent discharge in addition to pruritis and redness. Drainage from viral and bacterial conjunctivitis can also cause crusting or sticking of the eyelids. There is no information in the question to increase suspicion of gonococcal or chlamydial sources of infection, and further diagnostic testing or empiric treatment for these pathogens would not be warranted. Polymyxin B/trimethoprim eye drops are usually adequate for the management of bacterial conjunctivitis, but a fluoroquinolone is necessary to cover *Pseudomonas* in patients who wear contact lenses or have a history of diabetes.

Test-taking tip: The hint of unilateral eye involvement with discharge helps steer you to the diagnosis of bacterial conjunctivitis. You can then eliminate A and B and narrow down your choices.

17. ANSWER: A

This question relates to the diagnosis and management of acute angle closure glaucoma. Visual acuity deficits are sudden and caused by compression of the optic nerve by increased IOP. Patients may not always complain of eye pain. In glaucoma, IOP is increased because of abnormal outflow of aqueous humor, aqueous humor production, and/or aqueous humor volume. The mainstays of treatment in the acute setting are to consult ophthalmology and to correct the underlying processes that increase IOP and subsequent optic neuropathy.

Pilocarpine is a miotic agent that causes pupillary constriction and improved outflow of aqueous humor. Inhibiting humor production is achieved with either timolol 0.5%, a β-blocker, or with acetazolamide, a carbonic anhydrase inhibitor. Finally, reducing aqueous and vitreous humor volume is achieved with IV mannitol, which works to draw water out of the aqueous or vitreous humor. While institutional medication preferences will differ, the immediate treatment of acute angle closure glaucoma is to reduce IOP and consult ophthalmology.

Test-taking tip: All of the listed choices need to be done. However, consultation of ophthalmology needs to occur first.

18. ANSWER: D

Unilateral painful vision loss and afferent pupillary defect in a young female should raise the suspicion of optic neuritis as the initial presentation of multiple sclerosis. Optic neuritis is inflammation of the optic nerve, which can lead to visual acuity deficits as well as pain with eye movements. Optic neuritis is the initial presentation for 25% of individuals diagnosed with multiple sclerosis. The etiology of optic neuritis includes sarcoidosis, systemic lupus erythematosus, alcohol abuse, and infectious causes such as Lyme disease, syphilis, or meningitis.

Test-taking tip: You can eliminate B because there is no redness or swelling around the eye and A because the patient is young and has no temporal headache.

19. ANSWER: B

The goal of this question is to select the appropriate diagnosis among the differential for eyelid inflammation and skin lesions. Hordeolums are typically localized red, swollen, and tender skin lesions of the internal or external eyelid that most commonly arise from a staphylococcal infection of the meibomian glands. While chalazions may have a similar red appearance and often arise from granulomatous inflammation of a hordeolum, they are typically firm and not tender to palpation. The common way to distinguish hordeolum from chalazion is that hordeolums hurt. Management of these two skin lesions is also different: hordeolums may be treated conservatively with warm compresses but may need incision and drainage, and chalazions may need incision and curettage or steroid injection. Blepharitis is usually a chronic condition presenting with a spectrum of inflammatory symptoms and findings at the eyelid margins related to seborrheic glands (anterior blepharitis) or meibomian glands (posterior blepharitis). Signs and symptoms include burning pain and pruritis, red and scaly eyelids, and bilateral eyelid involvement. Treatment for blepharitis is usually conservative with warm compresses and/or baby shampoo to remove glandular debris, but suspicion for bacterial infection or inflammation extending beyond the eyelid margins warrants antibiotic treatment or additional evaluation if there is preseptal or septal involvement.

Test-taking tip: Brush up on the differences in common benign infections of the eyelids.

20. ANSWER: C

The goal of this question is to identify the diagnosis of hordeolum and select the most appropriate management option. The picture shows a hordeolum, which is typically a localized red, swollen, and tender skin lesion of the internal or external eyelid that most commonly arises from a staphylococcal infection of the meibomian glands. While chalazions may have a similar red appearance and often arise from granulomatous inflammation of a hordeolum, they are typically firm and not tender to palpation. The common way to distinguish hordeolum from chalazion is that hordeolums hurt.

This patient does not have vital signs or physical exam findings concerning for periorbital or orbital cellulitis. Conservative management of hordeolums is appropriate, but this patient has already used conservative treatment at home in the past 48 hours. I&D is appropriate, and additional treatment with outpatient antibiotics may be warranted.

Test-taking tip: Brush up on the differences in common benign infections of the eyelids.

21. ANSWER: B

This question concerns eyelid lacerations and the need for surgical consultation. The evaluation of patients with penetrating eyelid trauma should include a thorough search for foreign body, globe rupture, or damage to the orbit, lacrimal glands, and canaliculi. Deep lacerations through the eyelid margin require careful reapproximation when repaired with sutures, especially if the anatomic "gray line" is damaged. Consultation is necessary when there is clinical suspicion for injury of the lacrimal gland or medial canthal ligament (lacerations of the medial one-third of the eyelid or tearing), canthal ligament support (sometimes subtle rounding or widening of the eyelid margins), orbital septum (adipose tissue observed within the eyelid laceration), levator palpebrae superioris (ptosis of the eye), or supraorbital nerve (decreased sensation of the forehead on the side of injury).

Test-taking tip You can eliminate C because the patient has a normal pupil with no injury to the eyeball.

22. ANSWER: A

Figure 7.8 shows a picture of auricular perichondritis. This is infection and inflammation of the perichondrium.

It usually involves infection of the pinna. It presents as a painful, red, swollen pinna. The most likely causative organism is *Pseudomonas aeruginosa*. Because cartilage has poor blood supply, separation of the perichondrium from the cartilage can lead to avascular necrosis and a deformed ear ("cauliflower ear") in a short time. Rapid diagnosis and treatment are key.

Diabetes and immune suppression put patients at increased risk for this infection. Treatment is admission with IV antibiotics to cover both gram-negative and gram-positive organisms and to cover *Pseudomonas* (e.g., ciprofloxacin or piperacillin-tazobactam).

Test-taking tip: You can eliminate B and C because discharge home is not an option with this ear infection. That helps narrow your choices down by half.

23. ANSWER: B

This question concerns the presentation of ocular symptoms in an infant with no neonatal or maternal prenatal care. In the absence of prenatal testing, there should be increased suspicion for infectious etiologies, including *C. trachomatis, Neisseria gonorrhoeae,* and herpes simplex virus. The diagnosis of the patient in this question is ophthalmia neonatorium, or conjunctivitis in the newborn, which presents in the first month of life and is most commonly caused by *C. trachomatis* in developed countries.

Pediatric and ophthalmology consultation is highly recommended for this patient. Topical treatment with silver nitrate or antibiotic drops is not effective, and empiric treatment with oral erythromycin is recommended. Definitive diagnosis can be made by collecting a sample of the discharge for Gram stain, polymerase chain reaction amplification, and viral cultures.

Test-taking tip: Conjunctivitis in the neonate is *Chlamydia* until proved otherwise.

24. ANSWER: C

Otitis externa, also known as "swimmer's ear," is an inflammatory process that affects the external ear canal. Moisture and trauma can erode the skin/cerumen barrier of the external canal, allowing a local inflammatory process to ensue.

Acetic acid is a reasonable treatment option for mild otitis externa. This patient is presenting with moderate disease as evident with the moderate degree of pain, swelling, and discharge. Cortisporin is an otic suspension consisting of neomycin, polymyxin B sulfates, and hydrocortisone. Neomycin is an aminoglycoside and is known to be ototoxic and not recommended in the setting of tympanic membrane perforations. Despite the cost limitations associated with

fluoroquinolone otic preparations, they have excellent coverage against gram-negative and gram-positive organisms, including excellent coverage against *P. aeruginosa*. One must take into account appropriate antibiotic stewardship to minimize risk for resistance. The potential side effect of cartilaginous damage among pediatric patients is not a concern with topical preparations given there is no systemic absorption. Cipro HC Otic is contraindicated in the setting of a tympanic membrane perforation because its preparation yields a nonsterile product.

Test-taking tip: This is a "you know it or don't" kind of question. If you don't know it, choose an answer and move on. You can perhaps mark it for review when you are done at the end of the test. Don't, however, let these kinds of questions get you stuck and waste your time.

25. ANSWER: D

Staphylococcus, Streptococcus, Corynebacterium, and *Pseudomonas* organisms have all been described to naturally be present as normal otic flora. *H. influenzae* is a gram-negative coccobacillus found mainly in the respiratory system. Its prevalence has decreased in populations for which vaccination for this organism has been implemented.

Test-taking tip: This is a "you know it or don't" kind of question. If you don't know it, choose an answer and move on. You can perhaps mark it for review when you are done at the end of the test. Don't, however, let these kinds of questions get you stuck and waste your time.

26. ANSWER: A

AOM is a frequent infection in children and becomes less frequent in adults. *S. pneumoniae* and *H. influenzae* have been shown to account for more than 50% of AOM cases. Because *H. influenzae* is not listed as a possible answer, *S. pneumoniae* is the best answer.

Test-taking tip: This is a "you know it or don't" kind of question. If you don't know it, choose an answer and move on. You can perhaps mark it for review when you are done at the end of the test. Don't, however, let these kinds of questions get you stuck and waste your time.

27. ANSWER: A

The child in the question stem has conjunctivitis-otitis syndrome (COS). *H. influenzae* is the most common cause of COS. Concurrent otitis media has been reported in up to 73% of patients who had purulent conjunctivitis, of which

60% of patients did not complain of ear pain. Treatment for these patients consists of systemic coverage against β-lactamase producing organisms.

AOM is a frequent infection in children and becomes less frequent in adults. *S. pneumoniae* and *H. influenzae* have been shown to account for more than 50% of AOM cases.

Given decades of success and coverage against *S. pneumoniae, H. influenza,* and *M. catarrhalis,* amoxicillin is the initial medication of choice for both children and adults with AOM. The American Academy of Pediatrics 2013 guidelines for diagnosis and management of AOM allow for 48- to 72-hour observation versus immediate treatment in patients between 6 months and 2 years old.

Test-taking tip: You can eliminate C because *Chlamydia* is a sexually transmitted disease and not usually found in an ear.

28. ANSWER: A

Acute auricular hematoma of the pinna is common after blunt trauma to the ear whereby a collection of blood forms beneath the perichondrial layer of the pinna (Figure 7.14). If untreated it will ultimately result in a deformity of the ear

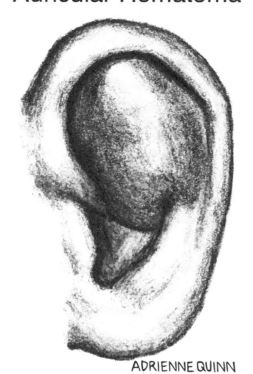

Auricular Hematoma

ADRIENNE QUINN

Figure 7.14 Auricular hematoma.

commonly known as "cauliflower ear." Various treatments including needle aspiration and scalpel I&D are employed to relieve the hematoma, but no clear consensus exists on the best way to do so in order to produce the best cosmetic result with the least permanent deformity. However, there is consensus that the hematoma does need to be drained.

Test-taking tip: You can eliminate D because the hematoma is not infected, and you can eliminate C because drainage of the hematoma is needed. This narrows your options down by two.

29. ANSWER: C

Aural foreign bodies commonly present to the ED. Organic foreign bodies are known to swell when irrigated with water, which may cause inflammation. Popcorn kernels have been studied and found to *not* swell sufficiently to lodge tightly in an ear canal of patients younger than 1 year. Other organic foreign bodies have been shown to have a substantial increase in size when in a moist environment. The use of isopropyl alcohol and water has been shown to result in more rapid evaporation, decreasing subsequent swelling and facilitating further extraction attempts. Irrigation is useful for small foreign bodies near the tympanic membrane and for smooth, round objects difficult to grasp. Multiple methods of foreign body retrieval are available, such as irrigation, suction, forceps, loops, and hooks. Consideration of which technique to use should take into account the shape, size, and position of the foreign body within the ear while trying to avoid potential complications.

Test-taking tip: This is a "you know it or don't" kind of question. If you don't know it, choose an answer and move on. You can perhaps mark it for review when you are done at the end of the test. Don't, however, let these kinds of questions get you stuck and waste your time.

30. ANSWER: D

Sudden sensorineural hearing loss as an otologic emergency. All of the answer choices are possible causes of sudden sensorineural hearing loss. Idiopathic hearing loss is "loss of hearing of 30 dB over three test frequencies within 3 days." The association between pregnancy and hearing loss has been described, but the exact mechanism for its occurrence is not understood. It has been hypothesized that it is associated with increased activation of both blood coagulation and fibrinolysis ("hypercoagulable state"), which occurs during normal pregnancy. Hormonal dysfunction, otosclerosis, changes in the cardiovascular/endocrine system, and fluid regulation, which can affect the circulation of cochlear fluid, have also been suggested as mechanisms.

Test-taking tip: This is a "you know it or don't" kind of question. If you don't know it, choose an answer and move on. You can perhaps mark it for review when you are done at the end of the test. Don't, however, let these kinds of questions get you stuck and waste your time.

31. ANSWER: B

With the incidence of nosebleed being 11% annually and with 6% of people seeking medical care, epistaxis is a common presentation to the ED. Myriad of options are available to providers in dealing with epistaxis. These include inflatable balloons, gauze packing on a string, and others. The big difference in packing is whether it is placed in the anterior nares or in the posterior nasopharynx.

Patients who require posterior packing (Figure 7.15) should be admitted to the hospital because of the risk for airway obstruction and subsequent hypoxemia and dysrhythmias and antibiotics should be given to prevent toxic shock syndrome, sinusitis, or nasopharyngitis. Antibiotics can include ceftriaxone, clindamycin, or Unasyn.

Admission is needed for posterior packing to monitor pulse oximetry and respirations. Patients may have respiratory difficulty because of the nasopulmonary reflex. Anterior packing does *not* require admission or antibiotics.

Test-taking tip: You can eliminate C and D because discharge is not an option after posterior packing is placed.

32. ANSWER: A

In the CT scan you see a nasal fracture with a collection of fluid in the nares. Septal hematomas appear as a purple to bluish mass on the septal surface of the nose and can be present unilaterally or bilaterally. Because of the potential for necrosis of the septal cartilage yielding asymmetry and/or a deformity of the nose, once identified they must be urgently drained. Pooled blood within the hematoma and moist environment of the nose is a potential for formation of an infection. One must also consider opening a hematoma in the setting of a nasal fracture might render it an open fracture, in which case antibiotics may be warranted.

Although a relatively rare injury, it is an important one to recognize because it can lead to significant morbidity, including abscesses, septal perforation, or saddle nose deformity if left untreated.

Given the potential morbidity of a septal hematoma, immediate treatment in the ED with I&D is the correct answer rather than referral to an ENT, which might lead to delay in care and complications.

Nasal packing is not indicated in septal hematoma but rather is used in epistaxis that cannot be managed by less invasive treatment (e.g., direct pressure, topical agents).

Test-taking tip: Try to eliminate the answers that are most likely incorrect, such as nasal packing (not used in this setting) and IV antibiotics (not usually indicated because no infection yet). This leaves you with an answer that requires action in the ED versus one that results in delay of care. Action in the ED will usually win out as the correct answer.

33. ANSWER: C

D-dimer does not rule out cerebral venous thrombosis. MRI/MRV is the imaging technique of choice for diagnosing and following up cavernous sinus thrombosis. CT venography appears to be a reasonable alternative to MRI/MRV if unable to obtain MRI/MRV and may have

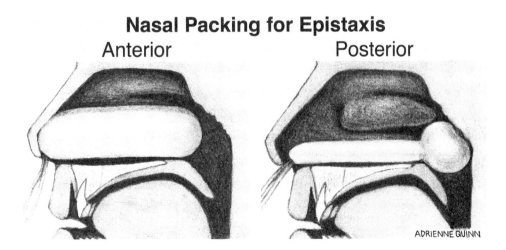

Figure 7.15 Nasal packing for epistaxis.

similar sensitivity. Noncontrast CT has no role in the evaluation or diagnosis of cavernous sinus thrombosis.

Veins afferent to the cavernous sinus drain the anterior face, nasal cavity, orbit, eye, paranasal sinuses, middle ear, mastoid region, cerebral cortex, and pituitary. It is usually a complication from a facial infection. It presents with nonspecific symptoms like headache, fever, and malaise but then can progress to a painful red eye or exophthalmos and facial edema.

MRI/MRV is the diagnostic test of choice.

Test-taking tip: This is a "you know it or don't" kind of question. If you don't know it, choose an answer and move on. You can perhaps mark it for review when you are done at the end of the test. Don't, however, let these kinds of questions get you stuck and waste your time.

34. ANSWER: D

Each of the answer choices are known causes of sialadenitis. Cat-scratch disease is caused by *Bartonella henselae*, is self-limited, and can involve the intraparotid lymph nodes and mimic a salivary gland tumor. IgG4-RS (Related Sialadenitis) is a systemic disease that is characterized by infiltration of IgG4-positive plasma cells and lymphocytes and is associated with fibrosis. CJRP is "10 times more common than adult chronic parotitis and mainly affects children 3–6 years old." Other causes include bacterial, viral, obstructive, lymphoepithelial, granulomatous, and post-treatment sialadenitis.

Test-taking tip: This is a "you know it or don't" kind of question. If you don't know it, choose an answer and move on. You can perhaps mark it for review when you are done at the end of the test. Don't, however, let these kinds of questions get you stuck and waste your time.

35. ANSWER: C

Technically, a complication can happen at any time, but there are three clinical stages that are present in both aspiration and ingestion of foreign bodies. The first stage is known as the initial stage and may present with choking, gagging, and episodes of coughing. This stage subsides, yielding to the second stage, also known as the asymptomatic phase, when cough/gag reflexes subside. Complications often occur within the third stage, also known as the complications stage, when one may see obstruction, erosion, infection, or perforation. These clinical stages illustrate the point that although a patient may be asymptomatic, aspiration and/or ingestion of a foreign body may still be present. Once the provider has recognized that a foreign body is within the airway, measures must be immediately put into place to retrieve the foreign body and secure the airway as needed.

Test-taking tip: You can eliminate D because there is no such thing as a fourth stage.

36. ANSWER: B

The foreign body (earring) seen in this radiograph is located above the hyoid bone, suggesting that it is likely in the vallecula, making bronchoscopy unnecessary at this time and direct visualization with a tongue blade less likely. You may be able to retrieve this foreign body with just a laryngoscope. However, video-assisted guidance has the advantages of good illumination, clear visualization, and precise extraction and is safe and generally well tolerated with a low morbidity rate.

Test-taking tip: You can eliminate A and D because bronchoscopy is not necessary with the foreign body above the hyoid. This narrows your choices down by two.

37. ANSWER: D

Each choice is a finding on radiograph in the setting of acute epiglottitis. This is a condition in which cellulitis of the epiglottis and adjacent tissues are present, which can rapidly become life-threatening because of compromise of the airway.

Epiglottis is an acute, life-threatening upper airway disease. It is most common in children 3 to 8 years old. *H. influenzae* was the most common pathogen causing the disease. However, with the invention of the Hib vaccine in 1985, it has become a much rarer disease in children. Pathogens can be *S. pneumoniae* and *Klebsiella pneumoniae*.

Local bacterial invasion of the glottic mucosa occurs, causing edema to the area. Symptoms are usually acute in onset and progress rapidly. The airway needs to be secured with intubation before any testing or imaging.

Test-taking tip: Common head, ears, eyes, nose, and throat (HEENT) infections like epiglottis and croup are easily testable. Try to brush up on these infections before the exam.

38. ANSWER: B

Croup is most commonly caused by parainfluenza virus. Other viruses, such as influenza A and B, RSV, measles, and adenovirus are less common causes.

Before the availability of the diphtheria vaccine, croup was commonly caused by diphtheria and was often fatal. Various treatment options such as warm and cold humidified air, racemic epinephrine, and steroids have been debated over time. Corticosteroids are routinely recommended for patients, with single-dose dexamethasone 0.6 mg/kg being the most practical.

Test-taking tip: Common HEENT infections like epiglottis and croup are easily testable. Try to brush up on these infections before the exam.

39. ANSWER: B

Croup is most commonly caused by parainfluenza virus. Other viruses such as influenza A and B, RSV, measles, and adenovirus are also less common causes. Before availability of the diphtheria vaccine, croup was commonly caused by diphtheria and was often fatal. Various treatment options such as warm and cold humidified air, racemic epinephrine, and steroids have been debated over time. Corticosteroids are routinely recommended for patients, with single-dose PO or IM dexamethasone 0.6 mg/kg being the most practical.

Test-taking tip: Common HEENT infections like epiglottis and croup are easily testable. Try to brush up on these infections before the exam.

40. ANSWER: D

Dental disease can easily erode into the mandible and invade the submandibular space, thus making dental disease the most common cause of Ludwig's angina. Other causes of this type of infection include mandibular fractures, foreign bodies, lacerations, tongue piercings, traumatic intubations/bronchoscopy, secondary infections of oral malignancy, osteomyelitis, otitis media, submandibular sialadenitis, peritonsillar abscess, furuncles, and infected thyroglossal cyst.

Ludwig's angina is cellulitis of the floor of the mouth involving the submandibular space. It is a rare infection but more common in older adults and debilitated people. It can become an airway emergency because it involves the floor of the mouth. On exam, you can see upward displacement of the tongue and feel a hard edema of the floor of the mouth (Figure 7.16). Treatment is admission, IV antibiotics, early intubation, and emergent surgical consult.

Test-taking tip: You can eliminate A because this infection involves the floor of the mouth and not the ear.

41. ANSWER: B

Uvulitis can be a result of various etiologies that can broadly be classified as infectious versus noninfectious causes. With vaccination against *H. influenza* type b (Hib), group A *Streptococcus* is generally thought to be the most common bacterial cause of uvulitis. Other infectious causes include *S. pneumoniae, Fusobacterium nucleatum, Prevotella intermedia,* and *Candida* and *Mycobacterium* species. Noninfectious causes of uvulitis include angioedema, allergic reactions, vasculitis, trauma, and inhalation of irritants, such as smoking crack cocaine and cannabis.

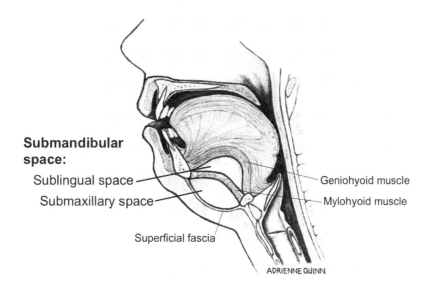

Figure 7.16 Ludwig's angina.

Edema of the uvula can occur in isolation or in conjunction of affected nearby counterparts. Management of the ABCs of emergency medicine should always be considered in the primary assessment of patients. Treatment should be directed at the causative agent of uvulitis when known. Antihistamines, epinephrine, steroids, fresh frozen plasma, purified C1E1, antibiotics, and surgical management have all be described as treatment options for uvulitis.

Test-taking tip: This is a "you know it or don't" kind of question. If you don't know it, choose an answer and move on. You can perhaps mark it for review when you are done at the end of the test. Don't, however, let these kinds of questions get you stuck and waste your time.

42. ANSWER: A

Edema of the uvula can occur in isolation or in conjunction with affected nearby counterparts. Treatment should be directed at the causative agent of uvulitis when known. Because this patient has fever and pharyngitis on exam, treatment should be aimed at the pharyngitis. Group A *Streptococcus* is the most common bacterial cause of uvulitis in the setting of pharyngitis.

Antihistamines, epinephrine, steroids, fresh frozen plasma, purified C1E1, antibiotics, and surgical management have all be described as treatment options for uvulitis.

Lateral neck radiographs may be warranted to exclude subclinical epiglottitis in patients with uvulitis without pharyngitis

Test-taking tip: You can eliminate B because the patient does not sound that sick in the question stem.

43. ANSWER: C

Peritonsillar abscess is most common among adults in their 20s and 30s. The internal carotid artery is situated approximately 2.5 cm posterolateral to the tonsil. Drainage of the peritonsillar abscess can be accomplished by needle aspiration or by I&D with a scalpel. False-negative needle aspiration can happen approximately 10% of the time. When suspected, despite a negative needle aspiration or I&D, patients should always be started on antibiotics to help treat peritonsillar cellulitis.

Test-taking tip: This is a "you know it or don't" kind of question. If you don't know it, choose an answer and move on. You can perhaps mark it for review when you are done at the end of the test. Don't, however, let these kinds of questions get you stuck and waste your time.

44. ANSWER: A

Retropharyngeal abscess is more common among pediatric patients than adults. The retropharyngeal space is found between the carotid sheaths, extending from the base of the skull to the mediastinum. In pediatric patients, distant infections seed lymph nodes in this region, which may induce liquefactive necrosis yielding cellulitis or as a result of direct trauma. In adults, this space becomes compromised by adjacent infections such as Ludwig's angina/dental infections or contaminated by direct trauma. When looking at soft tissue neck radiographs, normal prevertebral space should be less than 7 mm at C2, less than 14 mm at C6 in children, and less than 22 mm at C6 in adults. CT imaging of the neck has been reported to have sensitivity of more than 90% in confirming the diagnosis, but it is also thought to be only about 60% specific, often with difficulty distinguishing between a retropharyngeal abscess from cellulitis and lymphadenopathy or lymphadenitis. A patient's clinical condition guides management. One must always secure an airway when needed, but mild cases may often be managed with IV antibiotics and steroids.

Test-taking tip: This is a "you know it or don't" kind of question. If you don't know it, choose an answer and move on. You can perhaps mark it for review when you are done at the end of the test. Don't, however, let these kinds of questions get you stuck and waste your time.

45. ANSWER: B

Retropharyngeal abscess is more common among pediatric patients than adults. The retropharyngeal space is found between the carotid sheaths, extending from the base of the skull to the mediastinum. In pediatric patients distant infections seed lymph nodes in this region, which may induce liquefactive necrosis yielding cellulitis or as a result of direct trauma. In adults, this space becomes compromised by adjacent infections such as Ludwig's angina/dental infections or contaminated by direct trauma. When looking at soft tissue neck radiographs, normal prevertebral space should be less than 7 mm at C2, less than 14 mm at C6 in children, and less than 22 mm at C6 in adults. CT imaging of the neck has been reported to have sensitivity of more than 90% in confirming the diagnosis, but it is also thought to be only about 60% specific, often with difficulty distinguishing between a retropharyngeal abscess from cellulitis and lymphadenopathy or lymphadenitis. A patient's clinical condition guides management. One must always secure an airway when needed, but mild cases may often be managed with IV antibiotics and steroids.

CT scan of the neck with IV contrast is the imaging test of choice.

Test-taking tip: You can eliminate A because the radiograph is nonspecific to help determine whether the swelling is just inflammation or in fact an abscess.

46. ANSWER: C

Ideal storage medium is capable of maintaining periodontal ligament and pulp cell viability with compatible physiologic pH and osmolality, is readily accessible, and has low cost. With up to 94% cell viability in up to 24 hours of storage, HBSS is widely employed as a reference solution and has ideal properties to preserve viability of dental cells.

Saline has physiologic osmolality and pH, but it does not contain essential ions and glucose and, if used, is best used for less than 4 hours. Saliva is a contaminated media with various microbes and can cause rapid lysis of cell membranes. It also has pH and osmolality incompatible with dental cells.

Milk is an isotonic liquid with neutral pH and physiologic osmolality, has low to no bacterial content, contains growth factors and essential nutrients for cells, is a good alternative to HBSS, and is usually readily available in public places.

Test-taking tip: This is a "you know it or don't" kind of question. If you don't know it, choose an answer and move on. You can perhaps mark it for review when you are done at the end of the test. Don't, however, let these kinds of questions get you stuck and waste your time.

47. ANSWER: C

The patient has acute necrotizing ulcerative gingivitis (ANUG).

It is a rapid-onset infection of the gums that presents with mouth pain, halitosis, and increased pain with chewing. Physical exam will show gum bleeding and ulceration with sloughing of the gingiva. Patients can also have painful regional lymphadenopathy and systemic complaints like malaise and low-grade fever.

Patients are predisposed by immunodeficiency, poor oral hygiene, smoking, and trauma.

Treatment is with chlorhexidine rinse twice a day. Antibiotics are needed if there is excessive gingival involvement or systemic signs (fever).

Test-taking tip: You can exclude B and narrow your options because the patient is not systemically ill and does not require IV antibiotics.

48. ANSWER: C

Mucormycosis is a serious and often fatal fungal infection caused by a group of molds called mucoromycetes. These molds live throughout the environment. Mucormycosis mainly affects people with weakened immune systems like those with diabetes, those with HIV/AIDS, and patients receiving chemotherapy.

Affected skin may appear relatively normal during the earliest stages of infection. This skin quickly becomes reddened and may be edematous before eventually turning black because of tissue death. Treatment is IV amphotericin B and emergent surgical consult. In most cases, the prognosis of mucormycosis is poor, and mortality approaches 90%.

Test-taking tip: The presentation of a diabetic patient with a proptotic eye is mucormycosis until proved otherwise. These disease associations are high yield on standardized exams.

8.

HEMATOLOGIC AND ONCOLOGIC EMERGENCIES

James McCue

1. A 20-year-old man comes to the emergency department (ED) after falling while playing basketball onto his right knee. He has hemophilia B and is unable to bend his right knee because of the pain and swelling. While you are waiting for imaging to rule out bony injury, what is the next best step in management?

    A. Local measures: rest, elevate, ice, and compression
    B. Factor IX 50 IU/kg bolus
    C. Factor VIII 50 IU/kg
    D. Drain the palpable effusion

2. You have diagnosed a patient with severe sepsis due to an unknown source. While waiting for admission to the intensive care unit (ICU), the nurse approaches you stating that patient is bleeding from his IV sites and is not hemostatic with pressure. What is the mechanism behind the patient's bleeding?

    A. Disseminated intravascular coagulation (DIC)
    B. Patient is undergoing simultaneous thrombus formation and hemorrhage
    C. Platelets are inactive secondary to cyclooxygenase-2 (COX-2) inhibitor
    D. Von Willebrand factor (vWF) deficiency

3. A 35-year-old female with lymphoma who is undergoing chemotherapy presents with altered mental status after having progressive fatigue over the past week. She has a Glasgow Coma Scale (GCS) score of 13, and her vital signs include temperature 36.8° C, heart rate (HR) 130 bpm, blood pressure (BP) 130/90 mm Hg, and respiratory rate (RR) 28 breaths/min. Her husband states she has not been urinating much in the past 3 days. On physical exam, she is lethargic and has rales in all lung fields. Laboratory findings show that she is in acute renal failure, has hyperkalemia, and is acidotic. What is the best intervention to start at this time?

    A. IV hydration
    B. IV hydration with diuretic therapy

    C. Emergent hemodialysis
    D. Antibiotic therapy

4. A 4-year-old female presents to the ED with diffuse bruising after minimal trauma. She is well developed, nontoxic appearing, and afebrile. She was recently ill with a viral upper respiratory infection but otherwise has been well and has no past medical history. Laboratory testing reveals a platelet count of 4,000. While waiting for admission, what is the most appropriate initial therapy to get started?

    A. Antibiotics
    B. Platelet transfusion
    C. Steroids
    D. IV immunoglobulin

5. A 45-year-old male on warfarin for a recent pulmonary embolus presents with altered mental status to the ED. He has a GCS score of 6. After intubation and stabilization, he undergoes emergent head computed tomography (CT), which shows a profound subdural hematoma with shift. His laboratory results are significant for an international normalized ratio (INR) of 5. The neurosurgical consult wants to take the patient to the operating room but would like his coagulopathy treated. What is the best treatment for this patient?

    A. Vitamin K
    B. Platelets
    C. Fresh frozen plasma
    D. Vitamin K and fresh frozen plasma

6. A 26-year-old female with sickle cell disease presents to the ED with fever and malaise for the past 3 days. Her temperature in the ED is 38.5° C rectally, and her workup is significant for an elevated white blood cell (WBC) count and right lower lobe pneumonia. What is the most important organism to cover with antibiotics in this patient?

A. *Streptococcus pneumoniae*
B. Methicillin-resistant *Staphylococcus aureus* (MRSA)
C. *Candida albicans*
D. Herpes simplex

7. An adopted 2-year-old African American male is brought in by his parents to the ED because of excessive fussiness for 1 hour. On exam, you find he has priapism and no other findings. What is the best initial management of this patient?

A. Emergent urology consult for penile aspiration and irrigation
B. IV hydration, analgesia, and supplemental oxygen
C. Hydroxyurea
D. Observation for 4 hours

8. A 65-year-old man who is a heavy smoker presents with a hoarse voice, blurred vision, and dysphagia that has progressively worsened over the past 3 weeks. His vital signs are normal outside of some mild hypertension, with BP 149/90 mm Hg. On exam, he has prominent neck veins, and his symptoms are worsened by sitting him forward. A radiograph reveals a right upper lobe mass. Besides admission, what therapy should be started in the ED?

A. Phlebotomy
B. Elevation of the head of the bed, diuretics, and steroids
C. Administration of broad-spectrum antibiotics
D. Aggressive IV hydration

9. An 8-year-old boy undergoing chemotherapy for leukemia presents with a low-grade fever of 38.4° C with nausea, vomiting, and malaise. His exam is unremarkable, but his WBC count is 1,900 with an absolute neutrophil count (ANC) of 10%. He has a Mediport in place. What organisms should be covered for the treatment of this patient?

A. *Pseudomonas* and MRSA
B. Anaerobes and MRSA
C. Fungal
D. Viral

10. A 65-year-old female with multiple myeloma presents with anorexia, fatigue, and memory loss. Her electrocardiogram (EKG) shows a shortened QT interval. What laboratory value is elevated in this patient that could explain all of her findings?

A. Calcium
B. Phosphate
C. Sodium
D. Potassium

11. A 45-year-old woman with a history of breast cancer status post–bilateral mastectomy presents with atraumatic back pain, difficulty urinating, and bilateral leg numbness. Her exam is significant for bilateral lower extremity weakness and decreased rectal tone. While waiting for imaging, what is the next best step in the management of this patient?

A. Emergent neurosurgical consultation
B. Antibiotics
C. Foley placement
D. Steroids

12. A 58-year-old man presents to the ED with altered mental status, and he is not moving his left side on exam. His head CT is normal, and there are no acute findings on his EKG. His WBC count comes back at 150,000, and his lumbar puncture shows no signs of infection. You start empiric antibiotics and fluids for the patient. What is the best treatment to manage this patient?

A. Plasmapheresis
B. Exchange transfusion
C. Aggressive IV hydration
D. Aspirin

13. A 27-year-old man develops shortness of breath, chest pain, and headache after having a peritonsillar abscess drained with the use of Cetacaine as a topical anesthetic. He states the doctor "used a lot" of Cetacaine because his pain was poorly controlled. The phlebotomist reports that the patient's blood is "chocolate" in color. His EKG shows sinus tachycardia with signs of ischemia, and his lung exam is clear throughout. What is the best next step in the management of this patient?

A. Supplemental oxygen
B. Administer IV methylene blue
C. Administer sublingual nitroglycerin
D. Activate the catheterization lab

14. A 34-year-old woman presents to the ED for shortness of breath, vaginal bleeding, and generalized weakness. She is found to be anemic and is currently undergoing a blood transfusion. Halfway through the transfusion, she develops a fever but denies any other related symptoms. Her blood pressure is 128/62 mm Hg, and she her oxygen saturation is 98% on room air. What is the most appropriate treatment for this patient?

A. Acetaminophen
B. Discontinue the transfusion
C. Diphenhydramine
D. Continued observation

15. A 68-year-old man presents with blackening of his buttocks region for the past few days. He denies trauma or similar symptoms in the past. He also denies fevers, chills, or other constitutional symptoms. He was recently diagnosed with atrial fibrillation by his primary care doctor and was started on warfarin for treatment. What is the appropriate next step in caring for this patient?

A. Continue his current therapy
B. Consult plastic surgery
C. Start antibiotics and admit the patient
D. Discontinue the warfarin and start the patient on heparin with admission to the hospital

16. A 4-year-old Southeast Asian boy presents after having a fainting episode and has been having less energy than the other children at school for weeks. His vital signs are normal at this time, and his exam reveals pale conjunctiva and a cardiac flow murmur. His workup is significant for a microcytic anemia with a hemoglobin of 5.4. His rectal exam is negative for blood. What is the likely cause of his anemia?

A. Sickle cell anemia
B. Iron deficiency anemia
C. Thalassemia
D. Hemolytic uremic syndrome (HUS)

17. A 67-year-old woman with breast cancer presents 3 days after her last dose of chemotherapy with generalized weakness and fever for the past day. Her temperature is 38.6° C, and she has streaking redness to her right lower extremity. With what lab values would she be at most risk for a neutropenic fever?

A. WBC count of 20,000 and ANC of 50%
B. WBC count of 12,000 with ANC of 50%

C. WBC count of 3,000 with ANC of 60%
D. WBC count of 1,200 with ANC of 80%

18. A 24-year-old woman presents with abdominal pain, nausea, and vomiting for the past few days, and her family report that she has been having more trouble remembering things for the past week. Her temperature is 38.3° C. Her lactate dehydrogenase (LDH) is elevated, creatinine is 1.9, and platelets are 34,000. She has no intracranial hemorrhage on head CT. What is the next most appropriate step in the management of this patient?

A. Fresh frozen plasma
B. Steroids
C. Plasma exchange
D. Platelet transfusion

19. A 6-year-old boy who has not traveled outside of the United States is found to have HUS. What is the likely infectious cause for his presentation?

A. *Escherichia coli* O157:H7
B. Adenovirus
C. *Shigella*
D. *Enterovirus*

20. A 6-year-old boy presents with generalized weakness, bleeding of his gums with brushing, and diarrhea for the past 5 days. He is tachycardic on exam but otherwise has a normal exam. His platelets are 36,000, and his creatinine is 2.4. What is the likely diagnosis of this patient?

A. HUS
B. Thrombotic thrombocytopenic purpura (TTP)
C. Von Willebrand disease
D. Hemophilia A

ANSWERS

1. ANSWER: B

This patient has hemophilia B and presents with a hemarthrosis, which requires factor IX replacement. Hemarthroses without signs of compartment syndrome are considered minor bleeds and only require 20- to 60-IU/kg boluses initially. Factor VIII is used for replacement in patients with hemophilia A. Local measures are a good adjunct therapy but are not the definitive therapy for hemophilia. Draining the effusion is not indicated unless there is a concern for a septic joint.

Some factor replacement guidelines are as follows:

- Hemophilia A: factor VIII replacement
  - Minor (hemarthrosis, hematoma, minor lacerations, fracture): 40% to 50% correction
    - 20 to 50 IU/kg every 12 to 24 hours for one to three doses
  - Major (intracranial hemorrhage (ICH), preoperative, significant trauma severe joint/muscle bleed, compartment syndrome): 80% to 100% correction
    - 50 to 100 IU/kg every 8 to 12 hours, may consider infusion after initial bolus in severe cases
- Hemophilia B: factor IX replacement
  - Minor (hemarthrosis, hematoma, minor lacerations, fracture): 40% to 50% correction
    - 20 to 60 IU/kg every 24 hours for one to three doses
  - Major (ICH, preoperative, significant trauma severe joint/muscle bleed, compartment syndrome): 80% to 100% correction
    - 50 to 100 IU/kg every 12 to 24 hours, may consider infusion after initial bolus in severe cases
- Von Willebrand disease: recombinant vWF
  - Minor (hemarthrosis, hematoma, minor lacerations, fracture): 40% to 50% correction
    - Local measures, DDAVP
  - Major (ICH, preoperative, significant trauma severe joint/muscle bleed, compartment syndrome): 80% to 100% correction
    - 40 to 80 IU/kg loading dose, then 40 to 60 IU/kg every 8 to 12 hours

Test-taking tip: With patients who have hemophilia, you know that factor replacement is the definitive treatment, allowing you to eliminate A and D as correct answers.

2. ANSWER: B

This patient has DIC, but that is not the mechanism behind the patient's bleeding, just the condition. DIC is caused by the simultaneous formation of thrombus and hemorrhage. In DIC, the prothrombin time (PT) and partial thromboplastin time (PTT) are prolonged, platelets are low, D-dimer is elevated, and fibrinogen is low. An elevated LDH and creatinine may reflect end-organ damage and support the diagnosis of DIC. In very ill patients who start bleeding with minimal to no trauma, consider DIC. There is no specific treatment for DIC except for the treatment of the underlying cause. Sepsis, trauma, obstetric events, and cancer are the most common culprits for DIC.

Platelets are inactivated by aspirin-like products but not due to DIC. This patient may have von Willebrand disease, but in the setting of sepsis, DIC is more likely and more life-threatening.

Test-taking tip: The key word in the question is "mechanism," allowing you to focus on the answers that describe a mechanism like B and C.

3. ANSWER: C

This presentation is concerning for tumor lysis syndrome (TLS), which is an oncologic emergency. The key laboratory findings are hyperkalemia, hypercalcemia, hyperphosphatemia, and an elevate uric acid, which are all intracellular products that are released during TLS. Because of the patient's decreased urine output, acidosis, and hyperkalemia, the best treatment is emergent dialysis. The recommended treatment for TLS in patients who do not appear fluid overloaded and are still making urine is IV hydration, allopurinol, and possible urinary alkalization.

IV hydration is recommended, but in a patient who appears fluid overloaded (rales) and with decreased urine output, it is not the best indicated emergent therapy.

The patient is afebrile with no signs or symptoms of infection, making antibiotics less likely to be the most appropriate treatment.

Test-taking tip: Many of the answers may play a role in the management of the patient; however, when the question asks what is the "best intervention," think of what is the most definitive treatment.

4. ANSWER: C

This patient's presentation is consistent with idiopathic thrombocytopenic purpura (ITP). Most children have complete disease remission within 6 months, while less than 10% of adults have spontaneous remission. In the ED, administration of steroids is the treatment of choice.

Platelet transfusion has not been shown to decrease the incidence of intracranial hemorrhage, and unless the underlying autoimmune response is treated, the platelets from the transfusion will undergo the same fate as the patient's native platelets.

Fluids and antibiotics are not the mainstay treatment for ITP, and there are no signs of dehydration or infection in this child.

IV immunoglobulin is usually given under the direction of a hematologist, and there are significant risks to its administration, including severe allergic reactions, which makes it not the initial treatment of choice in the ED.

Test-taking tip: You can easily eliminate A as an answer because the patient has no infectious symptoms, and if you think about the last time you administered IV immunoglobulin in the ED, you can also eliminate choice D.

5. ANSWER: D

This is a devastating injury for this patient, requiring emergent surgical intervention. In life-threatening bleeds, it is recommended to reverse warfarin with vitamin K and fresh frozen plasma.

Platelets play no role in reversal of warfarin and are used for patients who are taking aspirin, Plavix, or other antiplatelet drugs. It is recommended to transfuse 5 to 10 units of platelets to raise platelets above 50,000 for major bleeds and to consider using DDAVP.

Regarding warfarin, the recommendations for reversal are as follows:

- No bleeding
  - *INR <4.5:* hold therapy for one to two doses or lower the dose and then recheck INR in 24 to 48 hours
  - *INR 4.5–10:* hold therapy for one to two doses and then recheck INR in 24 to 48 hours
  - *INR >10:* hold therapy, administer vitamin K 2 to 5 mg PO, recheck INR in 24 hours, and restart therapy at a lower dose once INR is therapeutic
- Life-threatening bleeds
  - *Any INR:* vitamin K 10 mg IV, fresh frozen plasma 2 to 4 units, consider cryoprecipitate (institution dependent)

Test-taking tip: This is a gravely ill patient, suggesting that you want to do more rather than less, pointing to the correct answer in which you give vitamin K and fresh frozen plasma.

6. ANSWER: A

Sickle cell patients are at an increased risk for infection because of encapsulated bacteria species secondary to autoinfarction of their spleens, which usually occurs by the time they reach school age. The most common bacterial species are *S. pneumoniae* and *Haemophilus influenzae*.

There is no mention of recent hospitalizations, dialysis, or residence at a nursing facility, making MRSA pneumonia less likely because it is usually associated with hospital-acquired pneumonia.

While viral and fungal infections are possible, they are less likely in this patient than encapsulated bacterial organisms.

Test-taking tip: When you hear splenectomy or a sickle cell patient in the same sentence with infection, think encapsulated organisms.

7. ANSWER: B

This child likely has sickle cell disease, and the priapism is his initially presentation. It is very uncommon for toddlers to have priapism, and sickle cell is the leading cause in children at 65%, followed by leukemia, trauma, and idiopathic causes at 10% each.

If the priapism is suspected to have been present for less than 3 hours, as in this child who has only been fussy for 1 hour, initial treatment should consist of IV hydration, analgesia, and supplemental oxygen. Frequently, this conservative approach will treat the priapism without invasive measures.

If there is no relief within 3 hours of onset of symptoms, urgent urology consultation should be obtained with the goal of penile aspiration and irrigation with epinephrine. Pediatric patients requiring aspiration and irrigation should be admitted for observation, even if the treatment is effective.

Prolonged observation alone of a pediatric patient with priapism is not acceptable because the longer the erection lasts, the great the risk for long-term injury and morbidity.

If the patient is ultimately diagnosed with sickle cell disease, long-term treatment with hydroxyurea may be warranted, but it is not indicated in the acute treatment of a pediatric patient with priapism.

Test-taking tip: The key to this question is to come to the conclusion that the patient has undiagnosed sickle cell disease. If you make this association, then the correct answer is easy because IV hydration, analgesia, and supplemental oxygen are the mainstay of the initial management of many of the complications of sickle cell disease.

8. ANSWER: B

This patient's presentation is concerning for superior vena cava syndrome. Cancer is the most common cause, accounting for 85% to 95% of cases. Treatment in the ED includes elevating the head of the bed, diuretics, and steroids to decrease venous pressure. Definitive treatment for this condition may include radiotherapy, stent placement, or chemotherapy.

Phlebotomy is an effective treatment for polycythemia vera but is not indicated for superior vena cava syndrome. This patient has no infectious symptoms and thus antibiotics are not necessary, nor is aggressive IV hydration because the patient is not hypotensive or volume depleted.

Test-taking tip: When an answer is very specific, such as "Elevation of the head of the bed, diuretics, and steroids," it has a high probability of being the correct answer.

9. ANSWER: A

This patient is suffering from neutropenic fever, which is an oncologic emergency that has a mortality rate as high as 20% to 50%. Gram-negative bacilli, especially *Pseudomonas,* are common causes of neutropenic fever; however, patients with indwelling lines have a higher likelihood of gram-positive organisms causing their infections. Because this patient has a Mediport, he should be treated to cover MRSA and *Pseudomonas.*

While anaerobes and fungal and viral infections are possible, they are not the most likely source of this patient's infection and would be low yield in initial treatment unless exam findings supported their presence.

The definition of a neutropenic fever includes temperature >38.3° C or at least 38° C for more than 1 hour with an ANC of <500 cells/microliter or <1000 cells/microliter with a predicted nadir of <500 cells/microliter.

Test-taking tip: The key to this question is the presence of a Mediport, suggesting that skin flora, or MRSA, may be a potential culprit.

10. ANSWER: A

Shortening of the QT interval on EKG raises the concern of hypercalcemia, and in the setting of multiple myeloma, it is high on the differential secondary to bone turnover due to the lytic lesions.

Elevated phosphate does not typically cause shortening of the QT interval. Hypernatremia is associated with the QRS interval, and not the QT interval. While potassium can prolong the QT interval when elevated, it does not cause shortening of it.

Treatments for hypercalcemia include the following:

- *Mild symptoms and level <13:* PO or IV hydration alone
- *Severe symptoms and/or level >13:* IV hydration, loop diuretics, and bisphosphonates

Test-taking tip: With cancers affecting the bones, like multiple myeloma and bony metastasis, think hypercalcemia.

11. ANSWER: A

The patient is presenting with signs and symptoms of a spinal cord compression, most likely secondary to metastatic disease to her spine. This requires an emergent neurosurgical consultation for possible surgical intervention.

Antibiotics are not needed for this patient because she has no signs or symptoms of infection. Although an epidural abscess is one cause of spinal cord compression, metastatic disease is more likely in this patient.

Placement of a Foley catheter is not a definitive treatment for this patient, and it could be argued that it not needed when the risks and benefits are weighed.

While steroids may be helpful at some point in the management of this patient, they are not the best immediate step in her management.

Test-taking tip: Motor weakness with suspected cord compression equals early neurosurgical consultation.

12. ANSWER: A

Hyperviscosity syndrome is very hard to diagnosis in the ED but is considered one of the true oncologic emergencies. While there is no one test that can diagnosis hyperviscosity syndrome, patients presenting with neurologic deficits, blurred vision, bleeding, or purpura, with a concern for a cancer diagnosis, should be considered for this diagnosis. Very few diagnoses give you a WBC count of 150,000, with cancer being high on that list. This patient is at risk for hyperviscosity syndrome and requires emergent plasmapheresis.

IV hydration is also necessary but is not the definitive treatment for this patient.

Exchange transfusion is not indicated in patients with hyperviscosity syndrome, although it is used in some conditions related to sickle cell disease.

This patient is possibly having a stroke, but it is most likely secondary to the hyperviscosity of his blood and not a thrombus that would benefit from aspirin.

Test-taking tip: An abnormally high WBC count should make you think of hyperviscosity syndrome. Many of the answers may play a role in the management of the patient; however, when the question asks what is the "best intervention," think of what is the most definitive treatment.

13. ANSWER: B

This patient's presentation is concerning for methemoglobinemia, and symptoms are directly correlated with methemoglobin levels:

- *3%–15%:* Slight discoloration (e.g., pale, gray, blue) of the skin
- *15%–20%:* Cyanosis, though patients may have few or no symptoms
- *25%–50%:* Headache, dyspnea, lightheadedness (even syncope), weakness, confusion, palpitations, chest pain
- *50%–70%:* Abnormal cardiac rhythms; altered mental status, delirium, seizures, coma; profound acidosis
- *>70%:* Death

Methylene blue is the antidote for methemoglobinemia. Methylene blue works by accelerating the enzymatic reduction of methemoglobin by NADPH-methemoglobin reductase, and it also reduces to leucomethylene blue that, in turn, reduces methemoglobin.

Oxygen administration may be indicated, but it will not treat the patient's underlying disease process.

The ischemia on the patient's EKG is caused by the methemoglobinemia, not coronary artery disease; thus administration of nitroglycerin or activation of the catheterization lab is not the most appropriate treatment for this patient.

Test-taking tip: Three of the four answers are traditional treatment for coronary artery disease. Only the correct answer, administering methylene blue, stands out as different, suggesting it is the correct answer.

14. ANSWER: A

This patient is having a simple febrile reaction to the blood transfusion, which can be treated with acetaminophen alone. The transfusion does not need to be discontinued for a simple febrile response, and diphenhydramine or continued observation will not treat the patient's fever. The progression of reactions to blood transfusions includes the following:

- Fever only—simple febrile fever: treat with acetaminophen
- Urticaria only—minor allergic reaction: treat with diphenhydramine
- *Dyspnea, rales, and hypertension—congestive heart failure versus transfusion-related acute lung injury:* obtain a chest radiograph; treat with oxygen, nitroglycerine, and furosemide

- *Flushing, urticaria, hypotension, and wheezing—anaphylaxis*: treat with epinephrine, steroids, diphenhydramine, and fluids
- *Fever, hypotension, and back pain—hemolysis versus sepsis:* treat with fluids, vasopressors as needed, broad-spectrum antibiotics for sepsis, and furosemide for hemolysis

Test-taking tip: Fever in a stable patient points to an antipyretic such as acetaminophen.

15. ANSWER: D

This patient is suffering from warfarin-induced skin necrosis secondary to protein C deficiency. This occurs when patients are placed on warfarin without proper bridging using heparin first.

The patient has no constitutional symptoms suggesting infection, so antibiotics are not indicated. It is not an infectious process, and surgical intervention is not indicated at this time. The patient needs to discontinue his warfarin and to be started on heparin for a bridging therapy. Warfarin-induced necrosis mainly affects areas with large amounts of subcutaneous fat, and peak incidence is 3 to 5 days after starting warfarin without proper bridging.

Test-taking tip: This is a "you know it or don't" kind of question. If you don't know it, choose an answer and move on. You can perhaps mark it for review when you are done at the end of the test. Don't, however, let these kinds of questions get you stuck and waste your time.

16. ANSWER: C

This question is about knowing the epidemiology of different causes of anemia. A young child of Southeast Asian descent presenting with a microcytic anemia should raise the concern for thalassemia.

The other most common environmental cause of anemia in this age group is anemia secondary to lead exposure. Sickle cell anemia is usually associated with African American individuals.

Iron deficiency anemia is more common with infants and toddlers who are bottle-fed with cow's milk or nonfortified formulas. By 4 years of age, the toddler should be getting a sufficient amount of iron from his diet. There is no mention of renal injury or failure, making HUS unlikely.

Test-taking question: Epidemiology questions are fair game on a standardized emergency medicine test, so brush up on who is at risk for particular disease processes.

17. ANSWER: D

The definition for neutropenic fever includes temperature >38.3° C or at least 38° C for more than 1 hour with an ANC of <500 cells/microliter or <1,000 cells/microliter with a predicted nadir of <500 cells/microliter. The nadir occurs 5 to 7 days after the last dose of chemotherapy. This patient has not reached her nadir, and her ANC is already <1,000, putting her at risk for neutropenic fever.

Test-taking tip: This is a "you know it or don't" kind of question. If you don't know it, choose an answer and move on. You can perhaps mark it for review when you are done at the end of the test. Don't, however, let these kinds of questions get you stuck and waste your time.

18. ANSWER: C

This woman's presentation is concerning for TTP. While the symptoms can vary, the classic pentad is thrombocytopenia, neurologic abnormalities, fever, renal dysfunction, and microangiopathic hemolytic anemia.

While HUS can present similarly to TTP, TTP is more commonly associated with neurologic findings without renal involvement, whereas HUS is more commonly associated with renal involvement without neurologic involvement. Plasma exchange is the mainstay of treatment for patients with TTP, secondary to the need to remove proteins from the blood, including metalloprotease inhibitors and unusually large vWF.

Platelet transfusion has no role in the treatment of TTP unless there is a life-threatening intracranial bleed present. There is not a role for fresh frozen plasma in the treatment of these patients, and steroids alone will not help treat the underlying disease process.

Test-taking tip: Brush up on classic presentations of diseases (TTP pentad, Beck's triad, etc.) because they are frequently tested on emergency medicine standardized exams.

19. ANSWER: A

HUS is often associated with a diarrheal illness and usually occurs at least 4 days after the onset of the diarrhea. It presents similarly to TTP with thrombocytopenia, neurologic abnormalities, fever, renal dysfunction, and microangiopathic hemolytic anemia.

HUS is associated with renal dysfunction without neurologic findings, whereas TTP is more often associated with neurologic findings without renal dysfunction. The most common causative agent of HUS is *E. coli* O157:H7. *Shigella* is the second leading infectious cause. Viruses are less likely to be the causative agent because HUS is caused by particular toxins released by bacteria.

Test-taking tip: This is a "you know it or don't" kind of question. If you don't know it, choose an answer and move on. You can perhaps mark it for review when you are done at the end of the test. Don't, however, let these kinds of questions get you stuck and waste your time.

20. ANSWER: A

Based on this child's presentation, HUS is the most likely diagnosis. HUS is often associated with a diarrheal illness and usually occurs at least 4 days after the onset of the diarrhea.

HUS is more associated with renal dysfunction without neurologic findings, while TTP is more associated with neurologic findings without renal dysfunction. The most common causative agent of HUS is *E. coli* O157:H7.

Because of the lack of neurologic symptoms, TTP is less likely. Hemophilia and vWD are usually not associated with thrombocytopenia but instead are associated with hemarthroses and easy bleeding after surgery, respectively.

Test-taking tip: You can easily eliminate C and D as correct answers because these diseases do not affect platelet counts, leaving you two to choose from.

9.

IMMUNOLOGIC EMERGENCIES

Deena Bengiamin and Jannifer Matos

1. A 29-year-old woman presents to the emergency department (ED) with a rapidly progressing rash and facial swelling after a bee sting at the park. She reports feeling light-headed and denies shortness of breath. Vital signs are temperature 37° C, blood pressure (BP) 90/64 mm Hg, heart rate (HR) 127 bpm, respiratory rate (RR) 18 breaths/min, and oxygen saturation 99%. A diffuse urticarial rash is present on the patient's extremities, neck, and chest, and swelling is noted on the patient's lips and tongue. Which of the following is the next best step in management?

  A. IM epinephrine
  B. Nebulized albuterol
  C. Observation
  D. PO diphenhydramine

2. A 34-year-old man with no significant past medical history presents to the ED with a severe rash on his lower legs. He states that a few days ago he went hiking through some thick brush in the woods behind his house near the foothills of the Sierra Mountains. He reports wearing only shorts for most of the hike and removed his T-shirt because of heat. On exam, you note similar lesions on his face, arms, and chest. The lesions appear erythematous with scattered plaques and vesicles in a linear distribution on the affected areas. The lesions are described as intensely pruritic. He denies any dyspnea or oral swelling. Which of the following is the most appropriate treatment?

  A. Trimethoprim-sulfamethoxazole for 7 days
  B. Diphenhydramine as needed
  C. Prednisone taper over 21 days
  D. Prednisone taper over 10 days

3. A 43-year-old man presents to the ED with sudden-onset swelling of his lips and face, associated with shortness of breath. The patient reports multiple episodes of lip swelling since his teens but has never sought medical treatment, and the swelling would resolve over time. His family history is unknown. On exam, you note significant tongue and face swelling. You plan and prepare that this patient will need a definitive airway. Which of the following treatments will have the most benefit for this condition?

  A. Angiotensin-converting enzyme (ACE) inhibitor
  B. C1-esterase inhibitor
  C. Diphenhydramine, methylprednisolone
  D. Epinephrine, nebulized β_2-agonist

4. A 7-year-old girl presents to the ED accompanied by her mother with a diffuse maculopapular rash that started last night. Her mother reports the patient was treated with a penicillin injection for a throat infection by the pediatrician 4 days ago. The rash has a target-lesion appearance throughout the body, including the palms and soles. No painful blisters on the lips or skin sloughing by gentle touch was noted. Which of the following treatments should most likely be initiated?

  A. Diphenhydramine
  B. Epinephrine
  C. Systemic corticosteroids
  D. Topical corticosteroids

5. A 6-year-old boy accompanied by his mother presents to the ED with abdominal pain for 2 days. She states her son has been complaining of abdominal pain and knee pain for the past 2 days; last night she noted a rash on his legs. The mother states he is otherwise healthy and up to date on vaccinations. She notes he did have a recent upper respiratory infection last week. He has been eating regularly and behaving normally. His vital signs are within normal limits. On exam, he has a diffusely tender abdomen, lower extremity edema, and a violaceous, raised, nonblanching rash, most notably on his extremities. His complete blood count test was normal.

His urinalysis is positive for trace blood and protein. What therapy should be initiated?

A. Azithromycin
B. Renal transplantation
C. High-dose prednisone
D. Nonsteroidal antiinflammatory drug (NSAID)

6. A 7-year-old girl presents to the ED accompanied by her father complaining of left knee pain for 2 days. Her father reports she visited her pediatrician last week and received an antibiotic medication for an earache. The father expresses concern that the patient awoke this morning with a rash all over her body and a fever. On exam, you note an ill-appearing child with a widespread morbilliform rash and a few tender joints. Her vital signs are BP 98/62 mm Hg, HR 98 bpm, temperature 39° C, and RR 20 breaths/min. Which of the following is the most likely diagnosis?

A. Still's disease
B. Henoch-Schönlein purpura
C. Systemic lupus erythematosus
D. Serum sickness

7. A 55-year-old man with a history of hypertension, seizures, gastroesophageal reflux disease (GERD), chronic obstructive pulmonary disease (COPD), and recent lung transplantation 5 months ago presents to the ED with shortness of breath for the past 2 days. He reports that symptoms started at rest and have persisted with associated dry cough and subjective fever. He endorses compliance with his prescribed cyclosporine. His vital signs are BP 104/60 mm Hg, HR 99 bpm, RR 24 breaths/min, oxygen saturation 93%, and temperature 37.9° C. On exam, you note a thin, ill-appearing male in mild respiratory distress. He exhibits poor inspiratory effort, a harsh and dry cough, and lungs clear to auscultation. You review his medication list and note that he takes various medications for his chronic conditions. Which of the following drugs would be expected to precipitate acute rejection in a lung transplant recipient taking cyclosporine?

A. Cimetidine
B. Erythromycin
C. Nifedipine
D. Phenytoin

8. A 4-year-old boy presents to the ED accompanied by his mother with fever, rash, and malaise for the past 6 days. The mother reports that the patient has had fever, malaise, and rash for 6 days with associated nausea, vomiting, and diarrhea. She reports treating the patient's fever with acetaminophen and thought the symptoms would resolve but became worried after his appetite decreased. His vital signs are BP 90/50 mm Hg, HR 130 bpm, RR 15 breaths/min, and temperature 38° C. Your examination reveals an uncomfortable-appearing child with cracked red lips, a swollen red tongue, cervical lymphadenopathy, bilateral conjunctivitis, edema, and erythema of the palms and soles with a generalized macular rash. Labs show leukocytosis, thrombocytosis, and elevated C-reactive protein (CRP) and erythrocyte sedimentation rate (ESR). Which therapy should be initiated?

A. IV immunoglobulin and aspirin
B. Amoxicillin–clavulanic acid
C. Glucocorticoids
D. Warfarin

9. A 13-year-old girl presents to the ED accompanied by her father with complaints of joint pain and stiffness in her hands. The patient describes the pain as intermittent and progressively worsening over the past 5 months. She attributed the pain to increased homework at school but is now worried the pain is getting worse, and she is feeling more tired throughout the day. She describes hand stiffness that is worse in the morning and relieved over time. Her father reports giving Tylenol for the pain with only minimal alleviation. Her vital signs are BP 113/78 mm Hg, HR 89 bpm, RR 14 breaths/min, and temperature 37.2° C. On examination, you note a nondistressed, well-developed adolescent with at least four symmetric swollen joints at the hands. The swelling is most prominent over the proximal interphalangeal and metacarpophalangeal joints, sparing the distal interphalangeal joints. The affected joints appear warm and are tender to palpation without obvious deformity. There is no evidence of erythema or fluctuating mass to the affected areas. Laboratory studies reveal a mild anemia, normal ESR, and a positive rheumatoid factor. Which of the following is the most likely diagnosis?

A. Reactive arthritis
B. Polyarticular juvenile rheumatoid arthritis (JRA)
C. Septic arthritis
D. Still's disease

10. A 9-year-old girl presents to the ED with her caregiver with fever, malaise, and joint pain for the past 2 days. The caregiver reports that the patient complained of sore throat 3 weeks ago, but she did not take her to the pediatrician. Currently it is reported that the patient has been more lethargic, complaining of intermittent knee, shoulder, and elbow pain. Her vital signs are notable for a temperature of 38.5° C. On examination, you note a young, ill-appearing girl with

tender knee and ankle joints. Auscultation reveals clear breath sounds and diastolic murmur heard best at the apex. Laboratory, electrocardiogram (EKG), and imaging studies are pending; however, your differential diagnosis includes rheumatic fever. Which of the following findings would allow you to make this diagnosis based on the modified Jones criteria?

A. Fever, arthralgia, and elevated ESR
B. Fever and arthralgia
C. Evidence of carditis with a prolonged P-R interval
D. Evidence of carditis with multiple tender and swollen joints

11. An 8-year-old boy is brought to the ED accompanied by his mother for bizarre behavior that started today. She reports this morning she observed her son writhing on the kitchen floor making purposeless uncontrollable movements. She states last week he had intermittent fevers and was complaining of joint pain and swelling of the knees and elbows. His vital signs are normal. On exam, the patient has a diastolic murmur best heard at the apex and has multiple swollen and tender joints. He is actively making choreiform movements. Which of the following tests is most likely to confirm the diagnosis?

A. Antistreptolysin titer
B. Complete blood count
C. EKG
D. Echocardiogram

12. A 12-year-old girl presents to the ED accompanied by her father with a rash. Her father reports she visited her pediatrician 7 days ago and received a 10-day course of Bactrim for a urinary tract infection. Father expresses concern that the patient awoke this morning with a rash all over her body and a fever. On exam you note an ill-appearing child with a nonpruritic, widespread morbilliform rash and a few tender joints. Her vital signs are BP 104/62 mm Hg, HR 98 bpm, temperature 39° C, and RR 20 breaths/min. What is the next best step in the treatment of her condition?

A. Oral diphenhydramine
B. Prescribe a prednisone taper
C. Stop trimethoprim-sulfamethoxazole
D. Switch drug to amoxicillin–clavulanic acid

13. A 59-year-old man presents to the ED for abdominal pain with associated diarrhea and emesis that started today. He reports a history of hypertension for which he takes a β-blocker and seasonal allergies managed with an histamine-2 receptor antagonist. His vital signs are normal. Your clinical exam warrants concern for diverticulitis. You order a contrast-enhanced computed

tomography (CT) scan of his abdomen. He denies any medication or food allergies, stating, "I don't like seafood, it smells weird, never had it." Moments later a rapid response alert is called to the CT room. You find your patient flushed, diaphoretic, and tachypneic. He states, "I feel a lump in my throat," with a hoarse voice. Repeat vital signs are temperature 37° C, BP 83/40 mm Hg, HR 120 bpm, RR 25 breaths/min, oxygen saturation 87% on room air. You examine the oropharynx and notice swelling. What is the next best step in management?

A. Obtain a definitive airway by endotracheal intubation
B. Administer 50 mg diphenhydramine IV
C. Administer 5 mL 1:1,000 epinephrine IM and complete the CT scan
D. Administer 1 mg glucagon IV every 6 minutes

14. A 65-year-old woman is brought in by ambulance to the ED with sudden-onset swelling of her tongue and lips. According to emergency medical services (EMS), a family member saw her take her medications this morning and an hour later noticed her lips were swelling. Of note, there was a new hypertension medication added to her medication list recently. Her vital signs are BP 156/90 mm Hg, HR 117 bpm, temperature 37° C, RR 30 breaths/min, and oxygen saturation 92%. On exam you find the patient in respiratory distress with prominent swelling of her lips and tongue. The patient is unable to speak, you are unable to exam the oral cavity because of the swelling, and auscultation reveals stridor. What is the next step in management?

A. Administer nebulized albuterol-ipratropium
B. Place patient on a non-rebreather mask with oxygen flow at 15 L
C. Obtain an emergent surgical airway
D. Administer diphenhydramine IV

15. A 50-year-old woman with a history of hypertension and polycystic kidney disease with recent kidney transplantation 3 months ago presents to the ED with fever, malaise, and oliguria. She reports having symptoms for the past 5 days but became worried when she noticed a decrease in her urine output today. She reports compliance with her immunosuppressant medications. You order laboratory studies and imaging. Which of the following findings is most indicative of acute renal transplant rejection?

A. Elevated creatinine level
B. Hypertension
C. Proteinuria
D. Leukocytosis

16. An 11-year-old girl presents to the ED accompanied by her mother with complaints of rash, joint pain, and joint stiffness. The patient describes the pain as intermittent and progressively worsening over the past 3 months. She describes hand stiffness that is worse in the morning and relieved over time. Her mother reports that she has had a fever every day for the past 2 weeks and has been taking acetaminophen. Her vital signs are BP 113/78 mm Hg, HR 104 bpm, RR 18 breaths/min, and temperature 38.8° C. On examination you note an ill-appearing adolescent with multiple symmetric swollen joints of the upper and lower extremities. The affected joints appear warm and are tender to palpation without obvious deformity. You note a diffuse salmon-colored rash throughout her entire body, and she has left upper quadrant tenderness and splenomegaly. Laboratory studies reveal a mild anemia, leukopenia, thrombocytopenia, elevated ESR, and a negative rheumatoid factor. What is the next best step in management?

A. Give oral NSAIDs and follow up with primary care provider
B. Administer corticosteroids and consult pediatrics for admission
C. Perform arthrocentesis of synovial fluid for analysis
D. Start vancomycin IV

17. A 5-year-old boy accompanied by his father presents to the ED with dark stools, abdominal pain, and a new rash. The father reports his son had an upper respiratory infection 2 weeks ago. Since then he has been complaining of joint pain and abdominal pain with a decreased appetite. He developed a dark-purple rash on his legs a few days ago, and this morning he noticed his son had dark-colored stool. The father reports he is up to date on vaccinations. His vital signs are BP 90/50 mm Hg, HR 120 bpm, RR 25 breaths/min, and temperature 37.9° C. On exam you note a mildly distressed boy with a diffusely tender abdomen, lower extremity edema, and a violaceous, raised, nonblanching rash most notably on his extremities. What is the most appropriate next step in management?

A. Prescribe topical corticosteroid preparation for the rash
B. Start oral acetaminophen therapy
C. Provide reassurance to the parent because this process is self-limited
D. Obtain an abdominal ultrasound

18. A 4-year-old boy presents to the ED accompanied by his mother with fever, rash, and malaise for the past 6 days. The mother reports the patient developed fever, malaise, and rash 6 days ago with associated nausea, vomiting, and diarrhea. She reports treating the patient's fever with acetaminophen and thought the symptoms would resolve but became worried after his appetite decreased. His vital signs are BP 90/50 mm Hg, HR 130 bpm, RR 15 breaths/min, and temperature 38° C. Your examination reveals an uncomfortable-appearing child with cracked red lips, a swollen red tongue, cervical lymphadenopathy, bilateral conjunctivitis, edema, and erythema of the palms and soles, with a generalized macular rash with some desquamation of the skin on the finger tips. Labs were ordered. All the following criteria support the child's diagnosis *except*:

A. Cervical lymphadenopathy
B. Fever for 6 days
C. Platelet count of 130,000/mL
D. Edema of the hands and feet

19. A 5-year-old boy presents to the ED accompanied by his mother for fever, rash, and malaise for the past 5 days. The mother reports that the patient developed fever, malaise, and rash 6 days ago, with associated nausea, vomiting, and diarrhea. She became concerned when the patient started refusing to eat. His vital signs are BP 90/50 mm Hg, HR 130 bpm, RR 15 breaths/min, and temperature 38° C. Your examination reveals an ill-appearing child with conjunctivitis, cracked red lips, a strawberry-red tongue, and cervical lymphadenopathy. On further examination you note a generalized macular rash. Labs show leukocytosis, thrombocytosis, and elevated CRP and ESR. You diagnose this patient with Kawasaki disease. The most important complications to identify early in Kawasaki disease are:

A. Gastrointestinal
B. Hematologic
C. Cardiovascular
D. Neurologic

20. A 19-year-old man with a history of seasonal allergies and asthma presents to the ED following a motorcycle collision. His vital signs are BP 104/56 mm Hg, HR 120 bpm, RR 20 breaths/min, oxygen saturation 98% on room air, and temperature 37.1° C. On examination you note a diffusely tender abdomen without obvious signs of trauma. You perform a FAST exam that is positive for a fluid collection within Morrison's pouch. The patient is taken immediately to the operating room for abdominal surgery

and is found to have a large splenic laceration. He is transfused three units of packed red blood cells of the appropriate blood typing. He suddenly develops respiratory distress and airway edema. Repeat vital signs are BP 88/40 mm Hg, HR 129 bpm, RR 30 breaths/min, and oxygen saturation 90%. His findings are consistent with anaphylaxis, and you prepare for a definitive airway. Which of the following preexisting conditions will best account for this patient's symptoms?

A. C1-esterase deficiency
B. DiGeorge's syndrome
C. Selective immunoglobulin A (IgA) deficiency
D. Down syndrome

ANSWERS

1. ANSWER: A

The patient's presentation is most concerning for anaphylactic reaction. Anaphylaxis presents as upper airway obstruction, bronchospasm, hypotension, and urticarial rash. IM 1:1,000 epinephrine is recommended in this case. IM epinephrine may be administered every 5 to 10 minutes. Oral diphenhydramine, a histamine-1 receptor antagonist, should be used, but onset of action will be delayed, and you do not want to give oral medications to a patient with airway compromise.

Patients can present with anaphylaxis with various allergens such as bee stings, peanuts, and shellfish. This reaction is classified as a type I hypersensitivity reaction that is IgE mediated, resulting in mast cell degranulation and histamine release.

Test-taking tip: You can immediately eliminate C and D because once the patient has oral swelling, oral medications and observation are no longer a treatment option.

2. ANSWER: C

This patient was exposed to poison oak and developed an allergic contact dermatitis. Treatment for moderate to severe outbreaks require systemic steroid taper that should be continued for 2 to 3 weeks. Systemic antihistamines can be taken concomitantly to help control the pruritus but are not indicated as the only treatment for moderate to severe cases.

Poison oak is part of the *Toxicodendron* genus, which includes poison ivy, poison oak, and sumac. The classic-appearing lesion of poison oak is a linear rash that occurs from the person brushing against the poison oak leaf. The rash usually appears 2 to 21 days after exposure and is associated with intense pruritus and possibly the formation of vesicles, plaques, or bullae. Other common causes of allergic contact dermatitis include rubber products, nickel, clothing, jewelry, soaps, cosmetics, and medications. Contact dermatitis is classified as a type IV hypersensitivity reaction. This type of reaction is T-cell mediated and antibody independent. It is an inflammatory reaction of the skin to a chemical, physical, or biologic agent causing sensitization to the irritant.

Test-taking tip: Choices C and D are very similar, just with different lengths of treatment. You can guess one of those will be the correct answer.

3. ANSWER: B

This patient is most likely suffering from an exacerbation of his hereditary angioedema. This condition is autosomal dominant and due to a deficiency in C1-esterase inhibitor, which is responsible for regulating the activity of vasoactive mediators. It manifests with recurrent airway edema that can be life-threatening and abdominal colic. It commonly presents first in adolescence, and typically there is a strong family history reported. Treatment of choice is to give a C1-esterase inhibitor, or alternatively fresh frozen plasma (FFP) because FFP contains some C1-esterase inhibitor along with other components of plasma.

Test-taking tip: You can easily eliminate C and D because these are treatments for allergy/anaphylaxis and not hereditary angioedema.

4. ANSWER: C

This patient presented with a classic presentation that is consistent with erythema multiforme (EM). EM is an acute self-limited disease caused by the sudden appearance of erythematous macules or papules in a target-like appearance. It is considered a type IV hypersensitivity reaction and is associated with certain infections, including herpes simplex virus, Epstein-Barr virus, and histoplasmosis. The rash is described as a central dark macule with surrounding pale area and surrounding halo of erythema. This rash involves the palms and soles and in severe cases may also involve the mucous membranes. Severe cases should be treated with systemic corticosteroids. Additionally, the patient should receive supportive care. Diphenhydramine may be used for symptom control but will not suffice in severe cases of EM.

Test-taking tip: You can eliminate A and B because there is no indication that the patient has pruritus or any signs of allergic reaction or airway compromise. The remaining answer choices are both steroids with a variation in route of administration, and because they are so similar, one is likely the correct answer.

5. ANSWER: D

This child is presenting with signs and symptoms consistent with Henoch-Schönlein purpura (HSP). HSP is an IgA-mediated vasculitis that occurs from the deposition of IgA and immune complexes into the small vessels of the body. Classic presentation begins with a history of recent upper respiratory infection followed by abdominal pain, joint pain, lower leg edema, and palpable purpuric rash. Diagnosis is based on clinical findings. Laboratory studies aid in supporting the diagnosis because blood and protein are often found on urinalysis.

Thrombocytopenia or coagulopathies usually do not occur, which can be misleading because the name of the condition contains the word purpura. Treatment for HSP is supportive in the form of NSAIDs for pain symptoms and adequate hydration. Azithromycin, an antibiotic, is not warranted in the treatment of HSP because despite a recent history of upper respiratory infection, the mechanism of HSP is not bacteria related.

Test-taking tip: You can eliminate A and C because the patient does not appear to have an infection and is not in septic shock or suffering from a condition requiring steroids. This helps narrow the answers down to two choices.

6. ANSWER: D

This patient developed a rash, arthralgia, and fever 1 week after starting antibiotic therapy. This presentation is consistent with serum sickness, a type III hypersensitivity reaction characterized by immune complex deposition disease. Serum sickness appears as erythema of the extremities that spreads proximally into a widespread morbilliform rash. Previous exposure to the offending agent may produce symptoms within 12 to 36 hours. Patients without prior exposure to the agent may have delayed symptoms starting 7 to 20 days after exposure. Treatment for serum sickness is supportive with symptom control.

Still's disease is rare autoimmune inflammatory disease that presents with a salmon-colored bumpy rash, spiking fevers, and joint pain. HSP presents with a palpable purpuric rash and typically develops after an upper respiratory infection. Systemic lupus erythematosus presents with a malar "butterfly" rash.

Test-taking tip: Based on the widespread nature of the rash, you can eliminate B and C, narrowing your options down to two.

7. ANSWER: D

Cyclosporine and phenytoin are both agents that induce the cytochrome P-450 pathway. Any agents that induce this pathway decrease the half-life of immunosuppressant agents such as cyclosporine and greatly increases the likelihood of acute organ rejection. Commonly used agents that induce the cytochrome P-450 pathway include nafcillin, rifampin, and phenobarbital. Acute lung rejection presents with symptoms of shortness of breath, cough, and low-grade fever. It is important to distinguish between acute rejection and infection because both are common in the first 6 month after transplantation. Patients presenting to the ED should be started on glucocorticoid therapy and admitted for further evaluation, including bronchoscopy.

Test-taking tip: This is a "you know it or don't" kind of question. If you don't know it, choose an answer and move on. You can perhaps mark it for review when you are done

at the end of the test. Don't, however, let these kinds of questions get you stuck and waste your time.

8. ANSWER: A

This patient presents with findings consistent with Kawasaki syndrome. The mainstay of therapy should include IV immunoglobulin. Kawasaki disease is an acute medium-sized vessel vasculitis that occurs commonly in children. Ninety percent of cases occur before the age of 5 years. Classic findings consist of a prolonged fever (>5 days) and at least four out of five clinical signs: unilateral cervical lymphadenopathy, strawberry tongue, cracked red lips, extremity edema and/or erythema, nonvesicular rash, and bilateral conjunctivitis.

Labs are nonspecific and may show thrombocytosis, leukocytosis, anemia, elevation of inflammatory markers (CRP, ESR), and elevated liver function tests. The mainstay of therapy for these cases includes high-dose aspirin and IV immunoglobulin. Complications include coronary artery aneurysms, and therefore a baseline echocardiography should be performed.

Currently, studies are limited in showing the benefits of glucocorticoid therapy in patients with Kawasaki disease. A randomized trial comparing standard therapy with standard therapy plus an initial dose of methylprednisolone did not demonstrate a benefit. However, post-analysis studies revealed some benefit for patients with Kawasaki disease refractory to initial IV immunoglobulin therapy showing a lower risk in the development of coronary artery aneurysms. Warfarin is indicated for patients with known Kawasaki disease who have developed giant coronary aneurysms (>8 mm), but it is not the mainstay of therapy and should not precede the administration of IV immunoglobulin and high-dose aspirin.

Test-taking tip: You can eliminate B and D given that the patient does not have an infection requiring antibiotics or a clotting disorder.

9. ANSWER: B

JRA presents as two variations of the disease: pauciarticular and polyarticular. Polyarticular JRA occurs in approximately 35% of patients with this disease, is characterized by symmetric joint involvement in more than five joints, and is most common in girls 10 to 15 years of age. Laboratory studies will reveal a positive rheumatoid factor in the polyarticular form and a positive antinuclear antibody in the pauciarticular form. Early radiographic imaging may reveal nonspecific findings such as soft tissue swelling or periarticular osteopenia or may be normal.

Reactive arthritis is related to a recent viral or bacterial infection that presents with the triad of arthritis, conjunctivitis, and urethritis. Septic arthritis more commonly presents as monoarticular and is usually acute in onset with associated erythema. Still's disease is also known as systemic JRA, and it is a less common form of JRA seen in approximately 15% of cases. It is characterized by daily intermittent fever spikes and a transient, nonpruritic, pale pink maculopapular rash on the trunk. Rheumatoid factor is typically negative in this type.

Test-taking tip: This is a "you know it or don't" kind of question. If you don't know it, choose an answer and move on. You can perhaps mark it for review when you are done at the end of the test. Don't, however, let these kinds of questions get you stuck and waste your time.

10. ANSWER: D

Rheumatic fever may be diagnosed on clinical grounds using the modified Jones criteria (Table 9.1) and historical evidence of prior streptococcal infection. This decision-making tool requires either two major or one major and two minor criteria to be met. Major criteria include evidence of carditis, polyarthritis, erythema marginatum, subcutaneous nodules, and/or Sydenham's chorea. Minor criteria include fever, arthralgia, prolonged PR interval, elevated ESR or CRP, and/or previous history of rheumatic fever.

Table 9.1 MODIFIED JONES CRITERIA FOR RHEUMATIC FEVER

Major	Polyarthritis
	Carditis
	Chorea
	Subcutaneous nodules
	Erythema marginatum
Minor	Fever
	Polyarthralgia
	Erythrocyte sedimentation rate, C-reactive protein, leukocytosis
	Electrocardiogram: prolonged PR interval
Evidence of preceding *Streptococcus* infection	Antistreptolysin O
	Positive throat cultures
	Positive rapid strep antigen test

Test-taking tip: This question will be easy to answer if you know the modified Jones criteria and the requirement of two major or one major and two minor criteria.

11. ANSWER: A

This patient's presentation is due to acute rheumatic fever, a systemic disease caused by an immune response to a preceding group A *Streptococcus* infection. This patient presents with chorea, carditis, and polyarthritis—three major manifestations outlined in the modified Jones criteria created by the American Heart Association (see Table 9.1). To fulfill the modified Jones criteria there must be evidence of recent streptococcal disease to support the diagnosis and either two major or one major and two minor criteria present. A positive antistreptolysin titer or rapid streptococcal antigen test will help confirm the diagnosis in this case.

Complete blood count may show thrombocytosis in acute rheumatic fever, but the presence of this finding is not confirmatory of the disease. EKG may show a prolonged PR interval or evidence of strain due to carditis but will not aid in confirming the diagnosis. Echocardiogram will be required to evaluate the extent of this patient's carditis but will not aid in confirming the diagnosis.

Test-taking tip: This is a "you know it or don't" kind of question. If you don't know it, choose an answer and move on. You can perhaps mark it for review when you are done at the end of the test. Don't, however, let these kinds of questions get you stuck and waste your time. The question is asking how to make the diagnosis of acute rheumatic fever and how to provide evidence of prior strep infection.

12. ANSWER: C

This patient is presenting with signs and symptoms of serum sickness, a type III hypersensitivity reaction characterized by immune complex deposition disease. The rash associated with serum sickness appears as erythema of the extremities that spreads proximally into a widespread morbilliform rash. Previous exposure to the offending agent may produce symptoms within 12 to 36 hours. Patients without prior exposure to the agent may have delayed symptoms starting 7 to 20 days after exposure. Treatment for serum sickness is supportive with symptom control, and mainstay of treatment is removal of the offending agent.

Oral diphenhydramine may be used in cases in which the patient's rash is pruritic or urticaria is present. Prednisone taper may be used in more severe cases of serum sickness, but ultimately the removal of the offending agent is the mainstay of therapy. Switching to amoxicillin–clavulanic acid would not help this patient's symptoms and is not a good antibiotic to treat urinary tract infection.

Test-taking tip: You can eliminate A and D because the patient's rash is not pruritic, and the antibiotic is the likely offending agent, so changing the antibiotic is not helpful.

13. ANSWER: A

This patient is likely suffering from an anaphylactoid reaction to contrast media. Airway management is the most appropriate next step in this hemodynamically unstable patient with impending respiratory failure. Oral intubation is the procedure of choice initially, but the provider may also perform transtracheal jet insufflation or cricothyroidotomy if other airway methods fail.

Anaphylactoid reactions resemble anaphylactic reactions but do not require prior exposure. Contrast media, aspirin, NSAIDs, and codeine are among the most common causes. People taking β-blockers who also have a history of allergies may have a higher risk for anaphylaxis.

Diphenhydramine, although appropriately dosed, will not immediately help this patient. Epinephrine should be administered in all cases of anaphylaxis but should not supersede the need for a definitive airway in severe cases like this. Glucagon may be helpful in anaphylactic cases in which the patient is persistently hypotensive and taking a β-blocker but is not first-line treatment and should not prevent the placement of a definitive airway.

Test-taking tip: All the answer choices except A involve delaying the definitive management of this unstable patient with airway compromise.

14. ANSWER: C

This patient is presenting with medication-induced angioedema. Her new hypertensive medication is likely an ACE inhibitor. Her signs and symptoms are suggestive of impending airway obstruction, and thus she requires an emergent surgical airway. ACE inhibitor–induced angioedema is mediated by increased levels of bradykinin. Clinical manifestations are characterized by swelling, most commonly of the upper airway, that occurs rapidly within minutes to hours and resolves spontaneously within 24 to 72 hours. Angioedema of this type may occur when medication is first introduced or after medication dose adjustment. Airway protection is the mainstay of treatment, and the patient should be monitored for early signs of obstruction such as hoarseness or inspiratory stridor.

Nebulized albuterol-ipratropium is a medication used for reactive airway disease, asthma, and COPD. Administering this medication will not improve swelling and thus is not indicated in angioedema.

Although this patient is in respiratory distress and becoming hypoxic, a non-rebreather mask will not be effective in maintaining oxygen flow in a patient with upper airway obstruction, and a surgical airway is needed. Diphenhydramine may be given in the emergent setting when treating the patient for all types of angioedema; this medication, however, should not precede obtaining a definitive airway. Antihistamines are not effective in treating ACE inhibitor–induced angioedema because they serve no role in altering levels of bradykinin.

Test-taking tip: This question is asking you to recognize an unstable airway and to know when to go right to a surgical airway.

15. ANSWER: A

This patient presents with signs and symptoms of acute renal transplant rejection. Renal transplant rejection most commonly occurs within the first 6 months after transplantation. Patients are typically placed on calcineurin inhibitors such as tacrolimus or cyclosporine. Patients with acute rejection commonly present with fever, malaise, and oliguria. A rise in creatinine levels is most specific for acute transplant rejection and is commonly a late finding indicative of significant histologic destruction.

Hypertension, proteinuria, and sterile pyuria can be present in acute kidney transplant rejection but are relatively nonspecific. Leukocytosis may be present because of an acute stress reaction but is not specific for acute rejection and may indicate infection or relate to another cause.

Test-taking tip: This is a "you know it or don't" kind of question. If you don't know it, choose an answer and move on. You can perhaps mark it for review when you are done at the end of the test. Don't, however, let these kinds of questions get you stuck and waste your time.

16. ANSWER: B

This patient is presenting with signs and symptoms of acute systemic JRA. This form of JRA presents with daily spiking fevers, salmon-colored rash, and multiple swollen and tender joints. Most concerning are the patient's laboratory findings, which are suggestive of macrophage activation syndrome (MAS), a rare complication in patients with systemic JRA. MAS should be treated as a rheumatologic emergency because it carries high mortality if untreated. Initial treatment includes administration of corticosteroids such as dexamethasone. This patient will require admission to a pediatric unit for further monitoring of disease progression and prevention of organ failure.

NSAIDs and primary care follow-up are adequate when treating mild systemic JRA disease, but this patient is presenting with concerning systemic manifestations and would benefit from an escalation in treatment. Arthrocentesis is not indicated in a patient with suspected rheumatoid arthritis. Vancomycin would be beneficial in a patient with a septic joint and risk factors for MRSA infection. This patient does not warrant antibiotic therapy.

Test-taking tip: You can eliminate choice A because the patient is in extremis and requires inpatient treatment. The patient has symmetric joint involvement, which does not support a diagnosis of septic joint, thus eliminating choices C and D.

17. ANSWER: D

This patient is presenting with signs and symptoms of Henoch-Schonlein Purpura (HSP), an IgA vasculitis of the medium-sized vessels. This disease is most commonly seen in children aged 3 to 15 years. Patients typically present with classic signs of recent upper respiratory infection, followed by abdominal pain, joint pain, lower extremity edema, and a palpable purpuric rash. Diagnosis is made clinically, but it is important to identify potential complications early. The patient described in the question reports abdominal pain, anorexia, and dark stools, which should raise suspicion for intussusception.

Intussusception is the most common gastrointestinal complication in patients with HSP. The diagnostic test of choice for intussusception in a hemodynamically stable patient is abdominal ultrasound. The classic finding on ultrasound for the diagnosis is the "target sign" or "bull's eye," representing a layer of intestine within another layer of intestine. Definitive treatment for intussusception in a hemodynamically stable patient is nonoperative reduction such as saline, contrast, or pneumatic enema. If the patient is unstable or there is high suspicion for bowel perforation, then definitive treatment is surgical.

Test-taking tip: You can eliminate A and B because neither topical nor oral medications help in the treatment of intussusception.

18. ANSWER: C

This patient presents with findings consistent with Kawasaki syndrome, and thrombocytopenia (platelet count <150,000/mL) is not characteristic of the disease. Kawasaki disease is an acute medium-sized vessel vasculitis that occurs commonly in children. There are five classic signs for this disease as outlined in Table 9.2. Ninety percent of cases occur before the age of 5 years.

Classic findings consist of a prolonged fever (>5 days) and at least four out of the five signs: unilateral cervical lymphadenopathy, strawberry tongue, cracked red lips, extremity edema and/or erythema, nonvesicular rash, and bilateral conjunctivitis.

Labs are nonspecific and may show thrombocytosis, leukocytosis, anemia, elevation of inflammatory markers

Table 9.2 KAWASAKI DISEASE SYMPTOMS AND SIGNS

Classic Kawasaki symptoms	Fever for 5 or more days
	Four of the five following symptoms:
	Extremity rash or swelling (involves palms and soles)
	Rash
	Bilateral conjunctivitis
	Lip/oral cavity redness/ swelling (strawberry tongue and fissured lips)
	Cervical lymphadenopathy
Classic Kawasaki laboratory signs	Elevated platelet count
	Elevated white blood cell count
	Elevated C-reactive protein and erythrocyte sedimentation rate

(CRP, ESR), and elevated liver function tests. The mainstay of therapy for these cases is high-dose aspirin and IV immunoglobulin. Complications include coronary artery aneurysms, and therefore a baseline echocardiography should be performed.

Test-taking tip: Choices A, B, and D are all classic signs of Kawasaki disease. This is a "you know it or don't" kind of question. If you don't know it, choose an answer and move on. You can perhaps mark it for review when you are done at the end of the test. Don't, however, let these kinds of questions get you stuck and waste your time.

19. ANSWER: C

Cardiovascular complications in Kawasaki disease are important to identify early to determine a child's prognosis and outcome. Approximately 25% of children will go on to develop coronary artery aneurysms if left untreated. Children younger than 12 months are at higher risk for complications. Early assessment of cardiac status with EKG, echocardiography, and chest radiography may help identify cardiac abnormalities in this disease. Early diagnosis and treatment have been shown to reduce incidence of coronary artery aneurysms to approximately 4%.

Gastrointestinal complications such as gallbladder hydrops, cholestasis, and ileus have been identified in patients during the acute of phase of Kawasaki disease. These typically resolve once IV immunoglobulin therapy is initiated and do not carry a higher mortality than the cardiovascular complications. Hematologic complications are rare and may be due to proliferation of macrophages and T lymphocytes seen in macrophage activation syndrome (MAS). This syndrome may lead to severe complications such as disseminated intravascular coagulation (DIC), cytopenia, and thromboses. This syndrome is more commonly noted in patients with prolonged fever despite IV immunoglobulin therapy. Neurologic complications have been poorly identified in cases of Kawasaki disease. Few studies describe hearing loss during the acute phase of the disease, with others noting possible long-term behavioral effects after resolution of the disease.

Test-taking tip: You can eliminate all answer choices except for choice C because the cardiovascular complications in Kawasaki disease are the most important complications to diagnose and treat.

20. ANSWER: C

Selective IgA deficiency is the most common type of immunologic defect in humans. It is considered a primary humoral immunodeficiency despite most commonly being asymptomatic. Other manifestations of selective IgA deficiency include recurrent sinus and pulmonary infections, allergic reactions, and anaphylactic reactions. Anaphylaxis has been reported in patients with IgA deficiency owing to the presence of IgA antibodies in the serum interacting with IgA in the blood products. Common transfusion products that contain IgA include whole blood, red blood cells, platelets, FFP, cryoprecipitate, and IV immunoglobulin.

C1-esterase deficiency is known to cause hereditary angioedema manifested by laryngeal edema and recurrent colic episodes. DiGeorge's syndrome is caused by a segment deletion at chromosome 22q11.2. Patients with this syndrome may develop thymic aplasia or hypoparathyroidism. They do not develop anaphylaxis. Down syndrome is caused by trisomy of chromosome 21. These patients are born with dysmorphic facial features, including brachycephaly, a large protruding tongue, narrow palate, short neck, and abnormal teeth that may make obtaining a definitive airway more difficult, but the condition is not associated with anaphylaxis.

Test-taking tip: Knowing that choice A is referencing hereditary angioedema, which is not associated with blood products, you can eliminate this answer choice.

10.

SYSTEMIC INFECTIOUS DISEASES

Leah Bauer, Carolyn Chooljian, and Whitney Johnson

1. A 35-year-old male who lives in a remote rural area of New Mexico presents to the emergency department (ED) with a cough and respiratory difficulty. He has been ill for 2 days with fever, chills, and myalgia and now has developed severe shortness of breath.

He is otherwise healthy. Vital signs are temperature 39° C, blood pressure (BP) 90/60 mm Hg, heart rate (HR) 120 bpm, respiratory rate (RR) 28 breaths/min, and oxygen saturation 90% on room air.

His physical exam reveals an ill-appearing male with difficulty breathing. Lungs have diffuse rales. Heart is tachycardic, and abdomen is soft and nontender. There is no rash or edema. Chest radiograph reveals bilateral interstitial infiltrates, white blood cell (WBC) count is $26,000 \times 10^{-3}/mm^3$ with predominant polymorphonuclear neutrophils (PMNs) and marked left shift. Other laboratory results include hematocrit 56.3%, platelets $64,000 \times 10^{-3}/mm^3$, lactate dehydrogenase (LDH) 568 IU/L, aspartate aminotransferase (AST) 148 IU/L, alanine aminotransferase (ALT) 63 IU/L, blood urea nitrogen (BUN) 17 g/dL, creatinine 1.4 mg/dL, and lactate 4.4 mmol/L.

Which statement about this illness is true?

A. The illness is caused by exposure to another infected individual, and this patient requires isolation
B. Doxycycline is the antibiotic of choice
C. Transmission is by aerosol of infected rodent urine, feces, or saliva
D. Ribavirin has been shown to be effective treatment

2. Each of the following statements about influenza are true *except*:

A. Influenza A is subject to antigenic shift of its hemagglutinin and neuraminidase envelope glycoproteins, producing the potential for severe pandemics; influenza B only undergoes antigenic drift

B. The treatment of choice is amantadine or rimantadine started within 48 hours of symptom onset
C. Influenza vaccine is developed each year to try to match the strain of influenza virus that is likely to be circulating; therefore annual vaccination is recommended
D. A positive rapid antigen test is most likely to be true positive during peak influenza season and a negative rapid antigen test is most likely to be false negative during peak influenza season

3. All of the following statements about infectious mononucleosis are true *except*:

A. It is caused by the Epstein-Barr virus
B. The classic diagnostic triad for infectious mononucleosis is fever, pharyngitis, and anterior cervical lymphadenopathy
C. It is characterized by lymphocytosis and atypical lymphocytes
D. Spontaneous splenic rupture is a potential complication

4. What is the most likely organism causing pneumonia in the stable transplant recipient 2 years after transplantation?

A. *Pneumocystis jirovecii*
B. Cytomegalovirus (CMV)
C. *Pneumococcus*
D. *Coccidioides immitis*

5. The most common opportunistic infection in the post-transplantation patient is:

A. *P. jirovecii*
B. CMV
C. *Coccidioides immitis*
D. Toxoplasmosis

6. The highest risk period for opportunistic infection in the post-transplantation patient is:

A. Early postoperative period
B. The first month after transplantation
C. 1–6 months after transplantation
D. >6–12 months after transplantation

7. A 67-year-old male presents to the ED with a 6-day history of intermittent fevers (temperatures to 39.4° C), headache, nausea, vomiting, and abdominal pain.

Physical examination is remarkable for temperature of 38.9° C, diffuse abdominal tenderness, and tachycardia. He is an avid golfer and lives in a golf-oriented retirement community bordering a wooded wildlife area in Eastern Tennessee noted to have many deer.

Laboratory results include WBC count 3,600/mm³ (abnormal <4,000/mm³), hematocrit 36.3%, platelets 59,000/mm³, AST 127 IU/L (abnormal >40 IU/L), ALT 280 IU/L (abnormal >40 IU/L), and creatinine 1.5 mg/dL.
Which antibiotic is most likely to be effective in the management of his illness?

A. Doxycycline
B. Ceftriaxone
C. Azithromycin
D. Levofloxacin

8. A 62-year-old woman from Connecticut presents with persistent fever, headache, and myalgias for 2 weeks. She saw her family physician a week earlier for an expanding red rash on her right volar forearm. She had gone hiking a week before the onset of the rash. The physician placed her on a 2-week course of amoxicillin, which she is still taking.

Her vital signs are temperature 39° C, BP 90/60 mm Hg, and HR 120 bpm. Her physical exam reveals conjunctival icterus and right upper quadrant tenderness. Her laboratory studies show WBC count 2,800/μL (2.8 × 10⁹/L), hemoglobin 9 g/dL (90 g/L), platelet count 30,000/μL (30 × 10⁹/L), ALT 500 U/L, and bilirubin 7.4 mg/dL .

What is the proper next step in the management of this patient?

A. Vancomycin
B. Ceftriaxone
C. Doxycycline
D. Vancomycin and ceftriaxone

9. A-30-year old male presents with fever, headache, nausea, vomiting, and cough for 3 days. He is an otherwise healthy individual. He works on a cattle ranch and recently aided in the delivery of a calf.

His temperature is 39.9° C, HR 130 bpm, RR 24 breaths/min, and BP 100/60 mm Hg. Physical exam reveals bilateral rales and mild right upper quadrant abdominal tenderness. He has no rash. Laboratory studies reveal platelet count 110,000, WBC count 8,000 × 10⁻³/mm³, and AST 90 IU/L.

All of the statements about this illness are true *except*:

A. Infection may occur by inhalation and/or ingestion
B. This illness may have a chronic phase
C. The treatment of choice is doxycycline
D. The causative agent is a spirochete

10. Which of the following is *not* a tick-borne illness?

A. Rocky Mountain spotted fever (RMSF)
B. Q Fever
C. Lyme disease
D. Human monocytic ehrlichiosis (HME)

11. Which of the illnesses is *not* caused by a rickettsial organism?

A. Lyme disease
B. HME
C. Human granulocytic anaplasmosis (HGA)
D. RMSF

12. A 39-year-old 20-week pregnant woman presents to the ED with 5 days of fever, headache, myalgias, abdominal pain, vomiting and diarrhea. She is an otherwise healthy person and takes no medications. Her recent travel includes a camping trip to the Blue Ridge Mountains of Virginia for 1 week. She has been home for 10 days. She does not recall a tick bite.

Physical examination shows a moderately ill individual mild abdominal discomfort. There is no rash.

Vital signs include temperature of 39.9° C, BP 125/65 mm Hg, HR 90 bpm, and RR 18 breaths/min.

Laboratory findings include hemoglobin 15 g/dL, WBC count 3,500/μL, platelet count 90,000/μL, AST 90 U/L, ALT 89 U/L, and sodium 130 mEq/L.

The next step in the management of this patient is:

A. Order indirect fluorescent antibody acute and convalescent serology and start ceftriaxone
B. Order indirect fluorescent antibody acute and convalescent serology and start doxycycline
C. Order indirect fluorescent antibody acute and convalescent serology and observe
D. Order indirect fluorescent antibody acute and convalescent serology and start chloramphenicol

13. A 73-year-old male patient is brought to the ED by his family for evaluation of increasing confusion and

weakness over the past 2 days. He has no significant past medical history and was well until the onset of these symptoms. He lives in an urban area. His wife recalls seeing a dead bird in their yard a week ago. He has evidence of recent mosquito bites.

Vital signs are temperature 39.1° C, HR 130 bpm, BP 120/70 mm Hg, and RR 28 breaths/min.

On physical exam he is somnolent with slurred speech, is disoriented, and does not follow commands well but is protecting his airway.

He has mild nuchal rigidity. His general neurologic exam reveals mild tremors, myoclonus, and flaccid paralysis of his extremities.

His lung, cardiac, and abdominal exams are unremarkable.

Laboratory studies reveal WBC count 11,000/mm³, hematocrit 44%, and platelet count 350,000/mm³. Serum chemistry and liver enzyme levels are normal.

A lumbar puncture is performed with the following results: WBC count 70/mm³ (81% PMNs, 10% monocytes, and 9% lymphocytes), glucose 60 mg/dL, protein 77 mg/dL, and Gram stain negative.

All of the following statements about this illness are true *except*:

A. It is associated with a high mortality
B. Advanced age, immunocompromised states, and malignancy increase the risk for neuroinvasive disease
C. Immunoglobulin M (IgM) in the cerebrospinal fluid (CSF) is diagnostic
D. Brain computed tomography (CT) is usually normal

14. A 70-year-old man presents to the ED with slurred speech, difficulty chewing, blurry vision, generalized weakness, and unsteady gait after awakening this morning. He denies trauma, fevers, headache, leg or arm weakness, difficulty swallowing, nausea, constipation, or diarrhea. His past medical history includes hypertension and hyperlipidemia.

Vital signs are temperature 36.4° C, BP 201/95 mm Hg, HR 85 bpm, RR 16 breaths/min, and oxygen saturation 98%.

The general physical exam is within normal limits. He is alert but his speech is dysarthric and almost unintelligible. The cranial nerve exam reveals weakness on abduction of the right eye. Pupillary responses to light are intact. There is bilateral rotary nystagmus. The rest of his neurologic exam is normal.

The patient's son stated that the patient had been eating home-preserved green beans and tomatoes in the 4 days.

Which of the following would be most important choice in managing this patient?

A. Stat head CT
B. Call the state health department
C. Tensilon test
D. Electromyography (EMG)

15. The following statements regarding methicillin-resistant *Staphylococcus aureus* (MRSA) are true *except*:

A. MRSA is susceptible to cephalosporins
B. Community-acquired MRSA is associated with the Panton-Valentine cytotoxin, which enhances its virulence
C. The mechanism of methicillin resistance is the presence of penicillin-binding protein 2a (PBP 2a) located on the bacterial membrane
D. Hospital-associated MRSA produces a biofilm on invasive foreign devices that enhances it persistence

16. The following statements about rabies are true *except*:

A. Rabies is a catastrophic viral illness caused by the *Lyssavirus*, which is transmitted by the bite of infected mammals
B. The most common source of rabies worldwide is rabid dogs
C. The most common source of rabies in the United States is raccoons
D. Early symptoms include paresthesias from the wound extending proximally

17. A 42-year-old male presents to the ED with a chief complaint of back pain. While lifting a heavy object 3 days before admission, he felt sudden onset of severe pain all over his middle back. He has been having back pain and spasms since then. He has had one episode of emesis but denies fever, chills, shortness of breath, or chest pain. He denies any past medical history and takes no medications but does endorse injection drug use of heroin. His vital signs are BP 143/98 mm Hg, HR 106 bpm, RR 20 breaths/min, and temperature 36° C.

He is alert and oriented. Physical exam is pertinent for diffuse muscle spasms throughout his upper and lower back with no point tenderness. He is unable to open his mouth completely and has a strange facial expression and is holding his arms up and out. He is sitting up on the gurney, and when he is given a tablet of valium, he is unable to swallow it. He has multiple scars on his extremities but no evidence of an abscess.

Which of the following is the most likely diagnosis?

A. Acute muscle strain
B. Epidural abscess
C. Generalized tetanus
D. Local tetanus

18. Meningococcemia has which of the following findings that occurs most often in patients?

A. Arthritis
B. Bilateral adrenal infarction
C. Seizures
D. Skin lesions

19. A 9-year-old girl was brought into the ED by her parents about 1 week after returning from India with reports of 3 days of fever, headache, malaise, nausea, and generalized abdominal pain. There have also been some loose stools without blood. All vaccinations are up to date, including vaccines for hepatitis A and yellow fever before the family trip. Throughout their vacation she was given prophylactic mefloquine for malaria. Vital signs are temperature 39.3° C, BP 90/50 mm Hg, HR 53 bpm, and RR 16 breaths/min. She appears lethargic with sunken eyes and delayed capillary refill. A faint, blanching, erythematous rash is noted over her anterior chest. Laboratory studies show anemia with a mild leukocytosis and elevated liver function tests (LFTs). Which of the following is true?

A. Admit for presumed dengue fever and start antibiotics
B. Child most likely contracted a strain of malaria that is resistant to mefloquine
C. Laboratory studies would likely reveal evidence of eosinophilia
D. The likely diagnosis is typhoid fever

20. A 21-year-old male presents to the ED with complaints of skin lesions. He reports that he and a group of friends were on a canoeing and camping trip in rural southern Georgia a few weeks ago. On examination, he has a serpiginous, raised, pruritic, erythematous eruption on the buttocks. During diagnostic testing, *Strongyloides* larvae are found in his stool. His friends were later also called in for evaluation. Despite being asymptomatic, these patients were are also found to have *Strongyloides* larvae in their stool. Regarding *Strongyloides* infections, what are the goals of care in an asymptomatic carrier?

A. Fluconazole
B. Ivermectin
C. Mebendazole
D. Mefloquine

21. In a patient who has traveled to Southeast Asia, which of the following is the most common cause of fever?

A. Dengue fever
B. Malaria
C. Salmonella
D. Yellow fever

22. A previously healthy 12-year-old boy was brought into the ED by his parents with a 2-day history of fevers, headache, and photophobia. The parents noted that the boy seemed to be increasingly confused as well. They report that they recently returned from a family vacation at a nearby lake where they grilled hamburgers for a picnic and swam in the freshwater lake. No other members of the family have been ill recently. On clinical examination the patient appears lethargic. Vital signs are temperature 39.5° C, BP 90/60 mm Hg, and HR 120 bpm. Patient is warm to touch with tachycardia, and nuchal rigidity is noted. Despite fluid resuscitation and empiric antibiotics, the patient dies. At autopsy, a brain biopsy shows evidence of trophozoites.

Which of the following is the most likely route of transmission of the infection acquired by this patient?

A. Ingestion of contaminated food
B. Ingestion of contaminated water
C. Mosquito bite
D. Penetration through the nasal mucosa

23. A 54-year-old female was brought into the ED with fever, productive cough, dyspnea with minimal exertion, and congestion for the past several days. She has also noted some general fatigue but no hemoptysis, headaches, dizziness, chest pain, or leg swelling. On clinical assessment, the patient's vital signs are temperature 39.3° C, HR 134 bpm, RR 16 breaths/min, BP 80/45 mm Hg, and oxygen saturation 80% on room air. Coarse breath sounds are noted in bilateral lung bases on auscultation. A chest radiograph shows a right lower lobe infiltrate. What is the first step in the initial management of this patient?

A. Antibiotic therapy
B. β-Blocker therapy to control heart rate
C. IV fluid resuscitation
D. Supplemental oxygen and airway management

24. Infection with which of the following helminths is known to cause a fatal hyperinfection in the immunocompromised patient?

A. *Ascaris lumbricoides*
B. *Enterobius vermicularis*
C. *Necator americanus*
D. *Strongyloides stercoralis*

25. A 28-year-old female with a history of HIV (CD4 count unknown; not on HAART) presents to the ED with increasing headaches for the past few weeks. Over the past 3 to 4 days she has also began experiencing high fevers, nausea, and vomiting. Vital signs at triage are temperature 41° C, BP 111/64 mm Hg, HR 130 bpm, and RR 16 breaths/min. On physical examination, the patient is lying in bed with the lights off and appears ill. There are no meningeal signs, and she has an essentially unremarkable neurologic exam. A lumbar puncture was performed with the following results: opening pressure 30 cm H_2O, CSF clear color, WBC count 17 cells/mm³ (lymphocytic predominance), red blood cell (RBC) count 1 cells/mm³, glucose 60 mg/dL, and protein 108 mg/dL.

Based on these findings, which test are you most likely to obtain?

   A. Cryptococcal antigen
   B. Herpes simplex virus (HSV) antigen
   C. Pneumococcal antigen
   D. Venereal Disease Research Laboratory (VDRL)

26. An 18-year-old male presents to the ED for evaluation of a skin wound on his left thigh. He explains that he recently returned from working in Saudi Arabia with the Peace Corp and that the ulcer has been present for the past 12 weeks despite wound care and repeated antibiotics. Which of the following is the most likely culprit?

   A. MRSA infection
   B. Leishmaniasis
   C. Onchocerciasis
   D. *Trypanosoma cruzi* infection

27. A 36-year-old HIV-positive male (CD4 count of 33) is brought to the ED by ambulance with 5 days of fever and headache. He has not had any primary care for more than 1 year and is not taking any medications. On physical exam, the patient appears lethargic. There are white patches on his tongue and buccal mucosa. Among diagnostic testing, magnetic resonance imaging (MRI) of the brain was completed. It demonstrates focal, enhancing lesions with surrounding edema in the right parietal lobe as well as the left basal ganglia. The best evaluation and treatment plan for this patient should be:

   A. Consult neurosurgery for brain biopsy
   B. Continue current regimen and supportive measures
   C. Obtain lumbar puncture to evaluate for cryptococcal meningitis
   D. Start pyrimethamine and sulfadiazine

28. A previously healthy 21-year-old male was brought into the ED after a sudden onset of severe headache, followed by vomiting and lethargy. On clinical evaluation, he was found to be responsive only to painful stimuli, with evidence of nuchal rigidity, normal optic fundi, and an otherwise normal neurologic examination. Blood cultures, WBC count, and differential were obtained and emergency CT requested before lumbar puncture. The decision to start antibiotics immediately was made. Which of the following regimens would be best for empiric therapy in this patient?

   A. Ceftriaxone alone
   B. Vancomycin, ampicillin, ceftriaxone, and dexamethasone
   C. Vancomycin and ceftriaxone
   D. Vancomycin, ceftriaxone, and dexamethasone

29. A 23-year-old, previously healthy male was brought into the ED with complaints of severe headache for the past 24 hours. He reports that he is visiting from Kentucky for vacation where his regular diet includes homemade cheese made from raw cow's milk. During his vacation, he has been camping and swimming with friends on a nearby human-made lake. On evaluation in the ED, the patient is alert and has some neck stiffness. No other focal findings or neurologic deficits were noted. His CSF showed the following: WBC count 1,740 cells/mm³ (82% neutrophils), RBC count 30 cells/mm³, glucose 18 mg/dL, protein 420 mg/dL, Gram stain negative.

Dexamethasone, vancomycin, and ceftriaxone are initiated for presumed bacterial meningitis. However, over the next 48 hours the patient shows some clinical decompensation with worsening mentation and persistent vomiting. Cultures of the blood and CSF had no growth at 72 hours. Which of the following would be the best addition to this patient's regimen to provide coverage for the likely pathogen causing his illness?

   A. Add amphotericin B
   B. Add ampicillin
   C. Add antituberculous therapy
   D. Add tetracycline

30. A 65-year-old male was brought into the ED with complaints of fever, cough, and diarrhea for the past 5 days. He reports that he recently returned from a 2-week cruise to the Bahamas. There is a documented history of chronic obstructive pulmonary disease (COPD), hypertension, and a 30 pack-year history of cigarette smoking. There were no other sick contacts that he could recall while on the cruise. Vital signs are as follows: temperature 39° C, BP 100/60 mm Hg, HR 90 bpm, RR 24 breaths/min, and oxygen saturation 87% on room air. On physical examination mucous membranes are dry, heart is tachycardic, and there is dullness to percussion at the left lung base. Chest radiograph demonstrates a left lobar infiltrate, with patchy opacities on the right. Laboratory studies are noteworthy for WBC count $18,000 \times 10^{-3}/mm^3$, sodium 130 mEq/L, serum creatinine 1.0 (baseline), and elevated AST/ALT. A urinary antigen test was positive. Which of the following regarding his suspected disease is *false*?

A. Can be acquired by drinking infected water
B. Hyponatremia is typical
C. Most cases are sporadic
D. Smokers are more susceptible

31. A 40-year-old female presents to the ED with complaints of fevers, diaphoresis, abdominal pain, and constipation for 3 days. She reports that she is from a remote Peruvian village. Vital signs show temperature 39.5° C, BP 111/70 mm Hg, HR 50 bpm, and RR 14 breaths/min. On examination, she is flushed and lying uncomfortably in bed. Lungs are clear to auscultation and heart sounds mildly bradycardic. She has diffuse abdominal tenderness to palpation with decreased bowel sounds and mild distention. No peritoneal signs are noted. There is no peripheral edema seen. Lab results show only an elevated WBC count and platelets of 50000 $\times 10^{-3}/mm^3$. Normal LFTs. The most likely diagnosis is:

A. Dengue fever
B. Hepatitis
C. Malaria
D. Typhoid fever

32. A 32-year-old man with no past medical history presents with a temperature of 38.5° C, tenosynovitis, polyarthritis, and a nonpruritic, pustular rash on his arms and legs. The most likely diagnosis is:

A. Secondary syphilis
B. Gout
C. HSV
D. Disseminated gonococcal infection (DGI)

33. A 40-year-old man with no past medical history and no allergies presents to the ED with fevers, chills, malaise, and a maculopapular rash involving his trunk and extremities, including his palms and soles (Figure 10.1). The most appropriate treatment is:

A. Oral doxycycline
B. IM benzathine penicillin G
C. Oral azithromycin
D. IV ceftriaxone

34. A 40-year-old homeless male with a history of HIV is sent to the ED from his primary care doctor's clinic

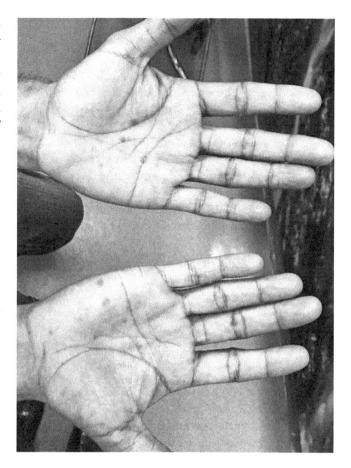

Figure 10.1 Rash.

with cough, fever, and shortness of breath for 1 week. He has not taken his medications for the past month because they were stolen. His most recent CD4 count is 100, and a chest radiograph done at the clinic shows bilateral interstitial infiltrates. On your assessment he is febrile, normotensive, and tachycardic with a SpO$_2$ of 91% on room air. You order an arterial blood gas (ABG) test, which shows pH 7.42, PCO$_2$ 36 mm Hg, and PaO$_2$ 68 mm Hg. Which of the following is the best choice of therapy?

A. Trimethoprim-sulfamethoxazole
B. Ceftriaxone, azithromycin, and prednisone
C. Levaquin and prednisone
D. Trimethoprim-sulfamethoxazole and prednisone

35. A 28-year-old woman is brought in by ambulance for altered mental status with abdominal pain, nausea, vomiting, and diarrhea. She is found to have a temperature of 40° C, BP 82/56 mm Hg, and HR 120 bpm. Physical exam reveals diffuse macular erythematous rash and nonpurulent conjunctivitis. Laboratory studies are remarkable for thrombocytopenia, markedly elevated creatinine, and pyuria. The most likely causative organism is:

A. *Escherichia coli*
B. *Neisseria meningitidis*
C. *S. aureus*
D. *Rickettsia rickettsia*

36. An 8-month-old girl is brought into the ED by her mother for 3 days of cough and fever with temperature up to 40° C. Physical exam reveals a fussy infant with injected conjunctiva, rhinorrhea, and inflamed nasal mucosa. Koplik spots are found on her buccal mucosa. Which of the following statements is *true?*

A. Those at high risk for complications include pregnant women, infants, children younger than 5 years, and immunocompromised persons
B. Transmission is airborne or by contact with infectious droplets
C. Patients are contagious 4 days before and 4 days after development of a maculopapular rash
D. All of the above

37. A 4-year-old boy is brought into the ED by his father for malaise, painful blisters in his mouth, and a nonpruritic vesicular rash on his palms and soles. He is fully vaccinated and otherwise healthy. His father reports that several other children at the group child care have been sick with similar symptoms. He has had no decrease in oral intake or urine output. Physical exam reveals a tired-appearing boy with painful, erythematous oral ulcerations and a vesicular rash involving his palms and soles. He is febrile with a temperature up to 38° C and with otherwise normal vital signs. The most appropriate management is

A. IV antibiotics
B. Topical steroids
C. PO antiviral
D. Hydration, antipyretic, topical oral pain relief

38. A 6-year-old girl presents with fever and facial rash for 2 days. Physical exam reveals a diffuse fiery red facial rash most prominent over the cheeks with perioral pallor and sparing of the chin and eyelids. The oropharynx is clear and moist without rash or exudate. The most likely causative organism is:

A. Parvovirus
B. *Candida* species
C. *Streptococcus* species
D. Coxsackie virus

39. A 13-year-old unvaccinated boy with no past medical history presents with low-grade fever and a diffuse, pruritic vesicular rash sparing his palms and soles. He is alert and oriented without neurologic deficits. A Tzanck

smear is performed and reveals giant cells with inclusion bodies. The most appropriate treatment is

A. Supportive care only
B. PO valacyclovir
C. Topical steroids
D. IV acyclovir

40. A 10-year-old female is brought into the ED by her mother for evaluation of a diffuse, blanching, papular, sandpaper-like rash that developed 2 days ago. The mother reports that the girl has been complaining of sore throat for the past 2 weeks with fevers for the past several days. You diagnose her with scarlet fever and decide to treat with penicillin. Which of the following has been shown to be a benefit of treatment?

A. Prevention of rheumatic fever
B. Shortening the duration of symptoms
C. Reducing the risk for transmission
D. All of the above

41. A 5-day-old male born at term by uncomplicated vaginal delivery is brought in for fever. Parents deny accompanying symptoms. Vital signs are temperature 39° C, HR 149 bpm, BP 80/40 mm Hg, RR 20 breaths/ min, and SPO_2 100%. Physical exam is unremarkable. Which of the following is the most appropriate initial treatment regimen?

A. Reassurance and supportive care
B. Vancomycin and ceftriaxone
C. Acyclovir, ampicillin, and cefotaxime
D. Ceftriaxone, vancomycin, and metronidazole

42. A 22-year-old female in her first trimester of pregnancy who recently emigrated from Ethiopia presents with arthralgias and a maculopapular rash from head to toe. She endorses a low-grade fever and upper respiratory symptoms for 3 days before development of the rash. Her fetus is at risk for which of the following?

A. Stillbirth
B. Cataracts
C. Deafness
D. All of the above

43. A 4-year-old girl is brought in by parents for fever and dry, barking cough. Her neck radiograph is shown in Figure 10.2. What is the most likely causative organism?

A. Group A *Streptococcus*
B. Parainfluenza virus

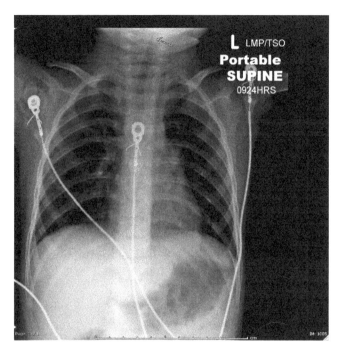

Figure 10.2 Chest radiograph.

C. *Haemophilus influenzae*
D. Influenza B

44. A 21-month-old girl who is up to date on vaccinations is brought in by her mother for a nonpainful, nonpruritic rash that developed abruptly this morning. Her mother reports she had been sick for the past week with cough, runny nose, and high temperatures. Two days ago she was seen by her pediatrician, who recommended Tylenol, hydration, and rest. According to the mother, the girl had started feeling better yesterday and hasn't had a fever in the past 24 hours. Physical exam reveals a happy, playful toddler with normal vital signs and a blanching, erythematous, macular rash over her trunk and buttocks. The most likely diagnosis is:

A. Roseola infantum
B. Measles
C. Chickenpox
D. Hand-foot-and-mouth disease

45. A 2-year-old boy with no past medical history is brought in by his parents for a 2-day history of sore throat and fever. He has never been immunized. He is febrile with temperatures up to 39° C, HR 151 bpm, BP 90/50 mm Hg, and oxygen saturation 92% on room air. On exam, he is distressed and drooling with nasal flaring and suprasternal retractions. Which of the following is the most appropriate next course of action?

A. Racemic epinephrine and IV antibiotics
B. IV steroids and nebulized albuterol
C. Prepare for intubation
D. Obtain a CT scan of the neck

46. A 47-year-old female with a history of HIV and a most recent CD4 count of 60 cells/μL presents for 3 days of headache, nausea, vomiting, and fever. She denies cough, shortness of breath, and hemoptysis. Her chest radiograph is normal. Her head CT is unremarkable, and CSF analysis reveals an opening pressure of 55 cm H_2O, glucose 30 mg/dL, protein 120 mg/dL, and WBC count 20 cells/μL with a mononuclear predominance. Which of the following is the most likely causative organism?

A. *H. influenzae*
B. *N. meningitidis*
C. *Cryptococcus neoformans*
D. HSV

ANSWERS

1. ANSWER: C

This patient has hantavirus cardiopulmonary syndrome, a viral illness that is transmitted by aerosol exposure to rodent urine, feces, or saliva. Antibiotics and antivirals are not effective in treating this illness. Treatment is supportive. No person-to-person transmission has been described.

Hantavirus is a genus of viruses of the order Bunyavirales. There are up to 30 different species. Hantavirus infection may be asymptomatic but is known for two major clinical syndromes: hantavirus cardiopulmonary syndrome (HCPS) and hantavirus fever with renal syndrome (HFRS). Rodents are the reservoir for these viruses, and aerosol exposure to rodent feces, urine, and saliva is the mode of transmission. Person-to-person transmission is not thought to occur.

The syndrome seen in North America is HCPS, caused by the Sin Nombre virus species carried by deer mice. Patients from rural areas with potential exposure to wild rodents are at risk for this illness. The incubation period is 1 to 6 weeks after exposure, with a median of 14 to 17 days. The prodrome is clinically nonspecific with fever, chills, and myalgias. The cardiopulmonary phase starts with a dry cough followed by a rapid onset of hypotension and noncardiogenic pulmonary edema.

HFRS is seen with exposure to other hantavirus species. The illness causes an acute tubulointerstitial nephritis with increased vascular permeability.

Prominent laboratory findings include thrombocytopenia, marked leukocytosis, elevated LDH, and elevated transaminases. These findings with bilateral interstitial infiltrates characterize HCPS, whereas proteinuria, hematuria, and reduced glomerular filtration rate (GFR) are seen in HFRS.

Antiviral antibodies of IgM and IgG class are present by the time the patient develops symptoms.

Treatment is supportive. Extracorporeal membrane oxygenation (ECMO) has been successfully used to manage those with severe heart failure.

Test-taking tip: Two big hints in this question stem are that the patient lives in rural New Mexico and that it is an acute onset of symptoms, which should lead you to conclude it is hantavirus.

2. ANSWER: B

Amantadine and rimantadine are only active against influenza A viruses, which have developed high levels of resistance to these drugs. They are no longer recommended as drugs of choice.

The neuraminidase inhibitors oseltamivir (oral) and zanamivir (inhaled) are active against influenza A and B viruses and are the current drugs of choice. They are recommended when a patient with influenza presents within 48 hours of symptom onset.

Influenza A and B are viruses that cause acute respiratory infections, usually in the winter. Clinical symptoms include fever, cough, rhinitis, headache, and myalgia. They are highly contagious and spread from person to person by contact with respiratory secretions.

The incubation period is 1 to 4 days, and viral shedding is highest at 24 to 48 hours of illness for influenza A. Influenza B begins shedding before clinical symptoms appear and lasts about 48 hours after symptoms.

Only influenza A undergoes antigenic shifts, a major change in the envelope glycoproteins hemagglutinin and/or neuraminidase, leading to epidemics and pandemics. Both influenza A and B viruses undergo antigenic drifts, which produce minor point mutations in the glycoproteins and less propensity to severe outbreaks.

A new vaccine is produced yearly to try to match the predicted influenza strains that will be circulating. Yearly vaccination is recommended.

The accuracy of rapid antigen tests depends on the likelihood of influenza activity at the time. In times of peak influenza activity, positive tests are likely to be true positive; however, negative tests are more likely to be false negative given the low sensitivity of the test.

Test-taking tip: All of the "except" questions are difficult. Treat each statement as a true/false question. This helps avoid confusion.

3. ANSWER: B

The lymphadenopathy for mononucleosis is more commonly posterior cervical, unlike streptococcal pharyngitis, which classically has anterior cervical lymphadenopathy.

Infectious mononucleosis is an infection caused by the Epstein-Barr virus, which is a herpesvirus. Epstein-Barr virus is also associated with B-cell lymphoma, T-cell lymphoma, Hodgkin's lymphoma, and nasopharyngeal lymphoma.

Infectious mononucleosis is usually transmitted by intimate contact. It is characterized by low-grade fever, malaise, headache, fatigue, tonsillitis, pharyngitis, and posterior cervical adenopathy. The lymphadenopathy can also be generalized. Characteristic laboratory findings include lymphocytosis (>4,500/μL, >50% of differential) and atypical lymphocytes (>10% of lymphocytes).

Most infections are subclinical, and 90% to 95% of adults worldwide are seropositive.

Three clinical patterns have been described:

1. The glandular form: lymph node enlargement out of proportion to pharyngitis
2. The systemic (typhoidal) form: fever and fatigue more prominent than lymphadenopathy and pharyngitis
3. The hepatitis form: hepatitis without the other manifestations of infectious mononucleosis

A morbilliform rash may develop in association with ampicillin treatment, but this does not indicate allergy to ampicillin.

Splenomegaly develops in 50% to 60% of patients, and splenic rupture can occur. About 50% of splenic ruptures are spontaneous, and they occur about 14 days after symptom onset. Rupture may be the presenting symptom. It is rare after 4 weeks of illness.

The treatment of infectious mononucleosis is generally supportive. Steroids may be needed for potential airway obstruction due to marked tonsillar enlargement. The Monospot test is a latex agglutination assay using horse erythrocytes and has a sensitivity and specificity of 85% and 100%, respectively, for mononucleosis, though it is less accurate in young children.

Test-taking tip: All of the "except" questions are difficult. Treat each statement as a true/false question. This helps avoid confusion.

4. ANSWER: C

Infections due to community-acquired organisms are seen more than 6 to 12 months after transplantation, when immunosuppression is stabilized. These include pneumonias due to respiratory viruses and common bacteria including *Pneumococcus* and *Legionella*.

Post-transplantation patients often receive prophylactic trimethoprim-sulfamethoxazole, which is effective in preventing *P. jirovecii*, *Toxoplasma gondii*, *Listeria monocytogenes,* and other pathogens.

CMV is the most common opportunistic infection after transplantation, and the highest risk for infection with this pathogen is in the recipient-negative, donor-positive setting. IV ganciclovir and oral acyclovir are used for prophylaxis of CMV.

Test-taking tip: In this question, both A and B are viruses and thus can be eliminated. That leaves C *(Pneumococcus)* and D *(Coccidioides)*. The question stem did not mention the patient living in an area where *Coccidioides* is endemic, so you can rule out D and pick the correct answer C.

5. ANSWER: B

CMV is the most common opportunistic infection after transplantation, and the highest risk for infection with this pathogen is in the recipient-negative, donor-positive setting. IV ganciclovir and oral acyclovir are used for prophylaxis of CMV.

Test-taking tip: This is a "you know it or don't" kind of question. If you don't know it, choose an answer and move on. You can perhaps mark it for review when you are done at the end of the test. Don't, however, let these kinds of questions get you stuck and waste your time.

6. ANSWER: C

Posttransplant infections are divided into three stages: (1) early postoperative period to first month, (2) 1 to 6 months after transplantation; and (3) more than 6 to 12 months after transplantation.

Two predominant causes of infection in the *first month after transplantation* are complications due to hospitalization and the surgery and donor- or recipient-derived infections. Infections involve nosocomial bacteria including *Legionella* species, *Pseudomonas aeruginosa,* MRSA, and vancomycin-resistant *Enterococcus* (VRE). Nosocomial fungi include *Aspergillus* and *Candida* species. Hepatitis B and C may reemerge. Graft-associated infections from viruses such as HIV, rabies, and parasites such as toxoplasmosis may be transmitted. Prolonged mechanical ventilation increases the risk. Nosocomial bacteria and fungi infect anastomotic sites and fluid collections.

In the period *1 to 6 months after transplantation,* immunosuppression is greatest and opportunistic infections become prevalent. These include *P. jirovecii* pneumonia; latent protozoal infections such as toxoplasmosis, leishmaniasis, and Chagas' disease; endemic fungi such as *Histoplasma, Coccidioides, Cryptococcus,* and *Blastomyces* species; viruses, particularly herpes group, hepatitis B, hepatitis C, BK polyomavirus, human herpesviruses 6 and 7, and Kaposi's sarcoma–associated herpesvirus; respiratory viruses including respiratory syncytial virus (RSV), influenza, parainfluenza, and adenovirus; *Mycobacterium tuberculosis* and nontuberculous mycobacteria; and gastrointestinal parasites and viruses including *Cryptosporidium* species, *Microsporidium* species, CMV, and rotavirus.

Test-taking tip: The question stem states opportunistic infections. This is a hint to the correct answer because it takes a few weeks for all of the immunosuppressants to take effect.

7. ANSWER: A

This patient is infected with *Ehrlichia chaffeensis,* a rickettsial-like obligate intracellular organism that is the agent of human monocytic ehrlichiosis (HME). It is transmitted to humans by the Lone Star tick *(Amblyomma americanum).* The reservoirs for HME are deer, dogs, and goats.

A similar illness is caused by *Anaplasma phagocytophilum,* another rickettsial-like organism transmitted by the *Ixodes scapularis* tick, the agent of human granulocytic anaplasmosis (HGA).

The clinical syndrome is nonspecific and similar for both organisms and typically includes fever, headache, and myalgia. Leukopenia, thrombocytopenia, and mild elevation of liver enzymes are characteristic of these illnesses.

Rash is less likely than in RMSF, though 40% of HME cases may have a nonspecific trunk rash.

The *I. scapularis* tick (vector for HGA) also carries *Babesia microti,* the cause of babesiosis, and *Borrelia burgdorferi,* the cause of Lyme disease. Simultaneous infection with more than one organism has been described. The differential diagnosis for HME and HGA includes RMSF, viral illnesses such as mononucleosis and West Nile virus, and thrombotic thrombocytopenic purpura. The diagnosis of HME and HGA may be confirmed with polymerase chain reaction (PCR) testing or indirect fluorescent antibody (IFA) serology, which requires acute and convalescent serum. Intracytoplasmic inclusions (morulae) are diagnostic but rarely found in HME mononuclear cells (≤20%). HGA neutrophils are more likely to have the detection of morulae (20%–80% positive.)

Culture of the organisms is difficult. The standard and preferred treatment is doxycycline. An alternative may be rifampin.

Test-taking tip: In the question stem, note the reference to Tennessee and wooded areas with deer. This is a huge hint that it is a tick-infested area because ticks live on deer.

8. ANSWER: C

The patient has a dual infection with the spirochete *B. burgdorferi,* the cause of Lyme disease, and the rickettsial-like organism *A. phagocytophilum,* the cause of human granulocytic anaplasmosis (HGA).

Both organisms are transmitted by the *I. scapularis* tick, which may also carry *B. microti,* the cause of babesiosis. The *I. scapularis* tick has been found to be co-infected with *B. burgdorferi* and *A. phagocytophilum* in 2.2% to 26% of samples in studies from different locations.

The treatment of Lyme disease with amoxicillin will not treat HGA. Both illnesses are responsive to doxycycline.

Lyme disease has three stages:

The first stage is characterized by the expanding rash of erythema migrans, which appears 5 to 14 days after inoculation. No rash may be apparent in 20% of patients. Mild systemic symptoms may accompany the rash in early Lyme disease, including fever, myalgia, and arthralgia.

The second stage is early disseminated Lyme disease, which occurs weeks to months after infection and is characterized by neurologic and cardiac manifestations. Aseptic meningitis, radiculopathies, and cranial nerve palsies are some of the neurologic syndromes possible. The cardiac syndromes include transient heart block and myocarditis.

Third-stage Lyme disease may occur months to years later with monoarthritis or oligoarthritis, usually of the knees. A subtle encephalopathy or polyneuropathy may also occur.

The treatment of Lyme disease is different according to stage.

Doxycycline, amoxicillin, and cefuroxime are the drugs of choice for early Lyme disease.

The clinical presentation of HGA is nonspecific with fever, headache, and myalgia. Laboratory findings of leukopenia, thrombocytopenia, and mild elevation of liver enzymes are characteristic.

HGA neutrophils with morulae (intracytoplasmic inclusions) are found in 20% to 80% of cases.

The preferred treatment of HGA is doxycycline, though rifampin may be effective.

B. microti, an intracellular protozoan, is the agent of babesiosis. It is transmitted by the *I. scapularis* tick to humans. The reservoir is cattle and rodents. Babesiosis can be subclinical or febrile with myalgias, arthralgias, nausea, and vomiting. Physical examination may reveal hepatomegaly, splenomegaly, and jaundice. Severe illness occurs in asplenic and immunosuppressed patients and may be life-threatening. Complications include acute respiratory distress syndrome, renal failure, congestive heart failure, and disseminated intravascular coagulation.

Co-infection with Lyme disease occurs in two-thirds of patients with babesiosis. One-third of patients with babesiosis are co-infected with HGA. Diagnosis of babesiosis is made by microscopy of thin blood smears demonstrating round, oval, or pear-shaped organisms, often in a ring form. PCR and IFA serology testing are also diagnostic tools. Treatment of babesiosis is with the combination of atovaquone and azithromycin or the combination of clindamycin and quinine.

Test-taking tip: In the question stem, note the reference to Connecticut and that the patient had gone hiking. This is a large clue that the question is asking about a tick-borne illness.

9. ANSWER: D

The illness is Q fever, which is caused by a gram-negative coccobacillus, *Coxiella burnetii.*

It is a zoonosis that is transmitted by exposure to infected cattle, sheep, and goats, though dogs, cats, rabbits, and pigeons can also be sources. The organism resides in the uterus and mammary glands of the infected animal and disperses to the environment during parturition, spreading by inhalation of infected material as well as through ingestion of contaminated milk.

Q fever can manifest as an acute or chronic infection. Acute Q fever has an incubation period of 3 to 30 days. The acute infection often presents as a flu-like illness with fever, headache, and myalgias. Nausea, vomiting, and diarrhea can occur. It can manifest with pneumonitis from inhalation or hepatitis if acquired through ingestion of raw contaminated milk.

In one case series, 40% of patients had both pneumonitis and hepatitis.

Nonspecific rash is seen in 4% to 18%. Infection during pregnancy can lead to spontaneous abortion.

Chronic Q fever is seen in patients with valvular heart disease, prosthetic heart valves, aneurysms, renal insufficiency, bone and joint disease, and immunosuppression. It is a cause of culture-negative endocarditis and culture-negative osteomyelitis.

Laboratory findings include thrombocytopenia in 25% and elevated liver transaminases. The WBC count is usually normal. People at high risk include abattoir workers, farmers, and veterinarians.

Test-taking tip: The question stem gives a large hint to a zoonotic illness when it states the patient works on a cattle ranch and recently delivered a calf.

10. ANSWER: B

Q fever is caused by a gram-negative coccobacillus, *C. burnetii*.

It is a zoonotic infection that is transmitted by exposure to infected cattle, sheep, and goats, though dogs, cats, rabbits, and pigeons can also be sources. The organism resides in the uterus and mammary glands of the infected animal and disperses to the environment during parturition, spreading by inhalation of infected material as well as through ingestion of contaminated milk.

Q fever can manifest as an acute or chronic infection.

Test-taking tip: This is a "you know it or don't" kind of question. If you don't know it, choose an answer and move on. You can perhaps mark it for review when you are done at the end of the test. Don't, however, let these kinds of questions get you stuck and waste your time.

11. ANSWER: A

Lyme disease is transmitted by the *I. scapularis* tick which carries *B. burgdorferi*.

The treatment of Lyme disease is with doxycycline.

Lyme disease has three stages:

The first stage is characterized by the expanding rash of erythema migrans, which appears 5 to 14 days after inoculation. No rash may be apparent in 20% of patients. Mild systemic symptoms may accompany the rash in early Lyme disease, including fever, myalgia, and arthralgia.

The second stage is early disseminated Lyme disease, which occurs weeks to months after infection and is characterized by neurologic and cardiac manifestations. Aseptic meningitis, radiculopathies, and cranial nerve palsies are some of the neurologic syndromes possible. The cardiac syndromes include transient heart block and myocarditis.

Third-stage Lyme disease may occur months to years later with monoarthritis or oligoarthritis, usually of the knees. A subtle encephalopathy or polyneuropathy may also occur.

Test-taking tip: This is a "you know it or don't" kind of question. If you don't know it, choose an answer and move on. You can perhaps mark it for review when you are done at the end of the test. Don't, however, let these kinds of questions get you stuck and waste your time.

12. ANSWER: D

This patient is very ill, and RMSF is a reasonable concern. Chloramphenicol is the only alternative to doxycycline in the treatment of RMSF. Tetracyclines such as doxycycline are generally contraindicated in pregnancy because of associated hepatoxicity in the mother and fetal teeth and bone abnormalities in the fetus.

Although chloramphenicol is associated with low risk for fatal aplastic anemia (1:25,000 to 1:40,000), it should be started in this ill patient with reasonable likelihood of RMSF. Delay in therapy (>5 days after onset of illness) is associated with increased mortality.

If chloramphenicol is not available, the patient should be started on doxycycline.

Chloramphenicol is associated with gray baby syndrome in the third trimester, and doxycycline is preferred at that stage of pregnancy.

RMSF is a rickettsial illness caused by the gram-negative obligate intracellular organism *R. rickettsii*. It has a hallmark petechial rash.

It is transmitted to humans by tick bite. The major vectors in the United States are the American dog tick *Dermacentor variabilis* in eastern and south central United States and the Rocky Mountain wood tick *Dermacentor andersoni* west of the Mississippi River. The common brown dog tick *Rhipicephalus sanguineus* is a vector in the southwest United States. One-third of patients do not recall a tick bite. The tick can transmit the organism successfully if attached for 6 to 10 hours.

Patients become symptomatic between 2 and 14 days after the bite.

The early phase of the clinical syndrome is nonspecific and resembles a flu-like illness with headache, fever, and myalgias. Nausea, vomiting, and abdominal pain may be present, especially in children.

A blanching erythematous evolving to petechial rash is the hallmark of this illness. It develops in 90% of patients but occurs in only 15% on presentation. The rash usually starts on the wrists and ankles, may involve the palms and soles, and spreads to the trunk. However, it may be atypical and confined to one body region.

Laboratory abnormalities often include thrombocytopenia, elevated liver transaminases, and hyponatremia. The WBC count is usually normal at presentation.

The case fatality rate was 20% to 30% in the preantibiotic era, and delay in therapy (>5 days after onset) leads to higher mortality (6.5% vs. 22.9% death rate in early vs. delayed therapy in one retrospective study).

The differential diagnosis of fever with a petechial rash includes meningococcemia, thrombotic thrombocytopenic purpura, ehrlichiosis, anaplasmosis, leptospirosis, bacterial sepsis, and vasculitis. The differential is broader before the onset of the rash. Thus consideration of RMSF is important in the setting of potential exposure to ticks because therapy is usually started empirically without diagnostic certainty.

Diagnostic tests include IFA testing, which requires acute and convalescent titers. Sensitivity of IFA is 95%. Because the antibodies are not detectable within the first 5 days of symptoms, treatment should be presumptive and not based on early IFA results.

Skin punch biopsy with direct immunofluorescence testing is 70% to 90% sensitive and can give rapid results.

The therapy of choice is doxycycline. In the pregnant patient, chloramphenicol is the preferred treatment except during the third trimester. It may not be available, and in a patient with life-threatening illness, doxycycline should be given.

Test-taking tip: The question stem referenced the Blue Ridge Mountains of Virginia and that the patient had been camping. This is a large clue that the question is asking about a tick-borne illness like RMSF.

13. ANSWER: A

This patient has neuroinvasive West Nile virus infection.

The mortality in this illness is 10% with good care.

West Nile virus infection is an arboviral infection caused by a single-stranded RNA flavivirus called West Nile virus. The illness is reported in nearly all states of the United States and is usually seen in late summer and early fall.

It is transmitted by mosquito bites and carried by many mosquito species. The *Culex* mosquito is the most common carrier. Birds are the main reservoir and amplifying host.

It can also be transmitted through blood transfusions, by organ transplantation, transplacentally, and by breastfeeding.

Most people who are infected are asymptomatic or have mild symptoms. About 20% have clinically apparent disease. The most feared clinical effect is neuroinvasive illness, which is seen in one of 150 to 250 of those infected. This manifests as meningitis, encephalitis, or meningoencephalitis in <1% and as acute flaccid paralysis (asymmetric limb weakness rapidly progressing to poliomyelitis-like flaccid paralysis) with or without meningitis or encephalitis, and it may be irreversible.

One-third of patients recover to near baseline.

Neuroinvasive illness can present with confusion, coma, parkinsonian features with tremors, myoclonus, and cogwheel rigidity. Advanced age, immunocompromised state, and malignancy increase the risk for neuroinvasive disease. The neuroinvasive form has a mortality rate of 10%. The incubation period is 2 to 14 days. A maculopapular or morbilliform rash may be seen in 20% (if a rash is present, there may be a lower chance of neuroinvasive disease).

Diagnostic studies include the serum IgM antibody capture enzyme-linked immunosorbent assay (MAC-ELISA). The serum MAC-ELISA test may remain positive for 6 months or longer.

The CSF in neuroinvasive West Nile virus usually has a lymphocytic pleocytosis, but 40% neutrophilic predominance. Positive IgM in CSF indicates intrathecal production of virus and is diagnostic of neuroinvasive disease because the virus does not cross the blood-brain barrier. (Ninety percent of patients with neuroinvasive disease will be positive for CSF IgM antibodies 8 to 10 days after symptom onset.)

CT of the brain is typically normal. Early MRI of the brain may appear normal, with abnormalities appearing later. MRI brain abnormalities include mixed-intensity or hypodense lesions on T1-weighted images of thalamus, basal ganglia, and midbrain, which are hyperintense on T2-weighted and fluid-attenuated inversion recovery (FLAIR) imaging.

Treatment is supportive. There is no effective therapy at this time.

Test-taking tip: The question stem mentions a dead bird and the presence of mosquito bites. This is a large clue that they are asking about a mosquito-borne illness.

14. ANSWER: B

This patient has the findings of botulism with cranial nerve palsies and the recent history of eating home-preserved vegetables. The suspicion of this diagnosis should lead to emergent acquisition of antitoxin through the state health department.

EMG findings will be characteristic. The Tensilon test to assess for myasthenia gravis may be false positive.

Botulism can be confirmed by analysis of serum, stool, and vomitus, but treatment must be started based on the clinical suspicion.

Botulism is a neuroparalytic disorder caused by a neurotoxin produced by spores of the bacterium *Clostridium botulinum*. *C. botulinum* is a gram-positive obligate anaerobic rod. The toxin affects the presynaptic cholinergic neuromuscular junction, blocking neurotransmitter release. There are eight toxins, named A to H, and all but C and D cause human disease. A and B cause food spoilage, but the others do not and are therefore odorless and tasteless. The botulinum toxin is the most potent poison known and is a potential inhalational bioterrorism weapon.

There are six types of botulism: infant (most common), food-borne, wound, adult enteric (like infant in adults), inhalational, and iatrogenic. Botulism spores are heat resistant but can be destroyed if heated to 120° C for 5 minutes. The toxin is heat labile and can be destroyed by boiling canned food for 10 minutes.

The diagnosis of botulism is initially based on clinical suspicion, and treatment must be initiated before confirmatory studies are available. The clinical presentation is that of acute bilateral cranial neuropathies with descending weakness. Important clinical features include blurred vision, normal mental status, no fever, normal heart rate or bradycardia, and nonspecific gastrointestinal symptoms if due to ingestion.

If a lumbar puncture is performed, CSF is normal.

Wound botulism is associated with the intramuscular or subcutaneous use of black tar heroin.

Infant botulism usually occurs is children younger than 12 months and is associated with the ingestion of raw honey. However, most cases are likely due to ingestion of the ubiquitous spores in the environment, including soil and surfaces of fruits and vegetable. The infant often presents with constipation followed by hypotonia, drooling, feeding difficulty, irritability, and weak cry.

Respiratory compromise is the usual cause of death. Vital capacity should be monitored, and early intubation should be considered if vital capacity is less than 30% and is indicated if there is respiratory distress.

Suspicion of botulism should prompt immediate contact with the state health department to acquire antitoxin.

Equine serum heptavalent botulism antitoxin should be given.

Infants younger than 12 months may receive human derived botulinum antitoxin.

Wound botulism is often treated with antibiotics as well, though efficacy is uncertain. Penicillin G and metronidazole are the choices used.

Aminoglycosides are contraindicated because of their possible potentiation of neuromuscular blockade.

Serum, stool, and vomitus toxin analyses are sent for food-borne botulism.

Wound botulism is assessed by wound toxin analysis.

Test-taking tip: Neurologic findings (especially bulbar findings) in an adult with a history of eating home canned goods is botulism until proved otherwise.

15. ANSWER: A

MRSA is resistant to all ß-lactams, which include the cephalosporins. Methicillin resistance is defined as an oxacillin maximal inhibitory concentration (MIC) of ≥4 mcg/mL. Resistance is due to the presence of the *mecA* gene, which encodes for penicillin-binding protein 2a (PBC2a), the source of the resistance.

MRSA causes skin and soft tissue infections, including cellulitis and abscesses.

Because of high community prevalence, empiric antibiotic treatment should be directed at MRSA.

Oral antibiotics of choice are trimethoprim-sulfamethoxazole, tetracyclines, and clindamycin. Alternative antibiotics include linezolid and vancomycin. Parenteral antibiotics of choice are vancomycin and daptomycin.

MRSA has been divided into community-associated (CA-MRSA) and health care–associated (HA-MRSA) infections (develop within 48 hours of hospitalization to within 12 months of exposure to health care, including long-term care facilities, dialysis, history of surgery, or hospitalization). HA-MRSA is associated with severe invasive infections of skin and soft tissue, bacteremia, and pneumonia. MRSA has the capacity to form biofilm on invasive foreign devices, which enhances its ability to persist. MRSA is associated with longer hospitalizations, increased mortality, and higher health care costs than methicillin-sensitive *S. aureus* (MSSA).

CA-MRSA soft tissue and skin infections occur in young healthy individuals not associated with health care exposure. Most CA-MRSA strains produce the Panton-Valentine cytotoxin, which enhances its virulence. CA-MRSA is the most frequent cause of skin infections seen in US EDs and clinics.

HA-MRSA is being seen in community settings more frequently. MRSA colonization increases the risk for staphylococcal infection after a procedure. Reasons that MRSA is increasing in prevalence include antibiotic use (cephalosporins and fluoroquinolones), HIV infection, hemodialysis, and long-term care facility residence.

MRSA is transmitted by health care workers to patients by direct contact and by contaminated fomites.

Test-taking tip: This is a "you know it or don't" kind of question. If you don't know it, choose an answer and move on. You can perhaps mark it for review when you are done at the end of the test. Don't, however, let these kinds of questions get you stuck and waste your time.

16. ANSWER: C

The most common source of rabies in the United States is bats, not raccoons, although raccoons are a source of rabies.

Rabies is a devastating illness caused by the neurotropic single-stranded RNA *Lyssavirus* of the Rhabdoviridae family. It is typically transmitted by the bite of an infected animal through infected saliva. All mammals are susceptible to rabies. Rabid dogs account for 90% of infections worldwide. In the United States, the major source is wildlife, with bats, skunks, foxes, coyotes, and raccoons being the most commonly infected animals. Bats are the most common source of human rabies in the United States, and many patients do not recall a bat bite. Transmission has occurred from tissue transplantation to recipients from unrecognized infected donors.

The virus travels up the peripheral nerves near the site of the bite and travels retrograde to the dorsal root ganglion of the spinal cord. From there it progresses to the brain, particularly the diencephalon, hippocampus, and brainstem.

Incubation is 1 to 3 months on average, though it has been described to be days to several years in some cases. The onset of illness is nonspecific with myalgias, weakness, fatigue, sore throat, low-grade fever, nausea, and vomiting. Paresthesias from the wound extending proximally is a concerning sign.

Two clinical syndromes are described: encephalitic rabies (most common) and paralytic ("dumb") rabies. Encephalitic rabies is characterized by fever, pharyngeal spasms, dysarthria, dysphagia, hydrophobia, and excitation, leading to paralysis and death. Paralytic rabies is an ascending paralysis resembling Guillain-Barré syndrome that leads to a flaccid paralysis.

The CSF will have a lymphocytic pleocytosis and elevated protein. Early CT scan of the brain may appear normal. Virus isolation from saliva, skin biopsy virus-specific immunofluorescent staining, and CSF or serum antirabies antibodies are diagnostic.

Wound care is important, and the wound should be thoroughly washed. Postexposure prophylaxis consists of administration of rabies immune globulin (RIG) and rabies vaccine. RIG is not indicated in previously vaccinated patients. RIG should be administered as close to the wound as possible, with excess given intramuscularly. Vaccine should be given intramuscularly at a different site from RIG, in the deltoid or anterior thigh. Vaccine is administered in a

schedule of four or five doses at days 0, 3, 7, 14, and ±28 and should be started as soon as possible.

Test-taking tip: This is a "you know it or don't" kind of question. If you don't know it, choose an answer and move on. You can perhaps mark it for review when you are done at the end of the test. Don't, however, let these kinds of questions get you stuck and waste your time.

17. ANSWER: C

This patient has diffuse muscle spasms of his back and extremities. The strange facial expression is risus sardonicus, which is due to the spasms of the masseter muscles of the face. His attribution of his pain to heavy lifting is his effort to explain his back pain. However, his findings are much more generalized, and he is a user of black tar heroin, which is associated with tetanus. Local tetanus begins in a localized area of the wound and may generalize, but his presentation is generalized. He is at risk for an epidural abscess because of his injection drug use as well but does not have the findings of that diagnosis. There is no point tenderness over his spine, and there are no signs of spinal cord compression.

Tetanus is a neuroexcitatory disease caused by the toxin tetanospasmin that is produced by the anaerobic bacterium *Clostridium tetani*. *C. tetani* is ubiquitous and is found in the soil. It produces the toxin in damaged tissues. The toxin spreads to the spinal cord and brainstem and irreversibly binds to receptors, causing disinhibition of anterior horn cells and autonomic neurons. This results in painful muscle spasms, increased tone, and autonomic instability.

The mean incubation period is 7 to 10 days. One million cases of tetanus are estimated to occur worldwide yearly.

There are four clinical syndromes described: generalized, local, cephalic, and neonatal.

Generalized is the most common and is characterized by severe muscle spasms and autonomic instability. Masseter muscle spasms are the cause of "lockjaw" and risus sardonicus. Patients may have rigidity of the abdominal wall, dysphagia, and opisthotonus. They are at risk for upper airway obstruction and apnea. Local tetanus affects the local muscles proximate to the wound but can evolve to a generalized form.

Cephalic tetanus initially involves the cranial nerves and occurs when the wounds are in the head and neck. It can also evolve to the generalized form.

Neonatal tetanus occurs in neonates of poorly immunized mothers who typically have an umbilical stump wound that is contaminated.

The key to prevention is good wound care and vaccination. If tetanus is suspected, actions need to be directed toward stopping toxin production and neutralizing unbound toxin. Wound debridement is essential. Metronidazole (preferred) and penicillin are the antibiotics of choice, though penicillin has a γ-aminobutyric acid (GABA) antagonist effect and may exacerbate central nervous system (CNS) excitability.

Tetanus immune globulin (TIG) will neutralize unbound toxin. Tetanus toxoid should be given at a site other than the TIG site, usually as Td or Tdap. Tdap is used only once in adults except in pregnant patients, who should receive it during each pregnancy.

Tetanus is uncommon in developed countries because of widespread vaccination.

In the management of patients with a wound, if less than three doses of tetanus toxoid have been received and the wound is minor, tetanus toxoid vaccine should be given. If three or more doses have been previously administered to the patient, a booster is recommended only if the last dose was given 10 years or more prior.

If the wound is dirty and tetanus prone, a booster is recommended if the prior dose was given 5 years ago or longer.

TIG is given to patients with tetanus-prone wounds who do not have a history of receiving three or more previous tetanus toxoid doses.

Test-taking tip: You can eliminate A and B and narrow down your choices. The patient is much sicker than just a back strain, and even though his risk for epidural abscess is high with a history of IV drug use, the muscle spasm of his face and limbs does not fit.

18. ANSWER: D

Meningococcemia is a systemic infection caused by *Neisseria meningitidis*, a gram-negative diplococcus. It has a high mortality rate from septic shock ultimately leading to multiorgan failure potentially within just a few hours of infection. Fever and rash occur in most patients. Fifty percent of patients present with petechiae, while 20% to 30% exhibit a maculopapular rash that later evolves into petechiae or purpura. Bilateral adrenal infarction, seen in *Waterhouse-Friderichsen syndrome*, only occurs in about 10% of patients. Hypothermia, seizure, and arthritis are among other symptoms noted. Laboratory studies show leukocytosis, thrombocytopenia, and disseminated intravascular coagulation. Therapy includes antibiotics with a third-generation cephalosporin and aggressive management of associated shock.

Test-taking tip: This is a "you know it or don't" kind of question. If you don't know it, choose an answer and move on. You can perhaps mark it for review when you are done at the end of the test. Don't, however, let these kinds of questions get you stuck and waste your time.

19. ANSWER: D

Typhoid fever is a bacterial infection caused by *Salmonella typhi* transmitted through ingestion of contaminated water or food. Symptoms manifest approximately 1 to 2 weeks after exposure and include fever, generalized fatigue/malaise, nausea, anorexia, diffuse abdominal pain, and a headache. Approximately 30% of patients develop "rose spots," which are blanching erythematous maculopapular rash, over the anterior trunk. On clinical assessment, affected patients will display paradoxical bradycardia in the setting of fever along with dehydration. Laboratory studies will reveal anemia with either a leukocytosis (more common in children) or a leukopenia (more common in adults). Approximately 80% of patients will also have a transaminitis. Fluoroquinolones are the first-line treatment for typhoid fever in adults. In pediatric populations, it is more appropriate to use a third-generation cephalosporin.

There are two vaccines against typhoid fever that collectively provide only 55% immunity. However, a vaccination against yellow fever will provide nearly complete immunity. This child's presentation also corresponds to malaria, but given her recent prophylactic treatment (which provides 91% protection against malaria), this is less likely. Dengue fever is a viral illness caused by mosquitoes resulting in fever, malaise, severe myalgias, arthralgias (also known as break-bone fever). This infection typically does not require antibiotic. If the patient were to develop an eosinophilia, one would suspect a helminthic infection as the culprit.

Test-taking tip: With infectious diseases, there are usually clues that go together. Low HR in the setting of sepsis, recent travel, and rash is typhoid until proved otherwise.

20. ANSWER: B

Strongyloides is a parasitic helminth infection transmitted when larvae in fecally contaminated soil penetrate the skin or mucous membranes. It is a blood-borne infection, but the larvae can traverse the lungs. They ultimately reach the small intestine, where they mature into adult worms, which penetrate the mucosa of the small intestine. Many patients are asymptomatic or have mild gastrointestinal symptoms. The cutaneous eruption described in the question stem is known as larval currens. Eosinophilia is common with all clinical manifestations. Most commonly it is immunocompromised patients who are susceptible to hyperinfection or dissemination; thus all patients, whether symptomatic or asymptomatic carriers, should be treated with ivermectin, which is more effective than albendazole. Fluconazole is used to treat candidal infections. Mebendazole is used to treat trichuriasis, enterobiasis (pinworm), ascariasis, and hookworm. Mefloquine is used for malaria prophylaxis.

Test-taking tip: This is a "you know it or don't" kind of question. If you don't know it, choose an answer and move on. You can perhaps mark it for review when you are done at the end of the test. Don't, however, let these kinds of questions get you stuck and waste your time.

21. ANSWER: A

Although the causes of febrile illness in travelers vary by geography, dengue is most common in Southeast Asia. Symptoms are self-limited and only require supportive therapy. Malaria is most prevalent in sub-Saharan African countries, so any febrile traveler from malaria-endemic regions should be assumed to have malaria until ruled out or another diagnosis established, especially because falciparum malaria may be life-threatening and effective therapy is available. Salmonella is prevalent in South Central Asia. Yellow fever has a predominance in Africa.

Test-taking tip: Infectious diseases in certain regions are very testable on standardized exams. Familiarize yourself with common traveler's diseases before the exam.

22. ANSWER: D

Primary amebic meningoencephalitis (PAM) is a disease caused by infection with *Naegleria fowleri*, a free-living ameba found in warm freshwater sources. The bacteria are transmitted to the brain through the olfactory nerves after penetrating the nasal mucosa. It carries a very high mortality rate of 99%. Ingestion of contaminated foods typically predisposes affected individuals to gastrointestinal symptoms and does not usually progress to CNS infections. Viral infections of the CNS that can be transmitted by mosquitoes include West Nile virus and St. Louis encephalitis. These infections would not show trophozoites on examination of the brain tissue. Ingestion of contaminated water causes *Giardia lamblia, Vibrio cholerae*, and hepatitis A virus, but like ingestion of contaminated food, these infections tend to cause gastrointestinal, rather than CNS, symptoms.

Test-taking tip: The presence of trophozoites indicates amebic disease. This association with warm freshwater swimming and penetration through the nasal mucosa has to be memorized for the exam.

23. ANSWER: D

The initial evaluation of any critically ill patient in shock should include algorithmic ABCs—assessing and establishing an airway, evaluating breathing, and restoring adequate circulation. Initial adequate oxygenation should be ensured with a goal of achieving an arterial oxygen saturation of 90% or greater. The other remaining options would be appropriate in ongoing management of sepsis, after components of hemodynamic instability are addressed.

Test-taking tip: You can eliminate B because β-blockers are not helpful in sepsis. Choices A, C, and D are all needed simultaneously, but D (oxygen) is needed first.

24. ANSWER: D

S. stercoralis is a parasite that is transmitted to the small intestine. Infection is caused when the larva passes through the skin causing allergic-type symptoms such as pruritus and erythematous rash. After the parasite embeds in the intestine, there are typically no associated symptoms. Eosinophilia is a feature of this infection. The resulting hyperinfection syndrome happens in patients who have an established *S. stercoralis* infection and concurrently become immunocompromised through debilitating illness, immunosuppressive therapies, or HIV infection. The numerous migrating larvae cause severe overwhelming infections in the affected organ systems such as pneumonia, meningitis, septicemia, or ileus.

Diagnosis is made from clinical gestalt because there is no evidence of eosinophilia in those affected by hyperinfection syndrome. *A. lumbricoides* causes infections through oral ingestion. Larvae will hatch in the stomach, migrate through the lungs, and then settle in the intestinal tract. Those infected will typically display respiratory and gastrointestinal symptoms like pneumonitis, small bowel obstruction, and biliary obstruction.

E. vermicularis is transmitted through the skin of the anus, leading to perianal itching. *N. americanus* and *Trichuris trichiura* are parasites that penetrate through the skin in patients who walk barefoot through soiled areas. These infections usually result in anemia from gradual blood loss due to the parasitic infestation.

Test-taking tip: This is a "you know it or don't" kind of question. If you don't know it, choose an answer and move on. You can perhaps mark it for review when you are done at the end of the test. Don't, however, let these kinds of questions get you stuck and waste your time.

25. ANSWER: A

Given the clinical presentation, the highest suspicion should be aimed at cryptococcal meningitis, which has been considered an AIDS-defining illness. It is characterized by a subacute headache coupled with fevers, nausea, vomiting, altered mental status, and focal neurologic deficits. On CSF studies, opening pressure is usually elevated, but there are only mild derangements on the other studies. There is a lymphocytic predominance. CSF cryptococcal antigen is nearly 100% sensitive for detection of illness. HSV antigen can be used to diagnose herpes encephalitis. The most common presentation for this illness describes a patient with headaches, personality changes, seizures, and altered mental status. VDRL would assist in diagnosis for suspicions of neurosyphilis; however, this patient's presentation and examination are not consistent with tertiary syphilis. Pneumococcal infections of CSF would have studies showing low glucose and a neutrophil predominance.

Test-taking tip: You can narrow down your choices by eliminating C because that is more common in the immunocompetent host. Because the patient in the question has untreated HIV, you need to think of illnesses that are more likely in AIDS patients.

26. ANSWER: B

Leishmaniasis is a parasitic protozoan infection that comes from getting bitten by the sandfly. The disease most commonly manifests with cutaneous symptoms. Early infection is characterized as skin papules and nodules at the site of inoculation. This progresses to an ulceration with raised borders. Ultimately diagnosis is made by skin biopsy with direct visualization of organisms or a positive fluorescent antibody test. MRSA infection is not a likely possibility because of slow temporal progression. It would be expected to have a progressive extension over the proposed length of time. It would also be expected to be responsive to appropriate courses of antibiotics.

T. cruzi is a parasitic infection that is carried by the reduviid bug. Characteristic features include fever, lymphadenopathy, myocarditis, megaesophagus, and cardiomegaly. This disease is typically diagnosed in later stages.

Onchocerciasis, also known as river blindness, is a filarial parasitic infection carried by black flies. It is characterized by skin nodules and eventual blindness from larvae invading the eye.

Test-taking tip: The clue of a visit to Saudi Arabia with a nonhealing ulcer is key. Review travel-related infections.

27. ANSWER: D

CNS toxoplasmosis is a disease caused by *T. gondii,* which is an obligatory intracellular pathogen that is transmitted by the oral or transplacental route. Consumption of raw or undercooked meat containing viable cysts, water contaminated with oocysts from cat feces, and unwashed vegetables is the primary route of oral transmission; improper handling of undercooked meat or contaminated soil also may lead to hand-to-mouth infection. Toxoplasmosis in HIV-infected patients is due to reactivation of chronic infection, and it usually presents as toxoplasmic encephalitis. In AIDS patients with CD4 counts greater than 100, *T. gondii* is the most common opportunistic infection that causes focal brain lesions. Common clinical features include fever, headache, altered mental status, focal neurologic deficits, and seizure. In patients with suspected toxoplasmosis, serology and neuroimaging are typically used to make the diagnosis.

Biopsy is reserved for uncertain diagnoses or for patients who fail empiric therapy. CSF analysis is rarely useful in the diagnosis of cerebral toxoplasmosis and is not performed routinely given the risk for increasing intracranial pressure with lumbar puncture. With high clinical suspicion and appropriate patient presentation, empiric therapy should be initiated as soon as possible. Treatment consists of administration of pyrimethamine/sulfadiazine and possible addition of leucovorin. Steroids such as dexamethasone should also be initiated for mass effect from cerebral edema; alternatives include pyrimethamine-clindamycin and Bactrim. With early detection and treatment, clinical and/or radiographic improvement is evident within 1 to 2 weeks.

Test-taking tip: Opportunistic infections in HIV/AIDS patients are a high-yield topic. Review these infections before the exam.

28. ANSWER: D

The majority of bacterial meningitis cases in adults is caused by *S. pneumoniae.* Meningococcal meningitis in adults is mostly found in adolescents and is mostly caused by serogroup B. Studies have shown that headache, fever, neck stiffness, and altered mental status are common signs and symptoms of meningitis in young adult and adult populations. The classic triad of fever, neck stiffness, and altered mental status, however, is reported in only 41% to 51% of patients.

Classic abnormalities of CSF composition in bacterial meningitis are a pleocytosis with PMN predominance as well as low glucose and elevated protein levels.

Because *S. pneumoniae* has shown reduced resistance to penicillin, it is appropriate to initiate empiric therapy that includes vancomycin and ceftriaxone. In this clinical presentation, there would be no need to include ampicillin. This regimen would be more appropriate for older adult, immunosuppressed patients, or alcoholic adults to ensure coverage for possible listeria. Addition of high-dose corticosteroid before or simultaneously with the administration of antibiotics has been shown to decrease mortality in patients with bacterial meningitis. In cases of viral or aseptic meningitis, there is no utility of steroids; thus these can be discontinued following results of CSF studies if needed.

Test-taking tip: This is a "you know it or don't" kind of question. If you don't know it, choose an answer and move on. You can perhaps mark it for review when you are done at the end of the test. Don't, however, let these kinds of questions get you stuck and waste your time.

29. ANSWER: A

The most likely diagnosis in this case is primary amebic meningoencephalitis, which is a deadly infection caused by *N. fowleri*. The ameba causes CNS infection after migrating through the olfactory nerves into the brain. This is a rapidly progressive disease. The CSF studies demonstrate findings similar to bacterial meningitis; thus diagnosis is made by identification of trophozoites on Giemsa or Wright stain of CSF. Because of the high mortality with this disease, a high clinical suspicion and aggressive therapy are necessary for survival. This includes intrathecal and IV administration of amphotericin B.

Addition of ampicillin would be appropriate for coverage of *Listeria* because the question stem does describe a history of consumption of unpasteurized dairy products. However, listeriosis is generally a disease of children, pregnant women, older adults, and immunocompromised patients. Tetracycline would be the best therapy in the setting of a rickettsial infection, which can cause CNS infections. However, low glucose and an elevated WBC count on CSF fluid studies would not be consistent with such infections. The fact that the CSF cultures had no growth over a 72-hour period would also exclude bacterial meningitis as the primary affliction; thus maintaining the current antibiotic regimen or even broadening the regimen would not be appropriate. The rapid progression of this patient's disease course makes tuberculosis less likely.

Test-taking tip: Reviewing infections in travelers is helpful for the exam. The association between swimming in a warm freshwater lake and this patient's sudden onset of symptoms is a huge clue for amebic disease.

30. ANSWER: A

This patient has Legionnaires' disease, which is an illness caused by *Legionella pneumophila,* a gram-negative bacterium that is found widely in water systems and is spread by droplet inhalation. Infection may be associated with inhalation of free-living amebae. It typically does not spread directly between people, and most people who are exposed do not become infected. Those at increased risk fir infection typically include older adult men, smokers, and immunocompromised patients.

The bacteria cause an atypical pneumonia approximately 2 to 10 days after exposure. Many infections are asymptomatic; however, clinical symptoms seen usually include fever, rigors, headache, myalgia, cough, and dyspnea. In more serious cases of the disease, there can also be gastrointestinal or CNS symptoms like altered mental status or diarrhea. Laboratory studies commonly show an elevated WBC count, hyponatremia, and a transaminitis. Diagnosis is usually confirmed by the detection of rising antibody titers in the serum. It may take 2 to 3 weeks for serology to become positive. Faster detection may be possible using urinary or sputum antigen testing.

Test-taking tip: The association between low sodium and a pneumonia on chest radiograph is a large hint that this is Legionnaires' disease. Use the clues in the question stem to help you.

31. ANSWER: D

Typhoid fever is a systemic, flu-like infection that is caused by *Salmonella typhi*. It is most prevalent and endemic in Mexico, Indonesia, Peru, and the Indian subcontinent. It is transmitted by contaminated food, drink, and water sources and has a variable incubation period ranging from 1 week to 1 month. The bacteria migrate to the bloodstream after ingestion into the intestines. It can then rapidly spread to other organs, including lymph nodes, gallbladder, liver, and spleen. Risk factors include poor sanitation and poor hygiene.

Onset and progression of symptoms are insidious and include fevers, chills, constipation, myalgias, hematochezia, and delirium. Classic symptoms noted on presentation to the ED can include bradycardia despite high fevers and sometimes a diffuse erythematous rash with rose-colored spots. Fever with temperatures greater than 39.5° C (103° F) and diarrhea are strong indicators of severe disease. Laboratory studies will show a leukocytosis and thrombocytopenia. Definitive diagnosis is possible with cultures of either blood, stools, or bone marrow. Treatment of disease is with azithromycin, fluoroquinolones, or third-generation cephalosporins

Test-taking tip: Review the differential of febrile illness in the traveler. The clue of the patient from Peru with a high fever and bradycardia is a hint at the diagnosis of typhoid.

32. ANSWER: D

DGI is the result of hematogenous spread of the sexually transmitted bacteria, *Neisseria gonorrhoeae*. Patients with DGI often do not present with simultaneous evidence of mucous membrane involvement. DGI typically presents in one of two forms: (1) arthritis-dermatitis syndrome characterized by fever/chills/malaise, polyarthralgia involving the small or large joints, tenosynovitis, and rash or (2) purulent arthritis without rash most commonly affecting the knee, elbow, or wrist. There is often overlap between the two forms.

Patients with DGI should be admitted with infectious disease specialist consultation and should be screened for other sexually transmitted infections including HIV, syphilis, and *Chlamydia trachomatis*. The recommended treatment regimen is ceftriaxone 1g IM or IV every 24 hours plus azithromycin 1g PO in a single dose.

Patients with gonococcemia need to be admitted for IV antibiotics and workup for endocarditis and meningitis. Those with gonococcal arthritis rarely require surgical drainage and irrigation.

Test-taking tip: You can eliminate A and B and narrow your choices down. Secondary syphilis rash is not pustular, and gout is monoarticular (not polyarticular).

33. ANSWER: B

The patient is presenting with secondary syphilis. Syphilis typically presents in three stages: primary, secondary, and tertiary. Primary is characterized by a painless genital chancre that resolves spontaneously. If untreated, progression to secondary syphilis occurs 3 to 6 weeks after resolution of the chancre and manifests as a light red, papular rash involving the palms and soles, lymphadenopathy, and nonspecific constitutional symptoms.

Tertiary or latent syphilis develops in approximately one-third of patients after secondary syphilis and can occur 20 years or later after the initial infection and present as dementia, meningitis, and tabes dorsalis. Penicillin G is the treatment for all stages of syphilis. Alternative regimens using PO doxycycline (A), PO azithromycin (C), or IV/IM ceftriaxone (D) have been described for persons with penicillin allergy but require careful clinical and serologic follow-up. Patients should be counseled regarding the Jarisch-Herxheimer reaction, which can occur 24 hours after any treatment for syphilis and is characterized by fever, headache, and myalgias. All patients diagnosed with syphilis should be screened for HIV.

Test-taking tip: This is a "you know it or don't" kind of question. If you don't know it, choose an answer and move on. You can perhaps mark it for review when you are done at the end of the test. Don't, however, let these kinds of questions get you stuck and waste your time. The clue of rash to the palms and soles is the huge hint at syphilis.

34. ANSWER: D

The patient is presenting with classic features of *Pneumocystis jiroveci* pneumonia (PCP pneumonia), which should be suspected in any patient with HIV and CD4 counts of <200 who presents with respiratory symptoms, particularly if the patient is noncompliant with medications. First-line treatment for PCP pneumonia is trimethoprim-sulfamethoxazole. Steroids should be added if the patient's PaO_2 is less than 70 or their arterial-alveolar gradient is greater than 35 mm Hg. Alternatives depending on severity for those with sulfa allergies include primaquine with clindamycin, pentamidine, dapsone with trimethoprim, and atovaquone.

Test-taking tip: This is a "you know it or don't" kind of question. If you don't know it, choose an answer and move on. You can perhaps mark it for review when you are done at the end of the test. Don't, however, let these kinds of questions get you stuck and waste your time. The low PaO_2 is the clue that steroids are also needed to treat this PCP pneumonia.

35. ANSWER: C

This patient's presentation meets Centers for Disease Control and Prevention (CDC) clinical criteria for toxic shock syndrome (TSS), which include temperature ≥38.9° C, rash, or desquamation 1 to 2 weeks after rash onset, hypotension, and evidence of multisystem involvement. TSS is caused by *S. aureus* and is mediated by exotoxin release. It has been associated with tampon use during menstruation, although many cases not related to menstruation have been reported, including wound infections and burns. TSS is a clinical diagnosis, and treatment includes IV fluid resuscitation, IV antibiotics, and source control if necessary.

Test-taking tip: You can eliminate B because the patient has no headache or rigidity. *E. coli* is unlikely because of the rash. This narrows your options down by half.

36. ANSWER: D

Measles is a highly contagious illness caused by paramyxovirus. It is a vaccine-preventable illness that has seen a recent surge in incidence with the increase in unvaccinated children in the United States. The illness classically presents as fever, malaise, coryza, and conjunctivitis followed by the development of rash. It is subdivided into four clinically relevant stages: incubation, prodrome, exanthem, and recovery. If present, Koplik spots can be found during the prodrome stage approximately 48 hours before the exanthem. Potential complications include secondary infections, pneumonia, gastrointestinal upset, and encephalitis. Definitive diagnosis is made with serologic testing, and treatment includes symptom management and vitamin A.

Test-taking tip: Infectious viral illnesses have certain signs or symptoms that are pathognomonic for the illness. Koplik spots are pathognomonic for measles.

37. ANSWER: D

This boy has hand-foot-and-mouth disease, caused by Coxsackie virus. It is typically a self-limited illness, and management is supportive. Some patients may require admission for IV hydration if they are unable to tolerate oral intake secondary to pain.

The rash can also involve the buttocks and usually has mouth involvement first. This is usually seen in children younger than 5 years, and it is transmitted by the fecal-oral or oral-oral route.

Test-taking tip: Classic childhood rashes are high yield to brush up on because they are commonly tested on standardized exams.

38. ANSWER: A

The patient in the question is presenting with classic erythema infectiosum, or fifth disease, which is caused by parvovirus B19. The disease is characterized by a unique exanthem that typically starts as a diffusely erythematous facial rash in a butterfly pattern, often referred to as slapped-cheek appearance. The rash usually follows the fever.

Transmission is respiratory, and treatment is supportive.

Test-taking tip: Classic childhood rashes are very high yield to brush up on because they are usually tested on standardized exams. You can narrow down your choices by eliminating B and C because you know this is a viral syndrome and can eliminate *Candida* and *Streptococcus*.

39. ANSWER: B

This patient has varicella-zoster virus (chickenpox), and because he is an unvaccinated adolescent he is at higher risk for developing complications including bacterial superinfection of skin lesions with or without bacterial sepsis, pneumonia, CNS involvement (acute cerebellar ataxia, encephalitis, stroke/vasculopathy), thrombocytopenia, and other rare complications, such as glomerulonephritis, arthritis, and hepatitis. The American Academy of Pediatrics recommends treating immunocompetent children 13 years and older who are unvaccinated with oral antiviral therapy. IV treatment is recommended in those who are immunocompromised and/or exhibit evidence of complications.

Test-taking tip: Review common associations; the Tzanck test is associated with chickenpox or herpes.

40. ANSWER: D

The patient has scarlet fever, which is caused by group A *Streptococcus* and usually occurs in conjunction with pharyngitis. It is characterized by an erythematous, sandpaper-like rash that usually begins on the face and spreads. First-line treatment is penicillin, the same as for strep pharyngitis. Treatment has been shown to prevent nonsuppurative complications, including acute rheumatic fever and glomerulonephritis, but not suppurative complications, which include peritonsillar abscess, retropharyngeal abscess, and suppurative adenitis.

Test-taking tip: This is a "you know it or don't" kind of question. If you don't know it, choose an answer and move on. You can perhaps mark it for review when you are done at the end of the test. Don't, however, let these kinds of questions get you stuck and waste your time.

41. ANSWER: C

All febrile infants younger than 28 days should undergo a complete sepsis evaluation because they are at high risk for bacterial infection. Workup should include complete blood count, blood cultures, urinalysis and culture, CSF studies, and chest radiograph. Broad-spectrum empiric antibiotics should be initiated immediately and should include coverage for group B *Streptococcus, Listeria,* and herpes infection, if suspected. The antibiotic regimen can be narrowed after a source has been identified and sensitivities are determined. Ceftriaxone should not be given to children in this age group because it can displace bilirubin, which may lead to kernicterus.

Test-taking tip: Review neonatal sepsis treatment. You can eliminate A because a febrile neonate is not discharged.

42. ANSWER: D

This woman is presenting with features characteristic of rubella (German measles). While considered eradicated in the United States, it is still endemic in many other parts of the world. It is moderately contagious and spread from person to person by airborne transmission or contact with respiratory droplets.

It is typically a self-limited illness in adults. In pregnant women, infection with the virus is most severe in the first trimester, and up to 85% of fetuses are affected if infection occurs during the first trimester. Congenital rubella syndrome (CRS) can affect every organ system, including the eyes, brain, heart, bones, liver, and spleen, and may lead to preterm birth or fetal demise. Deafness is the most common complication, and manifestations of CRS may be delayed for up to 4 years after birth. Diagnosis is made by isolation of virus from a clinical specimen or serologic testing.

"TORCH" is an acronym for a group of infections that are harmful to a fetus.
T = toxoplasmosis
O = other (syphilis, HIV, hepatitis)
R = rubella
C = CMV
H = herpes simplex

Test-taking tip: This is a "you know it or don't" kind of question. If you don't know it, choose an answer and move on. You can perhaps mark it for review when you are done at the end of the test. Don't, however, let these kinds of questions get you stuck and waste your time.

43. ANSWER: B

This patient has croup, which is an upper respiratory tract infection characterized by fever and barking cough and is caused most often by parainfluenza virus. Some cases may present with inspiratory stridor, hoarseness, or respiratory distress. It is typically a self-limited illness but can be complicated by airway obstruction secondary to inflammation. Imaging is not necessarily indicated, but plain films may demonstrate narrowing of the subglottic space, called the "steeple sign." Treatment includes dexamethasone and racemic epinephrine in moderate to severe cases. Albuterol should be avoided as it may worsen edema and airway obstruction.

Test-taking tip: Review common etiologies of common diseases. Example: croup = parainfluenza virus; RSV = bronchiolitis.

44. ANSWER: A

Roseola infantum is most commonly caused by human herpesvirus 6. It is characterized by abrupt onset of often high fevers that are accompanied by nonspecific symptoms lasting a few days. The rash appears after resolution of the fever and lasts 1 to 2 days. Measles and Chickenpox is caused by the varicella-zoster virus and is characterized by a pruritic vesicular rash that typically begins on the trunk and is often described as having a "dew drop on a rose petal" appearance. Hand-foot-and-mouth disease is caused by Coxsackie virus and classically presents as painful vesicular lesions involving the oral mucosa, palms of the hands, and soles of the feet that were preceded by fever and malaise.

Test-taking tip: Classic childhood rashes are high yield to brush up on because they are commonly tested on standardized exams.

45. ANSWER: C

The patient is presenting with epiglottitis (acute inflammation of the epiglottis), which can rapidly progress to total airway compromise in children. The fact that the patient is unvaccinated is important because the most common pathogens causing epiglottis are *H. influenzae, S. pneumoniae,* and *S. aureus.* Patients typically present with a history of sore throat and fever and may present with signs of respiratory distress, including stridor, muffled voice, and drooling. The most important step in managing epiglottitis is ensuring airway protection. If the patient is stable enough for imaging, radiograph of the neck may reveal the thumbprint sign.

Test-taking tip: You can eliminate D because the patient is too unstable to go to the CT scanner. The question is describing an unstable airway with "drooling" and a "distressed" patient. Airway management is key.

46. ANSWER: C

Although AIDS patients are certainly at risk for the most common bacterial etiologies of meningitis, this patient is presenting with classic cryptococcal meningitis. She is at increased risk given her low CD4 count. CSF in fungal meningitis typically has lymphocyte predominance, an elevated opening pressure, low glucose, and increased protein. These features, in addition to the mononuclear predominance in the CSF of this patient, are indicative of cryptococcal infection. Diagnosis can be made with India ink staining, and confirmatory testing includes cryptococcal antigen testing of the CSF, which is more sensitive and specific but may not be readily available. Treatment is with amphotericin.

Test-taking tip: The question gives a large hint with an AIDS patient with meningitis signs for 3 days. Most bacterial meningitis patients would be deceased after 3 days of infection. Answer C is the organism most associated with AIDS.

11.

NONTRAUMATIC MUSCULOSKELETAL DISORDERS

Brenna Jane McCarney Derksen

1. A 60-year-old male with a past medical history significant for diabetes, hypertension, and chronic kidney disease presents with 1 day of elbow pain with the findings shown in Figure 11.1. His elbow is exquisitely tender on exam. Synovial fluid analysis shows white blood cell (WBC) count of 5,000 cells/uL, polymorphonuclear neutrophils (PMNs) 50%, with negatively birefringent crystals, and cultures are pending. What is the most appropriate treatment?

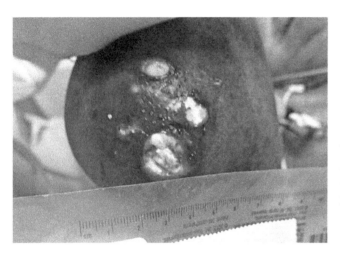

Figure 11.1 Elbow.

A. Operative washout, IV antibiotics, and admission with follow-up on synovial cultures
B. Incision and drainage (I&D), then discharge on oral antibiotics and follow-up wound check in 48 hours
C. Discharge home on allopurinol
D. Discharge home on prednisone taper

2. A 50-year-old male comes to emergency department (ED) complaining of a painful, swollen right knee that is gradually worsening over the last week. He has been taking ibuprofen daily with partial alleviation. He has had similar pain and swelling in his knees in the past. He is afebrile and otherwise well-appearing. Radiograph shows chondrocalcinosis. Arthrocentesis is performed with drainage of cloudy yellow fluid. What findings would you expect to find on synovial fluid analysis?

A. Weakly positive birefringent rhomboid-shaped crystals
B. Needle-like negatively birefringent crystal
C. Greater than 75% PMNs; fluid WBC 10,000 cells/uL, glucose less than 25
D. 5,000 WBCs, glucose of 70, no crystals

3. A 75-year-old female comes into the ED complaining of bilateral knee pain. She states she has had progressively worsening knee pain over the past few years but this week her symptoms are worse than normal after she implemented her new walking regimen. She denies recent falls or injury. On exam, she is afebrile, well-appearing, with mild bilateral knee swelling and mildly decreased range of motion of her knees. There is not overlying erythema or warmth. Radiographs show joint space narrowing and osteophytes. What is the best treatment for her condition?

A. Arthrocentesis to rule out pseudogout
B. Nonsteroidal antiinflammatory drugs (NSAIDs) and rest
C. Prednisone
D. Methotrexate and referral to rheumatologist

4. A 65-year-old female presents with a chief complaint of bilateral hand pain, swelling, warmth, and stiffness that is worse than her chronic pain for the past 3 days. Her medications include metformin, hydrochlorothiazide, methotrexate, and ibuprofen. She has had similar symptoms in the past and was treated with steroids. What findings are not consistent with her diagnosis?

A. Ulnar deviation of the metacarpophalangeal joints
B. Fatigue

C. Boggy, tender, swelling of the distal interphalangeal (DIP) joints
D. Morning stiffness

5. A 7-year-old previously healthy male presents for evaluation of joint pain and fatigue. He describes an aching pain that started in his knees and has progressed to his right ankle and right wrist. His knee pain and wrist pain resolved, but over the past few days he has developed ankle pain. His mother notes that he is typically healthy and active, but she does recall a febrile illness associated with a round rash he developed after a family camping trip in Connecticut a few months ago. What is the treatment?

A. Doxycycline IV for 2 weeks
B. Doxycycline PO for 4 weeks
C. Amoxicillin PO for 4 weeks
D. NSAIDs and supportive management

6. A 46-year-old female with a past medical history significant for type 2 diabetes presents to the ED for a painful, swollen right knee. Symptoms have been progressively worsening over the past few days. Last week she fell on her knee and sustained an abrasion; otherwise there is no history of trauma. On exam, she has a temperature of 38.6° C and appears uncomfortable. Her knee is erythematous, swollen, and warm. She is exquisitely tender to palpation throughout the knee and will not allow you to range her joint. Her radiograph is shown in Figure 11.2. What is the most likely pathogen causing her condition?

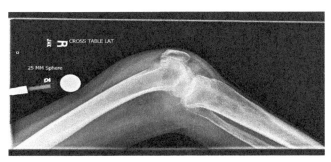

Figure 11.2 Knee radiograph.

A. *Staphylococcus aureus*
B. *Neisseria gonorrhoeae*
C. *Streptococcus*
D. Noninfectious inflammation of the bursa

7. A 20-year-old sexually active female presents to the ED with a painful swollen left knee. Last week she said she was sick with "the flu" and describes feeling warm, tired, and joint pain throughout her body that has since resolved except for her knee. What is the most likely infectious agent causing her symptoms?

A. *S. aureus*
B. *Streptococcus epididymis*
C. *N. gonorrhoeae*
D. *Borrelia burgdorferi*

8. A 62-year-old female with a past medical history significant for rheumatoid arthritis (RA) and hypertension presents with a bilateral knee pain and swelling, bilateral wrist pain, fatigue, and generalized body aches. Her knees are diffusely tender, boggy, and warm. Her right knee is pictured in Figure 11.3. What findings would you expect on synovial fluid analysis?

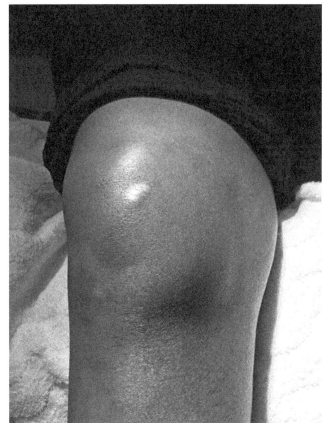

Figure 11.3 Knee.

A. WBCs 5,000 and 50% PMNs with weakly positive birefringent rhomboid-shaped crystals
B. WBCs 5,000 and 50% PMNs with negatively birefringent needle-shaped crystals
C. WBCs 5,100 and 50% PMNs, negative crystals, cultures pending
D. WBCs 51,000 and 75% PMNs, cultures pending

9. A 25-year-old male presents with right heel pain and swelling. He denies recent trauma or increased physical activity. On exam, he is tender over the Achilles tendon and heel with mild swelling. Range of motion, strength, and sensation are intact, and he has a negative Thompson test. He is normally healthy but notes that a few weeks ago he had a bout of diarrhea and some discomfort when urinating. What is the most likely cause of his symptoms?

A. Overuse injury causing strain of the Achilles tendon and plantar fasciitis
B. *Chlamydia trachomatis*
C. *S. aureus*
D. Antibiotic use

10. A 31-year-old male presents for evaluation of low back pain for the past 3 months. He describes bilateral low back pain that is aching and associated with stiffness. He says it is worst when he wakes up in the morning but improves as he moves throughout the day, although he has had less energy than normal lately. He denies history of trauma or heavy lifting. On exam, he is afebrile and has mild tenderness over bilateral sacroiliac joints; no midline pain; normal reflexes, strength, and sensation in his lower extremities; and negative straight-leg test. His radiograph is shown in Figure 11.4. What is the most likely diagnosis?

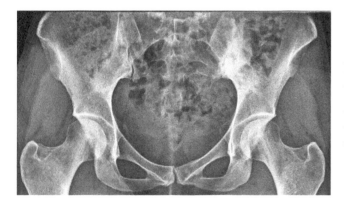

Figure 11.4 Pelvis radiograph.

A. Sacroiliitis
B. Lumbago
C. Spinal stenosis
D. Malignancy

11. A 34-year-old male with Crohn's disease presents for evaluation of atraumatic low back pain for the last 6 months. His radiograph is shown in Figure 11.5. Based on the findings seen in his lumbar radiograph, what other associated signs and symptoms who you expect with the cause of his back pain?

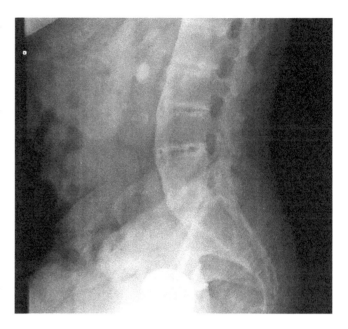

Figure 11.5 Spine radiograph.

A. Point midline tenderness over L5
B. Saddle anesthesia
C. Positive straight-leg test
D. Pain that is worse in the morning and improved with activity

12. A 29-year-old male with a past medical history of irritable bowel disease presents with 5 months of low back pain. His pain is most significant in his low back and over his sacroiliac joints. His symptoms are worse in the morning and when going to bed but improve throughout the day with activity. He has felt fatigued but denies fevers, saddle anesthesia, incontinence, IV drug use, or history of trauma. What is the most common extraarticular comorbidity associated with his condition?

A. Uveitis
B. Conjunctivitis
C. Aortic regurgitation
D. Urethritis

13. A 65-year-old male patient is sent over from urgent care for evaluation of low back pain. The referring physician was concerned for cauda equina syndrome. What is the most common associated symptom aside from back pain in patients presenting with cauda equina syndrome?

A. Fever
B. Urinary retention
C. Saddle anesthesia
D. Lower extremity weakness

14. In which of the following patients is emergent imaging indicated for their back pain?

A. A 20-year-old male presenting with 5 days of low back pain after lifting heavy boxes helping his friend move, alleviated with NSAIDs and rest

B. A 20-year-old female with fever, dysuria, and right-sided back pain for the past 3 days

C. A 48-year-old male with chronic low back pain and positive straight-leg test and normal lower extremity strength and sensation

D. A 48-year-old male with chronic low back pain and 3 days of difficulty walking secondary to bilateral leg weakness

15. A 71-year-old female with a past medical history significant for diabetes presents for evaluation of low back pain radiating down her legs. She says her pain feels slightly better when she bends forward during her morning stretching routine, but her back and leg pain are much worse during her morning walk. She says the pain is especially bad when walking down the hill by her house. She has had to sit and rest at the bottom of the hill until her pain resolves, and she notes the pain is less severe when she walks back up the hill home. On exam, she has reproducible pain with passive extension of her legs. She has strong distal pulses and intact strength and sensation in her lower extremities. On chart review, prior radiographs of her lumbar spine have shown degenerative disease. What is the most likely cause of her symptoms?

A. Spinal stenosis

B. Sciatica

C. Vascular claudication

D. Diabetic neuropathy

16. A 42-year-old male presents with acute exacerbation of his chronic low back pain. The patient works in construction and a few days ago noticed sudden worsening of pain in his low back that shoots down the side of his right leg. Although he has had similar exacerbations of pain in the past, he is particularly concerned because of numbness in his right leg and foot. On exam, the patient has a positive straight-leg test on the right and decreased sensation behind his calf and on the lateral aspect of his right foot but has intact sensation of his great toe. What nerve root is likely affected and what is the next best step in management?

A. L5 nerve root, no further imaging, activity as tolerated, and symptomatic treatment

B. L5 nerve root, emergent magnetic resonance imaging (MRI)

C. S1 nerve root, no further imaging, activity as tolerated, and symptomatic treatment

D. S1 nerve root, emergent MRI

17. A 32-year-old female presents with finger pain 5 days after getting a manicure at a nail salon. On exam, she has swelling, erythema, warmth, fluctuance, and severe tenderness over the soft tissue surrounding the ulnar side of the finger nail on her fourth digit. There is fluctuance and purulent drainage when the lateral nail is lifted. What is the best treatment for her symptoms?

A. Warm soaks

B. Oral antibiotics

C. I&D

D. Trephination of the nailbed

18. A 35-year-old male presents to the ED with right hand pain. He is a mechanic and thinks he may have cut his hand on something at work and has been unable to fix cars because of pain and swelling on his index finger and hand. His finger is pictured in Figure 11.6, and you notice that he holds his index finger in slight flexion. Which symptom is not consistent with his diagnosis?

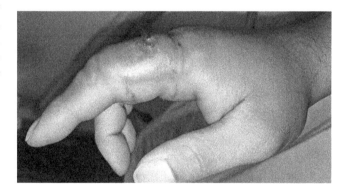

Figure 11.6 Finger.

A. Fusiform swelling of the digit

B. Pain with passive extension

C. Pain with passive flexion

D. Tenderness along the palmar aspect of his finger and hand

19. A 42-year-old with a history of IV drug use presents with 4 days of swelling in her left index finger. She denies fevers or any history of trauma. On exam, her finger is held in flexion, diffusely swollen, tender along the flexor tendon, and painful when you attempt to extend her finger. What is the next best step in management?

A. I&D at the bedside

B. Orthopedic consultation

C. Admission for IV antibiotics
D. Radiograph of the finger

20. A 72-year-old male with a past medical history significant for type 2 diabetes mellitus and hypertension was brought in by his concerned daughter for evaluation of weakness and thoracic back pain for the past month. She says her father has not been eating much and is having difficulty getting out of bed, walking, and caring for himself because of pain and weakness. The pain is located in the thoracic region and has been progressively worsening. The patient describes a dull, aching pain that is now interfering with his sleep. He also endorses fatigue, decreased appetite, nausea, and constipation. He denies fevers, urinary or bowel incontinence, and saddle anesthesia and has no history of falls or trauma. On exam, he appears dehydrated, has minimal generalized abdominal tenderness without rebound pain, and has mild weakness in his bilateral lower extremities. Radiograph of his thoracic spine shows a compression fracture at T8 concerning for a pathologic fracture. In addition to labs, symptom control, and IV fluids, what is the next best step in management of this patient?

A. Radiograph of the entire spine
B. MRI of the thoracic spine
C. MRI of the entire spine
D. Computed tomography (CT) of the abdomen and pelvis with contrast

21. A 6-year-old male present with knee and ankle pain and recent upper respiratory infection and pharyngitis. A week ago his mother noted he had a fever, headache, sore throat, and cough and has now developed joint pain and a rash on his legs. On exam, he has palpable purpura on his buttock and lower extremities bilaterally as well as edema and tenderness in his knees and ankles. What are the likely long-term effects of the patient's knee and ankle pain?

A. Most patients have complete resolution with no long-term effects
B. Chondrocalcinosis
C. Chronic arthritis
D. Recurrent hemorrhagic joint effusions

22. A 13-year-old boy presents with atraumatic leg pain, localized to the distal femur. Pain is aching and dull, ongoing for 3 weeks, and worse when he is sleeping. On exam, he has tenderness and swelling at the distal femur but is neurovascularly intact. What findings would you expect on radiograph?

A. Lytic lesion with periosteal reaction
B. Fragmented ossification of the tendon

C. Rate bite erosions
D. Chondrocalcinosis

23. A 13-year-old boy presents with left knee pain for the past month. He is a soccer player and says his coach wanted him evaluated because he has a mild limp after practice. Pain is worse after running drills and games. He has swelling and tenderness localized over the proximal tibia but full range of motion, strength, and sensation. What is the most likely etiology of his pain?

A. Osgood-Schlatter disease
B. Septic knee
C. Osteosarcoma
D. Pre-patellar bursitis

24. A 30-year-old homeless male with a past medical history significant for hepatitis C and polysubstance abuse is brought in by medics with complaints of weakness. He endorses generalized weakness, fatigue, fever, and body aches for the past week. He denies history of trauma but has some old abrasions on his hands, appears disheveled and tired, and has feces on his clothing. On exam, he has a temperature of 38° C, heart rate (HR) of 105 bpm, tenderness over the cervical and lumbar spine, weak grips bilaterally and bilateral lower extremity weakness, decreased rectal tone, and inability to ambulate. Radiographs are notable for degenerative changes. What is the next best step in management?

A. Lumbar puncture and broad-spectrum antibiotics
B. Neurosurgical consult, MRI of the spine, and broad-spectrum antibiotics
C. CT myelography, neurology consultation, high-dose steroids, and broad-spectrum antibiotics
D. Admission for broad-spectrum antibiotics and follow-up blood cultures

25. A 28-year-old male with hemophilia A presents with right knee pain and swelling 1 hour after a mechanical fall while playing basketball. His knee feels tense and is very painful. He describes a very uncomfortable pressure sensation. Which of the following is *not* a relative contraindication to performing arthrocentesis on a patient with a knee effusion?

A. Hemarthrosis in a hemophiliac patient before factor replacement
B. Overlying cellulitis
C. Prosthetic joint
D. Tricompartmental osteoarthritis (OA)

26. A 38-year-old male with a past medical history significant for hepatitis C virus (HCV) and HIV, not

compliant with his antiretroviral medication, presents with the painful, fluid-filled vesicles pictured in Figure 11.7 on his third digit. He denies any recent trauma, and there is no involvement of the pulp of his finger. What is the best management of this condition?

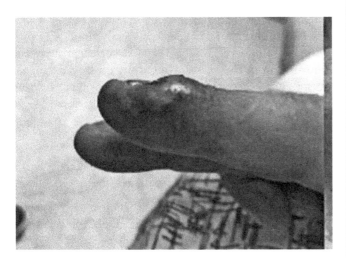

Figure 11.7 Finger.

A. I&D over the area of greatest fluctuance
B. I&D with high lateral incision and oral antibiotics
C. Oral antibiotics
D. Oral antivirals

27. A 4-year-old previously healthy male is brought into the ED by his concerned mother because her son has developed a limp. She states he was recently sick with an upper respiratory infection. On exam, the patient is well-appearing with a temperature of 38° C and nasal congestion. He begins to cry when you attempt to examine his hip. He ambulates with a slight limp. What is the treatment of his condition?

A. NSAIDs, rest, close follow-up
B. Joint aspiration and orthopedics consult
C. Orthopedics consult, non–weight bearing, eventual surgical stabilization
D. Orthopedics consult, bracing, eventual femoral osteotomy

28. A 31-year-old female presents with finger pain for 2 days. She admits she has the "bad habit" of biting her nails and picking at her cuticles. On exam, she has mild tenderness, no drainage or fluctuance, and the findings seen in Figure 11.8. What is the best initial treatment for her symptoms?

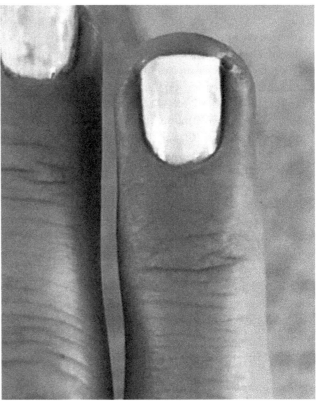

Figure 11.8 Finger.

A. Warm soaks and close follow-up with a primary care provider.
B. Oral antibiotics with removal of the proximal third of the nail
C. High lateral incision for drainage of abscess
D. Longitudinal incision near the eponychium directed away from the nail fold, directed over the area of greatest fluctuance

29. A 20-year-old male presents with atraumatic back pain and stiffness for the past 3 months that improves with activity. Radiograph shows squaring of the vertebral bodies. Which of the features below is not traditionally seen in this disorder?

A. Rash
B. Sacroiliitis
C. Uveitis
D. Negative rheumatoid factor

ANSWERS

1. ANSWER: D

The patient's presentation is consistent with gout, as evidenced by the negatively birefringent crystals seen on synovial fluid analysis as well as the tophi shown in the picture. Gout is typically seen in the middle-aged or older adults with a predilection for the lower extremity and first metatarsophalangeal (MTP) joint (podagra). Gout develops acutely with monoarticular joint pain associated with erythema, warmth, and joint effusion. There are multiple treatment options available for acute gout flairs such as NSAIDs, colchicine, or steroids. This patient has chronic kidney disease and will not be a candidate for colchicine or NSAIDs if there is evidence of significantly impaired renal function; thus steroids are the treatment of choice for his acute flair. Colchicine was once the treatment of choice for acute gout but is less commonly used because of its narrow therapeutic window and common adverse effects of diarrhea and vomiting. Colchicine must be renally dosed and avoided in cases of renal failure. NSAIDs would be another viable treatment strategy for an acute flair, but this is not an answer choice. NSAIDs should be avoided in cases of known peptic ulcer disease, gastrointestinal bleeds, or renal insufficiency. Corticosteroids can be given to patients with gout who cannot use NSAIDs or colchicine. Treatment of pseudogout is similar to the treatment of gout (Table 11.1).

Operative washout and admission for IV antibiotics is the treatment for a septic joint. It is difficult clinically to distinguish gout from infectious etiologies such as septic joint or bursitis, and arthrocentesis is necessary to differentiate between these diagnoses. Joint fluid showing crystals will differentiate a septic joint from gout or pseudogout. In gout and pseudogout the WBC count is typically elevated to between 2,000 and 50,000 compared with a septic joint, which typically shows WBC >50,000 with >75% PMNs.

Table 11.1 GOUT VERSUS PSEUDOGOUT

	GOUT	PSEUDOGOUT
Most common joint	First metatarsophalangeal	Knee, often multijoint
Crystals	Uric acid	Calcium pyrophosphate
Shape	Needle	Rhomboid
Microscope	Negatively birefringent	Positively birefringent
Imaging	Rat-bite erosions	Chondrocalcinosis
Treatment	NSAIDs, colchicine, steroids	NSAIDs

I&D would be appropriate treatment for an abscess, and antibiotics play no role in the treatment of gout.

Allopurinol helps to reduce tissue uric acid levels and can be used for prophylaxis in the management of chronic gout. Allopurinol should be avoided during acute gout attacks. This patient has gouty tophi and symptoms that are consistent with an acute attack, and thus allopurinol is not indicated in this patient.

Test-taking tip: Although a visual stimulus is provided, it is not necessary to choose the correct answer. The information in the question about negatively birefringent crystals is all that you need to know that you are treating acute gout, pointing you toward the correct answer.

2. ANSWER: A

The patient presentation is consistent with pseudogout, also known as calcium pyrophosphate deposition disease. Calcium pyrophosphate crystals appear as weakly positive birefringent rhomboid-shaped crystals on microscopy analysis of the synovial fluid. These calcium pyrophosphate crystals can be deposited, causing densities on articular cartilage, ligaments, tendons, soft tissues, and synovium, with the characteristic radiographic finding of chondrocalcinosis, which refers to densities in the cartilage and joint inflammation seen on radiographs. Patients with pseudogout may present with a monoarticular inflammatory arthropathy, and the knee is the most commonly affected joint.

The clinical symptoms of gout can present similarly to pseudogout, but the first MTP is the most commonly affected joint in gout (podagra) versus the knee in pseudogout. Classic radiographic findings of "rat-bite erosions" are seen in gout. The crystals seen in gout are needle-shaped, negatively birefringent crystals.

Greater than75% PMNs and 50,000 WBCs are consistent with a septic joint. It can be difficult to differentiate gout and pseudogout from septic joint. Yellow cloudy synovial fluid with elevated WBCs and PMN predominance can be seen in both infectious and other inflammatory conditions. Typically, inflammatory conditions have 3,000 to 50,000 WBCs and negative culture, whereas infectious conditions have >50,000 WBCs, low glucose, and possibly a positive culture. There must be a high index of suspicion when ruling out septic joint because there is a significant difference in management. The classic findings of chondrocalcinosis, lack of systemic symptoms, and repetitive nature of the patient's symptoms are consistent with pseudogout.

Laboratory findings of WBC count of 5,000, glucose 70, and no crystals are consistent with an inflammatory joint effusion, which can be seen in conditions such as RA, Lyme disease, spondyloarthropathies, gout, and pseudogout. These inflammatory conditions often present similarly to pseudogout (Table 11.2).

Table 11.2 CLASSIC FINDINGS OF COMMON ARTHROPATHIES

	SIGNS/SYMPTOMS	RADIOGRAPH FINDINGS	FLUID ANALYSIS
Gout	First metatarsophalangeal, tophi	Rat-bite erosions	Inflammatory, negatively birefringent, needle-shaped uric acid crystals
Pseudogout	Knee, can be polyarticular and symmetric	chondrocalcinosis	Inflammatory, positively birefringent, rhomboid calcium pyrophosphate crystals
Rheumatoid arthritis	Polyarticular, symmetric with sparing of distal interphalangeal joints, boggy, tender, morning stiffness	Joint space narrowing, ulnar deviation of the metacarpophalangeal joints, boutonniere and swan neck deformities	Inflammatory, no crystals
Osteoarthritis	Polyarticular, often asymmetric	Joint space narrowing, osteophytes, subchondral cysts	Noninflammatory, no crystals
Ankylosing spondylitis	Spine and pelvis, <40 years old, morning stiffness, HLA-B27	Squaring of vertebral bodies (bamboo spine), sacroiliitis	N/A

Test-taking tip: Brush up on the classic signs and symptoms, radiographic findings, and joint fluid analysis findings for common arthropathies.

3. ANSWER: B

The patient's presentation is consistent with OA, which is a degenerative breakdown of the articular cartilage in the synovial joints. Diagnosis is based on clinical and radiographic findings. Patients typically present with chronic and progressively worsening joint pain, stiffness, decreased range of motion, and crepitus. The most common joint affected is the knee, but joint destruction is typically polyarticular (Table 11.3). Radiographs may show joint space narrowing

Table 11.3 DISTRIBUTION OF DIFFERENT ARTHROPATHIES

NUMBER OF JOINTS AFFECTED	CONDITIONS
Monoarthritis (1)	Septic joint, trauma, crystal induced, acute osteoarthritis,* Lyme disease,* avascular necrosis, tumor
Oligoarthritis (2–3)	Reiter's syndrome, ankylosing spondylitis, rheumatic fever, gonococcal septic arthritis, Lyme disease*
Polyarthritis (>3)	Rheumatoid arthritis, systemic lupus erythematosus, chronic osteoarthritis*

*THESE conditions can affect a different number of joints.

due to destruction of articular cartilage, osteophytes, and subchondral cysts. Pain is typically relieved by rest and antiinflammatories.

Unless there is a large joint effusion or concern for an alternative etiology of the joint pain (such as septic joint, gout, or pseudogout), arthrocentesis is not necessary in the management of OA. OA may be associated with noninflammatory joint effusions, however, and removal of this fluid with arthrocentesis may provide some therapeutic relief for patients. Pseudogout has a predilection for the knee, but there is low concern for pseudogout in this patient given that there is no erythema, warmth, or obvious effusion.

Treatment consists of rest and topical or oral antiinflammatories. Intraarticular corticosteroid injections are sometimes used to provide pain relief and antiinflammatory effects, but NSAIDs are the first-line treatment. Systemic steroids are not indicated in treatment of OA.

Methotrexate is one of the treatments for RA that is characterized by tender, boggy, and warm joints with sparing of the DIP joints of the hand. This medication is typically initiated by a specialist.

Test-taking tip: Brush up on the different distributions of the arthropathies because they may help you narrow your differential, both in your practice and on the examination.

4. ANSWER: C

The patient in this question suffers from RA. RA is an autoimmune disorder with symmetric, polyarticular joint involvement. Patients typically present with boggy, tender, swelling joints. RA may be confused with other polyarticular joint diseases such as OA. Unlike OA,

RA does *not* involve the DIP joints of the hand, and symptoms are typically worse after periods of rest. Classic physical exam findings seen on the hands of patients with late-stage RA include ulnar deviation of the metacarpophalangeal joints, boutonniere deformity of the thumb, and swan neck deformity of the fifth digit, such as seen in Figure 11.9.

Other symptoms of RA may include morning stiffness, fever, myalgias, and extraarticular symptoms such as pericarditis, myocarditis, pleural effusion, and pneumonitis. Synovial fluid analysis will show an inflammatory profile without positive cultures or crystals. Treatment includes NSAIDs and disease-modifying antirheumatic drugs, such as methotrexate, steroids, and antimalarials.

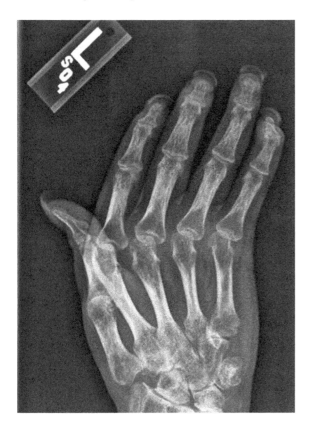

Figure 11.9 Hand radiograph.

Test-taking tip: Brush up on the difference between OA and RA because they are both chronic conditions with some similar features but very different treatments.

5. ANSWER: C

The patient is presenting with arthritis secondary to late Lyme disease, which is treated with amoxicillin 500 mg PO three times daily for 4 weeks in patients younger than 8 years and pregnant populations. Lyme disease is endemic to the northeast and is caused by *B. burgdorferi* transmitted through the *Ixodes* (also known as black-legged) tick. Lyme disease can manifest as a migratory, monoarticular or oligoarticular, asymmetric arthritis that often involves large joints secondary to hematogenous dissemination of the spirochete after initial infection. The arthritic manifestations are often delayed by weeks to months, as seen in this patient.

Acute Lyme disease typically presents with symptoms of fever, headache, fatigue, and erythema migrans, characterized by target lesions, that is classic for Lyme disease. Arthritic manifestations are often seen months later and usually present as brief exacerbations with complete remission. Patients may develop large effusions with synovial fluid analysis consistent with an inflammatory process and negative cultures. Patients will usually have a history of tick bite, erythema chronicum migrans rash, travel to endemic location, or other stage II or III findings such as fatigue, neurologic abnormalities, and cardiac conduction disturbances. Diagnosis is based on enzyme-linked immunosorbent assay (ELISA) titer or isolation of *B. burgdorferi* spirochete. If a high degree of clinical suspicion exists, patient should be treated empirically with antibiotics.

IV regimens are appropriate for patients with Lyme arthritis who also have neurologic involvement, which this patient does not have.

Doxycycline 100 mg PO for twice daily 4 weeks is the preferred treatment of choice for Lyme arthritis but is not recommended in patients younger than 8 years and pregnant women.

Supportive care and NSAIDs would be appropriate management of a simple viral illness or musculoskeletal pain from arthritis, trauma, or overuse but is not the appropriate treatment of arthritis associated with Lyme disease.

Test-taking tip: If you know that doxycycline is not usually recommended in the pediatric population because of the potential negative effect on cartilage development as well as teeth staining, it allows you to eliminate two of the possible answers.

6. ANSWER: A

This patient is presenting with a septic joint, and the most common cause in her age group is *S. aureus*. A septic joint presents as an exquisitely painful monoarthritis that is resistant to movement. The patient may have fevers or chills, but absence should not preclude the diagnosis of a septic joint, and if there is concern, arthrocentesis must be performed.

S. aureus infection is overall the most commonly cultured organism in acute septic arthritis in adults older than 35 years. Gonococcal arthritis is the most common cause in adolescents and young adults (<35 years old). Arthrocentesis in both types will show WBC counts >50,000 with >75% PMNs, but cultures may be negative in gonococcal arthritis.

Streptococcus species are a common cause of septic bursitis and may cause septic joint as well; however, *S. aureus* is the most common cause in this age group. Group A *Streptococcus* if left untreated can rarely cause rheumatic fever, which is associated with fever, muscle aches, and joint pain. This diagnosis is extremely rare, and although this patient has fever and joint pain, there is no history of strep throat or other symptoms associated with rheumatic fever.

Bursitis is a noninfectious inflammation of the bursa and is often secondary to local trauma or occupational risk factors (e.g., housemaid's knee, student's elbow). Bursitis is associated with swelling, pain, and decreased active range or motion but normal passive range of motion. Bursitis can become infected, causing septic bursitis, and the most common organisms include *S. aureus, Staphylococcus epidermidis,* and *Streptococcus.* It is usually treated initially with oral antibiotics. Arthrocentesis and imaging are not necessary unless there is concern for alternative etiology of symptoms.

Test-taking tip: Brush up on the pathogens that cause septic arthritis and differences depending on the patient's age.

7. ANSWER: C

The patient's presentation is consistent with a gonococcal septic joint.

Gonococcal arthritis is the most common cause of septic joint in adolescents and young adults. A septic joint is usually associated with a prodromal migratory arthritis and tenosynovitis, followed by a septic joint. Patients can also show evidence of vesiculopustular lesions on their fingers. Arthrocentesis should be performed, and fluid should be sent for analysis including culture and Gram stain. Arthrocentesis profile will be consistent with septic joint usually showing WBC counts >50,000 with >75% PMNs. Despite adequate fluid samples and active infection, synovial cultures are often negative in cases of *N. gonorrhoeae* infection. In addition to management of the septic joint and gonococcal infection, patients should be covered for possible co-infection with *Chlamydia.*

S. aureus infection is overall the most common cause of a septic joint in adults older than 35 years. *Streptococcus* species can also cause septic joint but are not the most common cause in this age group.

The *B. burgdorferi* spirochete is the cause of Lyme disease. Patients with Lyme disease develop migratory, asymmetric joint pain and effusions and may develop and inflammatory response that appears similar to septic joint. Typically, the large joints are affected. Although this patient describes a migratory and large joint distribution, Lyme disease is not the most common cause of joint pain or septic joint in this age group and therefore incorrect. If there is concern for Lyme disease, a Lyme titer may be sent. Treatment of Lyme disease includes doxycycline in adults or amoxicillin in pediatric and pregnant populations.

Test-taking tip: Look for clues in the question that will point you to the correct answer, in this case the term "sexually active."

8. ANSWER: C

This patient is presenting with an acute exacerbation of her RA and pictured is a swollen knee with a large effusion. RA is an autoimmune disorder with symmetric, polyarticular inflammatory joint involvement. Patients typically present with boggy, tender, swelling joints, as with this patient. RA may be confused with other joint diseases but is characterized by polyarticular and symmetric involvement with sparing of the DIP joint. Other symptoms of RA include fatigue, morning stiffness, fever, myalgias, and extraarticular symptoms such as pericarditis, myocarditis, pleural effusion, and pneumonitis (Table 11.4). Synovial fluid analysis will show an inflammatory profile with elevated WBC counts (usually 3,000–10,000) and PMNs >50%, but without positive cultures or crystals.

Table 11.4 RHEUMATOID ARTHRITIS AND OSTEOARTHRITIS SYMPTOMS

DISEASE	SYMPTOMS
Rheumatoid arthritis	Worse in the morning and with rest, tender and boggy, sparing of the distal interphalangeal joints, polyarticular, and symmetric
Osteoarthritis	Worse with use, improved with rest, acutely may have joint swelling, does not spare distal interphalangeal joints; chronic is polyarticular with monoarticular acute exacerbations

The presence of weakly birefringent crystals suggests the diagnosis of pseudogout, which usually presents as a monarticular arthropathy. The knee is the most commonly affected joint in pseudogout.

Negatively birefringent needle-shaped crystals would be seen in gout; they are caused by uric acid deposition. Similar to pseudogout, gout is a monoarticular inflammatory arthropathy with a predilection for the lower extremity and the MTP joint.

Septic joint will have an infectious profile on synovial fluid analysis with WBC counts >50,000 and >75% PMNs. Usually there will be a positive culture; however, in cases of gonococcal disease, culture is often negative (Table 11.5). Septic joint occurs secondary to hematogenous spread of bacteria from a focus contiguous to a joint or direct inoculation into the joint.

Table 11.5 FINDINGS IN SYNOVIAL FLUID WITH DIFFERENT CONDITIONS

	NORMAL FLUID	NONINFLAMMATORY	INFLAMMATORY	INFECTIOUS
Condition		Osteoarthritis, trauma, rheumatic fever	Gout, pseudogout, Lyme disease, spondyloarthropathies, systemic lupus erythematosus, rheumatoid arthritis	Septic, gonococcal in young, sexually active patients
Appearance	Colorless, transparent	Straw/yellow, transparent	Yellow, cloudy	Yellow, cloudy
WBC/μL	<200	<200–3,000	3,000–10,000	>50,000
Polymorphonuclear neutrophils	<25%	<25%	>50%	>75%
Culture	Negative	Negative	Negative	Positive (can be negative in gonococcal); *S. aureus*
Crystals	None	None	Positive in gout/pseudogout	None
Glucose	Normal	Normal	>25 (lower than serum)	<25 (lower than serum)
Treatment	N/A	NSAIDs	Disease specific	IV antibiotics, surgical washout

Test-taking tip: Brush up on the synovial fluid profiles for common arthropathies.

9. ANSWER: B

The patient is presenting with Reiter's syndrome, also known as reactive arthritis. Reactive arthritis is a seronegative spondyloarthropathy, associated with HLA-B27. Other HLA-B27 syndromes include ankylosing spondylitis (AS), irritable bowel syndrome, and psoriatic arthritis. Patients typically present with an acute, asymmetric oligoarthritis with a preceding infectious illness (typically urethritis or diarrhea). *Chlamydia* and *Ureaplasma* are the most common inciting infections. The arthritic symptoms usually involve the lower extremity, and the heels of the feet are commonly involved. The classic triad of symptoms associated with reactive arthritis is arthritis, urethritis, and conjunctivitis or uveitis, but you do not need all three for a diagnosis. The mnemonic, "can't see, can't pee, can't climb a tree," is often used to remember this triad. Treatment of pain is with NSAIDs as well as treatment of the underlying infection.

S. aureus is the most common cause of septic joint in adults, but gonococcal infection is the most common cause of septic joint in this patient's age group. Gonorrhea can be associated with joint effusion and dysuria but is not typically accompanied by diarrhea and does not typically affect the Achilles tendon like reactive arthritis does.

Fluoroquinolones have been associated with Achilles tendon rupture. The patient has a negative Thompson test, which is used to evaluate for ruptured Achilles tendon. He also has no history of antibiotic use, and given his young age and lack of comorbidities, he would be at low risk for Achilles tendon rupture even if he were to have taken a fluoroquinolone.

Test-taking tip: The question stem of "no recent trauma or increased physical activity" allows you to eliminate A, and with no history mentioned of recent antibiotic use or illness, you can eliminate D, giving you two answers to choose from.

10. ANSWER: A

The patient's symptoms and radiograph are consistent with sacroiliitis. The radiograph shows irregularity and sclerosis of articular surfaces of sacroiliac joints, here with preserved joint space, but more advanced stages can show joint space narrowing and severe sclerosis and ankylosis. Sacroiliitis is seen in AS, which is an autoimmune arthritis associated with HLA-B27. Patients are typically men younger than 40 years. Typical symptoms include more than 3 months of back pain that is worse in the morning and stiffness that improves with activity and is often accompanied by malaise and fatigue. Other radiographic findings of AS include squaring of the vertebral bodies known as "bamboo spine." Treatment includes NSAIDs and referral to rheumatology.

Lumbago refers to nonspecific back pain from sprain or mechanical injury such as lifting, but often patients do not remember an inciting event. Patients with lumbago will present with pain that is typically worse with movement and improves with rest. Most symptoms resolve within 6 weeks. Patients with lumbago should resume activity as tolerated, avoid exercise until acute pain improves, and take acetaminophen and NSAIDs for pain control.

Spinal stenosis presents as chronic back pain secondary to narrowing of the lumbar spine (spinal canal, nerve root canal, intervertebral foramina) and is usually caused by degenerative disease leading to compression of vascular and neural structures. Patients are typically older adults and will have back pain that is worse with standing and extension and better with flexion. Diagnosis is with CT or MRI, and patients should be referred to a surgeon. Our patient is young, with no mention of degenerative disease, and his symptoms and imaging findings are more consistent with sacroiliitis.

Metastatic disease can present as back pain. Typically, patients are older, and radiographs will show evidence of bony lesions, but MRI may be needed if it is not seen on radiographs. Patients may present with neurologic and compressive symptoms, in which case urgent MRI is needed. This patient is young and does not have any neurologic deficits or compressive symptoms, making this diagnosis unlikely.

Test-taking tip: Although a visual stimulus is provided, it is not necessary to choose the correct answer. The patient is young with no midline pain but with bilateral sacroiliac pain, pointing to the correct answer.

11. ANSWER: D

The radiograph shows squaring of the vertebral bodies and formation of syndesmophytes, longitudinal fibrous bands leading to ossification and fusion of the vertebrae. These changes lead to the classic "bamboo spine" appearance seen in AS. AS is an autoimmune, seronegative spondyloarthropathy associated with HLA-B27, most commonly affecting the spine and pelvis. Patients are typically younger than 40 years with an insidious onset of symptoms lasting greater than 3 months. Symptoms include back pain and stiffness, that improves with activity and is worse in the morning. Back pain is also associated with malaise, weakness, and fatigue. Treatment is with NSAIDs and referral to rheumatology.

Point tenderness is typically present with bony fractures and bacterial infections. Patients with AS may present with sacroiliitis as well as syndesmophytes and may present with tenderness over the sacroiliac joint. However, AS is not isolated to only one vertebral body, so point tenderness would not be expected

Saddle anesthesia can be seen in epidural compressive syndromes but is not a typical finding in AS. Epidural compressive syndromes can be caused by hemorrhage/

hematoma, infection, mass, or severe midline disk herniation. Symptoms may include back pain (duration is not helpful), saddle anesthesia, urinary retention or incontinence, reduced sphincter tone, and possible history of malignancy if from a tumor. Patients require an emergent MRI that includes the entire spine if there is concern for metastatic disease.

Positive straight-leg test is seen with sciatica. Sciatica can be secondary to disk herniation at the L4–5 or L5–S1 nerve root. Pain is burning, shooting, or sharp, beginning in the low back and radiating in dermatomal distribution to below the knee (Figure 11.10). The straight-leg test has a very high sensitivity and very low specificity (Table 11.6).

Test-taking tip: Brush up on the buzz words and common clinical presentations of conditions associated with back pain.

12. ANSWER: A

The patient presents with symptoms of AS, and the most common extraarticular manifestation seen is anterior uveitis. AS is an autoimmune arthritis associated with HLA-B27 and affecting the lower spine and hips but can involve peripheral joints (ankles and knees) and enthesitis (pain and stiffness at the insertion sites of ligaments and tendons). Patients are usually men younger than 40 years and will present with chronic (>3 months) back pain and stiffness that is worse in the morning and improves with activity. Radiographs may show sacroiliitis and squaring of vertebral bodies ("bamboo spine"). Patients can also have systemic symptoms of malaise and fatigue as well as extraarticular symptoms. The most common complication is anterior uveitis, but AS is also associated with irritable bowel syndrome (as seen in this patient), psoriasis, aortic regurgitation, and restrictive pulmonary disease.

AS can be easily confused for reactive arthritis (also known as Reiter's syndrome), which is commonly associated with conjunctivitis and urethritis. A popular mnemonic, "can't see, can't pee, can't climb a tree," refers to the classic triad of symptoms of arthritis, conjunctivitis, and urethritis associated with reactive arthritis. Similar to AS, patients with reactive arthritis are also young males, but they typically present with lower extremity oligoarthritis and myalgias a few weeks after a diarrheal illness or symptoms of dysuria and eye complaints. Although conjunctivitis may progress to uveitis, this patient's distribution of back pain and lack of dysuria is more consistent with AS, thus making choices B and D less likely.

Choice C refers to aortic regurgitation and aortic root disease, which are possible extraarticular comorbidities associated with AS, but uveitis is the most common.

Test-taking tip: This is a "you know it or you don't" kind of question. If you don't know it, choose an answer

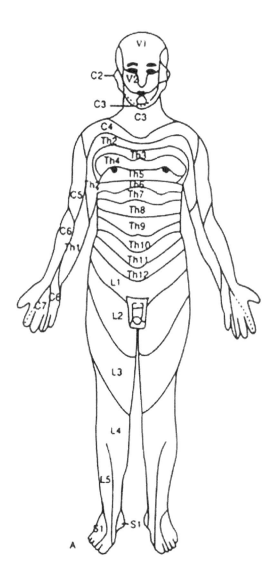

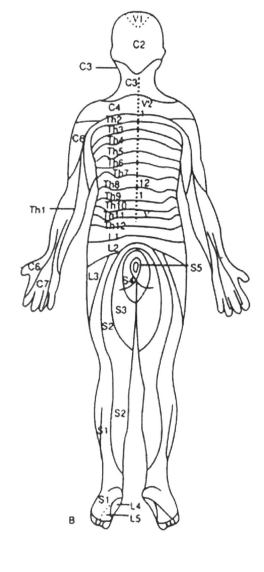

Figure 11.10 Dermatomes.

Table 11.6 BUZZ WORDS OF BACK PAIN

	BACK PAIN + MOST COMMON SYMPTOMS
Fracture	Acute bony tenderness
Malignancy	Night pain, weight loss
Spinal Stenosis	Pain with extension, relief with flexion
Sciatica	Shooting pain past knee, worse with bending and sitting, relief with lying
Reiter's syndrome	Worse in morning, polyarthritis, urethritis, conjunctivitis
Ankylosing spondylitis	Worse in morning, uveitis
Cauda equina syndrome	Urinary retention
Spinal epidural abscess	Fever, neurologic deficit

and move on. You can perhaps mark it for review when you are done at the end of the test. Don't however, let these kinds of questions get you stuck and waste your time.

13. ANSWER: B

Cauda equina syndrome is caused by compression of a collection of lumbosacral nerve roots below the level of the conus medullaris. The nerve roots distal to the conus medullaris (the most distal part of the spinal cord) resemble a horsetail, thus referred to as the cauda equine, which is Latin for horse's tail. When these nerve roots are compressed, they result in a myriad of lower motor neuron symptoms, including back pain, bladder and bowel dysfunction, saddle anesthesia, and lower extremity motor and sensory loss. Urinary retention is the most common symptom other than back pain in patients presenting with cauda equina syndrome. Urinary retention then progresses to overflow incontinence. Other associated symptoms that patients may present with include sciatica, saddle anesthesia, bowel disturbances, lower extremity motor and sensory weakness, and reduced lower extremity reflexes. All of the answer choices listed may be present in cases of cauda equina syndrome, but urinary retention is the most common. Cauda equina syndrome is a surgical emergency, and recognition in the ED is very important. There are many causes of cauda equina syndrome, including disk disease, spinal stenosis, trauma, tumors, infection, hemorrhage, and arteriovenous malformations.

Test-taking tip: This is a "you know it or you don't" kind of question. If you don't know it, choose an answer and move on. You can perhaps mark it for review when you are done at the end of the test. Don't, however, let these kinds of questions get you stuck and waste your time.

14. ANSWER: D

Patients presenting with "red flags" associated with back pain, such as the patient in choice D, should have further imaging to evaluate their pain. Red-flag symptoms in the setting of back pain include fever (especially if history of IV drug use), neurologic deficits, acute bony tenderness, age <18 or >50 years with night pain and/or weight loss, history of malignancy, bowel and/or bladder involvement, and morning stiffness in a young adult.

The patient in scenario D has symptoms concerning for compression of the cauda equina nerve roots and is displaying motor deficits that are impairing his ability to walk. Patients presenting in this manner must have an emergent MRI. Cauda equina syndrome is caused by compression of a collection of lumbosacral nerve roots below the level of the conus medullaris. There are many causes of cauda equina syndrome, including disk disease, spinal stenosis, trauma, tumors, infection, hemorrhage, and arteriovenous malformation. This patient has a history of chronic back pain suggesting progression of disk disease or spinal stenosis. Patients may also present with saddle anesthesia, bowel and bladder disturbances, lower extremity sensory deficits, and reduced lower extremity reflexes. Cauda equina syndrome is a surgical emergency, and recognition in the ED is critical.

Choice A is consistent with lumbago or back strain. The patient does not have red-flag symptoms and thus dos not require further imaging and can be managed symptomatically with the resumption of usual daily activities as tolerated. Most nonspecific back pain resolves in 4 to 6 weeks.

Choice B is consistent with pyelonephritis, which can be diagnosed clinically with urinalysis. Although this patient has a fever, which may be a red-flag symptom in cases of back pain, her pain is in the costovertebral angle (CVA) region and secondary to her infection. Imaging may be indicated if there is concern for an obstructing kidney stone or if she has pain consistent with osteomyelitis or an abscess.

Choice C is consistent with sciatica or radiculopathy usually secondary to disk herniation, most commonly at the L4–5 nerve root. Imaging in the ED is not indicated for uncomplicated radiculopathy in the abscess of red-flag symptoms. If symptoms do not resolve over time, an MRI may later be indicated on a nonemergent basis.

Test-taking tip: The use of the words "emergent imaging" suggests the need to make a diagnosis rapidly. Only the patient described in D with new bilateral weakness fits this scenario.

15. ANSWER: A

The patient's symptoms are consistent with neurogenic claudication, which is seen in spinal stenosis. Spinal stenosis is usually seen in older adult patients and is caused by narrowing of the lumbar spine (spinal canal, nerve root canal, intervertebral foramina), usually secondary to degenerative disease and leading to compression of vascular and neural structures. Symptoms include back and radicular pain that are worse with exertion, standing, and extension of the back but improved with back flexion and rest. Bending forward at the waist causes an increase in the diameter of the spinal canal diameter, thus reducing tension on the spinal cord and decreasing pain. Walking uphill causes a slightly flexed position which may improve symptoms, while walking downhill results in slight extension and thus increases pain. Improvement with flexion is characteristic of spinal stenosis. Diagnosis is with CT or MRI, and patients should be referred to a surgeon.

Sciatica presents as back and radicular pain described as burning, shooting, or sharp pain beginning in the low back and radiating down the leg past the knee. Sciatic pain is typically worse with bending, straining, or sitting and relieved with lying supine. On exam, patients with sciatica may have tenderness in the sciatic notch and positive straight-leg test. Our patient reports improvement with flexion and sitting, which is characteristic of spinal stenosis, not sciatica.

Because of the exertional component of symptoms, this is sometimes referred to as pseudo-claudication and is secondary to neurologic compression. Vascular claudication is also exertional and improved with rest but is secondary to arterial occlusion. Patients with vascular claudication would not experience relief with bending forward, and you can assess distal pulses and check ankle-brachial index, and if <0.9, this would be consistent with vascular claudication.

Diabetic neuropathy can present as lower extremity pain, but you would expect a symmetric, stocking-and-glove distribution and likely sensory deficits. Diabetic neuropathy is also not associated with back pain and should not be exertional or alleviated with flexion as seen in our patient.

Test-taking tip: This is a "you know it or you don't" kind of question. If you don't know it, choose an answer and move on. You can perhaps mark it for review when you are done at the end of the test. Don't however, let these kinds of questions get you stuck and waste your time.

16. ANSWER: C

The patient presents with symptoms of sciatica consistent with compression of the S1 nerve root. Uncomplicated sciatica does not require emergent imaging even if paresthesias are present, making this answer choice correct. About 95% of patients with a symptomatic herniated disk will endorse symptoms of sciatica. Sciatica typically involves L4–5 disk disease resulting in L5 nerve root compression or L5–S1 disc disease resulting in S1 nerve root compression. Symptoms are often described as burning, shooting, or sharp pain beginning in the low back and radiating down the leg past the knee in a dermatomal distribution depending on which nerve root is affected. Our patient's distribution of paresthesias to the back of the leg and lateral foot are consistent with S1 nerve root compression.

L5 nerve root compression is commonly seen in sciatica and may present similarly, but you would expect paresthesias to the lateral leg and medial foot, including the great toe. The question stem explicitly states intact sensation over the great toe, suggesting intact sensation in the L5 dermatomal distribution.

As mentioned earlier, uncomplicated sciatica does not require emergent imaging even in the setting of paresthesias. The patient has a history of chronic back pain and works in construction, suggesting likely disk disease as the cause of his symptoms. If there is concern for a more worrisome etiology such as spinal epidural abscess (SEA), spinal cord compression, fracture, or malignancy, further imaging would be indicated.

Test-taking tip: Brush up on your sensory and motor function dermatomes before the test.

17. ANSWER: C

The patient presents with a paronychia and has signs of purulent discharge concerning for an abscess formation. Paronychia is a localized infection of the proximal or lateral nail folds, causing pain and swelling of the paronychial tissues of the hands or feet. Typical inciting events include aggressive manicuring, nail biting, finger sucking, a hang nail, or trauma. Symptoms begin as a mild infection but can progress to abscess formation at the nail folds.

Warm soaks and trimming of the nail may be adequate treatment for minor or early cases of paronychia, but this patient has fluctuance and purulent discharge and thus requires I&D.

Oral antibiotics are indicated for cellulitis, but pus and abscess must be drained.

Trephination of the nailbed is the treatment of subungual hematoma usually secondary to trauma causing bleeding under the fingernail. This bleeding can cause pressure and pain, which can be relieved by draining through a hole placed with either a needle or electrocautery. It is not an appropriate treatment for paronychia.

Test-taking tip: Pus on the finger must be drained, whether it be a felon, paronychia, or abscess. The question, which describes fluctuance and drainage, points to the need for I&D.

18. ANSWER: C

The patient presents with symptoms concerning for flexor tenosynovitis (FTS). FTS is an infection of the flexor tendon sheath usually secondary to penetrating trauma or hematogenous spread. The patient is a mechanic and sustained an injury to his finger which likely served as the inciting event leading to spread of his infection to the tendon sheath of his finger.

Patient's with FTS will have clinical evidence of the four Kanavel's signs, which include fusiform swelling of the digit (sausage digit), finger held in flexion, pain with passive extension, and tenderness along flexor tendon. Fusiform swelling and finger held in flexion are evident on the image provided. You would also expect the patient to have pain with passive extension and tenderness along the tendon sheath with palpation of the palmar aspect of his finger and hand. Pain with passive flexion is not one of Kanavel's signs used in the diagnosis of FTS.

Test-taking tip: Brush up on signs and symptom complexes (Kanavel's signs, Beck's triad, etc.) because they are frequently tested on standardized emergency medicine examinations.

19. ANSWER: B

The patient presents with symptoms concerning for flexor tenosynovitis (FTS). FTS is an infection of the flexor tendon sheath usually secondary to penetrating trauma or hematogenous spread of bacteria. Patient displays all four of Kanavel's criteria: fusiform swelling of the digit, finger held in flexion, pain with passive extension, and tenderness along the flexor tendon. FTS is an orthopedic emergency, and requires emergent orthopedic consultation.

Treatment includes orthopedics consultation in the ED, IV antibiotics, and often surgical I&D. The most common isolate is *S. aureus*, but infections are often polymicrobial. Suspect *Pasteurella multocida* if FTS develops after a cat bite and *Eikenella corrodens* after a human bite.

In mild cases you can consult orthopedic surgery and start initially with IV antibiotics and monitor symptoms, but this patient displays all four of Kanavel's criteria and likely needs surgical I&D in addition to IV antibiotics.

Bedside I&D in the ED is not adequate treatment for FTS. Patients can have extensive infection along the tendon sheath, requiring surgical I&D by a specialist.

Test-taking tip: Serious infections of the hand have a high rate of morbidity, so when in doubt, surgical consultation is probably the correct answer.

20. ANSWER: C

This patients' symptoms and presentation are concerning for metastatic disease. An MRI should be obtained in patients presenting with signs and symptoms of bony metastases with evidence of bony lesions on radiograph and acute neurologic symptoms. Neurologic symptoms may be signs of epidural compression syndrome, in which case patients should receive dexamethasone and then emergent MRI of the entire spine to evaluate for metastatic disease in the rest of the spine.

Primary malignancies that commonly metastasize to bones include lung, breast, prostate, renal, and melanoma. Patients may present with pain and pathologic fractures. This patient is also showing signs of hypercalcemia, which may be seen in malignancies affecting the bone. Symptoms of metastatic hypercalcemia include bone pain, muscle weakness, abdominal pain, kidney stones, dehydration, nausea, depression, and confusion. Symptoms of hypercalcemia can be remembered with the mnemonic "painful bones, renal stones, abdominal groans, and psychiatric moans." Red-flag symptoms for malignancy, which this patient endorses, in the setting of back pain include night pain, weight loss, age younger than 18 years or older than 50 years, and acute bony tenderness.

Although it is not unreasonable to obtain a radiograph of the entire spine, ultimately this patient needs emergent MRI of his entire spine (not just thoracic spine) because of the concern for metastatic lesions and signs of compressive symptoms. CT of the abdomen and pelvis should be obtained if there is concern for metastasis to the abdomen, obstruction, or surgical pathology, but our patient's abdominal symptoms are more consistent with hypercalcemia, which can be diagnosed with labs and does not necessitate CT.

Test-taking tip: The immediate concern is lower extremity weakness, which raises the concern for cord compression, so it is easy to eliminate A and D because these imaging modalities will not help you manage the most emergent condition.

21. ANSWER: A

This patient is presenting with Henoch-Schönlein purpura (HSP). HSP is an acute immunoglobulin A–mediated disorder characterized by a generalized vasculitis involving the small vessels of the skin, gastrointestinal tract, kidneys, and large joints.

Large joints, such as the knees and ankles, are the most commonly involved, and generally the arthritis resolves completely over several days without permanent articular damage. This is not a true arthritis, and joint effusions are rare, but if arthrocentesis is performed, synovial fluid is serous, not hemorrhagic. Joint pain may be the only presenting symptoms, making this sometimes a difficult diagnosis.

Most patients present with a myriad of symptoms, usually preceded by a recent upper respiratory infection. Gastrointestinal manifestations may include colicky abdominal pain and heme-positive diarrhea. Kidney involvement may present as hematuria or decreased renal function. HSP is associated with intussusception in the ileoileal location.

HSP is generally a benign disease with an excellent prognosis. Diagnosis is usually made clinically. Workup is often nonspecific and may show thrombocytosis and leukocytosis, blood and protein on urinalysis, and impaired renal function. Treatment is supportive, and spontaneous resolution of symptoms usually occurs within 8 weeks.

Although patients presenting with joint pain may experience recurrent symptoms up to 50% of the time, joint effusions are rare and serous in nature, and symptoms are transient without permanent damage. Chondrocalcinosis is seen in pseudogout. Hemorrhagic effusions are from hemarthrosis in cases such as hemophilia, coagulopathy, anticoagulation medication, and trauma.

Test-taking tip: Brush up on common and interesting syndromes such as HSP, thrombocytopenic purpura, idiopathic thrombocytopenic purpura because they are frequently tested on emergency medicine examinations.

22. ANSWER: A

This patient is presenting with symptoms concerning for osteosarcoma, which appears as lytic lesions with periosteal reaction causing a sunburst appearance on radiograph.

Osteosarcoma is the most common primary bone tumor in patients 10 to 15 years old. It typically peaks in adolescence after a growth spurt. Symptoms include persistent bone pain that is worse at night and with activity. There is often swelling and tenderness to palpation at the involved site. The most commonly involved areas include the distal femur, proximal tibia, and proximal humerus. Labs may show elevated alkaline phosphatase and lactate dehydrogenase. Definitive diagnosis is achieved through bone biopsy.

Osgood-Schlatter disease is an apophysitis of the tibial tubercle seen in children usually 10 to 15 years old. It is caused by repetitive stress or overuse that results in microavulsion of the ossification center of the tibial tuberosity. Patients have tenderness over the tibial tuberosity, but our patient is describing pain at the distal femur that is worse at night without a history of repetitive overuse, making this answer choice less likely.

Rat-bite erosions are seen in chronic gout, and chondrocalcinosis is seen in pseudogout.

Test-taking tip: Brush up on the common causes of leg pain in the pediatric population, including common presenting signs and symptoms.

23. ANSWER: A

Osgood-Schlatter disease is an apophysitis of the tibial tubercle seen in pediatric patients usually between 10 and 15 years old. It is caused by repetitive stress or overuse that results in microavulsion of the ossification center of the tibial tuberosity. Patients have tenderness over the tibial tuberosity, such as that described in the question stem.

Septic knee would present with a painful knee, associated with swelling, erythema, warmth, and possible systemic symptoms and fever. Range of motion is limited in patients with septic knee and it is not secondary to overuse.

Osteosarcoma can present similarly, given the patient's age and area of pain, but typically is not associated with overuse and often presents with nighttime pain. Osteosarcoma is the most common primary bone tumor in pediatric patients, peaks in adolescence, and presents as persistent bone pain that is worse at night and with activity. The most commonly involved areas include the distal femur, proximal tibia, and proximal humerus. If there is concern for malignancy, labs and imaging should be obtained. Definitive diagnosis is achieved through bone biopsy.

Pre-patellar bursitis can occur in the pediatric population and presents with pain and swelling in the front of the knee with associated tenderness, warmth, and erythema. It can be associated with a direct blow to the patella while playing sports or can be due to infection.

Test-taking tip: Brush up on the common causes of leg pain in the pediatric population, including common presenting signs and symptoms.

24. ANSWER: B

The patient is presenting with symptoms concerning for SEA, and emergent neurosurgical consult and broad-spectrum IV antibiotics are indicated before obtaining definitive imaging. The patient is also displaying signs of spinal cord compression, which can lead to permanent neurologic deficits, so emergent neurosurgical consultation is warranted.

SEA is an infection in the epidural space from either direct or hematogenous spread and can lead to cord compression. This patient presents with multiple red-flag symptoms of back pain, including stool incontinence, spine point tenderness, history of IV drug use, immunocompromised state, and fever. Patients with SEA will present with fever, back pain, and neurologic deficit. Risk factors include IV drug use, immunocompromised state, recent spinal instrumentation, and concurrent infection. Radiographs may be normal, as in this case, unless demineralization of bone has occurred because of prolonged infection, so MRI is often needed for diagnosis. Labs may show leukocytosis or elevated erythrocyte sedimentation rate (ESR). Treatment includes broad-spectrum antibiotics that cover *S. aureus* as well as immediate neurosurgery consult because the patient may require decompression through drainage and laminectomy. Spinal osteomyelitis may also present similarly and has similar management.

Lumbar puncture and broad-spectrum antibiotics are indicated in patients presenting with symptoms concerning for meningitis, which include fever and neck pain. Lumbar puncture should not be performed in patients with a history concerning for SEA because this may risk spreading bacteria into the subarachnoid space.

CT myelography is an alternative imaging modality with a high sensitivity in diagnosing SEA when MRI is not immediately available, but neurology is not the appropriate consulting service because this patient is showing signs of compression and may need emergent surgical decompression.

Lastly, this patient will require broad-spectrum antibiotics, admission, and follow-up on blood cultures, but neurosurgery involvement is also necessary.

Test-taking tip: There may be multiple right answers, but pay attention to key words in the question stem such as "most common" and "next step." Know the standard-of-care treatment options and the alternative options if the preferred method is not available.

25. ANSWER: D

This patient presents with hemarthrosis secondary to trauma in the setting of underlying hemophilia A before factor replacement. Hemarthrosis in a hemophiliac patient before factor replacement is one of the *relative* contraindications to arthrocentesis.

Arthrocentesis is often an important diagnostic tool in differentiating the etiology of many common causes of joint effusion. The most concerning diagnosis of acute joint pain is septic arthritis due to bacterial invasion, so the decision to perform arthrocentesis often focuses on ruling in or out a septic joint. The two most important diagnostic considerations for acute nontraumatic monoarthritis are nongonococcal or gonococcal septic arthritis contrasted with crystal-induced arthropathy (gout and pseudogout); however, patient age, gender, and comorbid illnesses also play a role in the decision to perform arthrocentesis and the likely cause of the patient's symptoms.

Relative contraindications to performing arthrocentesis in addition to hemarthrosis in a hemophiliac patient before factor replacement include overlying cellulitis, coagulopathy, and prosthetic joint.

Tricompartmental OA may present with a noninflammatory joint effusion and, although arthrocentesis usually is not required, it is not a relative contraindication to arthrocentesis.

Test-taking tip: Choices A and B are obvious relative contraindications to arthrocentesis, leaving two answers to choose from.

26. ANSWER: D

This patient presents with herpetic whitlow. Herpetic whitlow is a viral hand infection from autoinoculation of herpes simplex virus 1 or 2. Acyclovir may be indicated in the treatment of herpetic whitlow, which is often confused for paronychia and felon. Symptoms initially begin as small, clear vesicles that progress to cloudy fluid and can mimic a pyogenic bacterial infection such as a felon or paronychia.

You want to avoid I&D in cases of herpetic whitlow because this may spread the virus. Symptoms are usually self-limited, but acyclovir may be used, especially in cases of immunocompromised patients, such as the patient in the question stem.

Volar longitudinal and high lateral incision techniques are the treatment of a felon. A felon is an infection of the pulp of the distal finger forming multiple abscesses within the septa of the pulp of the finger.

Paronychia, infections around the fingernail usually after nail trauma, are treated with I&D versus conservative management depending on severity.

Felons may also be confused for paronychia, which will present as swelling, erythema, and tenderness at the nail fold. Treatment of paronychia involves I&D as well, but the incision is typically made parallel to the nail bed under the eponychium and does not involve the septa of the pulp of the finger.

Test-taking tip: Vesicular lesions should make you think viral infection, pointing you to the correct answer.

27. ANSWER: A

This patient is presenting with transient synovitis, which is treated with rest and NSAIDs. Transient synovitis is a noninfectious, self-limited inflammatory process of the hip and is the most common cause of acute hip pain in children 3 to 10 years old (Table 11.7). Most cases are thought to be postviral and are managed with rest and NSAIDs.

The presentation can be very difficult to differentiate from septic joint. Kocher's criteria can help differentiate septic joint from transient synovitis. These criteria can be applied to all pediatric patients with acute hip pain if septic arthritis and transient synovitis are on the differential diagnosis. Patients falling on either extreme of the criteria can be readily ruled in or out for septic arthritis in the right clinical setting. Patients in the intermediate range may need further work-up or intervention. Kocher's criteria are as follows:

+1 Non–weight bearing

+1 Temperature >38.5° C

+1 ESR >40 mm/hour

+1 WBC count >12,000

If one or two of the criteria are met, the patient is in the indeterminate zone and may need imaging or orthopedics consult. If none are met, there is low concern for septic joint, and the patient can be discharged with close monitoring. If three or four are met, the patient needs imaging, orthopedic consult, and likely surgical

Table 11.7 COMMON CAUSES OF NONTRAUMATIC HIP PAIN IN CHILDREN

SYNDROME	CHARACTERISTICS	TREATMENT
Septic hip	Fever >38.5° C, limp	Ortho, aspiration, antibiotics
Transient synovitis	Hip pain and recent viral illness	NSAIDs, rest
Slipped capital femoral epiphysis	Obese, limp, "ice cream falling off cone:	Ortho, non–weight bearing, surgery
Legg-Calvé-Perthes disease	Age 4–9 years, normal weight, limp, avascular necrosis	Ortho, splinting or surgery

aspiration of the joint. This patient has no criteria, making the most likely diagnosis transient synovitis, and discharge with observation and conservative management is appropriate.

Orthopedics consult, non–weight bearing, and eventual operative stabilization are the treatment of slipped capital femoral epiphysis, which is typically seen in overweight adolescents. Radiographs may show posterior displacement of the epiphysis from the femoral neck resembling ice cream falling off a cone.

Orthopedics consult, bracing, and eventual femoral osteotomy are the potential treatment for avascular necrosis of the femoral head (Legg-Calvé-Perthes disease). Patients are typically between 4 and 9 years old and present with hip pain and limp.

Test-taking tip: Brush up on the common causes of leg pain in the pediatric population, including common presenting signs and symptoms and treatment.

28. ANSWER: A

The patient presents with a mild paronychial infection without signs of abscess formation. Paronychia is a localized infection of the proximal or lateral nail folds, causing pain and swelling of the paronychial tissues of the hands or feet. Typical inciting events include aggressive manicuring, nail biting, finger sucking, a hang nail, or trauma. Symptoms begin as a mild infection but can progress to abscess formation at the nail folds. Warm soaks are adequate initial treatment for minor or early cases of paronychia with appropriate follow-up.

Oral antibiotics are indicated for cellulitis, but if there is evidence of abscess, it must be drained. Removal of the proximal third of the nail is often warranted in cases in which I&D is required.

A high lateral incision to drain the abscess is one of the methods of I&D of a felon. This can be confusing if not read carefully because drainage of paronychia involves either bluntly elevating the eponychial fold from the nail or through I&D near the eponychium directed away from the nail fold and directed over the area of greatest fluctuance. The wound should then be irrigated and packed, and oral antibiotics should be started for a week.

Test-taking tip: Mild, early presentations of disease processes often only need minimal conservative therapy.

29. ANSWER: A

The presentation and radiographic findings of squaring of the vertebral bodies is consistent with the diagnosis of AS, which typically does not involve a rash. Patients with AS suffer from back pain secondary to the formation of longitudinal fibrous bands along the spine, leading to ossification and fusion of the vertebrae (bamboo spine).

Young patients presenting with joint pain and rash should increase suspicion for infectious causes such as Lyme disease or gonococcal arthritis.

Both AS and reactive arthritis are autoimmune, seronegative spondyloarthropathies associated with HLA-B27. AS most commonly affects the spine and pelvis, and reactive arthritis has a predilection for the heel and lower extremity. Patients with AS are typically younger than 40 years with an insidious onset of symptoms lasting more than 3 months. Symptoms include back pain and stiffness that improve with activity and are worse in the morning. Back pain is also associated with malaise, weakness, and fatigue. Treatment is with NSAIDs and referral to rheumatology.

Test-taking tip: This is a "you know it or you don't" kind of question. If you don't know it, choose an answer and move on. You can perhaps mark it for review when you are done at the end of the test. Don't however, let these kinds of questions get you stuck and waste your time.

12.

NERVOUS SYSTEM EMERGENCIES

Amy Briggs and Brandon Chalfin

1. A 57-year-old male with a history of diabetes, hypertension, and high cholesterol presents to the emergency department (ED) with acute onset of weakness. He was watching TV and at 3 PM he developed right-sided weakness and numbness with slurred speech. His wife immediately called 911, and it is currently 3:30 PM. His point-of-care glucose is normal. His vital signs are blood pressure (BP) 160/100 mm Hg, heart rate (HR) 92 bpm, respiratory rate (RR) 18 breaths/min, oxygen saturation 97% on room air, and oral temperature 37° C (98.8° F). His neurologic exam is remarkable for right-sided upper and lower extremity weakness and numbness with slurred speech. His pupils are equally round and reactive to light. What is the most appropriate initial management of this patient?

A. Order IV tissue plasminogen activator (tPA) without further testing and consult neurology and admit to the intensive care unit (ICU)
B. Order a noncontrast computed tomography (CT) scan of the head and, if normal, consult neurology and consent for IV tPA if no contraindications
C. Decrease patient's blood pressure to 140/90 mm Hg before any other workup
D. Order a CT angiogram of the head and neck and consult neurointerventional radiology before any other intervention

2. A 98-year-old female with a history of dementia and atrial fibrillation on warfarin, with baseline Glasgow Coma Scale (GCS) score of 14, presents from a nursing home with altered mental status and weakness. The staff at her nursing home noticed that she was confused and weak on her right side since she woke up today. She was last seen normal before going to bed about 10 hours ago. She is hypertensive with a systolic blood pressure of about 200 mm Hg. She is intubated for inability to protect her airway. A stat noncontrast CT scan of her brain is done and shown in Figure 12.1. She is beginning to show signs of impending brain herniation. Her

international normalized ratio (INR) is 8.9. She does not have an advance directive, and her family is in the waiting room asking to speak with the doctor to discuss the patient's wishes. Neurosurgery is consulted, and they state that her hemorrhagic stroke is nonoperable and she will not survive longer than 24 hours. What is the most appropriate management for this patient?

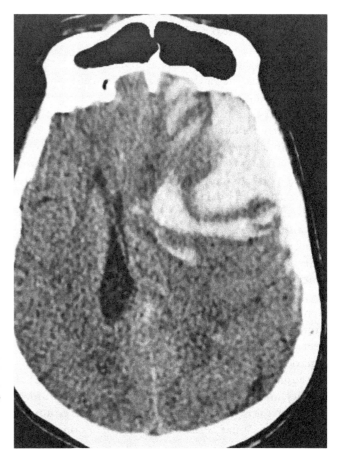

Figure 12.1 Head computed tomography.

A. Start a nicardipine drip and admit the patient to the ICU

B. Give the patient vitamin K and fresh frozen plasma (FFP) and admit her to the ICU

C. Given that the patient is having a stroke, order IV tPA and admit to ICU

D. Meet with the family to discuss goals of care; explain that her condition is terminal and offer the option to transition the patient to comfort care

3. A 25-year-old male with a history of epilepsy presents to the ED with complaint of seizures. He states that his seizures always involve involuntary movements of his entire right arm. He does not become confused during these events, and they are over within a few minutes. These seizures have been increasing in frequency over the past week. He has no other associated neurologic deficits during these events. He has no recent trauma or illness. He has returned completely to his baseline. He has no fever or nuchal rigidity. His neurologic exam and vital signs are unremarkable. You call the patient's neurologist, who confirms that this is the patient's typical seizure activity and that the patient has had advanced imaging recently. Basic labs and antiepileptic levels are within normal limits. What is the most appropriate management for this patient?

A. Order a stat electroencephalogram (EEG)

B. Discharge the patient with return precautions and follow-up with his neurologist

C. Order a non-contrast head CT and consent the patient for lumbar puncture (LP)

D. Admit the patient to the hospital

4. A 34-year-old male presents to the ED with a first-time seizure. His wife is with him and had witnessed the event. He has no past medical history and has never had a seizure before. He does not drink, use tobacco, or use any other drugs. His wife describes an event of generalized shaking with tongue biting and incontinence that lasted for about 2 minutes. He was in bed at the time, and she denies any associated trauma with the event. She states that he was confused for about an hour after, but now on your evaluation in the ED he is awake, alert, and without complaints. His physical exam is unremarkable with a normal neurologic exam and no signs of trauma or tenderness. He has no neck pain or nuchal rigidity, and his vital signs are all within normal limits. His seizure is reported to the county, and he is educated not to drive. What is the best course of action for this patient?

A. Order a basic metabolic panel and a noncontrast head CT and ,if normal, discharge the patient to primary physician and/or neurology follow-up

B. Order a basic metabolic panel and a noncontrast head CT and, if normal, discharge the patient to primary physician and/or neurology follow-up and start the patient on an antiepileptic medication

C. Order a basic metabolic panel and a noncontrast head CT and, if normal, admit the patient for stat neurology consult, magnetic resonance imaging (MRI), and EEG

D. Discharge the patient without any testing and have him follow-up with a neurologist in 1 month

5. An 18 year-old-female with no reported past medical history is brought in by emergency medical services (EMS) with uncontrolled seizures for the past 30 minutes. The medics have given her oxygen and 4 mg IV lorazepam but have been unable to stop her seizures. You ask the medics for any additional information, and they state that while that family on scene was in a panic, one of them mentioned that she may have taken a bottle of pills. The family was not sure of the names of the pills but says she has been on them for months because of some "silent" lung infection that she tested positive for. Which of the following is the next best course of action?

A. Intubate the patient and admit her to the ICU

B. Load the patient with IV Dilantin and wait 20 minutes for a clinical response

C. Administer pyridoxine (vitamin B$_6$) and more lorazepam

D. Order a stat MRI and tell the technician that she needs to go now before any further treatment

6. A 38-year-old male with a history of AIDS presents to the ED with complaints of fever and headache. He reports that his symptoms have been present over the past few days and he has started to develop weakness in his right arm and blurry vision. While in the ED he has a generalized tonic-clonic seizure for 2 minutes but continues to protect his airway. A CT scan is done that shows a hypodense center with a surrounding ring and edema. What is the most likely diagnosis?

A. Viral meningitis

B. Bacterial meningitis

C. Acute stoke

D. Brain abscess

7. A 29-year-old male presents to the ED with new-onset seizure. He is visiting his family from India. He has no history of seizures but has been getting headaches recently. His seizure was described as only affecting part of his body. He denies any headache, neck pain, numbness, weakness, or confusion. His vital signs and physical exam are unremarkable. A CT scan of the brain shows multiple cystic lesions with peripheral dots consistent with a scolex. What is the most likely diagnosis for this patient?

A. Brain abscess
B. Bacterial meningitis
C. Neurocysticercosis
D. Alcohol withdrawal seizure

8. A 19-year-old female presents to the ED with complaints of fever. She is in college and notes that everyone is sick around her. Yesterday she started to develop headache and fevers. She notes that it is extremely painful to move her neck around as well. She has no confusion but notes that she has been vomiting and the lights are bothering her. Her vital signs are BP 95/60 mm Hg, HR 130 bpm, RR 26 breaths/min, oxygen saturation 98% on room air, and temperature 39° C (102.3° F). Her physical exam is remarkable for nuchal rigidity. She has no rashes and a nonfocal neurologic exam. Which of the following is the most emergent management decision for this patient?

A. Noncontrast CT scan of the head
B. IV antibiotics with meningitis dosing
C. LP
D. MRI head with and without contrast

9. A 27-year-old previously healthy male presents to the ED for confusion. He is accompanied by his girlfriend who provides the history because the patient is unable to. She reports that over the past few days he had a headache and fevers, which they thought was from the flu. However, today he has become increasingly confused and engaging in bizarre behavior. The patient is started on IV antibiotics and antivirals. He has a noncontrast head CT and undergoes LP that shows 127 white blood cells (WBCs) with a lymphocytic predominance, 437 red blood cells (RBCs), mildly increased protein, and a normal glucose. An MRI shows hyperintensities in the limbic and hypothalamic areas on the T2-weighted and fluid-attenuated inversion recovery (FLAIR) sequences. What is the most likely pathogen?

A. *Haemophilus influenzae* type b
B. *Neisseria meningitidis*
C. Herpes simplex virus (HSV)
D. West Nile virus

10. A 26-year-old female with a history of ventriculoperitoneal (VP) shunt placement as an infant for congenital hydrocephalus presents with headache. Her shunt was revised 2 months ago. She reports that she gets occasional headaches, but this one is different. It has been increasing in intensity over the past few days. She has started to feel feverish, is having blurry vision, and at times feels confused. Her physical exam does not demonstrate any focal neurologic abnormality. Her neck demonstrates nuchal rigidity. A radiograph of

the shunt is done along its path and is read as normal. The patient is given pain medication and fluids and feels like her headache is improving. What is the most appropriate initial management in this patient?

A. Discharge the patient with outpatient follow-up with her neurosurgeon in 2 days
B. Perform an LP
C. Order a noncontrast head CT
D. Order an MRI with and without contrast to evaluate for encephalitis

11. A 35-year-old male presents to the ED with complaint of headache. The headache started last night, about 16 hours ago. He has a history of migraines, but states that this headache feels different. The headache started while he was running on the treadmill and reached maximal intensity within one minute. He has some associated neck discomfort, but no other neurologic complaint. He reports nausea and vomiting and has not taken any treatment. Physical exam reveals no acute neurologic deficit. What is the best management for this patient?

A. Give the patient IV prochlorperazine and IV diphenhydramine and discharge him if his headache improves.
B. Order a non-contrast head CT and, if normal, reassure him that his headache is benign
C. Order a CT angiogram head and neck before any other testing to look for aneurysm
D. Order a non-contrast head CT and, if normal, perform an LP

12. A 38-year-old previously healthy female presents to the ED with complaint of gradually worsening headache for the past month. She notes that the headache is worse in the morning when she wakes up and gets better after standing. Today the headache became so severe that she could not take the pain anymore. Her headache is associated with nausea and intermittent vomiting. Today she has been unable to stop vomiting. She reports intermittent blurry vision but denies any focal weakness or numbness. She does not report any fevers. She is awake and alert but in moderate distress because of pain. Her neurologic exam exhibits normal strength, sensation, and gait. Her pupils are equally round and reactive to light. Her visual exam is remarkable for papilledema. A noncontrast CT of her head is done with results concerning for obstructive hydrocephalus secondary to a tumor compressing the ventricular system. What is the next best course of action?

A. Consult neurosurgery for emergent evaluation for surgical intervention

B. Consult ophthalmology for further management of the papilledema
C. Proceed with LP to evaluate the patient's cerebrospinal fluid (CSF)
D. Start IV mannitol for increased intracranial pressure (ICP)

13. A 78-year-old female presents to the ED with complaint of right-sided headache for the past few days. She tried to see her primary care doctor but was unable to. The pain starts in her right eye and radiates posteriorly. She does not wear glasses but states that her vision in the right eye has been a little blurry recently. She has also noted that it is painful for her to chew for extended periods of time. She denies any fever, neck pain, or confusion. Her physical exam reveals normal cranial nerves, a normal-appearing anterior chamber of both eyes, pressures in both eyes of 15, and a normal fundoscopic exam. Her right eye vision is slightly diminished when compared with her left. What is the best management for this patient?

A. Treat her for acute angle glaucoma and call ophthalmology for a stat consult
B. Order an erythrocyte sedimentation rate (ESR) and discharge her if it is less than 60 mm/hr
C. Get a stat noncontrast head CT and, if negative, consent from the patient for IV tPA
D. Start the patient on steroids and consult surgery for a temporal artery biopsy

14. A 37-year-old male presents to the ED with complaints of left-sided weakness that he woke up with. Last night he went to bed early because he was having right-sided neck pain. He regularly sees a chiropractor. He denies fever, confusion, headache, or neck stiffness. His weakness is causing him difficulty walking, and it did not get better, so he came to the ED. It has been 6 hours since he woke up. He was previously healthy and does not take any medications. His physical exam is remarkable for left-sided weakness. He has no nuchal rigidity. His vital signs are within normal limits. A noncontrast head CT scan is done and read as negative. His electrocardiogram (EKG), chest radiograph, complete blood count (CBC), basic metabolic panel (BMP), and coagulation profile are all within normal limits. What is the most appropriate next step in management for his patient?

A. Reassure him that his workup, including a head CT, is negative and discharge him with neurology follow-up and a diagnosis of a transient ischemic attack (TIA)
B. Perform an LP to evaluate for meningitis or encephalitis

C. Get the patient's consent for IV tPA
D. Order a CT angiogram of the neck and consult neurology

15. A 25-year-old male presents to the ED with headache. He was seen 2 days early in the same ED. At that time, he had presented with a rapid, new-onset headache with associated nausea and vomiting that began 14 hours before presentation to the ED. The patient had a normal noncontrast CT scan and underwent LP, which showed no WBCs and no RBCs without xanthochromia. His headache improved with IV medication, and he was discharged. The next day the patient noticed that when he got out of bed and stood up, he developed another headache. The headache improved again with lying down. The patient denies fevers, neck pain, or any other new symptoms. He has a completely normal neurologic exam. What is the best management for this patient?

A. Consult anesthesia for a blood patch
B. Order an MRI to evaluate for stroke
C. Consult neurology for further recommendations
D. Reassure the patient and discharge him

16. A 30-year-old female presents to the ED with complaint of headache. She denies any past medical history and is not taking any medications. She does not have any allergies. Over the past 2 days she developed a gradual onset and progression of left-sided headache that is similar to prior headaches and pulsating in nature. It is associated with nausea but no vomiting, and she denies any visual changes. She states that she has gotten these headaches about five times per year since she was a teenager. She has tried acetaminophen at home without results. Her vital signs are BP 134/79 mm Hg, HR 94 bpm, RR 16 breaths/min, oxygen saturation 98% on room air, and oral temperature 36.9° C (98.5° F). Her neurologic exam is unremarkable with normal cranial nerves, normal strength, normal sensation, normal gait, and normal reflexes. A rapid pregnancy test is negative. What workup should be done on this patient?

A. Order a noncontrast head CT and, if negative, proceed with LP
B. Order IV prochlorperazine and IV diphenhydramine and reassess the patient for symptomatic improvement
C. Order magnetic resonance venography (MRV)
D. Order IV fluids and discharge the patient with reassurance

17. A 39-year-old male presents to the ED with a chief complaint of headache. The pain is behind his right eye, and he has noticed that his eye tears and his nose is running. He denies any blurry vision, weakness, or numbness. The pain is severe. For the past 3 days, he has had three to five episodes of these per day, each lasting about 30 minutes. He also reports similar grouped episodes in the past. His neurologic exam is unremarkable, and his eye pressures are read as normal. What is the next best action in the management of this patient?

A. Order a noncontrast head CT and, if negative, proceed with LP
B. Order IV morphine and IV fluids
C. Consult neurology for further recommendations
D. Order high-flow oxygen by way of non-rebreather mask

18. A 24-year-old male is brought into the ED by EMS. He was found on the sidewalk, when a bystander called EMS. No further history is available. He was just minutes away from the hospital, so no intervention was given other than oxygen. He has no signs of trauma and has a normal core temperature and fingerstick glucose. His vital signs are BP 100/60 mm Hg, HR 95 bpm, RR 6 breaths/min, and oxygen saturation 95% on nasal cannula. His pupils are 2 mm bilaterally. He appears to be protecting his airway, and nursing establishes IV access. What is the most appropriate next step in management of this patient?

A. Give the patient IV naloxone
B. Give the patient IV D50
C. Intubate the patient
D. Give IV thiamine

19. A 91-year-old male with a history of dementia presents to the ED with cough and fever. A workup is done, and a diagnosis of pneumonia is made. His vital signs are stable. Appropriate treatment is started, and the patient is admitted to the hospital. Which of the following is the best way to prevent development of delirium during his hospital stay?

A. Restrain the patient so that he is not able to wander around
B. Schedule benzodiazepines to keep him sedated
C. Place a urinary catheter for patient comfort
D. Encourage familiar family to stay with the patient and reduce lights at night

20. A 68-year-old male is brought into the ED by EMS with decreased level of consciousness after being found on the ground at home. He is being bagged by EMS because he is not currently taking any spontaneous breaths. He was last seen normal 5 hours ago. The patient is not moving any extremities or making any noises. You

prepare to intubate the patient, but as the nurses are drawing up medications you notice the patient looking up at you at the head of the bed and then back down to the nurses at the foot of the bed. Nevertheless, he is intubated for airway protection. What is the most likely etiology for this patient's condition?

A. Opioid overdose
B. Basilar artery occlusion
C. Wernicke's encephalopathy
D. Conversion disorder

21. An 82-year-old male presents to the ED with complaint of fall. He has had trouble walking over the past few months and has been falling. He also reports that over the past few months he has become increasingly confused. He has seen his primary care doctor but was told it was just normal aging. The family member at the bedside expresses concern that he has trouble with day-to-day tasks and keeping track of finances. Physical exam reveals a pleasant gentleman with mild confusion and a wide-based shuffling gait. The nurses report that they have to clean the patient because of urinary incontinence, for which the patient states that his doctor had started him on a medication for benign prostatic hypertrophy (BPH) but it is not helping. Which of the following statements is true?

A. The patient should be referred to his primary care doctor to start medications for Alzheimer's disease
B. Advanced brain imaging is likely to show hydrocephalus in this condition
C. If the patient's radiographs are negative, he should be reassured that his primary care doctor is managing him well and that no further workup is indicated for his symptoms
D. There is no treatment for this condition

22. A 26-year-old female presents to the ED with complaints of dizziness. She reports that she woke up this morning and felt the room spinning. She became nauseated and vomited. Her symptoms lasted for less than a minute and resolved. Every time she moves her head in a certain direction her symptoms return, but they are short-lived. She has no other associated neurologic symptoms. Her neurologic exam is unremarkable. She is able to walk. Her pregnancy test is negative. Which of the following is true regarding the most likely etiology of the patient's symptoms?

A. She has vestibular neuronitis
B. The best treatment for her is acetazolamide
C. She will have an abnormal head impulse test
D. The Epley maneuver is indicated as a potential treatment if her Dix-Hallpike test is positive

23. A 76-year-old female with a history of diabetes, hypertension, and dyslipidemia presents to the ED with complaints of dizziness. She woke up this morning with dizziness that has been constant and is described as the room spinning. This has never happened to her before. She does not have any focal weakness or numbness on exam, but she is unable to ambulate. She has positive skew deviation of her eyes. Which of the following is true her most likely diagnosis?

A. She will have an abnormal head impulse test
B. An MRI is indicated in her workup at this time
C. If her symptoms improve with meclizine, she can be safely discharged
D. She can be safely discharged if her noncontrast head CT is negative

24. A 42-year-old previously healthy male presents to the ED with facial weakness. He reports that he went to bed last night at about 10 PM feeling fine, and when he woke up and looked in the mirror at 7 AM he noticed that the right side of his face looked funny. He denies any other weakness or numbness. He has no trouble walking, speaking, or swallowing. He denies any pain or blurry vision. His neurologic exam is remarkable for right-sided facial paralysis including his forehead, and he has difficulty closing his eye on his right side. The remainder of his cranial nerves are intact, as are his gait and upper and lower extremity strength and sensation. What is the most appropriate management for this patient?

A. Discharge the patient with reassurance and have him see his doctor in 3 days for follow-up
B. Order a noncontrast head CT and, if negative, admit for MRI and stroke workup
C. Order a noncontrast head CT and, if negative, consult neurology for IV tPA consideration
D. Reassure the patient and discharge him with an eye patch/artificial tears, antivirals, and potentially steroids

25. A 52-year-old man with no significant past medical history presents complaining of five to six short episodes of shooting right-sided facial pain. The first episode occurred last night when he turned over in bed, and it has seemed to happen whenever he touches his face since then. His vital signs are stable, and he appears comfortable on your initial interview; however, when you touch his right cheek to test his facial sensation, he becomes extremely uncomfortable, complaining of 10/10 facial pain, which resolves after 30 seconds. What is the appropriate initial pharmacologic treatment for this condition?

A. Sumatriptan
B. Oxygen
C. Carbamazepine
D. Prednisone

26. A 52-year-old male presents with right-sided hearing loss for the past 18 months. He also complains of intermittent tinnitus and feeling "off balance" for approximately the past 6 months. On physical exam, his tympanic membranes are clear bilaterally, and he has decreased sensation in the distribution of V_2 and V_3, right-sided sensorineural hearing loss, and a slightly ataxic gait. He has no nystagmus, and his Dix-Hallpike test is negative. Which of the following is the most appropriate next step in management?

A. Trial of meclizine
B. MRI of the brain
C. Refer for hearing aid evaluation
D. Administer streptokinase

27. A 78-year-old male with a history of atrial fibrillation presents with complaints of low back pain, bilateral lower extremity pain, and numbness. Symptoms have been slowly worsening over the past 2 days; 2 days ago a box fell on his back while he was moving things in his garage. He is compliant with his warfarin therapy. On physical exam he has decreased strength and sensation to his lower extremities and decreased perianal sensation. What is the most appropriate next step in management?

A. Order labs including prothrombin time (PT) and INR
B. Start IV vancomycin and ceftriaxone
C. Give protamine sulfate IV
D. Emergent neurosurgical consultation

28. A 28-year-old woman presents with altered mental status. She is febrile and tachycardic and has multiple marks on her extremities consistent with IV drug use. She localizes pain in her upper extremities but does not move her lower extremities. She has poor rectal tone and a distended bladder. Which of the following is the most likely diagnosis?

A. Traumatic spinal injury
B. Opioid overdose
C. Spinal epidural abscess
D. Guillain-Barré syndrome

29. A 65-year-old male presents to the ED with back pain plus bowel and bladder incontinence that started earlier today. Radiographs of the lumbar spine that

were done at triage are normal by your read. On physical exam, there is loss of sensation in the "saddle" region and no tone on rectal exam. The MRI is completed. What is the next step?

A. Steroids, analgesics, and follow-up with neurosurgery in 2 weeks
B. Immediate neurosurgical consultation
C. Bedrest for 2 days with muscle relaxants and analgesia
D. CT scan of spine because MRI is inconclusive

30. A 52-year-old man with a history of HIV and IV drug abuse presents with a chief complaint of back pain that has been slowly worsening over the past month. He has no weakness, saddle anesthesia, or incontinence. He has midline tenderness to palpation at L2. His vital sign are stable. ESR and C-reactive protein (CRP) are elevated, and blood and urine cultures are pending. What is the most appropriate next step?

A. Order IV ceftriaxone and vancomycin
B. Consult neurosurgery
C. Order MRI of the lumbar spine
D. Trial of nonsteroidal antiinflammatory drugs (NSAIDs) and physical therapy

31. A 64-year-old man with a history of coronary artery disease (CAD), cirrhosis, and prostate cancer with known metastases to the lumbar spine presents with back pain, lower extremity weakness, and bowel and bladder incontinence. He is DNR/DNI and does not want any aggressive surgical interventions. MRI shows a metastatic mass compressing the spinal cord. What is the most appropriate next step in management?

A. Transfuse platelets and consult neurosurgery
B. Give dexamethasone and consult radiation oncology
C. Give dexamethasone and consult medical oncology
D. Start morphine infusion and consult palliative care

32. A 45-year-old female with a history of rheumatoid arthritis presents with a chief complaint of bilateral lower extremity weakness and bowel and bladder incontinence, which have progressed over the past 14 days. She reports paresthesias below the level of T6. MRI without gadolinium shows no evidence of cord compression. She is afebrile. CSF shows 80/mm³ lymphocytes and 110 mg/dL protein. What is the most appropriate therapy for this patient?

A IV ceftriaxone and vancomycin
B. IV methylprednisolone
C. PO prednisone
D. IV cyclophosphamide

33. A 68-year-old man presents with a chief complaint of paresthesias and decreased sensation to the backs of his shoulders and arms over the past year. He also feels like his hands have been "losing strength" over the past year. On physical exam, he has decreased sensation to pain and temperature in a cape-like distribution to his upper extremities, and upper extremity strength is four out of five. Which of the following preceding events or conditions may have contributed to the development of these symptoms?

A. Caudal descent of the cerebellar tonsils into the foramen magnum
B. Motor vehicle collision with hyperextension injury to neck 14 months ago
C. Both A and B
D. Vitamin A deficiency

34. A 40-year-old male presents with a chief complaint of bilateral leg weakness and difficulty walking. He also complains of some tingling to his bilateral feet. Last week he had bloody diarrhea, which self-resolved. On exam, he is afebrile, HR is 110 bpm, and strength is four out of five in the lower extremities. Which organism is likely responsible for his symptoms?

A. *Borrelia burgdorferi*
B. *Shigella* species
C. *Campylobacter jejuni*
D. *N. meningitidis*

35. A 50-year-old previously healthy female presents complaining of generalized weakness more severe in the lower extremities that started 1 week ago and has been progressively getting worse. Her breathing is rapid and shallow, and she is somnolent. Strength is two out of five in her lower extremities and three out of five in her upper extremities. She is subsequently intubated for respiratory failure. What is the most appropriate next step in treatment of the underlying cause?

A. IV corticosteroids
B. IV immunoglobulin
C. Plasmapheresis
D. Either B or C

36. A 40-year-old male visiting from Eastern Europe presents with a chief complaint of difficulty walking. He is unsure of when he last received any vaccinations. He eats a lot of canned goods. He had a severe sore throat 8 weeks ago. He also reports a recent hoarse voice, difficulty swallowing, and tongue numbness for 2 weeks, which seems to be improving. On physical exam, he has marked proximal muscle weakness of the lower extremities, decreased lower extremity reflexes,

and a hoarse voice. Which of the following might have prevented the development of his symptoms?

    A. Making sure the canned goods were properly canned
    B. Early administration of diphtheria antitoxin
    C. Early administration of IV penicillin
    D. Early initiation of immunosuppression with azathioprine

37. A 25-year-old female presents complaining of double vision, difficulty chewing, and exertional dyspnea. The symptoms are less severe in the morning and worsen throughout the day. She has had these symptoms on and off for about a year, but this episode has been acutely worsening over the past 3 days and has not improved on its own. Her symptoms are worse in the evening. On physical exam, she has obvious ptosis and mild tachypnea. Which diagnostic test is most likely to aid in correctly diagnosing this patient?

    A. Noncontrast head CT
    B. Ice-pack test
    C. Forced vital capacity and negative inspiratory force
    D. Chest CT with contrast

38. A 58-year-old male with a past medical history of myasthenia gravis (MG) presents with 2 days of cough productive of green sputum and fever. His physical exam reveals rhonchi in the left lung fields. He has a temperature of 39° C and pulse oximetry of 92% on room air. Which of the following medications should be avoided when treating this patient's pneumonia?

    A. Levofloxacin
    B. Vancomycin
    C. Clindamycin
    D. All of the above

39. A 55-year-old woman presents complaining of difficulty getting up from bed in the morning and bilateral arm weakness, but her symptoms improve throughout the day. On physical exam, she has proximal muscle weakness of her upper and lower extremities, which improves with repeated movement. Which of the following is associated with this condition?

    A. Pancreatic cancer
    B. Thymoma
    C. Small cell lung cancer
    D. Insulinoma

40. A 10-month-old girl is brought to your ED by her mother for acting sleepy and floppy. Her mother notes that she can barely open her eyes and hasn't been able

to eat or drink much today. Before today she had been trying new foods every day; yesterday's new food was yogurt with honey. Her father works at a dusty construction site. On physical exam you note a very lethargic 10-month-old female with rapid, shallow, noisy breathing, who does not open her eyes and who withdraws and cries weakly to painful stimuli. What is the most appropriate next step in management?

    A. Give naloxone
    B. Give the appropriate antitoxin
    C. Intubate
    D. Start IV fluids and antibiotics

41. A 9-year-old boy starts experiencing lower extremity weakness 5 days into a backpacking trip with his Boy Scouts troop. He presents to your ED after having just come from the trail. On your exam, his dorsiflexion and plantar flexion are three out of five, and knee flexion and extension are four out of five. He has had no preceding illness. He has no back pain or tenderness and does not complain of saddle anesthesia or bowel or bladder incontinence. Which of the following is the most appropriate next step in management?

    A. Removal of all clothing and full skin exam, with removal of any ticks
    B. Start plasmapheresis and admit to a monitored setting
    C. Check serum creatine kinase and start corticosteroids
    D. Consult neurosurgery and order MRI of the lumbar spine

42. A 17-year-old previously healthy male presents with episodic generalized weakness. He has noticed that these episodes occur several hours after basketball practice or in the morning on awakening, usually lasting 3 to 4 hours. His diet consists mostly of bread, pizza, rice, and oatmeal. His first-degree relatives are unaffected, but he thinks his grandfather might have a "muscle problem." On physical exam, his respiratory status is stable, and you note no facial involvement, but he has objective weakness of his proximal muscles, more pronounced in his lower extremities. Which of the following lab abnormalities would you expect to find?

    A. Potassium level of 2.4
    B. Elevated ESR
    C. Hemoglobin of 8.5
    D. Thyroid-stimulating hormone (TSH) level of 0.1

43. A 19-year-old woman presents complaining of left eye pain for 3 days and vision loss that began today. She

has never had these symptoms before but last year had an episode of mild foot drop lasting 1 month, for which she did not seek care. On physical exam, she has some tenderness to gentle palpation of the left eye, and when you swing your light source from her right to her left eye, her left pupil dilates. Which of the following tests or exams is most appropriate?

A. MRI of the brain
B. Dilated funduscopic exam
C. Edrophonium test
D. LP

44. A 35-year-old woman with a past medical history of multiple sclerosis (MS) presents with 1 day of sharp, left-sided facial pain occurring in episodes lasting 3 to 5 minutes, with complete resolution between episodes. She also complains of some weakness of her right leg. On physical exam she appears comfortable, until you touch her face, at which time she develops obvious severe pain and left facial spasm. Right quadriceps strength is four out of five. Which of the following is the most appropriate next step in management?

A. Prescribe carbamazepine and discharge with neurology follow-up
B. MRI of the brain, neurology consult, and IV methylprednisolone
C. Give sumatriptan and 1 L normal saline and observe for 2 hours
D. Prescribe prednisone and acyclovir and discharge with primary care follow-up

45. A 62-year-old man presents with a chief complaint of vomiting. His grandchildren recently visited, and they both had a "stomach bug" while they were with him. He has "some medical problems" and takes a medicine "to help with my walking," but he isn't sure of the name. On physical exam, you notice a slight resting tremor in his right arm, cogwheel rigidity of his arms, and a shuffling gait. His abdomen is benign. Which of the following medications should be avoided in this patient?

A. Meclizine
B. Prochlorperazine
C. Ondansetron
D. Diazepam

46. An 18-month-old girl is brought in by her mother after an episode of generalized shaking that lasted approximately 2 minutes. She is developmentally normal and has no past medical history. For the past 2 days, the patient has had temperatures up to 38.9° C (102° F) at home with a mild stuffy nose and mild cough. The patient's 3-year-old brother recently had a fever, which has resolved, but he now has a whole-body, erythematous, maculopapular rash. The girl is fully vaccinated and now is acting normally, appears well, and has a normal physical exam with the exception of a fever of 38.7° C (101.6) and nasal congestion. What is the most appropriate next step in management?

A. Acetaminophen, reassurance, and discharge with primary care doctor follow-up
B. Urinalysis, chest radiograph, head CT, and LP
C. Admit for MRI of the brain and neurology consult
D. Observe in the ED for 24 hours and discharge if no recurrence

47. A 6-month-old girl is brought in by her mother after an episode of generalized shaking lasting 6 minutes at home. The patient had been previously healthy, with no prior seizures. The mother reports that the patient had been crying a lot today but otherwise had no symptoms. On physical exam the patient is afebrile and listless, has a slightly bulging fontanelle and bruising to her upper arms of different ages, and is moving her right arm less than her other extremities. What finding would you expect to see on head CT of this patient?

A. Intracerebral abscess
B. Subdural hematoma
C. Normal head CT
D. Epidural hematoma

48. A 25-day-old male arrives by EMS with persistent eye deviation to the right and lip smacking for the past 15 minutes. He received one dose of midazolam in the field. You give two more doses of midazolam in the ED, but he continues to seize. What is the most appropriate next step in management?

A. Administer a dose of lorazepam
B. Administer a loading dose of levetiracetam
C. Administer a loading dose of phenytoin
D. Administer a loading dose of phenobarbital

49. A previously healthy 18-month-old girl is brought in by ambulance after an episode of apnea. Her mother reports that immediately before the episode the girl's brother hit her with a toy, after which she cried, fell to the ground, stopped breathing, and had abnormal movements of her arms and legs. The episode resolved after 1 minute, and the child started acting normally immediately afterward. She is afebrile. Which of the following is the most likely diagnosis?

A. Generalized tonic-clonic seizure
B. Cardiac arrhythmia
C. Breath-holding spell
D. Narcolepsy

ANSWERS

1. ANSWER: B

This patient has classic signs and symptoms of an ischemic stroke. The patient's symptoms were of acute onset and consistent with a middle cerebral artery clot on the left side of the brain given the right-sided weakness and difficulty speaking. tPA is the standard of care for ischemic strokes to be given within the determined time frame of symptom onset (in most cases 4.5 hours). Hemorrhagic stroke must be ruled out before administration of tPA (A). Post-tPA patients require ICU care. Neurology should be consulted to assist in the decision to give tPA. Patients must meet all of the inclusion criteria and none of the exclusion criteria. Patients should give consent, and if they are unable to do so, then the family should give consent. The National Institute of Neurological Disorders and Stroke (NINDS) trial demonstrated a number needed to treat of eight and a number needed to harm of 17.

Strict blood pressure control (C) is not recommended in patients with ischemic stroke, and the general guideline for tPA is BP <185/110 mm Hg before administration of tPA, which can be done with the use of antihypertensive medications. New research suggests that patients with large vessel occlusion presenting within 6 hours should be considered for thrombectomy but not without first evaluating for and potentially giving tPA (D).

Test-taking tip: Reading the subtle differences in answers carefully can help you find the right answer. The question is asking what to do first in an acute stroke. The answer is always noncontrast head CT first (choice B).

2. ANSWER: D

This patient has advanced dementia with a nonsurvivable hemorrhagic stroke. Neurosurgery has confirmed this, as do her signs of herniation. While answers A and B would be correct in a patient being treated for a hemorrhagic stroke with an elevated BP and INR, they are not the best answer for this patient. The patient does not have an advance directive and should not be extubated and designated for comfort care without a discussion with the family. While there may be some confusion about providing maximal therapy for a patient until the patient's wishes are known, this patient has family in the waiting room, and they are asking to speak with the doctor to make her wishes known. Choice C is wrong for many reasons, including that this patient is *not* having an ischemic stroke, is out of the tPA window, would require consent before initiation, and tPA would make the head bleed worse.

Test-taking tip: If two answers seem right, go back and read the question again. In this case, choices A and B would be correct in a patient with a hemorrhagic stroke that is being treated with maximal medical management. In our case, the stroke is nonsurvivable and the patient is beginning to herniate, so maximal medical management is not indicated.

3. ANSWER: B

This patient has a history of recurrent focal (partial) seizures. Although the International League Against Epilepsy has revised their classification of seizures, their original classification system is still used and is worth reviewing. Partial seizures were classified as simple partial (our patient) with a focal seizure and retained consciousness, whereas complex partial seizures occurred with impaired consciousness. Partial seizures could also evolve into generalized seizures described by the term secondary generalization. A generalized seizure also had multiple types, with the common theme being that the first clinical symptom involved both sides of the brain with impaired consciousness. This patient has an established diagnosis without change in anything except his seizure frequency, and therefore no additional workup (thus choices A, C, and D are incorrect) is required because the patient will have close follow-up with his neurologist.

Test-taking tip: This patient has an established history of partial seizures and because his labs are normal and he has had recent imaging, he does not need repeat imaging or testing. This helps you eliminate answers A and C.

4. ANSWER: A

This patient is presenting with a new-onset, unprovoked generalized tonic-clonic seizure with return to his baseline neurologic status. A provoked seizure is defined as occurring within 7 days of an insult, including a neurologic, toxic, systemic, or metabolic process. Unprovoked seizures occur without an insult in the past 7 days and include idiopathic seizures. Reporting the seizure as a lapse of consciousness to the county/Department of Motor Vehicles (DMV) is an important step. Per the American College of Emergency Physicians (ACEP) Clinical Policy, patients with a new-onset, unprovoked seizure with return to baseline neurologic status should have sodium, glucose, and pregnancy (if childbearing age) tests and neuroimaging if possible; or neuroimaging can be deferred with close, reliable follow-up. This makes choice A the most correct answer.

Choice B is incorrect because previously healthy patients with a new-onset, unprovoked seizure with return to baseline neurologic status do not need to be started on an antiepileptic medication. Choice C is incorrect because previously healthy patients with a new-onset, unprovoked seizure with return to baseline neurologic status do not require admission for monitoring. Choice D is incorrect because the patient should have his glucose and sodium checked, and while neuroimaging can be deferred, it should not be for 1 month.

Test-taking tip: When multiple answers have identical text, be sure to read each carefully to ensure the correct answer is selected. With A and B having almost identical answers, it is likely that one of those is the correct answer.

5. ANSWER: C

This question is asking about the treatment of a specific cause of status epilepticus: isoniazid toxicity. This patient needs pyridoxine (vitamin B_6). With an unknown ingestion, the initial dose is 70 mg/kg for a maximum of 5 g. While it is acceptable to simultaneously treat with benzodiazepines and antiepileptics, the ultimate treatment is pyridoxine. Choice A is incorrect because while the patient may ultimately need to go to the ICU, it does not mention anything about treatment. Choice B does not address the underlying problem, and waiting 20 minutes for a response is unacceptable.

The 2014 ACEP Clinical Policy on seizures defines status epilepticus as a seizure lasting more than 20 minutes. Patients in status epilepticus should be treated in a systematic manner, including ABCs, IV line, oxygen, monitor, glucose, benzodiazepines, antiepileptics, barbiturates, and general anesthesia. Patients should be considered for continuous EEG monitoring, may require intubation, and usually need ICU level of care. Special causes like isoniazid toxicity or overdose should be considered, as should other causes such as central nervous system (CNS) infection.

Test-taking tip: This is a "you know it or don't" kind of question. If you don't know it, choose an answer and move on. You can perhaps mark it for review when you are done at the end of the test. Don't, however, let these kinds of questions get you stuck and waste your time.

6. ANSWER: D

Given the patient's history of AIDS, clinical symptoms, and CT findings, the most likely diagnosis is a brain abscess. Risk factors for brain abscesses include immunosuppression, bacteremia, and infection in the surrounding structures of the brain, trauma, or prior instrumentation. The classic findings of headache, fever, and focal neurologic deficit occur in about 20% of patients. Seizures can occur in about 25% of patients with a brain abscess. A T1-weighted MRI with contrast will show a necrotic center and ring-shaped enhancement of the abscess wall and surrounding edema. Neurosurgery should be consulted for possible aspiration of the abscess and cultures. As with most CNS infections, antibiotic administration should not be delayed for further imaging. Empiric antimicrobial therapy includes ceftriaxone and metronidazole with or without vancomycin. Isolated meningitis should not have positive brain imaging (A, B). Acute stroke (D) is unlikely to have positive imaging findings and is not the leading diagnosis in an AIDS patient with fever, headache, and focal neurologic symptoms.

Test-taking tip: Risk factors and clinical presentation play an important role in determining the most likely cause of an illness when multiple answers seem appropriate.

7. ANSWER: C

This patient is presenting with symptoms and imaging findings consistent with neurocysticercosis, with the risk factor of visiting from a foreign country. Neurocysticercosis is a common cause of seizures in the developing world and the most common parasite to infect the brain. It is caused by the parasite *Taenia solium* or pork tapeworm. Like in our patient, symptoms of neurocysticercosis include headache and seizures (usually focal) and sometimes focal neurologic deficits that can mimic stroke. Neuroimaging can reveal different findings based on the stage of the disease, but the findings of a cystic lesion with a peripheral dot or scolex, such as in our patient, are highly suggestive of neurocysticercosis. The definitive diagnosis and treatment of neurocysticercosis can be challenging and should be done with neurosurgical and infectious disease consultation.

Isolated meningitis should not have positive brain imaging (B). The same is true for an alcohol withdrawal seizure (D). The imaging finding is more suggestive of neurocysticercosis than brain abscess (A).

Test-taking tip: Pay close attention to information like foreign travel or other risk factors that would make a certain diagnosis more likely.

8. ANSWER: B

Meningitis is an inflammation of the meninges. This patient has signs and symptoms of meningitis. The most common causes of bacterial meningitis are *H. influenzae* type b (Hib), *N. meningitidis*, and *Streptococcus pneumoniae*. *N. meningitidis* classically has outbreaks that occur in people who live in close proximity to each other (e.g., in college dorms or military housing). Prognosis is improved by early recognition and treatment; therefore antibiotic administration should never be delayed for other management decisions. Dexamethasone should also be considered in addition to antibiotics, especially in children. LP is the diagnosis of choice, with noncontrast head CT done before LP when there is concern for a possible space-occupying lesion. Head CT (A) can often delay LP (C), which will delay antibiotic administration if you wait for LP to administer antibiotics. Patients are usually given vancomycin and a third-generation cephalosporin, with ampicillin added for older adult or alcoholic patients. MRI with contrast (D) can be abnormal in encephalitis, but it is certainly not the most emergent management decision.

Test-taking tip: If a question asks about the most important or best answer, multiple answers may be part of the patient's management. For the correct answer, think about which answer will have the most effect on the patient and the outcome.

9. ANSWER: C

This patient is presenting with signs and symptoms of encephalitis. Signs and symptoms of encephalitis include confusion, fever, headache, focal weakness, seizures, and "psychiatric changes" because the infection is within the brain. HSV is estimated to cause up to 20% of viral encephalitis cases. HSV-1 accounts for 95% of the herpesvirus cases. HSV encephalitis has the characteristic findings seen on the MRI of our patient along with a corresponding hypointense appearance of the limbic and hypothalamic areas on T1-weighted imaging. CSF studies of HSV show increased WBCs, often with a lymphocytic predominance, and increased RBCs. Glucose is often normal, and protein can be mildly increased, with a normal to mildly increased pressure. HSV encephalitis is treated with IV acyclovir, and treatment should not be delayed. Other causes of viral encephalitis include varicella, enterovirus, other herpesviruses, and arboviruses, including West Nile virus (but they are not likely to have his MRI findings) (E). Choices A and B are causes of bacterial meningitis that would likely include a polymorphonuclear neutrophil (PMN) predominance in the WBC count of the CSF and low glucose levels.

Test-taking tip: Although it may be difficult to diagnose a specific bacteria or virus, there are classic findings associated with certain ones that make good test questions. HSV encephalitis classically can be associated with increased RBCs on CSF analysis.

10. ANSWER: C

Obstructive hydrocephalus is treated with VP shunt placement. Patients with VP shunts placed are at risk for complications and shunt failure. Shunt failure was reported to be as high as 50% in the past, but recent studies find rates closer to 15%, with a median time of 3 to 4 months. This patient's recent shunt revision puts her at risk for shunt complications. She is demonstrating symptoms of shunt failure and recurrence of hydrocephalus, likely secondary to an infectious process in the CSF. Although the patient's headache improved with treatment, discharge without a workup is not appropriate (A). LP should not be done without first obtaining a CT scan and then discussing the case with neurosurgery (B). While an MRI could eventually be useful, at this point it will delay the diagnosis (D). Patients with prolonged hospital stay, older age, lower baseline GCS score, shunt placement for brain tumor, or extraventricular drains are more likely to have shunt malfunction.

Test-taking tip: Patients on standardized test questions are different from patients seen in the ED. Most information is presented for a reason, and they often exhibit classic pathology. Recent VP shunt placement with headache is shunt malfunction until proved otherwise.

11. ANSWER: D

This patient has a concerning story for nontraumatic subarachnoid hemorrhage. Although he has a history of migraines, this headache is different than his previous headaches and reached maximal intensity within 1 minute. These are all features concerning for subarachnoid hemorrhage. If the patient does not have any of the Ottawa Subarachnoid Hemorrhage Rule features, including age greater than 40 years, neck pain or stiffness, limited neck flexion on exam, thunderclap description, loss of consciousness, and onset during exertion, then the patient is extremely low risk for subarachnoid hemorrhage.

Choice A is just treating the patient symptomatically to determine the course of action. Response of the headache to medication has not been shown to be reassuring that the headache is benign. Choice B is incorrect because the patient requires LP after a normal noncontrast head CT, particularly if the headache has been present for more than 6 hours. Choice D could be part of the patient's workup if he does have a subarachnoid hemorrhage to determine whether it is aneurysmal, but it should not be the first test that is done.

Test-taking tip: If two answers look similar, read them both carefully because their differences may give you some insight into what the test writer is asking (B, C).

12. ANSWER: A

The history of this patient's headache is concerning for tumor/mass ,and her physical exam is remarkable for papilledema, which is consistent with increased ICP. Her

CT scan shows obstructive hydrocephalus. This is a neurosurgical emergency, and neurosurgery should be consulted immediately for potential surgical intervention for the hydrocephalus. Common causes of adult acquired hydrocephalus include brain tumors, postmeningitic scaring, and sequalae of head trauma.

Ophthalmology consult (B) is not the best next course of action because the etiology of papilledema has already been determined and the patient needs neurosurgery. LP (C) is likely contraindicated in this patient given her increased ICP and concern for subsequent herniation. Mannitol (D) is given for increased ICP in the setting of impending herniation, which you would give after discussion with neurosurgery.

Test-taking tip: While some answers may be tempting and not necessarily wrong, the correct answer is often the best answer to address the immediate emergency.

13. ANSWER: D

This patient is presenting with signs and symptoms concerning for temporal arteritis that is progressing and starting to involve her vision. While glaucoma (A) is appropriate to keep on the differential, it is unlikely given the normal appearance of her eye and normal eye pressures. While B may seem like a reasonable answer and temporal arteritis is typically associated with an elevated ESR, there are cases of temporal arteritis with near-normal ESR. This patient does not have features classically associated with ischemic stroke, and symptoms have been present for more than 4.5 hours; therefore choice C is not the right answer.

Temporal arteritis, also known as giant cell arteritis, is a vasculitis that usually affects arteries of the head and neck. It has an association with polymyalgia rheumatica. Patients with concern for temporal arteritis should be treated with steroids, and a temporal biopsy should be obtained to support the diagnosis. Temporal arteritis patients are usually older, may have jaw claudication, and can even present with a nodular appearance of the temporal artery on physical exam.

Test-taking tip: If a patient has a high probability of a disease based on clinical history and physical exam, a single lab test (in this case an ESR of less than 60) should not eliminate your clinical suspicion for the disease.

14. ANSWER: D

This patient is presenting with signs and symptoms of a stroke. Although this patient is young, his symptoms and physical exam should not be disregarded because they are concerning for stroke. Stroke in a young patient is a rare

diagnosis but not exceedingly rare because 15% of all ischemic strokes are estimated to occur in young adults and adolescents. Causes of stroke in the young include categories like arterial pathology (including carotid artery dissection, the most likely cause of stroke in our patient given the history of recent chiropractor use), cardiac pathology, and hematologic etiology. Cervical artery dissection includes dissection of the carotid and vertebral arteries. The classic triad of this disease includes Horner's syndrome, unilateral head or neck pain, and ischemia of the brain or retina but is present in less than one-third of patients. Carotid artery dissections result in anterior circulation pathology, and vertebral artery dissections result in the posterior circulation pathology.

He does not have a TIA because his symptoms are not transient (A). This patient does not have signs or symptoms of meningitis (B), and while he does have neck pain, carotid artery dissection is more likely. This patient is out of the window for tPA because his symptoms have been present for greater than 4.5 hours (C).

Test-taking tip: The clue in the question stem of the patient seeing a chiropractor and then having neck pain is the key to the diagnosis. The best next step is to confirm the diagnosis of carotid artery dissection (with a CT angiogram of the neck).

15. ANSWER: A

This patient has classic signs and symptoms of post-LP headache. Blood patches have a success rate of over 75%. The patient had a LP 2 days prior and has a headache that is worse with standing and improves with lying down. This is the classic description of a post-LP headache, and the diagnosis should be made clinically. He does not have any new symptoms to warrant an MRI (B) in the ED and has a normal neurologic examination. The patient should not just be reassured and discharged without treatment (D) because possible complications include seizures and subdural hematoma. Factors that could decrease the incidence of post-LP headache include smaller needle size, use of atraumatic needle, fewer attempts, and use of a stylet for removal of the needle.

Test-taking tip: Be wary of an answer that just involves consulting an expert (C, in this case). While neurology could be involved in this case, it is not the best answer.

16. ANSWER: B

Headache is an extremely common presentation to the ED. As emergency medicine providers, it is our job to consider emergent causes of headache and provide symptomatic relief. Although this patient does not carry a formal diagnosis of migraines, her signs and symptoms are consistent with migraine. Her headache meets criteria for migraine without aura from the second edition of the *International Classification of Headache Disorders*. This requires at least five lifetime headaches like this one; two of the following features of headache: unilateral, moderate to severe intensity, exacerbated by physical activity, or throbbing; and headache lasting 4 to 72 hours without treatment or without relief with treatment. The patient does not have a history or physical exam consistent with subarachnoid hemorrhage (A). An MRV for venous sinus thrombosis (C) is not indicated at this time because she does not have focal neurologic findings or risk factors including pregnancy or other prothrombotic state or a recent facial infection. Choice D is incorrect because it does not provide symptomatic relief with monotherapy of IV fluids.

Test-taking tip: Symptomatic relief of patients is just as much our job as ruling out emergencies. Even though a patient does not appear to have an emergency, the patient's symptoms should be addressed.

17. ANSWER: D

This patient has the classic symptoms of a cluster headache. His pain is periorbital and unilateral, and his attacks occur in clusters. Attacks can last 15 to 180 minutes and can occur up to eight times per day. Associated symptoms include lacrimation, miosis, rhinorrhea, focal diaphoresis, and eyelid changes. First-line therapy is high-flow oxygen; further treatment includes subcutaneous triptans and dihydroergotamine. The patient should be referred to a neurologist for outpatient preventative therapy, and the next best action for this patient would not be neurology consult without implementing therapy (C). The patient does not have signs or symptoms of subarachnoid hemorrhage (A). Morphine and fluids are not first-line treatment for cluster headaches (B).

Test-taking tip: Even if you had forgotten that cluster headaches are treated with oxygen, all of the rest of the answers could be eliminated on their own. Process of elimination is an important test-taking tool.

18. ANSWER: A

This patient is presenting with altered mental status. While the differential is broad, there are some diagnoses that we can't miss. Our patient has one of them: opioid overdose. While he does not have any reported track marks, he is breathing slowly and has pinpoint pupils. He should immediately be given naloxone by IV, IM, or intranasal route (or theoretically through an endotracheal tube if one is in place). A second diagnosis would be hypoglycemia (B), but our patient had a normal fingerstick glucose. The patient is protecting his airway and should not be intubated (C), especially if his mental status will immediately improve with naloxone. Thiamine (D) is given for Wernicke's encephalopathy, which is typically represented by the triad of eye muscle weakness, trouble walking, and confusion, which does not fit this patient's constellation of symptoms. Vital signs must be carefully analyzed because they can give us significant information about what diagnosis could be causing the change in mental status. Core temperature, when feasible, is preferred. After an initial evaluation is done, an extensive physical exam must be done to look for focal neurologic deficits, pupil abnormalities, abnormal skin findings, murmurs, abdominal tenderness, edema, abnormal breath sounds, and potentially rectal bleeding. It is often useful to approach altered mental status in a systematic way. Broad categories include systemic disease (like infections or hypoxia), CNS disease (like brain hemorrhage or masses), and drugs and medications (like our patient). Mnemonics can be used that further subdivide these broad categories.

Test-taking tip: When approaching a broad differential on a test, like altered mental status, look for clues (like low RR and pinpoint pupils) that will almost always guide you in the right direction of the diagnosis.

19. ANSWER: D

Risk factors for delirium include older age, male sex, comorbid diseases (including dementia), and multiple medications. When patients with dementia must be hospitalized, certain things can increase their risk for developing delirium. Physical restraints (A) and urinary catheters (C) increase a patient's risk for development of delirium. When possible, vital sign monitoring devices should be removed from the patient's bedside when they are not in use. Attempting to maintain a proper sleep-wake cycle in the ED should be done to minimize delirium. Scheduled benzodiazepines (B) will increase his risk for developing delirium as well.

Test-taking tip: Even if you have not memorized all of the information about a certain disease or risk factors (in this case risk factors for development of delirium), some answers inherently seem wrong and can be eliminated.

20. ANSWER: B

Coma is achieved with disruption of the ascending reticular activating system–thalamic–cortical pathway. Coma results from structural causes like tumors that physically block this pathway and toxins (like alcohol) or metabolic derangements (like hypoglycemia) that cause global dysfunction of the neurons involved in this pathway. Coma is often evaluated using the GCS, which assigns four points to eye opening, five points to verbal performance, and six points to motor responsiveness. Although the scale was originally designed in the 1970s for head trauma patients, its use has been expanded to many different clinical scenarios as an evaluation of consciousness.

Locked-in syndrome is defined as quadriplegia with the inability to speak while the person is still conscious and able to the eyes. This patient has signs and symptoms of locked-in syndrome. While it is a rare diagnosis, it demonstrates the subtleties that exist in the diagnosis of coma. Our patient would score six out of 15 GCS points because the minimum in each category is one (four for eyes, one for verbal, and one for motor). However, he is not technically in a coma because his consciousness is preserved. Patients with basilar artery occlusion often have a hyperdense basilar artery sign on noncontrast CT and should be considered for tPA/endovascular intervention, when appropriate. Opioid overdose (A) would present with true coma. Be cautious of selecting an answer like choice E of conversion disorder because the patient is not breathing, which is not suggestive of this diagnosis. Lastly, Wernicke's encephalopathy is typically represented by the triad of eye muscle weakness, trouble walking, and confusion, which does not fit this patient's constellation of symptoms (C).

Test-taking tip: For rare diagnoses that you may not be familiar with, it is essential to eliminate other answers that you are familiar with but that do not fit the clinical presentation.

21. ANSWER: B

This patient is presenting with signs and symptoms of normal pressure hydrocephalus (NPH). See Figure 12.2, which shows hydrocephalus. NPH is a reversible type of dementia (D) that is often misdiagnosed (like in our patient) and classically has the triad of gait instability, dementia, and urinary incontinence. However, patients with symmetric gait instability should be considered for NPH because the triad is not required for diagnosis. LP is part of the workup in which a tap test is done to demonstrate improvement in gait after removal of about 30 to 50 mL of CSF. Given the patient's history, physical exam, and imaging, Alzheimer's disease (A) is not the most likely diagnosis. Choice C is incorrect for the same reason.

Ataxia can result from damage to the spinal cord, peripheral sensory nervous system, and brain (including the cerebellum). Cerebellar ataxia can result from a variety of causes, including hereditary, immunologic, metabolic

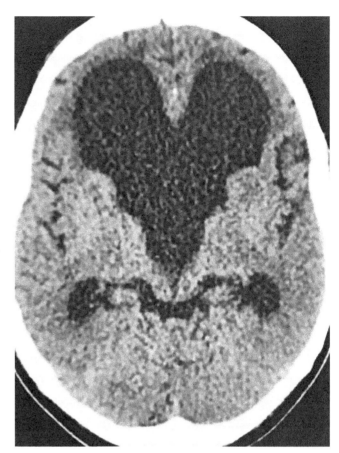

Figure 12.2 Head computed tomography.

derangements, and drugs. Injury to the cerebellum can cause problems with walking, coordination, speaking, muscle tone, and eye movement.

Test-taking tip: Some questions may involve multiple steps to arrive at the correct answer. In this case, the clinical presentation was consistent with NPH. Knowing this, you have to select an answer that is true of NPH. Keep track of this sequential information to avoid being tricked.

22. ANSWER: D

This patient is presenting with dizziness in the form of vertigo because of the sense that the room is spinning. Patients often have difficulty describing their dizziness, and a broader differential should be considered that includes vertigo, syncope, and presyncope. Vertigo traditionally can be classified into two broad categories: peripheral and central. Central causes are in the brain and generally dangerous (like posterior stroke), and peripheral causes are in the peripheral vestibular system (like benign paroxysmal positional vertigo [BPPV]) and usually benign.

However, a new approach involves the patient's symptoms being classified as continuous or intermittent and as triggered or spontaneous. Acute vestibular syndrome is a syndrome of acute-onset vertigo that is persistent and includes posterior circulation stroke and vestibular neuronitis. BPPV is triggered and episodic, meaning that it is not constant and is triggered by a specific head movement. This is most consistent with our patient's presentation as well. The Epley maneuver can be used to treat BPPV in patients with a positive Dix-Hallpike test. BPPV is a disorder in which otoconial debris break off and stimulate receptors of motion in the semicircular canals of the inner ear in certain positions. The last category is spontaneous and episodic, meaning that it is intermittent vertigo that is not triggered by anything. This includes vestibular migraine and TIA.

Our patient has intermittent vertigo, making choice A wrong. The head impulse test is positive in patients with vestibular neuronitis, and therefore C is wrong. It is done by asking the patient to focus on the examiner's face while moving the head left to central and right to central, no more than 20 degrees. A positive test is seen when the patient cannot continuously track the examiner's face and does a corrective saccade. Acetazolamide (B) is a common treatment for Ménière's disease, which is defined by episodes of spontaneous vertigo and hearing loss and symptoms of tinnitus and ear fullness.

Test-taking tip: Vertigo can get confusing. Breaking the symptoms into persistent vertigo, triggered episodic vertigo, and untriggered episodic vertigo allows for symptom-based classification to focus on certain diagnoses.

23. ANSWER: B

This patient is presenting with constant vertigo or an acute vestibular syndrome. Acute vestibular syndrome is a syndrome of acute-onset vertigo that is persistent and includes posterior circulation stroke and vestibular neuronitis. Our patient is an older adult with stroke risk factors, is unable to ambulate, and has a positive test of skew. The test of skew is 98% specific for a brainstem lesion and is done by having the patient look at your nose while you alternatively cover each eye. The test is positive when there is a vertical correction of the eye that occurs when switching from one to the other. Taking this all into account, her presentation is concerning for posterior circulation stroke. Her head impulse testing will likely be normal (A) because it is abnormal in vestibular neuronitis. A noncontrast head CT (D) is not reassuring for excluding stroke in the acute setting and, if done, should not be used to falsely reassure you that there is unlikely to be a central process occurring. Lastly, meclizine (C) is sometimes used for symptomatic treatment in vestibular neuronitis, and response to treatment should not be used diagnostically.

Test-taking tip: Persistent vertigo in older adults with an inability to ambulate is concerning for stroke and should be taken seriously even without other neurologic symptoms.

24. ANSWER: D

This is a classic case of Bell's palsy. Patients often present with concern for stroke. Bell's palsy is an acute-onset, unilateral paralysis of the facial nerve. The cause is not entirely known, and it is thought to be associated with HSV. The key to making the diagnosis involves the weakness of the entire unilateral facial nerve, including the forehead. Paresis sparing the forehead would be concerning for an upper motor problem and requires further workup. This patient was having a stroke, he would not be in the tPA window (C). There is evidence that steroids given early improve resolution of facial weakness, but the addition of antivirals is more controversial. Complications can develop from an inability to close the eye, so an eye patch and artificial tears are important, and patients should not just be discharged with reassurance (A).

Test-taking tip: Although it may be tempting to do a more extensive workup (like an MRI), when it is not indicated and the diagnosis is clear, it should not be done.

25. ANSWER: C

This patient presents with classic trigeminal neuralgia ("tic douloureux"), which is treated with carbamazepine. The differential diagnosis for this condition includes classic trigeminal neuralgia, secondary trigeminal neuralgia, acute herpes zoster, postherpetic neuropathy, and post-traumatic neuropathy. The determination of trigeminal neuralgia as classic or secondary is as follows: classic trigeminal neuralgia is either idiopathic or caused by microvascular compression, whereas secondary trigeminal neuralgia is caused by MS plaques or pathologic compressive lesions (e.g., tumor). Patients with classic trigeminal neuralgia typically are older than 40 years and have no history of malignancy or MS, and the neuralgia is typically unilateral in a full or partial distribution of the trigeminal nerve (Figure 12.3). Episodes last less than 2 minutes, are severe, and are described as sharp, shock-like, stabbing, or shooting. Patients must not have any neurologic deficits to fit the diagnosis of classic trigeminal neuralgia.

First-line treatment for classic trigeminal neuralgia includes carbamazepine 100 mg PO twice daily, with increases as needed to control symptoms. Outpatient referral to a neurologist is appropriate for these patients, and brain MRI with and without contrast can be obtained on an outpatient basis.

Cranial Nerve V (Trigeminal Nerve) Distribution

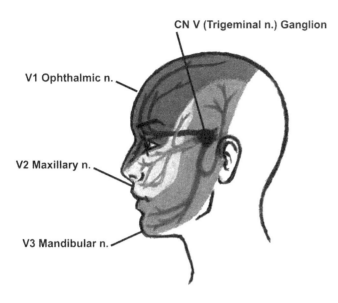

CN V (Trigeminal n.) Ganglion

V1 Ophthalmic n.

V2 Maxillary n.

V3 Mandibular n.

Figure 12.3 Distribution of the three branches of cranial nerve V.

Test-taking tip: If you are unsure of the diagnosis, consider what about the presentation is inconsistent with each diagnosis you are considering: for example, this pain is brief, and a migraine or cluster headache would last longer, ruling out A and B (sumatriptan for migraine, oxygen for cluster headache), and there are no motor deficits, ruling out Bell's palsy (D, prednisone).

26. ANSWER: B

This patient needs an MRI of the brain. This patient has a presentation concerning for a vestibular schwannoma (acoustic neuroma), which is a tumor arising from cranial nerve VIII. The duration of his symptoms (18 months) is longer than would be expected with any of the purely peripheral causes of dizziness such as vestibular neuritis. He also has additional neurologic deficits (decreased sensation in V_2 and V_3, ataxia), which should prompt additional imaging rather than symptomatic management alone (A). The patient might benefit from hearing aids (C), but this would not be appropriate until more serious causes of hearing loss have been ruled out. Administering streptokinase (D) would also not be appropriate in this patient because he is not having an acute cerebral infarction.

About 95% of patients with vestibular schwannoma complain of hearing loss. Other common symptoms include unsteadiness while walking (61%) and facial pain, decreased sensation, or paresthesias (9%). Bilateral vestibular schwannomas have been described in association with neurofibromatosis type 2. Patients with signs and symptoms of vestibular schwannoma need prompt diagnostic imaging (MRI is more sensitive than CT for posterior fossa lesions) and referral to neurosurgery.

The evaluation of patients with vague dizziness can be very challenging. After it has been determined that the patient is experiencing vertigo (rather than syncope/near syncope, orthostatic hypotension, or hypoglycemia), the next step is determining whether the cause is central or peripheral. Cerebellopontine angle tumors can be particularly challenging because they can have features of both a peripheral and central cause from their impingement on cranial nerve VIII and/or the cerebellum. Table 12.1 lists some of the elements that may help distinguish between central and peripheral causes of vertigo.

Table 12.1 CENTRAL VERSUS PERIPHERAL VERTIGO

Diagnoses	Vertebrobasilar insufficiency	Ménière's disease
	Tumor	Labyrinthitis
	Stroke/transient ischemic attack	Benign paroxysmal positional vertigo (BPPV)
	Multiple sclerosis	Vestibular neuritis
	Toxicologic causes	
	Basilar migraine	
	Seizure	
Symptoms	Gradual (tumor) or sudden (cerebrovascular accident) onset	Gradual (labyrinthitis) or sudden (BPPV) onset
	Continuous	Continuous or intermittent
	Usually no tinnitus	May have tinnitus
	Additional neurologic symptoms	No other neurologic symptoms
	Dysarthria	
	Diplopia	
	Dysphagia	
Exam findings	Dysmetria	No additional neurologic deficits
	Dysdiadochokinesia	Nystagmus: fatigable, horizontal
	Nystagmus: not fatigable, may be vertical/rotatory	
	Ataxia	

Test-taking tip: In a patient with no known diagnosis and any alarm signs (e.g., new objective neurologic deficits), symptomatic management alone will never be the right answer.

27. ANSWER: D

This patient's presentation is concerning for spinal epidural hematoma, which necessitates neurosurgical consultation.

In patients with signs of spinal cord, conus medullaris, or cauda equina compression (bilateral lower extremity numbness, weakness, pain, bowel or bladder incontinence, saddle anesthesia), neurosurgical consultation should not be delayed for labs (A) or imaging tests. Though nonsurgical management of spinal epidural hematomas has been described when deficits are mild and stable, the mainstay of treatment remains surgical decompression.

Choice B would be appropriate (after neurosurgical consultation) if spinal epidural abscess were suspected, though that is less likely in this patient because he is afebrile, and no history of intravascular procedures/devices or IV drug use was given. Warfarin reversal with vitamin K or prothrombin complex concentrate would be reasonable, but protamine sulfate (C) would reverse heparin, not warfarin.

Test-taking tip: This patient has signs of cord compression. If you know the patient has a condition with significant morbidity that is time sensitive (like this one), the correct answer choice will be the one that will decrease morbidity and mortality the most, which in this case is emergent neurosurgical consultation.

28. ANSWER: C

This patient has physical exam findings consistent with spinal cord compression (apparent lower extremity paralysis, bladder distention, and poor rectal tone). The presence of fever suggests an infectious etiology, and IV drug use is a risk factor for epidural abscess. Spinal injury (A) is also possible but is less likely without a history of trauma or physical exam findings suggestive of a significant trauma, and it would not explain the fever. Opioid overdose (B) could cause altered mental status but would not explain the fever or neurologic deficits. Guillain-Barré syndrome (D) does present with ascending paralysis, so epidural abscess is more likely in this case.

Spinal epidural abscess is an abscess between the dura mater and the periosteum of the vertebrae. Since the 1970s, the incidence of this diagnosis has been increasing, likely owing to increasing rates of IV drug use, invasive vascular access, intravascular procedures, and spinal instrumentation. Older adult patients, patients with multiple comorbidities, and immunocompromised patients are at higher risk for this disease. Symptoms include fever and signs of spinal cord compression (e.g., lower extremity weakness, saddle anesthesia). Initial management should include IV antibiotics and neurosurgical consultation.

Test-taking tip: Often more than one answer choice will be reasonable for the case presented. Look at all the data points given in the question stem and weigh them against each answer choice—unless you are given a pathognomonic finding, the one diagnosis that explains all the findings (in this case, neurologic deficits *and* fever) will be the best one.

29. ANSWER: B

The case in the question stem is one of a neurosurgical emergency. The differential diagnosis for this presentation includes the following:

1. Cauda equina syndrome—results from large midline disk herniation, can have urinary incontinence or retention, and will progress to lower extremity weakness. This is the likely correct answer.
2. Epidural hematoma—hints in the question stem for this would be anticoagulation, recent spinal surgery, and LP.
3. Epidural abscess—risk factors in the patient are IV drug use, diabetes or other immunocompromised state, and sometimes fever on presentation.
4. Spinal metastasis—hints in the question stem are cancer in past medical history of the patient, atypical night pain, and sweating/weight loss on review of symptoms.
5. Pott's disease (tuberculosis [TB] of the spine)—is possible in patients with a history of active TB or a history of recently treated TB who present with back pain.

All of these etiologies, if causing saddle anesthesia and no rectal tone, are neurosurgical emergencies and need a neurosurgical consult right away. MRI of the spine will confirm the diagnosis.

Test-taking tip: If you did not know the correct answer, try to figure out what the question stem is describing. It is describing a patient with a numb groin and no rectal tone. Both are ominous signs. Neurosurgery needs to be called regardless of the official diagnosis.

30. ANSWER: C

This patient has a presentation concerning for vertebral osteomyelitis or diskitis, which would be confirmed with MRI of the lumbar spine. Ceftriaxone and vancomycin (IV) are appropriate empiric treatment, but the patient is stable and has no evidence of cord compression, so antibiotics should be deferred until a pathogen is isolated (as long as he remains stable), either from blood cultures or biopsy of infected tissue. Consulting neurosurgery (B) would be appropriate if he had a known epidural abscess or any evidence of cord compression, which he does not. A trial of NSAIDs and physical therapy (D) is inappropriate in this patient because of his multiple risk factors and presentation concerning for infection.

Vertebral osteomyelitis and diskitis (Figure 12.4) most commonly occur in patients older than 50 years and have three potential paths for development: hematogenous spread, inoculation during surgery or invasive procedures, and spread from adjacent infection. Immunocompromised states, diabetes, heart disease, cancer, end-stage renal disease, and IV drug use are all risk factors for vertebral osteomyelitis and diskitis. Diagnosis should be confirmed with MRI before treatment initiation if the patient is not septic and does not have neurologic deficits or evidence of cord compression. Treatment consists of prolonged antibiotics, which should be tailored based on culture results, as well as treatment of endocarditis if present and removal of any source of infection (e.g., abscesses, infected indwelling catheters).

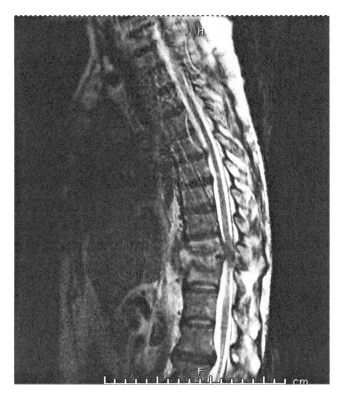

Figure 12.4 Spine magnetic resonance imaging.

Test-taking tip: In the ED, treatment is often initiated before all diagnostic tests have been obtained. This is appropriate in many situations. However, be sure to think carefully about the impact on the patient's long-term treatment, in this case, the possibility of obtaining negative cultures that would help to tailor antibiotic treatment.

31. ANSWER: B

This patient has spinal cord compression from a prostate metastasis, which would likely respond well to radiation therapy. Prostate cancer, breast cancer, and multiple myeloma are three of the most responsive malignancies to

radiation, and in many cases neurologic function can be preserved with prompt radiation therapy.

Dexamethasone is recommended to decrease inflammation in the interim until radiation or surgical therapy can be initiated. Choice A is incorrect because this patient does not desire surgery, so radiation oncology consultation should be prioritized. If the patient was uremic, had low platelets, or there was concern for hemorrhage into the tumor, platelet transfusion might be appropriate. Choice C is inappropriate again because radiation therapy takes priority over any chemotherapeutic intervention. Choice D is incorrect because although he is DNR/DNI, he will likely benefit from noninvasive radiation therapy.

Test-taking tip: You may have been tempted to jump to neurosurgical consultation after reading the beginning of the case. Make sure to read the entire question stem before choosing an answer. This patient does not desire surgery, and radiation therapy is an excellent option for prostate cancer, making choice B the best answer.

32. ANSWER: B

This patient has transverse myelitis (TM), which is a neuroinflammatory disorder that presents with acute-onset neurologic deficits, including weakness, sensory deficits, and bowel and bladder dysfunction, and can appear very similar to spinal cord compression. TM can be idiopathic or associated with autoimmune diseases such as sarcoidosis, lupus, and rheumatoid arthritis (which this patient has). The initial treatment for TM is IV methylprednisolone. Addition of cyclophosphamide (D) has also been described in the literature but is not first line. PO prednisone (C) would not be appropriate for this patient. If there was evidence of epidural abscess causing cord compression on MRI, IV antibiotics (A) might be appropriate while awaiting neurosurgical intervention. Although the presentation is very concerning for spinal cord compression, MRI without gadolinium rules this out. MRI with gadolinium should also be ordered for evaluation and would reveal inflammation of the cord, confirming the diagnosis of TM.

In addition to TM, other diagnostic considerations for this presentation (other than compressive lesions, which would be shown on MRI without gadolinium), include the following:

1. Vascular infarct—suggested by a history of recent vascular instrumentation, straining before symptom onset, age >50 years, and onset to nadir in <4 hours
2. Traumatic myelopathy—suggested by preceding trauma
3. Radiation myelopathy—suggested by history of radiation therapy

4. Congestive venous myelopathy (Foix-Alajouanine syndrome)—suggested by worsening symptoms with exertion and improvement with rest
5. MS—suggested by history of previous episodic neurologic deficits, previous diagnosis of MS or optic neuritis, multiple plaques on CNS imaging separated by time and space
6. Nutritional deficiencies (B$_{12}$, copper)—suggested by history of bariatric surgery, dietary restrictions, malnutrition

Test-taking tip: It can be challenging when a question stem changes direction mid-paragraph, eliminating the top differential diagnosis (in this case, a compressive lesion of the cord or cauda equina, eliminated by MRI). Don't be thrown off; reevaluate and rebroaden the differential.

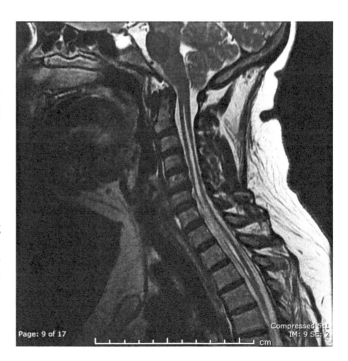

Figure 12.5 Cervical spine magnetic resonance imaging.

33. ANSWER: C

This patient has a gradual-onset central cord syndrome (cape-like loss of pain and temperature sensation with progressive upper extremity motor deficits) caused by syringomyelia. Syringomyelia is the presence of a fluid-filled cavity within the spinal cord, typically communicating with the CSF space. Syringomyelia may occur in patients of any age and is commonly associated with Chiari I malformations (elongated cerebellar tonsils with chronic herniation into the foramen magnum, choice A). It may also occur after trauma, such as a hyperextension injury from a motor vehicle accident (B). Without any prior history of trauma or known Chiari I malformation, it is impossible to know which of these contributed to his condition, and because both are possible, the correct answer choice is C. The diagnostic test of choice for syringomyelia is MRI (Figure 12.5), and treatment options include VP shunts, intracavitary shunts, and other neurosurgical procedures.

Vitamin B$_{12}$ deficiency can cause a peripheral neuropathy, but vitamin A (choice D) is not known to cause this. With B$_{12}$ deficiency the distribution is typically stocking and glove, which differs from this patient's presentation because only his upper extremities are affected. He has no history of veganism or atrophic gastritis, which would be the two major causes of vitamin B$_{12}$ deficiency.

Test-taking tip: Don't be distracted by answer choices that are intended to confuse you, like the vitamin deficiency option. If you know that the patient has symptoms consistent with central cord syndrome, make choosing the answer that causes central cord syndrome your focus, rather than trying to remember what vitamin deficiency causes what random constellation of symptoms.

34. ANSWER: C

The correct answer is *C. jejuni* (choice C). This patient has Guillain-Barré syndrome, a symmetric ascending polyneuropathy. A preceding infection by *C. jejuni* or other infections leads to an inappropriate autoimmune response mediated by antibodies and complement proteins, which leads to eventual damage of myelin sheaths or peripheral nerve axons. Choices A (*B. burgdorferi*), B (*Shigella species*), and D (*N. meningitidis*) are not known to be associated with Guillain-Barré syndrome.

Patients typically present complaining of ascending lower extremity weakness, which may be accompanied by paresthesias, or back or extremity pain. About 70% of patients will develop dysautonomia, most commonly tachycardia. Weakness will be evident on exam, and deep tendon reflexes will be diminished or absent. The incidence of Guillain-Barré syndrome increases with age and is slightly more common in males. Diagnosis is made initially by history and physical exam, followed by confirmatory studies including CSF analysis. In most cases CSF will show elevated protein and a normal WBC count. Nerve conduction studies and electromyography may also be used to confirm the diagnosis.

Test-taking tip: Some questions, like this one, are about memorization. The first step is recognizing the syndrome (Guillain-Barré syndrome), but if you have not memorized what organism is most commonly associated with it, don't waste time on the question. Pick an answer and move on to the next question.

35. ANSWER: D

This patient has Guillain-Barré syndrome. Treatment of Guillain-Barré syndrome involves supportive care as well as disease-modifying therapy. Disease-modifying therapy involves either administration of IV immunoglobulin or plasmapheresis because early treatment with these therapies shortens the disease course if initiated early. Respiratory failure should be addressed with intubation if warranted as in this patient, and care should be taken to prevent sequelae such as decubitus ulcers and deep venous thromboses while patients are immobilized.

Test-taking tip: If there are two answers that are relatively similar as in this question (IV immunoglobulin and plasma exchange, which are often both efficacious for the same condition), an answer grouping them together is likely to be correct.

36. ANSWER: B

This patient needs diphtheria antitoxin. Although the patient eats canned goods, his presentation is not consistent with botulism (A), which causes a descending weakness. Although penicillin (C) would have likely been administered if the diagnosis of diphtheria had been made earlier, this is mostly to prevent transmission rather than to stave off neurologic sequelae. Choice D would have been correct in a patient with MG, but we are not given a history of weakness throughout the day, and the improving bulbar symptoms with worsening extremity symptoms is not consistent with MG.

Diphtheria is an infection caused by the bacteria *Corynebacterium diphtheriae*, of which there are toxin-producing and non–toxin-producing strains. Non–toxin-producing strains often cause cutaneous diphtheria. Toxin-producing strains cause a pharyngeal infection that forms a pseudomembrane and can cause "bull neck" as a result of cervical lymphadenopathy. Sequelae of infection include cardiomyopathy, toxic shock, and diphtheric polyneuropathy.

Classically, diphtheric polyneuropathy presents 3 to 6 weeks after the initial infection and starts locally at the area of infection (e.g., the oropharynx) with symptoms such as dysphonia, palatal paralysis, and tongue numbness; other cranial nerves may be involved as well. These oral and bulbar symptoms improve as proximal motor weakness of the extremities begins, approximately 5 to 8 weeks after initial infection, leading to a "biphasic" symptom curve. Tachycardia, arrhythmias, and hypotension may also be seen as a result of autonomic dysfunction from the polyneuropathy or accompanying myocarditis. There were several recent outbreaks in Eastern Europe (notably Latvia and Belarus) among adults who had lost immunity from their childhood vaccination because they had not received boosters.

Treatment for diphtheria consists of early administration of IV penicillin and diphtheritic antitoxin. The purpose of antibiotic treatment is to prevent transmission to others, while the purpose of antitoxin treatment is to prevent cells from binding and taking up the toxin. The antitoxin may only be effective if administered early. Recovery of strength and sensation typically starts 2 to 3 months after symptom onset.

Test-taking tip: Several conditions can cause bulbar weakness that may be very similar in presentation. Among these are botulism, diphtheria, MG, and Guillain-Barré syndrome. The time course, muscles affected, and ascending versus descending weakness can help differentiate between them.

37. ANSWER: B

This patient's presentation is consistent with MG, and she may be having a myasthenic crisis as evidenced by her ptosis and tachypnea. MG typically presents with fluctuating weakness that worsens with use and often involves the ocular muscles. It is an autoimmune condition caused by antibodies to the acetylcholine receptor. Other potential diagnoses include Lambert-Eaton myasthenic syndrome (LEMS) or amyotrophic lateral sclerosis. The ice-pack test (Figure 12.6) is performed by placing an ice pack on the eyes of a patient with obvious ptosis (such as this patient), which improves the ptosis in patients with MG with a sensitivity of approximately 80%. The edrophonium test is another bedside test that can be used in patients with suspected MG and visible ptosis.

While forced vital capacity and negative inspiratory force (choice C) can help with the decision of when to electively intubate, these metrics are nonspecific, and the decision to intubate should not be based on a single value but rather on the overall clinical picture. It would be appropriate to take these measurements in this patient because she is tachypneic, but they will not help with the diagnosis.

Head CT (A) might be appropriate in this patient, but her presentation is not consistent with a stroke, hemorrhage, or intracranial tumor, so this test is also unlikely to confirm the diagnosis. Choice D, chest CT with contrast, may be appropriate at a later time to evaluate for a thymoma, which is frequently associated with MG.

Test-taking tip: Always be sure to fully read what the question is asking you—in this patient, many clinicians would first measure respiratory metrics (C) before performing the ice-pack test, which would be acceptable because the patient may require intubation. However, that is not what the question is asking; it asked which test would help make the diagnosis.

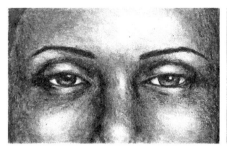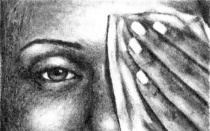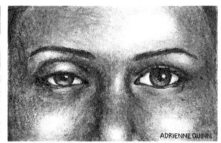

Figure 12.6 Myasthenia gravis ice-pack test.

38. ANSWER: D

All of the antibiotics listed (choices A, B, and C) can exacerbate the symptoms of MG.

MG is an autoimmune neurologic condition caused by antibodies to acetylcholine receptors. The main treatment strategies for this condition include symptomatic management with acetylcholinesterase inhibitors, short-term treatment with IV immunoglobulin or plasmapheresis, immunosuppressants and steroids for longer term therapy, and thymectomy. Patients with MG are also uniquely sensitive to many other medications, including antibiotics, which may worsen their symptoms and should be avoided because they can precipitate a myasthenic crisis (Table 12.2).

Test-taking tip: Process of elimination is again helpful in answering this question. If you know that both clindamycin and levofloxacin can worsen MG, you can

Table 12.2 MEDICATIONS REPORTED TO WORSEN MYASTHENIC SYMPTOMS

	SOME RISK FOR WORSENING SYMPTOMS	HIGHER RISK FOR WORSENING SYMPTOMS
Antibiotics	Macrolides	Fluoroquinolones
	Tetracyclines	Aminoglycosides
	Metronidazole	Ketolides
	Nitrofurantoin	Vancomycin
	Antiretrovirals	Clindamycin
Cardiac medications	Calcium channel blockers	β-Blockers
	Statins	Class Ia antiarrhythmics (e.g., procainamide)
Anesthetics	Local anesthetics (e.g., lidocaine) when injected intravenously	Neuromuscular blockers
Other	Glucocorticoids	Botulinum toxin
	Antiepileptics (e.g., phenytoin)	Magnesium

effectively eliminate each of them as the right answer because you are looking for a choice that includes both.

39. ANSWER: C

This patient's presentation is consistent with LEMS, which is often associated with malignancy, most commonly small cell lung cancer. Pancreatic cancer (A) has been associated with a migratory thrombophlebitis (Trousseau's syndrome), but not LEMS. Thymomas (B) are associated with MG, not LEMS. Insulinomas (D) would be associated with hypoglycemic episodes.

LEMS is characterized by proximal muscle weakness of the upper and lower extremities, which improves with repeated activity, unlike MG, which causes weakness that fatigues with repetition. LEMS is also less likely to have ocular involvement, which is a hallmark of MG. LEMS patients may have autonomic dysfunction and depressed deep tendon reflexes, which are less common in MG. Confirmatory electrophysiologic testing can be performed by a neurologist to definitively distinguish between the two.

LEMS is caused by an antibody to the voltage-gated calcium channel present at the neuromuscular junction. The antibody prevents calcium influx, which triggers acetylcholine release; the end result is less acetylcholine release and muscle weakness. The treatment involves identifying and treating the underlying cancer if present. If no cancer is identified, patients can be treated with immunosuppressants and acetylcholinesterase inhibitors, with chest CT scans every 6 months to evaluate for lung cancer.

Test-taking tip: This question has two steps—first identifying the condition described, and then matching it with a malignancy. If you are unsure of the condition being described, work backward from each answer choice (e.g., are there any conditions with fluctuating weakness associated with pancreatic cancer?) to match it to the condition in the question stem. This can help eliminate some of the choices.

40. ANSWER: C

This child has a presentation classic for infant botulism; however, she is breathing rapid shallow breaths and her pediatric GCS score is 7 or 8. After stabilizing the child's respiratory status with intubation, one would proceed to giving the appropriate antitoxin (B), in this case botulism immunoglobulin. If the patient had a history of ingesting opioids, a trial of naloxone would be indicated before intubation (A). If sepsis were suspected, starting IV fluids and antibiotics would be appropriate (D) after securing the airway.

Botulism is caused by *Clostridium botulinum*, a spore-forming bacteria that makes a variety of toxins (A–G) that bind the presynaptic membrane and prevent acetylcholine release. The clinical manifestations of this are symmetric cranial nerve palsies, followed by symmetric descending weakness and respiratory compromise. In infants, this presents as generalized weakness, poor feeding, a "floppy" baby, and even obstructive apnea from tongue weakness. Patients may also experience urinary retention and constipation. Toxins cannot cross blood-brain barrier, so the sensorium is unaffected.

There are a few important differences in the presentation of infant and adult botulism. Infant botulism accounts for the majority (70%) of botulism cases in the United States and results from the germination of ingested *C. botulinum* spores. Honey consumption has been linked to 20% of cases; other risk factors have not been quantified but may include exposure to vacuum cleaner dust, soil, or nearby construction. The higher pH of the infant gastrointestinal tract permits germination of these spores and toxin production, leading to botulism. Adult botulism is typically the result of exposure to *C. botulinum* through wound infection (most commonly from IV drug use) or less commonly from ingestion of improperly canned food or homemade prison alcohol ("pruno"). Treatment of both adult and infantile botulism involves supportive care with ventilatory support as needed and administration of equine antitoxin or human botulism immunoglobulin.

Test-taking tip: The challenge of this question is to identify the most urgent need of the patient. There are many clues in the question stem to lead you toward botulism (the patient's age, history of honey consumption, bulbar weakness), but her respiratory status is clearly compromised. Act first to stabilize the patient with intubation, and then treat her specific diagnosis.

41. ANSWER: A

This patient has tick paralysis. Tick paralysis is caused by gravid female ticks, most commonly of the genus *Dermacentor* in North America and *Ixodes* in Australia (Figure 12.7). Children are more frequently affected than adults, and ticks most frequently attach on the scalp or behind the ears. Onset of flaccid paralysis is rapid (<24 hours), may be preceded by a prodromal period of lethargy and muscle pain, and typically occurs between 3 and 7 days after tick attachment. The treatment is prompt removal of the offending tick, which leads to expeditious relief of symptoms (within 1.5 days), with excellent prognosis.

The differential diagnosis for symmetric ascending paralysis includes tick paralysis, Guillain-Barré syndrome, spinal cord lesions, and diphtheria. Botulism and poliomyelitis may also be considered, though botulism is typically descending in nature, and polio is generally asymmetric. There have been cases in the United States in which children were misdiagnosed with Guillain-Barré syndrome and even received plasmapheresis (B) and IV immunoglobulin before the tick was discovered. Checking a serum creatine kinase and starting corticosteroids would be the correct answer if polymyositis or dermatomyositis were suspected; however, muscle pain and rash were not mentioned, and weakness in these conditions is typically proximal. MRI of the lumbar spine and neurosurgical consult (D) are reasonable in a patient with symmetric lower extremity weakness because these can be signs of spinal cord compression or cauda equina syndrome, but should not be conducted before a full physical exam.

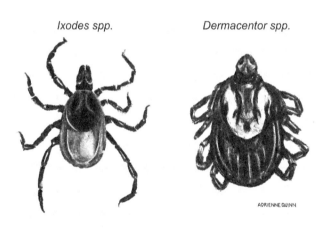

Ixodes spp.   *Dermacentor spp.*

ADRIENNE QUINN

Figure 12.7 Ticks.

Test-taking tip: In the absence of an unstable patient requiring immediate life-saving intervention, completing a full physical exam is likely to be the correct answer, particularly when coupled with a potentially curative intervention (tick removal).

42. ANSWER: A

There are four types of periodic paralysis (PP): hypokalemic, hyperkalemic, thyrotoxic, and Andersen-Tawil syndrome. The most common type is familial hypokalemic PP, which is caused by defective calcium channels. Attacks happen after a period of rest following vigorous exercise or during the night and early morning and can be provoked by carbohydrate-rich meals. Presentation is typically in the second decade of life. Serum potassium during an attack is low, but total body potassium is unaffected. Inheritance is autosomal dominant, with decreased penetrance in women. Affected individuals develop fixed proximal muscle weakness later in life (as in this patient's grandfather), but attacks decrease with age. Thyroid studies must be performed to evaluate for thyrotoxic PP, which should also be suspected in a patient with hypokalemia and PP. Treatment for acute episodes of hypokalemic PP is aimed at normalizing serum potassium with oral potassium supplementation. Patients should be counseled to avoid large carbohydrate loads to prevent future attacks. The carbonic anhydrase inhibitor dichlorphenamide has also been shown to decrease the frequency and severity of attacks.

Hyperkalemic PP is much less common than hypokalemic PP, usually presents in the first decade of life, and is characterized by muscle stiffness or weakness. It is the result of a sodium channelopathy. Potassium levels are usually elevated but may be normal during an attack. Attacks can be precipitated by rest following exercise and can be treated by carbohydrate-rich foods, inhaled ß-agonists, and light activity. Lifestyle modifications for hyperkalemic PP include avoiding potassium-rich foods and medications that increase serum potassium.

Andersen-Tawil syndrome is a genetic disorder characterized by the triad of PP, ventricular ectopy, and skeletal abnormalities and is caused by a defective potassium channel. These patients can have EKG abnormalities, including prolonged a QTc interval, U waves, premature ventricular contractions, ventricular bigeminy, and polymorphic ventricular tachycardia, and may even be asymptomatic from intermittent ventricular arrhythmias. Serum potassium can be elevated, low, or normal. Skeletal abnormalities include a small mandible, wide-set eyes, and low-set ears.

Test-taking tip: The PPs share many characteristics. Instead of trying to memorize each of the individual features of each type, remember that they are frequently associated with potassium derangements, and it is important to screen for thyroid abnormalities and long QT syndrome.

43. ANSWER: A

This patient has a presentation concerning for MS with optic neuritis, and MRI of the brain is the most appropriate test to support the diagnosis. If the presentation were consistent with MG, the edrophonium test (C) might be appropriate. A dilated funduscopic exam (B) would not be indicated unless an isolated ophthalmologic cause was suspected, and this exam should be performed only by an ophthalmologist.

MS is an autoimmune demyelinating disorder affecting the CNS, causing variable neurologic deficits. Common presentations include optic neuritis, focal weakness or paresthesias, urinary retention or incontinence, and constipation or fecal incontinence. Symptoms typically have their onset over a course of hours to days and improve or completely resolve over weeks to months, and they follow a relapsing and remitting course over the patient's lifetime. Physical exam may reveal an afferent pupillary defect (Marcus Gunn pupil, Figure 12.8), weakness or sensory loss, and upper motor neuron signs such as increased tone, hyperreflexia, positive Babinski's sign, and clonus.

The initial diagnostic test of choice after history and physical exam is MRI with contrast. MRI will usually reveal plaques in MS-typical locations (periventricular, juxtacortical, infratentorial, spinal cord). To fully confirm the diagnosis of MS, patients must have evidence of two different lesions separated by both space (CNS location) and time (two or more episodes). If the diagnosis cannot be made by history and MRI, LP (D) can be obtained, which would show oligoclonal bands or an increased CSF immunoglobulin G index.

Test-taking tip: Use process of elimination. Consider which diagnosis would be revealed by each answer choice and work backward—in this case, the edrophonium test and a funduscopic exam would not help with the diagnosis of MS, and LP should come after MRI when pursuing an MS diagnosis.

44. ANSWER: B

This patient has a presentation consistent with trigeminal neuralgia; however, in this patient with a history of MS, this likely represents an MS flare. The right leg weakness is another sign that this presentation is an MS flare.

Neurology consultation should be obtained for patients with suspected MS flares. Treatment of acute MS flares typically involves glucocorticoids, often IV methylprednisolone, which has been shown to shorten the duration of exacerbations. Immunomodulators, including natalizumab and interferon-ß, may be prescribed by neurologists. Special treatment considerations in the ED include monitoring for worsening respiratory status, testing for urinary tract infection/pyelonephritis in patients with urinary retention, and preparing for hypotension and aspiration if intubating because MS patients can be autonomically labile and have decreased gastric motility.

Test-taking tip: Think worst first. The trigeminal neuralgia described in this question is intended to distract you from the more serious diagnosis of an MS flare.

Afferent Pupillary Defect (Marcus-Gunn Pupil)

Left Eye Affected

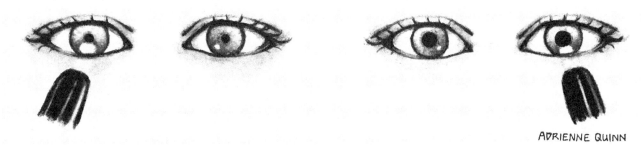

ADRIENNE QUINN

Figure 12.8 Marcus Gunn pupil: an afferent pupillary defect, demonstrated by dilation of the ipsilateral pupil when the light source is moved from the contralateral eye onto the ipsilateral eye.

45. ANSWER: B

This patient has Parkinson's disease (PD), as evidenced by his shuffling gait, tremor, and cogwheel rigidity. Prochlorperazine has antidopaminergic action and can worsen the symptoms of PD and so should not be given to this patient. Meclizine (A) would probably be safe for this patient, but his vomiting is not likely to be caused by vertigo because no dizziness is reported and he has had recent sick contacts. Ondansetron would also likely be safe. Diazepam has antiemetic effects and should be used with caution in those older than 65 years but would not be as dangerous for this patient (who is 62 years old) as prochlorperazine.

Parkinson's disease is a neurologic movement disorder thought to be caused by an imbalance of dopamine and acetylcholine in the CNS. The major symptoms of PD can be memorized with the pneumonic TRAP given in Table 12.3.

Table 12.3 MAJOR FEATURES OF PARKINSON'S DISEASE

Tremor	More severe at rest, described as "pill rolling," starts unilaterally, may be intermittent early in course of disease
Rigidity	Lead-pipe or cogwheel rigidity, may be unilateral or bilateral but asymmetric
Akinesia (bradykinesia)	Slowed movements, difficulty initiating movement, dragging or shuffling steps, "freezing"
Postural instability	Loss of postural reflexes, occurs late in disease, positive "pull test" (examiner pulls patient backward by shoulders, normal patient should be able to correct balance with one step)

Additional symptoms of parkinsonism include "mask facies," anosmia, constipation, sleep disturbance, cognitive dysfunction, hallucinations, and mood disorders. Treatment generally consists of direct dopaminergic agonists, medications that increase central dopamine levels, and anticholinergics. Patients with a history of PD on dopaminergic therapy may present to the ED with arrhythmias, orthostatic hypotension, dyskinesias, and dystonic reactions. Any adjustment of medication should be done in conjunction with the patient's primary care provider or neurologist.

Test-taking tip: Reading the last line of the question stem and the answer choices before reading the full question stem can help improve efficiency. In this case, reading the answer choices and last line would prime you to be searching for a condition that interacts with one of the medications, making you more likely to pick up on the Parkinson's diagnosis.

46. ANSWER: A

This patient has a simple febrile seizure and should be given acetaminophen for the fever and discharge with follow-up with the primary pediatrician. Further diagnostic workup (B, C) is not indicated in this patient with a clear history of simple febrile seizure, who is behaving normally, and who likely has roseola (her brother's presentation is consistent with roseola). Observation for 24 hours is not necessary. LP is appropriate in patients with simple febrile seizure if they have meningeal signs, are younger than 1 year and are not fully vaccinated, or have been taking antibiotics, which may mask infectious symptoms.

The decision of when to pursue further laboratory workup for complex febrile seizures is more difficult and is based on clinical suspicion, though it can safely be deferred if the patient returns to baseline in the ED. Parents should be educated about febrile seizures before discharge, particularly about the fact that patients with simple febrile seizures are not at higher risk for lifelong epilepsy.

The follow criteria define a *febrile seizure*:

1. The patient must be 6 months to 5 years of age.
2. The patient may not have a history of afebrile seizures.
3. The patient may not have intracranial infection or metabolic derangement.
4. The patient must have a temperature >38° C (100.4° F).

If the following criteria are present, the seizure is classified as a *simple febrile seizure*:

1. The patient must have had only one seizure within a 24-hour period.
2. The seizure must be generalized tonic-clonic.
3. The seizure must last <15 minutes.
4. There must be no persistence of neurologic deficit beyond post-ictal state.
5. The patient may not have had any previous neurologic problems.

If the following are present, the seizure is classified as a *complex febrile seizure*:

1. Recurrent within 24 hours
2. Focal seizure activity
3. Lasts >15 minutes
4. Persistence of neurologic deficit (e.g., Todd's paresis) beyond post-ictal state

Test-taking tip: The challenge in this case is determining that this patient is not sick. Seizures can be very frightening to parents, but knowing that the patient is well-appearing and back to baseline with a normal neurologic exam can reassure the clinician and parent that this was a simple febrile seizure (if the previous criteria are met) and that the patient is safe to go home.

47. ANSWER: B

This patient has shaken baby syndrome, which is associated with subdural hematomas. Neuroimaging is indicated in this case because the patient does not have a history of seizure, has a neurologic deficit (listless and decreased movement of right arm), and has signs of trauma (arm bruising). The absence of any history of trauma despite physical exam findings should raise suspicion for nonaccidental trauma. Epidural hematoma (D) is also possible but is more likely in the case of accidental trauma. Intracerebral abscess (A) and

normal head CT (C) might also be possible but are less likely in a patient with this presentation.

The most common type of seizure in the pediatric population is the febrile seizure. For pediatric patients presenting with a first afebrile seizure, a fingerstick glucose and EKG should be obtained to evaluate for hypoglycemia or arrhythmia. If these are unremarkable, most of these patients can be managed with referral for outpatient EEG and primary care physician follow-up if they are back to baseline in the ED, and emergent neuroimaging is not recommended. Almost 50% of them will never have another seizure. However, there are certain features that may increase the suspicion for a focal intracranial process and lead clinicians to obtain emergent neuroimaging, which are described in Table 12.4. If available, MRI is more sensitive for intracranial abnormalities, though it also requires patients to lie still for a prolonged period and may be logistically challenging to obtain.

Table 12.4 ELEMENTS THAT LOWER THE THRESHOLD FOR EMERGENT NEUROIMAGING

HISTORY OF PRESENT ILLNESS	PAST MEDICAL HISTORY	PHYSICAL
Age <6 months	Hematologic disorder	Altered level of consciousness
Focal seizure, age <3 years	Malignancy	Persistent post-ictal state
Seizure lasting >15 minutes	HIV	Focal neurologic deficit
Closed head injury	Ventriculoperitoneal shunt	Evidence of trauma
Travel to area with endemic cysticercosis	Known neurologic disorder	Any other abnormality

Test-taking tip: Sometimes more than one answer choice is reasonable, and a determination must be made based on the likelihood of each condition. The more elements in the question stem indicating a particular answer choice, the more likely it will that that choice is the correct one.

48. ANSWER: D

This patient is actively seizing. In neonates, the preferred agent for seizure after three doses of benzodiazepines is phenobarbital. The other agents mentioned are all reasonable choices for older children in status epilepticus.

Neonatal seizures often present with only subtle findings such as eye deviation or lip smacking. The most common cause for neonatal seizures is hypoxic-ischemic encephalopathy, and these patients usually present in the first 48 hours after birth. Intracranial hemorrhage is also a common cause for neonatal seizure, accounting for about 10% of seizures. Premature infants are at higher risk for intracranial hemorrhage.

Table 12.5 SEIZURE MIMICS

PATIENT AGE	SIGNS/SYMPTOMS	ELEMENTS SUGGESTIVE OF DIAGNOSIS
Any age	Arrhythmia	Family history of sudden cardiac death
	Syncope	
	Dystonic reaction	
Infant to toddler	Benign sleep myoclonus	Jerky movements in sleep without arousal
	Hyperekplexia	Exaggerated startle to touch/sound
	Jitteriness	Symmetric tremor improving with restraint
	Shuddering attacks	Rapid shivering of head/trunk/shoulder
	Breath-holding spells	Occurs after minor injury or emotional upset
	Opsoclonus-myoclonus-ataxia syndrome	Palpable abdominal mass crossing midline
	Self-gratification disorder	Self-stimulation or repeated thigh adduction
Children	Psychogenic nonepileptic seizures	Incontinence rare, tongue biting rare, last >2 minutes, comorbid psychiatric conditions
	Migraines (confusional, basilar)	
	Sleep disorders (night terrors, sleepwalking, narcolepsy)	
	Tics	Repetitive nonrhythmic movements or vocalizations, onset age 6–7 years
	Stereotypies	Repetitive movements that can be voluntarily suppressed, no evolution over time, resolve with distraction, onset <3 years of age
	Paroxysmal dyskinesia	Choreoathetosis or dystonia precipitated by exercise, movement, or other stressors

As with older children, a glucose level should be rapidly obtained. In neonates, lab workup is more likely to be helpful than in older children, and it is reasonable to check electrolytes and blood counts because these may guide therapy. Emergent neuroimaging should be obtained to evaluate for hemorrhage or congenital malformations, and the modality of choice is CT (though MRI may be higher yield if rapidly available and the patient is stable). Initial treatment should include stabilization of airway, breathing, and circulation and administration of benzodiazepines. If the patient continues to seize after three doses of benzodiazepines, phenobarbital should be initiated (for neonates). Phenobarbital can cause significant respiratory depression, so intubation may be necessary. Starting antibiotic therapy early and obtaining cultures are also indicated because sepsis/meningitis is possible.

49. ANSWER: C

Breath-holding spells are very common and occur in up to 5% of children aged 6 months to 5 years, usually following a minor injury or emotional upset. They can be associated with abnormal movements mimicking seizure-like activity (Table 12.5), but unlike seizures, breath-holding spells have no post-ictal period. Breath-holding spells can be associated with iron deficiency, so checking a hemoglobin and providing iron supplementation if indicated can help reduce the frequency of attacks.

If the patient had a significant post-ictal period, the diagnosis of generalized tonic-clonic seizure would be more likely (A). Cardiac arrhythmia (B) remains on the differential but would be much less likely than a breath-holding spell. Narcolepsy (D) would more likely present as a "drop attack," or sudden loss of tone, than with the described presentation and would likely present at an older age (5–6 years).

Test-taking tip: This is another question for which process of elimination helps you. If it had been a seizure, she would have been post-ictal, and you might have also expected a fever (because febrile seizure is the most common seizure type in this age group), eliminating option A. The description does not sound like the child fell asleep suddenly, eliminating D. When comparing B and C, you must then choose which is more common (in the absence of any cardiac history or other clues to point you toward arrhythmia), which is C, breath-holding spell.

13.

OBSTETRICS AND GYNECOLOGIC EMERGENCIES

Deena Bengiamin and Miranda Lewis

1. A 36-year-old G5P4 female at 32 weeks' gestation presents with vaginal bleeding for 6 hours. She denies any pain or leakage of fluids. There was no recent trauma. Vital signs are heart rate (HR) 86 bpm, blood pressure (BP) 106/64 mm Hg, temperature 37.7° C, respiratory rate (RR) 14 breaths/min, and SpO$_2$ 98%. Two large-bore IV lines are placed, and blood type and screen are obtained. What is the next best step in management?

A. Perform a sterile speculum exam
B. Obtain a transvaginal obstetric (OB) ultrasound
C. Perform a sterile digital vaginal exam
D. Obtain a ferning and Nitrazine test

2. A 35-year-old female presents with sudden-onset, severe, 10/10 right lower quadrant (RLQ) pain with associated nausea and emesis. On exam, the patient has RLQ tenderness. A transvaginal ultrasound is performed and shows normal adnexa bilaterally with normal arterial flow to both ovaries and a 5.2-cm cystic mass. Urine pregnancy test is negative. What is the next best step in management?

A. Discharge the patient home with strict return precautions and gynecology follow-up
B. Obtain a urinalysis
C. Obtain a computed tomography (CT) scan of the abdomen and pelvis
D. Urgent gynecology consult

3. A 30-year-old female, postpartum day 2 after normal spontaneous vaginal delivery, presents with seizure activity and hypertension. She was treated for presumptive eclamptic seizure with 4 g IV magnesium and started on a magnesium infusion at 2 g/hr. Which of the following is *not* a potential symptom of magnesium toxicity?

A. Hyperactive patellar reflexes
B. Respiratory depression
C. Hypothermia
D. Cardiac conduction abnormalities

4. A 28-year-old female presents in active labor. The fetal head is delivered, but repeated attempts at downward traction fail to deliver the anterior shoulder, and the head is tightly compressed against the perineum. McRobert's maneuver is performed with no progression of fetal movement. Which of the following maneuvers should be attempted next?

A. Apply firm downward fundal pressure
B. Perform posterior midline episiotomy
C. Apply steady downward suprapubic pressure
D. Fracture the anterior fetal clavicle using steady posterior pressure

5. A 27-year-old pregnant female at 26 weeks' gestation presents with mild periumbilical abdominal pain after being involved in a motor vehicle collision. She was the restrained passenger in a motor vehicle traveling 40 mph, which was struck on the rear passenger's side of the vehicle. On arrival to the emergency department (ED), she is alert and oriented with HR 90 bpm, BP 106/84 mm Hg, and RR 16 breaths/min. The patient has abdominal tenderness and a small amount of vaginal bleeding. Which of the following is true regarding this patient's presentation and probable diagnosis?

A. A normal ultrasound essentially rules out this diagnosis
B. A period of at least 4 hours of fetal monitoring is warranted for all patients suspected of having this diagnosis
C. This diagnosis is almost always precipitated by trauma
D. Patients with this diagnosis classically present with painless vaginal bleeding

6. A 25-year-old G3P2 female at 36 weeks' gestation presents with right upper quadrant (RUQ) pain that has been progressively worsening for 2 days with associated nausea, emesis, and malaise. Initial vital signs

are HR 86 bpm, BP 144/92 mm Hg, RR 18 breaths/min, and temperature 37° C. Initial labs show hematocrit 32%, platelets 88,000, aspartate aminotransferase (AST) 313 U/L, total bilirubin 1.5 mg/dL, and elevated lactate dehydrogenase (LDH) at 720. What is the most likely diagnosis?

A. Viral hepatitis
B. Cholestasis of pregnancy
C. HELLP syndrome
D. Preeclampsia

7. A 18-year-old female postpartum day 2 after cesarean delivery presents with abdominal pain and uterine tenderness. She is exclusively breastfeeding and denies any breast tenderness or discharge. Initial vital signs are HR 110 bpm, BP 94/60 mm Hg, temperature 39° C, RR 20 breaths/min, and SpO$_2$ 97%. Examination reveals uterine fundal tenderness and foul-smelling lochia. Breast examination is unremarkable. What is the most likely diagnosis and appropriate empiric treatment?

A. Pyelonephritis; ciprofloxacin
B. Normal postpartum fever; no treatment needed
C. Endometritis; doxycycline and metronidazole
D. Endometritis; clindamycin, gentamycin, and vancomycin

8. A 25-year-old G1P0 female presents at 36 weeks' gestation with regular contractions every 5 minutes. She reports a gush of watery discharge just before arrival. What steps should be taken to evaluate for preterm labor and premature rupture of membranes?

A. Obtain ferning and Nitrazine tests
B. Perform digital cervical examination to evaluate for dilation, effacement, and station
C. Perform non-sterile speculum exam to visualize the cervix
D. OB consult

9. Which of the following is *not* an appropriate dose/indication for the use of RhoGAM to prevent alloimmunization in an Rh-negative pregnant woman?

A. One 50-mcg dose for ectopic pregnancy in an 8-week gestation
B. One 300-mcg dose for ectopic pregnancy in an 8-week gestation
C. One 50-mcg dose for blunt abdominal trauma in a 32-week gestation
D. One 300-mcg dose for blunt abdominal trauma in a 32-week gestation

10. A 36-year-old G3P2 female who is 32 weeks' pregnant and has a history of gestational hypertension presents with RUQ pain for 1 day. Pain is 7/10, constant, nonradiating, and associated with headache, nausea, and emesis. Physical examination reveals tenderness in the RUQ and epigastric region and 2+ pitting edema bilaterally. Vital signs are BP 142/94 mm Hg, HR 88 bpm, RR 18 breaths/min, and SpO$_2$ 97% on room air. Which laboratory abnormalities would be expected based on the most likely diagnosis?

A. AST 290, alanine aminotransferase (ALT) 253, total bilirubin 2.2, platelets 90,000, schistocytes on peripheral smear, LDH 700, creatinine 0.9
B. AST 290, ALT 253, total bilirubin 2.2, platelets 200,000, normal red blood cells (RBCs) on peripheral smear, LDH 200, creatinine 0.9
C. AST 38, ALT 30, total bilirubin 1.0, platelets 90,000, schistocytes on peripheral smear, LDH 700, creatinine 1.5
D. AST 38, ALT 30, total bilirubin 1.0, platelets 200,000, schistocytes on peripheral smear, LDH 700, creatinine 1.5

11. A 20-year-old female patient at 32 weeks' gestation presents with malodorous vaginal discharge for 5 days. Vital signs are within normal limits, and speculum examination reveals copious thin, malodorous, homogenous, white vaginal discharge. Clue cells are seen on wet mount. Which of the following is an acceptable approach to management of bacterial vaginosis in this patient?

A. Defer treatment until after delivery
B. Metronidazole 500 mg twice daily for 7 days
C. Topical 2% clindamycin cream intravaginally once daily for 5 days
D. All of the above are acceptable treatment options

12. A 20-year-old female presents with vaginal discharge and lower abdominal pain for 5 days. She reports yellowish discharge with 6/10, cramping, suprapubic pain. She is sexually active with one male partner and uses condoms intermittently. Last menstrual period (LMP) was 10 days ago. Vital signs are HR 102 bpm, BP 124/76 mm Hg, RR 16 breaths/min, and temperature 37.1° C. On pelvic exam, there is copious mucopurulent discharge and cervical motion tenderness. She has suprapubic tenderness on abdominal exam. Labs reveal negative quantitative β-human chorionic gonadotropin (β-hCG), no leukocytosis, and normal wet mount, and gonorrhea and chlamydia by amplified DNA are pending. Urinalysis shows no evidence of infection. Transvaginal ultrasound with Doppler is normal. What is the appropriate empiric treatment for this patient?

A. Ceftriaxone 250 mg IM once and azithromycin 1 g PO once

B. Ceftriaxone 250 mg IM once and doxycycline 100 mg twice daily for 14 days

C. Metronidazole 500 mg twice daily for 7 days

D. Both A and B are acceptable

13. A 30-year-old female with no significant medical history presents with intermittent right-sided pelvic pain for 2 days. Pain is aching, 3/10, and nonradiating and is exacerbated with sexual intercourse. There is no associated fever, nausea, emesis, or diarrhea. LMP was approximately 2 weeks ago. Vital signs are HR 82 bpm, BP 114/74 mm Hg, RR 16 beats/min, temperature 36.9° C, and SpO₂ 98%. Labs are obtained, and quantitative β-hCG is negative, urinalysis is normal, and hemoglobin is 13.2. Pelvic ultrasound is performed and shows a 3-cm, thin-walled unilocular cyst in the right adnexa. There is normal Doppler flow to bilateral ovaries. What is the most appropriate management for this patient?

A. Admit for management of complicated cyst rupture

B. Refer to outpatient gynecology for follow-up

C. Obtain pelvic magnetic resonance imaging (MRI)

D. Immediate OB consultation

14. A 23-year-old female at 10 weeks' gestation presents with vaginal bleeding for 3 hours. She reports some mild cramping with a small amount of vaginal bleeding and has not noted any passage of large clots or tissue. Vaginal exam shows minimal blood in the vaginal vault and dilation of the cervix. A transabdominal ultrasound is obtained, and findings are shown in Figure 13.1. There is no fetal heart activity. What is the diagnosis?

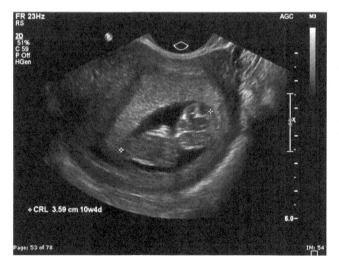

Figure 13.1 Transabdominal ultrasound.

A. Threatened abortion

B. Incomplete abortion

C. Inevitable abortion

D. Complete abortion

15. A 37-year-old female presents with fever and abdominal pain that has been progressively worsening for 2 days. She recently underwent a dilation and curettage for a spontaneous abortion at 13 week' gestation. Ultrasound shows retained products of conception. On pelvic exam, the patient is noted to have malodorous vaginal discharge and uterine tenderness with an open cervical os. Vital signs are BP 110/72 mm Hg, HR 108 bpm, RR 20 breaths/min, temperature 38.9° C. In addition to OB consultation, what is the appropriate treatment for this patient?

A. Ampicillin/sulbactam IV, gentamycin IV, and misoprostol PO

B. Ampicillin/sulbactam IV, gentamycin IV, and misoprostol intravaginal

C. Ampicillin/sulbactam IV, gentamycin IV, and expectant management

D. Ampicillin/sulbactam IV, gentamycin IV, and dilation and curettage

16. You are the only physician in a small rural hospital with no OB capabilities. A 20-year-old female at 11 weeks' gestation presents with worsening nausea and emesis since the beginning of her pregnancy. She reports frequent bouts of emesis and states that she has been unable to keep any fluids or foods down for the past several days. Additionally, she reports RUQ and epigastric pain for 3 days. Initial vital signs are BP 94/62 mm Hg, HR 102 bpm, RR 16 breaths/min, and temperature 37.1° C. On initial urinalysis the patient is noted to have 3+ ketones without evidence of infection. Complete blood count (CBC) shows white blood cells (WBCs) 8.2 and hemoglobin (Hgb) 15.6. Blood chemistry shows potassium 3.0.

The patient is given 2 L of lactated Ringer's solution, electrolytes are repleted, and she is given 8 mg Zofran IV with resolution of hypokalemia and ketonuria. Nausea is somewhat improved with Zofran, and there are no further bouts of emesis in the ED. What is the most appropriate disposition for this patient at this time?

A. Discharge home with obstetrician follow-up

B. Continue workup in the ED

C. Admit for observation

D. Transfer to a facility with OB capabilities

17. Which of the following statements is *false* regarding hydatidiform mole (gestational trophoblastic disease)?

A. β-hCG levels are often >100,000
B. In cases in which there is progression to choriocarcinoma, the prognosis is generally good
C. Symptoms include hyperemesis, vaginal bleeding, and pregnancy-induced hypertension
D. Vaginal bleeding in a Rh(D)-negative woman with a molar pregnancy does not warrant RhoGAM administration because hydatidiform mole arises from maternal tissue
E. All of the above are true

18. A 26-year-old G4P3 female at 38 weeks' gestation presents with regular uterine contractions that are approximately 2 minutes apart. Examination reveals a fully dilated cervix, complete effacement, and +1 station. What stage of labor is this patient in?

A. Latent phase
B. Active phase
C. Second stage
D. Third stage

19. A 30-year-old female at 39 weeks' gestation presents in active labor. Bimanual examination reveals a pulsatile cord in the vaginal vault and the fetal head at 0 station. What is the next best step in management?

A. Using two Kelly forceps, clamp the umbilical cord and cut between the clamps
B. Attempt to reduce the cord using firm, steady pressure
C. Insert a hand into the vagina and attempt to elevate the fetal head
D. Place the patient in reverse Trendelenburg position

20. A 29-year-old G5P4 female with a history of polysubstance abuse and asthma presents at 32 weeks' gestation in active labor. She felt a gush of fluid approximately 1 hour ago and has since been experiencing contractions of increasing intensity. Sterile speculum exam is performed and reveals what appears to be a fetal buttock and a cervix that is 10 cm dilated. Bedside ultrasound confirms that the fetal presentation is frank breech. Stat OB consultation is requested and is pending, but there is no in-house obstetrician, and estimated arrival time is 15 minutes. What is the appropriate management of this delivery?

A. Allow delivery to proceed spontaneously; deliver the head by placing the fingers on the maxillary bone to produce slight flexion of the fetal head, keeping the body in a horizontal plane while a delivery assistant applies suprapubic pressure
B. Administer tocolytics as a temporizing measure while awaiting emergency cesarean delivery

C. Allow delivery to proceed spontaneously; deliver the head with gentle steady traction in the horizontal plane while a delivery assistant applies suprapubic pressure
D. Allow delivery to proceed spontaneously; deliver the head by applying gentle pressure on the occiput to slightly extend the neck while a delivery assistant applies suprapubic pressure.

21. A 25-year-old G1P0 female at 38 weeks' gestation presents in active labor. The patient is completely dilated, 100% effaced, and at 1+ station, and delivery is imminent. Initial vital signs are HR 98 bpm, BP 126/78 mm Hg, RR 18 breaths/min, and SpO$_2$ 98% on room air. The patient reports that she has no significant medical history and no allergies. As labor progresses and the patient begins to push, she becomes increasingly agitated and confused. The patient suddenly develops severe respiratory distress, and oxygen saturations are 88% on a non-rebreather mask at 15 L/min. Blood pressure is 86/44 mm Hg. The patient subsequently develops significant vaginal bleeding. What findings are expected based on the most likely diagnosis?

A. Bedside echocardiogram demonstrating severely dilated, hypokinetic right ventricle
B. Elevated D-dimer, low fibrinogen, prolonged partial thromboplastin time (PTT)
C. Chest radiograph showing diffuse pulmonary edema
D. All of the above

22. A 26-year-old female presents in labor. Delivery is progressing normally. After the delivery of the fetal head, a nuchal cord is palpated. What should be the first step in management?

A. Clamp and cut the cord
B. Slip the loop of umbilical cord over the infant's head
C. Apply forceful traction to the umbilical cord to lengthen the cord for reduction
D. Stat OB consult

23. All but which of the following medications have known teratogenic effects in pregnancy?

A. Ondansetron
B. Warfarin
C. Phenytoin
D. Lisinopril

24. A 38-year-old G7P6 female presents on postpartum day 0 with heavy vaginal bleeding. She delivered a 3,900-g full-term infant 2 hours ago at home. Thirty minutes before arrival, she began to experience heavy vaginal bleeding. She had a normal pregnancy and has no

underlying medical conditions. Examination reveals a first-degree perineal laceration, heavy vaginal bleeding, and a soft uterine fundus. Vital signs are HR 114 bpm, BP 104/76 mm Hg, RR 18 breaths/min, and temperature 37.1° C. Initial resuscitation is initiated with IV fluids, and the patient is typed and crossmatched for 2 units of blood. The patient continues to have heavy bleeding with a soft uterine fundus despite bimanual uterine massage. What is the next step in management?

A. Repair the perineal laceration
B. Misoprostol 1,000 mcg rectally
C. Balloon tamponade with a Bakri catheter
D. Oxytocin 10 units intramuscular

25. A 20-year-old female at 12 weeks' gestation presents with dysuria and increased vaginal discharge for 3 days. On pelvic examination, the cervical os is closed, and there is thin white discharge in the vaginal vault with no bleeding. The patient is diagnosed with bacterial vaginosis, and treatment is initiated. In the course of her ED evaluation, an ultrasound is performed that shows an intrauterine pregnancy with size that is consistent with a 12-week gestation, shown in Figure 13.2, and absent fetal heart tones. The patient has normal vital signs with no abdominal pain. Which of the following is *not* an acceptable option for the management of this patient?

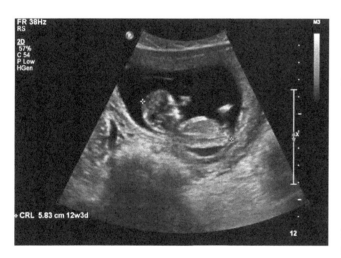

Figure 13.2. Transvaginal ultrasound.

A. Discharge to home with intravaginal misoprostol and OB follow=up in 5 days
B. Admission for dilation and curettage
C. Discharge to home with buccal misoprostol and OB follow=up in 5 days
D. All of the above are acceptable treatment options

26. A 19-year-old G2P1 female presents to the ED with vaginal bleeding and pelvic pain for 8 hours. Pain is cramping, 8/10, left-sided, and nonradiating. The patient reports that the amount of vaginal bleeding is consistent with a mild period. The patient denies passage of tissue. LMP was approximately 5 weeks ago. Physical exam reveals suprapubic and left lower quadrant tenderness. Vital signs are HR 102 bpm, BP 120/76 mm Hg, RR 16 breaths/min, temperature 37.4° C, SpO$_2$ 98% on room air. Quantitative hCG is 54.6 mIU/mL. Hemoglobin is 11.6 g/dL. Transvaginal ultrasound is obtained as shown in Figure 13.3. There is a 2-cm adnexal mass visualized. No gestational sac or fetal pole is seen, and there is no intrauterine pregnancy seen. What is the most appropriate management for this patient?

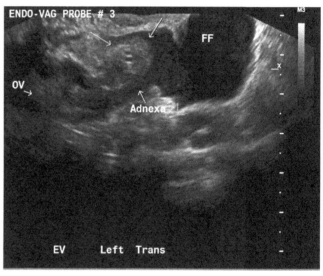

Figure 13.3 Transvaginal ultrasound.

A. Discharge home and have the patient return in 48 hours for a repeat quantitative β-hCG level
B. Immediate gynecologic consultation in the ED
C. Discharge home with methotrexate and gynecologic follow-up
D. Admit for serial abdominal exams and hemograms

27. A 27-year-old female at 24 weeks and 6 days of gestation presents with flank pain and dysuria for 4 days. She reports nausea and one episode of emesis before arrival. Vital signs are HR 98 bpm, BP 110/74 mm Hg, RR 18 breaths/min, temperature 38.3° C, and SpO$_2$ 99% on room air. On exam, the patient has left costovertebral angle tenderness and no abdominal or uterine tenderness. CBC and chemistry are normal. Urinalysis is remarkable for 1+ nitrites, 2+ leukocyte esterase, 10 WBCs, 3 RBCs, and many bacteria. What is the most appropriate treatment and disposition for this patient?

A. Admit to the hospital and initiate treatment with IV Rocephin

B. Discharge home with 10 days of oral cephalexin and prompt OB follow-up

C. Admit to the hospital and initiate treatment with IV ciprofloxacin

D. Discharge home with 10 days of oral nitrofurantoin and prompt OB follow-up

28. An 18-year-old female at 26 weeks' gestation presents with RLQ abdominal pain, nausea, malaise, and fever progressively worsening for 1 day. She denies any emesis, diarrhea, or dysuria. Her pregnancy has been uncomplicated to date. She has no significant prior medical history and has never had surgery before. Vital signs are HR 102 bpm, BP 106/72 mm Hg, RR 18 breaths/min, temperature 38.4° C, and SpO$_2$ 99% on room air. On exam, the patient is noted to be in moderate distress. Abdominal exam reveals a gravid uterus with no fundal tenderness and RLQ rebound tenderness. There is no costovertebral angle tenderness. Labs are obtained and are notable for WBCs 13.6; normal lactic acid, lipase, and liver function tests; and urinalysis showing no bacteria. Abdominal ultrasound is obtained and shows normal kidneys without hydronephrosis, normal gallbladder without stones or sludge, and a fetus whose size is consistent with a 26-week gestation with a HR of 150 bpm. The appendix is not visualized. What is the most appropriate next step in diagnosis?

A. MRI

B. Radiograph

C. Repeat ultrasound

D. Consult surgery

29. A 20-year-old female presents with malodorous discharge for the past 2 weeks. She endorses burning vaginal pain, pruritus, and dysuria. She is sexually active with two male partners and uses condoms intermittently. LMP was approximately 3 weeks ago. Vital signs are HR 86 bpm, BP 118/76 mm Hg, RR 16 breaths/min, temperature 37.1° C, and SpO$_2$ 99% on room air. Pelvic examination reveals vulvar erythema and thin malodorous discharge. Wet mount demonstrates motile trichomonads. Which of the following is *false* regarding *Trichomonas* infection?

A. Oral metronidazole is the treatment of choice for symptomatic pregnant and nonpregnant patients

B. Sexual partners generally do not need to be treated unless they are symptomatic

C. Wet mount is not very sensitive for detection of *Trichomonas vaginalis*

D. Infection with *T. vaginalis* significantly increases the risk for HIV transmission

30. A 23-year-old female presents with burning vaginal pain and dysuria for 3 days, now with subjective fever and malaise that started today. The patient denies vaginal discharge, bleeding, abdominal pain, nausea, vomiting, or diarrhea. She is sexually active with one male partner and does not use condoms. LMP was 20 days ago. Vital signs are HR 96 bpm, BP 114/72 mm Hg, RR 18 breaths/min, temperature 38.2° C, and SpO$_2$ 98% on room air. On exam, the patient has no abdominal tenderness. Pelvic exam reveals grouped vesicular lesions on an erythematous base over the vulva and tender inguinal lymphadenopathy. Which of the following is *true* regarding diagnosis of this infection?

A. The Tzanck test is the most reliable for diagnosing this condition given its high sensitivity and specificity

B. Viral culture is highly sensitive, especially in recurrent infections

C. Patients with positive type-specific herpes simplex virus type 1 (HSV-1) antibodies most likely have anogenital infection

D. Negative viral culture and polymerase chain reaction (PCR) do not indicate absence of infection

31. A 20-year-old female presents with painful genital ulcers and lymphadenopathy for 1 week. The patient states that the lesion started out as a tender "bump," which then eroded, and she subsequently developed purulent discharge. She also reports tender lymphadenopathy bilaterally. She denies any fever, chills, abdominal pain, or malaise. She is sexually active with multiple male partners and uses condoms intermittently. Vital signs are HR 86 bpm, BP 122/78 mm Hg, RR 16 breaths/min, temperature 37.2° C, and SpO$_2$ 98% on room air. On examination, the patient has two 1-cm ulcers present bilaterally and symmetrically near the vaginal introitus. The margins of the ulcers are sharp and undermined. The ulcer base is covered with purulent exudate. There are tender palpable inguinal lymph nodes. Darkfield examination and serologic tests for *Treponema pallidum* is negative, and HSV PCR is negative. What is the most likely diagnosis?

A. Bartholin's abscess

B. Primary syphilis

C. Chancroid

D. Lymphogranuloma venereum (LGV)

32. A 36-year-old female with a history of diabetes presents with left-sided tender inguinal lymphadenopathy for 2 weeks. She also reports chills and decreased appetite. On review of systems, the patient does recall that she had a painless vaginal lesion several weeks ago

that spontaneously resolved. She denies any vaginal discharge, abdominal pain, night sweats, or weight loss. Vital signs are HR 90 bpm, BP 110/72 mm Hg, RR 16 breaths/min, temperature 38.2° C, and SpO₂ 99% on room air. On exam, tender and firm inguinal lymph nodes are palpable with no fluctuance. There are no lower extremity lesions or edema. Vaginal exam is unremarkable. There is no rash. CBC, chemistry, and urinalysis are unremarkable. Rapid plasma reagin (RPR) and rapid treponemal testing are negative. What is the most likely causative agent?

A. *Chlamydia trachomatis,* L1, L2, or L3 serovars
B. *Haemophilus ducreyi*
C. *T. pallidum*
D. Polymicrobial infection

33. A 26-year-old G3P2 female at 12 weeks' gestation presents with rash for several days. She endorses some low-grade fever and mild headache. She denies any pruritis. She has no significant medical history and reports a severe penicillin allergy. On exam, the patient is noted to have a diffuse papulosquamous rash involving the palms of the hands and lymphadenopathy. RPR and rapid treponemal assay tests are positive. What are the appropriate disposition and treatment for this patient?

A. Admit to the hospital and treat with parenteral doxycycline
B. Admit to the hospital for penicillin desensitization and treat with parenteral penicillin G
C. Discharge home with a course of oral doxycycline and follow-up testing for nontreponemal antibody titers
D. Discharge home with a course of oral azithromycin and follow-up testing for nontreponemal antibody titers

34. A 20-year-old female presents with abnormal vaginal discharge and vaginal pain for the past 3 days. She denies any fever, dysuria, urinary frequency, nausea, or emesis. She is sexually active with one new male partner and uses condoms intermittently. She has no significant medical history. Vital signs are HR 82 bpm, BP 118/66 mm Hg, RR 18 breaths/min, SpO₂ 98%, and temperature 37° C. Abdominal exam reveals a soft and nontender abdomen with normal bowel tones. Pelvic exam reveals a friable cervix and mucopurulent cervical discharge. There is no cervical motion tenderness. Wet mount shows no clue cells, no fungal elements, and no trichomonads. Urinalysis shows 10 WBCs per high-power field, 2 RBCs per high-power field, no bacteria, and no squamous cells. CBC is unremarkable.

Gonorrhea and chlamydia tests are obtained, but results will not be available for about 24 hours. What are the most appropriate disposition and treatment of this patient?

A. Admit and treat empirically with parenteral azithromycin pending gonorrhea and chlamydia test results
B. Treat presumptively with a single dose of 1g PO azithromycin and 250 mg IM ceftriaxone and discharge home with plan for primary care physician follow-up
C. Defer treatment until the results of the gonorrhea and chlamydia tests are available and discharge home with plan for follow-up
D. Treat presumptively with oral metronidazole 500 mg twice daily for 7 days and PO doxycycline 100 mg twice daily for 7 days and discharge home with plan for primary care physician follow-up.

35. Which of the following describes the correct procedure for managing a Bartholin's abscess?

A. Clean and prepare the area, infiltrate with local anesthetic, make a small linear stab incision from the mucosal surface of the labia, break apart loculations using hemostats, insert and inflate a Word catheter
B. Clean and prepare the area, infiltrate with local anesthetic, make a small linear stab incision from the cutaneous surface of the labia, break apart loculations using hemostats, insert and inflate a Word catheter
C. Clean and prepare the area, infiltrate with local anesthetic, make bilateral small linear incisions from the cutaneous and mucosal surfaces of the labia, break apart loculations using hemostats, insert and inflate a Word catheter
D. The procedure for Bartholin's abscess drainage is the same as that for any cutaneous abscess

36. A 37-year-old female presents with worsening pelvic pain. She relates that she has had severe dysmenorrhea for several years and she came to the ED today because she "just couldn't take it anymore." She further reports that she has dyspareunia and pain with defecation. Pain is cyclic and worse with menstruation. Vital signs are HR 88 bpm, BP 132/80 mm Hg, RR 18 breaths/min, SpO₂ 99% on room air, and temperature 37° C. Exam shows some uterine tenderness but is otherwise unremarkable with no vaginal discharge and no cervical motion tenderness. Urinalysis, CBC, and chemistry are unremarkable. Gonorrhea and chlamydia testing is negative, and wet mount is normal. A pelvic ultrasound is performed

and is normal. You suspect that the patient may have endometriosis. All but which of the following are possible complications of endometriosis?

A. Infertility
B. Catamenial pneumothorax
C. Disseminated intravascular coagulation
D. Bowel perforation

37. A 48-year-old female with a history of diabetes mellitus and hypertension presents with vaginal bleeding for 1 week. She has not had a period for approximately 1 year and complains of ongoing hot flashes. She has not been sexually active since the death of her husband 1 year ago. She describes the vaginal bleeding as similar to a regular period. She denies any abdominopelvic pain, vaginal pain, dyspnea, dizziness, or other vaginal discharge. Vital signs are HR 88 bpm, BP 154/92 mm Hg, RR 16 breaths/min, temperature 37.1° C, and SpO$_2$ 98% on room air. Abdominal exam is unremarkable. Pelvic exam reveals a small amount of blood in the vaginal vault. The cervix and vaginal mucosa appear normal. There is no uterine or cervical motion tenderness. What is the most appropriate management for this patient?

A. Provide reassurance and discharge home
B. Discharge home with plan for prompt follow-up for endometrial biopsy and outpatient ultrasound

C. Initiate hormone replacement therapy and discharge home with plan for prompt follow-up for endometrial biopsy and outpatient ultrasound
D. Urgent gynecology consult

38. A 38-year-old female presents with heavy vaginal bleeding. The patient reports a history of heavy and irregular periods. She reports heavy vaginal bleeding for the past week. For the past 8 hours, she reports a significant increase in bleeding and has been soaking through three pads per hour. She reports cramping pelvic pain. She denies trauma or history of bleeding disorder. LMP was 5 weeks ago. She has no significant past medical history. Vital signs are HR 108 bpm, BP 96/68 mm Hg, RR 18 breaths/min, temperature 37.2° C, and SpO$_2$ 99% on room air. There is mild suprapubic tenderness on abdominal exam. On pelvic exam, there is significant pooling of blood in the vaginal vault. Pregnancy test is negative. Hemoglobin is 10.6. Two large-bore IV lines are established, and fluid resuscitation is initiated. The patient is typed and crossmatched for 2 units of packed RBCs. Urgent gynecologic consult is called. What is the next step in management?

A. Apply vaginal packing to control the hemorrhage
B. Give tranexamic acid 10 mg/kg IV
C. Give conjugated estrogen 25 mg IV every 4 to 6 hours
D. Interventional radiology consult for uterine artery embolization

ANSWERS

1. ANSWER: B

Any patient greater than 20 weeks' gestation with painless vaginal bleeding should be treated as having placenta previa until transvaginal ultrasound can be obtained to determine the position of the placenta relative to the cervix. Transvaginal ultrasound is the imaging modality of choice because it has been shown to be more accurate than transabdominal ultrasound in the diagnosis of placenta previa. Transvaginal ultrasound should be performed carefully and by an experienced sonographer so as not to disrupt the placenta and precipitate hemorrhage.

Test-taking tip: Digital (C) or speculum exam (A) should never be done in any patient suspected of having placenta previa because of the risk for catastrophic hemorrhage. Choice D can be eliminated next given that the patient has had no leakage of fluid and does not appear to be in labor

2. ANSWER: D

This patient presents with a large adnexal mass and history features concerning for ovarian torsion. Patients with adnexal masses greater than 4 cm are at increased risk for ovarian torsion. While an abnormal Doppler ultrasound has a high positive predictive value for ovarian torsion, the presence of normal Doppler flow on ultrasound does not exclude the diagnosis. In patients for whom there is a high clinical suspicion for ovarian torsion, urgent gynecology consult is warranted, even in the presence of normal imaging.

Test-taking tip: You can eliminate B and C because they would not improve the diagnostic yield for ovarian torsion and would create a delay in definitive treatment. Given the acuity of the patient's presentation, choice A can also be eliminated.

3. ANSWER: A

Early side effects of magnesium administration include nausea, flushing, hypothermia, and headache. The first sign of magnesium toxicity is diminished deep tendon reflexes, which occurs at a serum magnesium concentration of 3.5 to 5 mmol/L. Respiratory depression occurs at serum concentrations of 5 to 6.5 mmol/L, and cardiac conduction abnormalities occur at concentrations greater than 7.5 mmol/L. Patients receiving magnesium for treatment of eclampsia should be monitored carefully for signs of toxicity, with special attention paid to deep tendon reflexes, urinary output, and respiratory rate.

Test-taking tip: It is important to know the symptoms of magnesium toxicity. All the answer choices except A show a slowing down of bodily functions, and the odd one out can be picked as the answer if the symptoms of magnesium toxicity aren't known.

4. ANSWER: C

The patient is presenting with turtle sign (retraction of the fetal head against the perineum) indicating shoulder dystocia. Shoulder dystocia is an OB emergency and may result in fetal hypoxia. In cases of suspected shoulder dystocia, McRobert's maneuver should be performed first, whereby the maternal legs are hyperflexed against the abdomen with knees held far apart in the lithotomy position. Next, firm downward suprapubic pressure should be applied in an attempt to dislodge the anterior shoulder. If the patient is able, attempt to move her to the all-fours position (Gaskin maneuver) and apply downward traction to the fetal head.

Test-taking tip: Corkscrew maneuvers can be employed, in which the fetal shoulders are manually rotated. These maneuvers may require episiotomy (B) to allow for introduction of the fingers into the vaginal canal. Fundal pressure (A) should never be applied in cases of suspected shoulder dystocia because this may worsen the dystocia. Choice D is a complication of shoulder dystocia and should not be the next step in management of this patient.

5. ANSWER: B

OB consultation and fetal monitoring are warranted in the pregnant trauma patient with suspected placental abruption. The American College of Obstetrics and Gynecology recommends a minimum of 4 hours of fetal monitoring following maternal trauma, and longer periods of monitoring are indicated when there are signs and symptoms of abruption. Patients with placental abruption classically present with abdominal pain and vaginal bleeding, but the presentation may be variable, and some patients may present with back pain or even no pain at all. The patient in this question presents with placental abruption precipitated by trauma, but abruption frequently occurs in the absence of trauma.

Test-taking tip: A normal ultrasound (A) does not rule out the diagnosis of placental abruption, and sensitivity of ultrasound for abruption ranges from only 24% to 57%. Choice (D) can be eliminated because the patient has had trauma and has painful vaginal bleeding. Risk factors for atraumatic placental abruption include chronic hypertension, cigarette smoking, cocaine use, multiple gestations, maternal age, premature rupture of membranes, oligohydramnios, and chorioamnionitis. This eliminates choice C.

6. ANSWER: C

HELLP syndrome is characterized by hemolysis, elevated liver enzymes, and low platelets. Patients often present with hypertension, but this is not required to make the diagnosis. The common presentation for HELLP syndrome is RUQ or epigastric pain, nausea, vomiting, and lethargy, which may be erroneously diagnosed as a viral syndrome or other hepatobiliary disease. HELLP syndrome occurs most frequently in the antepartum period, but a significant minority of patients present postpartum. The laboratory criteria for diagnosis of HELLP syndrome includes platelets £100,000/L, AST ≥70 IU/L, and LDH ≥600 IU/L. Prompt recognition and treatment of HELLP syndrome is important to reduce the risk for morbidity and mortality due to associated disseminated intravascular coagulation (DIC), hepatic rupture, acute renal failure, pulmonary edema, and placental abruption.

Test-taking tip: Choices A and D can be eliminated given that neither viral hepatitis nor preeclampsia has signs of thrombocytopenia. Cholestasis (B) usually occurs in the third trimester, which could make it a likely answer; however, ALT is usually elevated, not AST, which is mentioned in this question, eliminating this answer choice.

7. ANSWER: D

The most likely diagnosis is postpartum endometritis, which is characterized by uterine tenderness, foul-smelling lochia, and fever in a postpartum patient. The most significant risk factor for postpartum endometritis is cesarean delivery. This patient presents with findings concerning for severe disease, warranting inpatient treatment with broad-spectrum IV antibiotics. Clindamycin, gentamycin, and vancomycin provide appropriate broad-spectrum coverage.

Test-taking tip: Choices A and B can be eliminated given that there is no mention of urinary symptoms and there is no such concept as normal postpartum fever. The difference between choices C and D is the antibiotic choice. Give that doxycycline (C) is contraindicated in breastfeeding women, the answer choice is eliminated.

8. ANSWER: A

Preterm labor is defined as onset of labor before 37 weeks' gestation. It often occurs with preterm premature rupture of membranes, which is rupture of the amniotic membrane before 37 weeks' gestation. OB consultation is required. Sterile speculum exam may be carefully performed to evaluate for dilation of the cervix but Ferning and Nitrazine tests are used to evaluate for the presence of amniotic fluid with pre-term rupture of membranes.

Test-taking tip: Digital cervical exam (B) and nonsterile speculum exam (C) should be avoided in a patient with suspected premature rupture of membranes because of increased risk for infection.

9. ANSWER: C

During the first trimester, the amount of circulating fetal blood present is relatively small. In women less than 12 weeks' gestation, a 50-mcg dose of RhoGAM is adequate to prevent alloimmunization; however, there is no harm in administering the standard 300-mcg dose. In any gestation greater than 12 weeks, the 300-mcg dose should always be used. Additional doses may be needed depending on the volume of fetal-maternal hemorrhage, and determination of further dosage should be performed in conjunction with OB and blood bank consultation.

Test-taking tip: Remember to pick the answer that is *not* true. At any time in pregnancy, there is no harm in administering RhoGAM 300 mcg, eliminating choices B and D because both are true. Before 12 weeks' gestation, RhoGAM 50 mcg can be administered, eliminating choice A, which is also a true statement.

10. ANSWER: A

The patient in this vignette presents with signs and symptoms of HELLP syndrome, characterized by hemolysis, elevated liver enzymes, and low platelets. The Tennessee criteria are frequently used to make the diagnosis of HELLP syndrome based on the criteria listed in Table 13.1. It is important to consider this diagnosis in any patient 20 weeks' gestation or greater presenting with abdominal pain because this disease entity has high morbidity and mortality. Classically, pain is located in the RUQ or epigastric region and may be associated with hypertension, headache, nausea, and emesis. In patients with suspicion for HELLP syndrome, rapid OB consultation and admission or transfer to a facility with capabilities for managing high-risk pregnancies is warranted.

Test-taking tip: Choices C and D can both be eliminated given the elevated kidney function, which is not a part of the HELLP syndrome criteria. Between choices A and B, the differences are platelet count, peripheral

Table 13.1 LABORATORY ABNORMALITIES IN HELLP SYNDROME ACCORDING TO THE TENNESSEE CRITERIA

LABORATORY TEST	RESULT
Serum aspartate aminotransferase	>70 U/L
Peripheral blood smear	Schistocytes
Platelet count	<100,000 cells/μL
Total bilirubin	>1.2 mg/dL

smear, and LDH level. Given that the diagnosis of HELLP includes thrombocytopenia and schistocytes to indicate hemolysis, choice B can be eliminated,

11. ANSWER: B

All symptomatic pregnant women with bacterial vaginosis should be treated. In women at high risk for preterm delivery, treatment of bacterial vaginosis may reduce the risk of preterm labor. For those patients not at risk for preterm labor, treatment is appropriate for symptom control. Oral metronidazole or oral clindamycin is the treatment of choice for bacterial vaginosis in pregnant women. Prior studies showed an increase in adverse events with the use of intravaginal clindamycin in the second half of pregnancy, but newer evidence suggests that intravaginal clindamycin may be safe in late pregnancy. Still, there is concern that intravaginal clindamycin may not effectively eradicate bacteria in the upper genital tract, and there have been studies that suggest that there may be improved neonatal outcomes in patients treated with oral regimens.

Test-taking tip: Eliminating choice A helps eliminate choice D, which includes all answer choices. This pregnant patient is symptomatic and therefore deferring treatment is not appropriate management. Between choices B and C, metronidazole (B) is the more effective treatment.

12. ANSWER: B

This patient presents with symptoms concerning for pelvic inflammatory disease (PID). Sexually active women who present with uterine tenderness, cervical motion tenderness, or adnexal tenderness, for whom no other cause of their symptoms is found, should be treated empirically for PID. The presence of mucopurulent discharge, fever, confirmed infection with *Neisseria gonorrhoeae* or *C. trachomatis*, increased erythrocyte sedimentation

rate and/or C-reactive protein, or abundant WBCs on wet mount should further increase suspicion for PID. It is appropriate to treat patients with mild suspected PID on an outpatient basis with close follow-up and return precautions. Treatment options for outpatient management of PID are listed in Table 13.2.

Table 13.2 OUTPATIENT TREATMENT OPTIONS FOR PELVIC INFLAMMATORY DISEASE

- Ceftriaxone 250 mg IM once *plus* doxycycline 100 mg PO twice daily for 14 days *with or without* metronidazole 500 mg twice daily for 14 days
- Cefoxitin 2 g IM once *plus* probenecid 1 g PO once *plus* doxycycline 100 mg PO twice daily for 14 days *with or without* metronidazole 500 mg twice daily for 14 days
- Other third-generation parenteral cephalosporin *plus* doxycycline 100 mg PO twice daily for 14 days *with or without* metronidazole 500 mg twice daily for 14 days

Test-taking tip: You can start by eliminating choice C, which is not adequate treatment alone for PID, although metronidazole can be used in conjunction with a cephalosporin and doxycycline if concurrent bacterial vaginosis is found. Choice A is the empiric treatment of choice for suspected *N. gonorrhoeae* or *C. trachomatis* cervicitis and is not adequate to treat PID. This helps eliminate choices A and D.

13. ANSWER: B

This patient presents with unilateral pain and dyspareunia and is found to have a simple cyst on ultrasound. All patients with ovarian cysts found during ED evaluation should be referred for gynecologic or primary care follow-up. The presence of ovarian cysts greater than 4 cm in diameter increase the risk for ovarian torsion, a condition that requires immediate OB consultation. This patient's presentation, with mild intermittent pain, dyspareunia, and normal Doppler flow on pelvic ultrasound, is less concerning for the diagnosis of ovarian torsion. In this case, it is appropriate to refer this patient for outpatient follow-up.

Test-taking tip: Consider resource utilization when choosing the best management option. Extensive diagnostic testing is often not indicated for benign findings in a well-appearing patient. MRI (C) may be performed on an outpatient basis to better characterize the cyst in those patients with a persistent large ovarian cyst, but ED MRI is not necessary. Emergency OB consultation (D) is not indicated in the management of a simple cyst. Choice A is also not indicated given that the patient has a simple unruptured ovarian cyst.

14. ANSWER: C

The diagnosis in this case is inevitable abortion, which is defined as vaginal bleeding in the presence of a dilated cervix. Inevitable abortion may be managed expectantly, but it is important to ensure follow-up within 1 week of diagnosis and give strict return precautions for heavy bleeding or fever.

Test-taking tip: The terminology of spontaneous abortion can be difficult to recall (Table 13.3). Start first by eliminating the obvious answer choices that do not fit the clinical situation, such as complete abortion (D) and threatened abortion (A). The main difference between inevitable and incomplete abortion is whether some or all of the products of conception are present, in both cases the cervical os is open (think "I" abortion has an open eye of the os).

Table 13.3 CLASSIFICATION OF THE SPECTRUM OF SPONTANEOUS ABORTION

CLASSIFICATION	DEFINITION
Threatened abortion	Vaginal bleeding in the first 20 weeks of pregnancy in the presence of a closed cervical os
Inevitable abortion	Vaginal bleeding in the first trimester in the presence of an open cervical os and products of conception within the uterine or cervical canal
Missed abortion	Nonviable fetus in the first 20 weeks of pregnancy with a closed cervical os and no vaginal bleeding
Incomplete abortion	Vaginal bleeding with partial expulsion of products of conception
Complete abortion	Empty uterus with no retained products of conception

15. ANSWER: D

Septic abortion should be suspected in patients with signs of infection and a history of recent abortion. The mainstays of treatment are broad-spectrum IV antibiotics and surgical evacuation of the retained products of conception. The source of infection in septic abortion is often retained products of conception, and source control consists of dilation and curettage. OB consultation should be obtained as early as possible so that surgical intervention is expedited. Misoprostol and expectant management are not reasonable options for patients with suspected septic abortion.

Test-taking tip: Briefly consider the consequences of each management option when asked to determine the most appropriate treatment. If the source of infection is the products of conception, then the management option that most effectively and expeditiously removes the nidus for infection is the correct answer. In this case, surgical dilation and curettage is the fastest way to achieve source control. Choices A, B, and C do not remove the nidus of infection fast enough.

16. ANSWER: B

At first glance, this may seem like a straightforward case of hyperemesis gravidarum. Typical symptoms and lab findings in hyperemesis gravidarum include severe nausea and emesis with ketonuria, hypokalemia, and clinical signs of dehydration. Abdominal pain, however, is not typical of hyperemesis gravidarum. In patients who present with symptoms of hyperemesis gravidarum and abdominal pain, the clinician must look for other potential etiologies of the patient's symptoms, including HELLP syndrome, peptic ulcer disease, gastritis, cholecystitis, and pancreatitis. In this case, there should be further investigation into the cause of the patient's abdominal pain before a final disposition decision is made.

Test-taking tip: Be sure not to fall into the trap of premature diagnostic closure. If a given symptom does not fit with a diagnosis, continue the workup until you have a unifying diagnosis or you are confident that there is not another dangerous cause of the patient's symptoms.

17. ANSWER: D

Hydatidiform molar pregnancy consists of two separate disease entities, complete mole and partial mole, both of which arise from abnormal trophoblastic tissue. The trophoblast forms the outer layer of cells in an early embryo and goes on to form much of the placenta. A complete mole consists of only abnormal trophoblastic tissue (fetal in origin) but no fetus, while in a partial mole a nonviable fetus is present. The molar pregnancy arises from fetal tissue, so Rh-negative women with vaginal bleeding are at risk for alloimmunization and should receive RhoGAM. Most women with molar pregnancy will present with vaginal bleeding early in pregnancy with excessively high β-hCG levels. Hyperemesis, uterine size greater than expected for dates, and pregnancy-induced hypertension may also be present. Ultrasound will show a characteristic "bunch of grapes" or "snowstorm" appearance of a heterogeneous mass with many cystic-appearing trophoblastic villi within the uterine cavity. Approximately 15% of complete moles and less than 1% of partial moles will progress to malignancy. Fortunately, with treatment, the prognosis for these patients is very good.

Test-taking tip: The answer to this question is embedded within the question stem but requires understanding that the trophoblast is fetal in origin. From this, you can deduce the correct *false* answer as the one that incorrectly identifies hydatidiform mole as maternal tissue, even if you aren't sure whether RhoGAM should be administered to these patients.

18. ANSWER: C

The process of labor is divided into three stages. The first stage of labor is subdivided into the latent phase and the active phase. The stages (and phases) of labor are defined as follows:

- *First stage:* commences with the beginning of uterine contraction and lasts until the cervix is fully dilated
  - *Latent phase:* characterized by early contractions that are spread far apart and are irregular
  - *Active phase:* begins when the cervix is dilated to 3 to 4 cm and ends when the cervix is fully dilated
- *Second stage:* begins when the cervix is fully dilated and ends when the fetus is delivered
- *Third stage:* begins when the fetus is delivered and ends when the placenta is delivered

Test-taking tip: Pay attention to the wording used in the answer choices. The question stem asks which stage of labor the patient is in. The latent and active phases of labor are actually part of the first stage. The patient has clearly progressed through the early stage of labor because delivery is imminent.

19. ANSWER: C

Umbilical cord prolapse is an OB emergency and requires emergent cesarean delivery because compression of the cord can compromise fetal blood supply. Initial steps in management include elevation of the presenting fetal part, placement of the patient in Trendelenburg position, and immediate urgent OB consultation. The physician should keep the hand in the vagina to prevent the presenting fetal part from compressing the cord until the patient is ready for surgery. Attempts at reducing the cord should never be made.

Test-taking tip: If an answer suggests that two of the answer choices may be correct, there is a good chance that at least one of them is. In this case, you could eliminate choices A and B and then focus your attention on the remaining choices.

20. ANSWER: A

There are several types of breech presentation, and management depends on fetal positioning. In the frank breech position, the buttocks are the presenting part, and the hips are flexed with legs stretched in front of the fetus so that the feet are in front of the fetal head. In complete breech position, the buttocks are the presenting part, and the hips and legs are flexed in a folded leg position. In footling breech, one or both feet are the presenting part.

In any breech presentation, OB consultation should be called for immediately. Only in complete or frank breech should the delivery be allowed to proceed spontaneously. The primary concern in footling delivery is that the cervix will not completely dilate, causing the fetal head to become stuck. In the event of frank or complete breech presentation, delivery should proceed according to the following steps:

1. Allow maternal efforts to deliver the fetus to the level of the umbilicus. If the legs are still extended, apply pressure to the back of the knee with one finger in order to flex the knee and allow delivery of the first leg and then repeat for the other
2. Rotate the sacrum anteriorly and allow the fetus to deliver to the level of the scapulae
3. Allow the shoulders to deliver spontaneously. If the shoulders do not deliver, rotate the infant counterclockwise until the shoulder becomes visible, and then sweep the arm out by flexing at the antecubital fossa
4. After the anterior arm is delivered, turn the baby clockwise and deliver the other arm in a similar fashion
5. To deliver the head, place the index and middle finger over the maxillary bone and provide gentle flexion of the fetal head while keeping the body in a horizontal plane

It is important to never apply traction to the fetal head because this could cause the head to become impacted.

Test taking tip: When attempting to answer this question, try to imagine or visualize how the fetus moves through the birth canal. In frank breech presentation, spontaneous delivery should be attempted, eliminating choice B. Extension of the fetal neck will lead to increased anterior-posterior diameter of the head as it passes through the birth canal, making delivery more difficult, eliminating choice D. Visualization is much more likely to elucidate the correct answer than simple memorization. Choice C does not adequately explain how to deliver the head.

21. ANSWER: D

The patient is presenting with symptoms concerning for amniotic fluid embolus. Amniotic fluid embolus occurs when amniotic fluid enters the maternal circulation, typically during the labor or in the immediate postpartum period. The cardinal symptoms of amniotic fluid embolus are sudden onset of altered mental status, hypoxemia, shock, and DIC.

The early phase of amniotic fluid embolism is characterized by both obstructive shock and cardiogenic shock. During the early phase, there is right ventricular failure, which manifests as dilated and hypokinetic right ventricle on echocardiogram. This may later progress to left ventricular failure. Pulmonary edema is commonly seen with the progression to left ventricular failure and may occur minutes to hours after the onset of symptoms. Most cases of amniotic fluid embolism have associated DIC as a result of circulating substances in the amniotic fluid. DIC may present early or late in the disease course.

Treatment involves supportive care, including oxygen, vasopressors, inotropes, and treatment of coagulopathy with fresh frozen plasma/cryoprecipitate. Unfortunately, mortality is high even with supportive care.

Test-taking tip: Each of the lab and imaging findings in the answers is supported by the patient's presentation. Even if you are not sure what imaging or lab findings are suggestive of amniotic fluid embolus, you can correlate the patient's symptoms with the findings of the supportive studies. The patient is hemodynamically unstable, which would support cardiovascular and pulmonary collapse.

22. ANSWER: B

Nuchal cord is common, occurring in one-third of deliveries. In most cases, the cord is loose and can be easily passed over the infant's head. This should be the first step in management because most cases can be managed with this simple maneuver alone. In cases in which there is a tight nuchal cord, it is important to avoid forceful reduction because of risk for cord avulsion. In the event of a nuchal cord that cannot be reduced, the next step is to clamp the cord with two Kelly forceps and then make a cut between the clamps. Clamping and cutting the cord should not be the first step in management. This maneuver should be reserved only for cases in which the cord cannot be manually reduced because early cord clamping is associated with increased rates of fetal anemia. Management of the nuchal cord should not be delayed while awaiting OB consult.

Test-taking tip: When considering management options, the first step will likely be the one that is effective but has the lowest risk for harm to the patient and baby. Choice A is the next step if the nuchal cord is tight; choices C and D could pose harm to the baby.

23. ANSWER: A

Of the drugs listed in the answers, all but ondansetron have known teratogenic effects. Until 2014, pharmaceutical drugs were labeled according to pregnancy risk categories A, B, C, D, and X. However, these categories were deemed to be difficult to interpret and apply given the paucity of human studies on drug safety in human pregnancy. The US Food and Drug Administration (FDA) has now removed the pregnancy risk category labels from pharmaceutical labeling. Instead, the FDA has established rules that require pharmaceutical companies to summarize the risks during pregnancy along with supportive data in labeling drugs. Table 13.4 provides a list of pharmaceutical drugs commonly encountered in the ED with known or potential teratogenic and adverse effects in pregnancy.

Table 13.4 TERATOGENIC MEDICATIONS IN PREGNANCY

MEDICATION	KNOWN OR POTENTIAL TERATOGENIC EFFECTS
Lisinopril	Oligohydramnios, decreased fetal renal function
Warfarin	Spontaneous abortion, congenital malformation
Phenytoin	Congenital malformations
Valproic acid	Neural tube defects
Aminoglycosides	Ototoxicity
Tetracycline	Tooth discoloration, skeletal abnormalities
Trimethoprim	Neural tube defects, congenital malformations
Haloperidol	Limb malformations (first trimester)
Lithium	Cardiac malformations
Nonsteroidal antiinflammatory drugs	Premature closure of ductus arteriosus, third trimester

Test-taking tip: It would be helpful to know the medications that are safe in pregnancy and use the process of elimination when faced with questions like this one.

24. ANSWER: D

As resuscitation is initiated in the patient with postpartum hemorrhage, the physician should attempt to identify the underlying cause of hemorrhage. The "four Ts" can be used to help recall the common causes of postpartum hemorrhage:

- Tone (uterine atony)
- Trauma
- Tissue (retained placental tissue)
- Thrombin (DIC)

The most common cause of postpartum hemorrhage is uterine atony, and this is the most likely cause of bleeding in the patient in the question. After delivery, the uterus contracts to decrease flow to the uterine vessels, and the uterine fundus should feel firm. Uterine atony should be suspected in the postpartum patient with a soft uterine fundus. Risk factors for uterine atony include nulliparity, fetal macrosomia, use of oxytocin for labor augmentation, preeclampsia, prolonged labor, and precipitous labor. The first-line treatment for postpartum hemorrhage secondary to uterine atony is oxytocin. Other agents that may be used include carboprost, misoprostol, and methylergonovine (Methergine). Carboprost and methylergonovine should be avoided in patients with hypertension.

Other causes for postpartum hemorrhage include lacerations and uterine inversion or rupture. The patient in the question has a first-degree perineal laceration and loss of uterine tone, and the more likely cause of bleeding is uterine atony. Repair should be performed immediately when the suspected source of bleeding is laceration. In cases of suspected uterine inversion, the uterus should be manually replaced. Surgery is indicated for cases of suspected uterine rupture.

Retained placental tissue or placenta accreta can also cause severe postpartum hemorrhage. If the placenta is available, it should be inspected. If portions of the placenta are missing, the uterus should be manually evacuated.

In patients with suspected DIC, coagulopathy should be corrected.

Test-taking tip: When considering the most appropriate treatment, it is important to consider the underlying cause for the patient's symptoms. In this case, the initial treatment beyond resuscitation will differ depending on the etiology. Choices B and E are possibilities after oxytocin is used or if it is not available.

25. ANSWER: D

In missed abortion, there is fetal demise but no cervical dilation, vaginal bleeding, or uterine activity to expel the fetus. Management decisions should be based on patient preference and access to follow-up. Medical management, surgical management, and expectant management are all appropriate options for patients who are hemodynamically

stable and able to obtain OB follow-up within a week. Intravaginal and buccal misoprostol are the mainstays of medical management, and both have similar efficacy. In all cases, strict return precautions should be given for heavy vaginal bleeding or signs/symptoms of septic abortion.

Test-taking tip: When a question asks you to make a disposition decision, pay special attention to clues indicating that a patient might not be safe for discharge home. Abnormal vital signs, severe pain, and inability to obtain appropriate follow-up are examples of cases in which discharge home may not be appropriate. This patient is appropriate for discharge home based on the information given.

26. ANSWER: B

The patient presents with ultrasound findings of adnexal mass and free fluid concerning for possible rupture of an ectopic pregnancy. She requires immediate gynecologic consultation in the ED. The discriminatory zone is the β-hCG level at which an intrauterine pregnancy should be visualized on ultrasound. The discriminatory zone for transvaginal ultrasound is 1,500 mlU/mL and for transabdominal ultrasound is 6,000 mlU/mL. The patient has a β-hCG level below the discriminatory zone, and as such there is no gestational sac or fetal pole visualized on ultrasound. Although no gestational sac or fetal pole is visualized, the patient has a concerning adnexal mass with free fluid, and this warrants immediate gynecologic consultation in the ED.

In patients with a completely normal ultrasound but exam and history findings concerning for ectopic pregnancy, management decisions may be more difficult. Hemodynamically stable patients with a normal ultrasound and a quantitative β-hCG level below the discriminatory zone may be appropriate for discharge home with plan for repeat β-hCG in 48 hours. In a normal intrauterine pregnancy, the β-hCG level should double every 48 hours. If the β-hCG level does not increase by at least 66%, abnormal pregnancy is likely, and further workup is needed. If the β-hCG level doubles appropriately in 48 hours, repeat ultrasound should be performed when the β-hCG level is above the discriminatory zone. Providers should have a low threshold to obtain ED gynecology consult given the potential morbidity and mortality associated with ectopic pregnancy. Patients with unruptured ectopic pregnancy may be managed medically with methotrexate, but this management decision should be made in conjunction with a gynecologist. Medical management is not appropriate for this patient because she has ultrasound findings concerning for rupture.

Test-taking tip: Pay attention to "red flags" on imaging. In this case, although there is no definite gestational sac, there is free fluid and an adnexal mass that are suspicious for ectopic pregnancy. Choices A and C can be eliminated because discharging a patient with concern for ruptured ectopic pregnancy is not appropriate management. The patient needs immediate gynecologic consultation, making B the better answer choice.

27. ANSWER: A

Pregnant patients with pyelonephritis should be admitted to the hospital and treated with IV antibiotics until afebrile for 48 hours, then discharged with a 10- to 14-day course of PO antibiotics. The antibiotic of choice for empiric treatment of pyelonephritis in pregnancy is a second- or third-generation cephalosporin such as ceftriaxone or cefazolin. Ampicillin plus gentamycin is also an acceptable parenteral treatment option. Ciprofloxacin use is generally not recommended in pregnancy, especially given the safety and efficacy of cephalosporins.

Given the risk for complications from pyelonephritis in pregnant patients, outpatient treatment is not recommended. Pyelonephritis is the number one cause of septic shock in pregnancy, and clinical course may be complicated by renal impairment, acute respiratory distress syndrome, and bacteremia. Oral nitrofurantoin and cephalexin are appropriate for outpatient treatment of cystitis or asymptomatic bacteriuria but are not appropriate for initial treatment of pyelonephritis.

Test-taking tip: Take a stepwise approach to problem-solving. The first step in solving this question is identifying that the patient has pyelonephritis. Next, recognize that pregnancy is considered a "complicating" factor for many disease states, including pyelonephritis, and admission is warranted. Choices B and D can be eliminated because the patient should not be discharged. You are left with choices A and C and the antibiotic that is safe to use in pregnancy.

28. ANSWER: A

Ultrasound is the preferred initial diagnostic test for appendicitis in pregnancy because it is inexpensive, it acts relatively quickly, and there is no fetal exposure to radiation. Ultrasound is reported to have good sensitivity and specificity for diagnosis of appendicitis, but detection is very operator dependent. In the question vignette, repeat ultrasound will likely lead to further delay in diagnosis. In cases in which the ultrasound is inconclusive, either MRI or CT can be used. MRI has the advantage of no radiation exposure. The major disadvantage of CT is fetal exposure to ionizing radiation.

Test-taking tip: In situations in which diagnostic testing and treatment may be harmful to the fetus,

clinical suspicion and gestational age should be factored into decision-making. There is a high clinical suspicion for appendicitis in this patient, so MRI is the diagnostic test of choice.

29. ANSWER: B

Trichomoniasis is the most common nonviral sexually transmitted infection in the United States, and most patients with trichomonal infection do not have symptoms. The sensitivity of wet mount for diagnosis of trichomonal infection is poor because motility of the protozoans is only apparent for about 20 minutes after specimen collection. Culture, nucleic acid amplification tests, and antigen detection tests are alternative tests with higher sensitivity.

Oral metronidazole is appropriate for treatment of *T. vaginalis* infection in pregnant and nonpregnant patients. Single-dose oral tinidazole is also very effective and can be used in nonpregnant patients. All sexual partners of patients diagnosed with *T. vaginalis* should be treated to prevent reinfection. Infection with *T. vaginalis* is associated with an increased risk for HIV infection, and trichomonal infection is present in up to half of HIV-infected women.

Test-taking tip: First read the question stem, then go back and read the vignette, making a mental note of the pertinent information. In this instance, the information in the vignette is not needed to answer the question. By reading the question stem first, you can save precious time on the exam.

30. ANSWER: D

This patient presents with symptoms concerning for primary HSV infection. Primary infection is often more severe than recurrences, and patients may have systemic symptoms such as fever, headache, malaise, and lymphadenopathy.

Genital herpes is common, and most affected individuals have never been diagnosed. It is a chronic infection characterized by recurrences and intermittent viral shedding, which makes diagnosis challenging. The diagnosis of HSV infection is made primarily based on clinical exam, and laboratory diagnosis of HSV infection can be challenging because of the intermittent nature of viral shedding. The Tzanck test is used to detect cellular changes associated with HSV infection, but it is neither sensitive nor specific. Viral culture is also insensitive, especially in the setting of recurrent infection, owing again to the intermittent nature of viral shedding. Nucleic acid amplification testing, such as DNA PCR, is more sensitive, but a negative PCR test still does not rule out infection, especially in the absence of active lesions.

HSV-2 is responsible for most cases of anogenital herpes, with HSV-1 causing most cases of oral herpes. Serologic testing for type-specific antibodies to HSV-1 and HSV-2 is available. Because most HSV 2 infections are sexually transmitted, a patient with a positive HSV-2 antibody test can be assumed to have anogenital infection. HSV-1 serologic tests are more difficult to interpret because many people have positive HSV-1 serology as a result of prior oral infection and have no anogenital infection.

Test-taking tip: Remember the definitions of sensitivity and specificity. A highly sensitive test has few false-negative results. A highly specific test has few false-positive results. Try to identify the one answer choice that is not like the others. In this question, choice D indicates that viral culture and PCR are insensitive and may lead to false-negative results. The other answer choices suggest high sensitivity and specificity of the tests.

31. ANSWER: C

The most likely diagnosis in this case is chancroid. Chancroid is caused by the bacterium *H. ducreyi* and is characterized by painful genital ulcer with lymphadenopathy. Patients may have "kissing lesions" in adjacent areas, as described in the patient in this vignette, due to autoinoculation. Chancroid is uncommon in the United States, but sporadic outbreaks do occur.

Diagnosis may be challenging because special media is required for culture that is typically not readily available and there are no available PCR tests. A presumptive diagnosis of chancroid can be made if the patient has painful genital ulcers with clinical presentation and lymphadenopathy characteristic of chancroid, and if syphilis and HSV have effectively been ruled out.

LGV also presents with genital ulcer and lymphadenopathy, but the ulcer associated with LGV is typically painless. Similarly, the chancre associated with primary syphilis is typically painless. This patient also had microscopic and serologic testing for syphilis, which was negative.

Ulceration and bilateral lesions as described in the vignette are not typical of Bartholin's abscess. Because this patient meets presumptive diagnostic criteria, it is appropriate to treat empirically. A single dose of azithromycin 1 g PO, a single dose of ceftriaxone 250 mg IM, ciprofloxacin 500 mg PO twice daily for 3 days, and erythromycin 500 mg PO three times daily for 7 days are all appropriate treatment regimens. Symptoms should improve within 3 days of treatment.

Test-taking tip: Pay close attention to the description of the lesions in the vignette and whether the ulcer is painful. Only one of the answer choices typically presents with painful ulcer. Choices B and D can be eliminated

because the primary lesion is painless. Choice D does not match the description in this vignette.

32. ANSWER: A

LGV is caused by the L1, L2, and L3 serovars of *C. trachomatis*. Infection usually begins with a painless chancre, followed by tender, usually unilateral, inguinal lymphadenopathy. Rectal exposure can cause proctitis. Patients may have systemic symptoms, including fever, chills, and arthralgias. LGV is not common in the United States, and diagnostic testing is not readily available at many facilities. Diagnosis is generally made based on clinical suspicion and epidemiologic information. Treatment with 21 days of doxycycline 100 mg twice daily is the preferred regimen.

H. ducreyi is the causative agent of chancroid. Chancroid may present similarly with lymphadenopathy, but ulceration is typically more prominent and painful. *T. pallidum* is the causative agent of syphilis. Primary syphilis presents with painless chancre. Secondary syphilis subsequently develops 3 to 6 weeks later, and patients may have rash and lymphadenopathy. This patient has negative treponemal and nontreponemal serologies, making the diagnosis of syphilis unlikely.

Test-taking tip: Pay attention to clues in the question stem that may help eliminate answer choices. In this question stem, it is noted that rapid treponemal testing is negative, making the diagnosis of *T. pallidum,* choice C, unlikely. Choice B presents with a painful lesion.

33. ANSWER: B

Penicillin G is the preferred treatment for all stages of syphilis and is the only antibiotic that has been shown to be effective in treating syphilis in pregnancy. Pregnant women with a documented allergy to penicillin should be admitted for penicillin desensitization and treatment. Duration of treatment depends on the stage of the disease. Doxycycline is the preferred alternative treatment for penicillin-allergic patients, but it is not recommended in pregnancy. Azithromycin can be used as an alternative treatment in nonpregnant patients if penicillin and doxycycline are not options, but resistance to azithromycin has been documented, and close follow-up is needed to ensure treatment efficacy. Azithromycin is not recommended for treatment of pregnant patients. There have been limited studies to suggest that ceftriaxone is effective in treating primary and secondary syphilis, but the dose and duration of treatment are not known, and it is not recommended for treatment of syphilis in pregnancy.

Test-taking tip: Pregnancy often requires special management given risks to the fetus and restrictions on the types of medications that can be used to treat infections. Be alert that typical management will not likely apply for pregnant patients, as is the case in this vignette. Choices C and D are eliminated because the patient cannot be discharged home with a severe penicillin allergy.

34. ANSWER: B

This patient presents with symptoms and exam findings concerning for cervicitis. The most common organisms isolated in cervicitis are *N. gonorrhoeae* and *C. trachomatis*. Patients at increased risk for cervicitis such as those younger than 25 years of age and patients with a new sexual partner, multiple sexual partners, or a sexual partner diagnosed with a sexually transmitted infection should be treated presumptively. Treatment may be deferred until test results are available in low-risk patients not meeting the previous criteria.

Presumptive treatment for chlamydia is with single-dose azithromycin 1 g PO or doxycycline 100 mg twice daily for 7 days. Presumptive treatment with gonorrhea is with single-dose ceftriaxone 250 mg IM. Metronidazole would be appropriate if there were concurrent bacterial vaginosis or infection with trichomonas, but this is not typically included in presumptive treatment for cervicitis. Cervicitis may be present in PID, and admission for parenteral antibiotics should be considered for patients with signs of severe PID. However, this patient is well-appearing with normal vital signs and no signs of PID and thus does not meet admission criteria.

Test-taking tip: When deciding the appropriate disposition for a patient, pay attention to clues that indicate whether the patient is sick or not sick. This patient is overall well-appearing, with normal vital signs and no risk factors for rapid dissemination of infection. Choices A and C can be eliminated because the patient does not need admission but requires treatment. Choice D adds treatment for *Trichomonas,* which the patient does not have on wet mount.

35. ANSWER: A

Bartholin's glands are located at the 4-o'clock and 8-o'clock positions at the vaginal vestibule. When the duct to the gland becomes blocked, Bartholin's cysts may form. Bartholin's abscess results from infection of the Bartholin's gland. The procedure for managing a Bartholin's abscess is described in choice A. The abscess should be incised from the mucosal side of the lesion. Incision from the cutaneous surface may lead to permanent fistula formation and should be avoided. The Word catheter is inserted to prevent recurrence of the abscess. Patients should be referred to gynecology for follow-up within 5 to 7 days.

Test-taking tip: If you are unsure of the correct procedural approach, it may be helpful to try to simplify the question to eliminate answer choices. In its simplest form, this question is asking the test taker, "Should a Bartholin's abscess be incised from the mucosal surface or the cutaneous surface?"

36. ANSWER: C

Endometriosis is caused by endometrial implants that grow outside of the uterus in response to hormonal stimulation. The pain associated with endometriosis is classically cyclic in nature and correlates with the menstrual cycle. Women may have dysmenorrhea, dyspareunia, dysuria, pain with defecation, chronic pelvic pain, and infertility. Endometriosis is common, affecting between 3% and 10% of reproductive-age women.

Most endometrial implants typically occur in the pelvis, but implants can be found in the lungs and bowels in severe disease, leading to spontaneous catamenial pneumothorax, bowel perforation, and bowel obstruction. DIC is not a known complication of endometriosis.

Test-taking tip: Try to think about the pathophysiology of the disease when reasoning through answer choices. In this case, if you understand that endometriosis is a process whereby endometrial cells implant outside the uterus and sometimes in distant sites, you may be able to reason through the answer choices, eliminating A, B, and D because those are all possible complications of endometriosis.

37. ANSWER: B

Vaginal bleeding in the postmenopausal patient should raise suspicion for endometrial hyperplasia and endometrial cancer. These patients should be referred for prompt outpatient follow-up. Outpatient evaluation of postmenopausal bleeding should include endometrial biopsy and ultrasound.

Postmenopausal bleeding should always be further evaluated and discharge home with only reassurance is not appropriate. Hormone therapy is the first-line treatment for patients with abnormal uterine bleeding, but hormone therapy should not be initiated in a postmenopausal patient before endometrial biopsy. Urgent gynecologic consult is not indicated for this hemodynamically stable patient.

Test-taking tip: Consider the spectrum of management possibilities in the context of the patient's presentation. The two extremes of management, to do nothing (A) and to call an urgent consult (D), can readily be eliminated based on the patient's symptoms and presentation. Choice C is not the appropriate treatment until a diagnosis is made.

38. ANSWER: C

Hormone therapy is the first-line medical treatment of acute uterine bleeding in patients without a known bleeding disorder. Options for hormone therapy include conjugated estrogen, combined oral contraceptives, and progestin. In patients with severe bleeding, 25 mg IV conjugated estrogen should be given every 4 to 6 hours until bleeding is controlled. Contraindications to estrogen use include history of thromboembolic disease, breast cancer, and liver disease.

Test-taking tip: Consider the consequences of each treatment when deciding on the most appropriate step in management. Vaginal packing (A) should not be attempted because of risk for infection and potential for masking ongoing bleeding. Tranexamic acid (B) has been shown to be effective for patients with abnormal uterine bleeding, but it is not first-line treatment. Surgical management (D) of abnormal uterine bleeding such as uterine artery embolization, hysterectomy, and dilation and curettage should be considered in consultation with a gynecologist and depends on the stability of the patient, effectiveness of medical management, and desire for fertility, among other factors.

14.

PSYCHOBEHAVIORAL DISORDERS

Shawn Hersevoort, Stephen Hurwitz, and Stephen Thornton

1. A 45-year-old female presents to the emergency department (ED) with acute onset of altered mental status and bizarre movements. She has a history of diabetes and depression and takes glipizide and citalopram. She was seen the day before by her primary care doctor, diagnosed with cellulitis, and started on linezolid. Her heart rate (HR) is 129 bpm, blood pressure (BP) 133/65 mm Hg, temperature 38.8° C, respiratory rate (RR) 18 breaths/min, and oxygen saturation 99%. Laboratory evaluation is normal, including white blood cell (WBC) count and serum lactate. Which of the following physical exam findings is considered pathognomonic for her condition?

    A. Hyperthermia
    B. Xanthopsia
    C. Torticollis
    D. Spontaneous clonus

2. Substance abuse in the geriatric population is an underappreciated problem in the ED. What substance is most commonly abused by those older than 65 years of age?

    A. Ethanol
    B. Heroin
    C. Marijuana
    D. Cocaine

3. A 25-year-old female with a past psychiatric condition presents to the ED acutely mute, staring, and immobile. Her family says she has not been eating or drinking for several days. What is the preferred pharmacologic treatment for her condition?

    A. IV lorazepam
    B. IM haloperidol
    C. IM olanzapine
    D. IV valproic acid

4. A 24-year-female is brought in by ambulance for acute onset of altered mental status. She has a history of depression and is on phenelzine and, per the emergency medical services (EMS) report, recently used cocaine. On exam, she is hyperthermic, tachycardic, and agitated. She has hyperreflexia in all extremities and has clonus in her lower extremities. Head computed tomography (CT), lumbar puncture, and laboratory workup are unremarkable. Cooling procedures are implemented. What is the next most appropriate intervention?

    A. Dantrolene
    B. Bromocriptine
    C. Lorazepam
    D. Fentanyl

5. An otherwise healthy 16-year-old female with a body mass index (BMI) of 17 presents after near-syncope at school. On examination she is bradycardic and appears slightly dehydrated, and her basic labs demonstrate markers for mild malnutrition. On further examination you see fine, downy hair on her face and arms. When asked about her weight she cheerfully says that she has never been able to gain weight no matter how much she eats. What is the most likely diagnosis?

    A. Age-appropriate behavior
    B. Anorexia nervosa
    C. Binge-eating disorder
    D. Bulimia nervosa

6. A 25-year-male presents to the ED for "not feeling right" for 1 day. He is normally on sertraline for depression and started taking dextromethorphan for a cough 2 days ago. He has a HR of 110 bpm, temperature 38.8° C, and BP 140/89 mm Hg. On exam, he is alert but anxious. Rigidity is not present, but he has hyperreflexia, tremor, and inducible clonus. He improves slightly with diazepam. What is the next most appropriate intervention?

  A. Rocuronium
  B. Cyproheptadine
  C. Dantrolene
  D. Meperidine

7. A sullen and overweight 13-year-old boy taking methylphenidate for attention deficit hyperactivity disorder (ADHD) presents for the third time in a year with a possible arm fracture. The boy is somewhat tearful and reluctant to answer questions, preferring to let his mother answer for him. When asked about other bruises on the child's body, his mother somewhat defensively says that he is very clumsy and always running into things. What is the most likely cause of the frequent injuries?

  A. Medication side effects
  B. Child abuse
  C. ADHD
  D. Normal childhood behavior

8. A 45-year-old male presents for management of left lower extremity cellulitis and endorses auditory and visual hallucinations of several days' duration. He gives no psychiatric history but describes heavy long-standing alcohol use. He is cognitively intact, organized in his thinking, and has no autonomic symptoms of alcohol withdrawal. What is the most likely cause of the hallucinations?

  A. Schizophrenia or a mood disorder with psychotic features
  B. Antibiotic use
  C. Alcohol use
  D. Malingering

9. A 65-year-old male presents following a failed suicide attempt by prescription medication overdose. He cites several social and financial stressors as causative. He currently expresses regret over the attempt and denies further suicidal intent. What symptoms would confer the greatest acute risk for another suicide attempt?

  A. The expression of hopelessness about his situation
  B. An absence of anxiety features
  C. Long-standing use of sertraline at the upper limit of dose
  D. Low energy

10. A 34-year-old female presents to the ED with right knee pain. She recalls twisting the knee awkwardly 1 day ago. She denies fevers or erythema of the knee. She has a history of depression, which is treated with

fluoxetine. She is diagnosed with an acute right knee sprain and placed in a knee immobilizer. Which of the following analgesics would be contraindicated in treating this patient's condition?

  A. Tramadol
  B. Oxycodone
  C. Ibuprofen
  D. Acetaminophen

11. A 45-year-old male with schizophrenia is brought in by family for several days of progressively worsening altered mental status. They note he is confused and unable to walk. He has been on haloperidol for 2 years and has compliant with his medication because it is given to him by his family. His vital signs demonstrate HR 124 bpm, BP 110/67 mm Hg, and core temperature 39.5° C. He is noted to have rigidity in all extremities and a decreased mental status on physical exam. Head CT is normal, as is a lumbar puncture. His diagnosis is characterized by which of the following?

  A. Rapid onset
  B. Spontaneous clonus
  C. Elevated serum creatine kinase
  D. Improvement with cyproheptadine

12. A 25-year-male arrives by ambulance for altered mental status. He has a core temperature of 41° C, HR 152 bpm, and BP 90/50 mm Hg. The medical record states he has a mood disorder and is on quetiapine and lithium. On exam, he is obtunded and does not respond to voice or pain. Lead-pipe muscle rigidity is noted in all extremities. His neck is stiff as well. Head CT and lumbar puncture are normal. A serum lithium level is undetectable. What pharmacologic treatment is most indicated first?

  A. Lithium
  B. Rocuronium
  C. Haloperidol
  D. Dantrolene

13. A 48-year-old female has frequently visited the ED for a variety of physical complaints. On each occasion she has been medically cleared without any significant medical findings. Psychiatric consultation concluded the likelihood of a somatic symptom disorder. She earnestly asks for your conclusions. What is the most appropriate initial response?

  A. "Fortunately, there is nothing wrong with you. You are cleared for discharge."
  B. "All the test results are negative, so you don't need to worry anymore."

C. "Your symptoms are psychological, so I encourage you to see a therapist for treatment."
D. "We have not found anything life-threatening, although I see that you are still suffering."

14. A 29-year-old woman with a BMI of 29 presents dehydrated with a mild metabolic alkalosis. She states that she must have a stomach bug. When examining her oral cavity, you notice significant erosion of tooth enamel. When asked about her diet and exercise patterns, she states that she focuses much of her energy on eating healthily and exercises daily. What is the most likely diagnosis?

A. Anorexia nervosa
B. Binge-eating disorder
C. Bulimia nervosa
D. Factitious disorder

15. A 78-year-old male presents with fever and altered mental status for 2 days. He has a history of Parkinson's disease and normally takes levodopa, but per his family, he ran out of his medications 1 week ago. He has a HR of 140 bpm, BP 95/40 mm Hg, temperature 41° C, RR 20 breaths/min, and oxygen saturation 95%. On exam, he is obtunded and rigid. He is paralyzed and endotracheally intubated, and IV fluid resuscitation is started. Head CT is normal. A lumbar puncture, chest radiograph, and urinalysis are normal. What is the next step in his management?

A. Levodopa
B. Cyproheptadine
C. Haloperidol
D. Benztropine

16. A 28-year-old male presented to the ED complaining of nausea, vomiting, and diarrhea for 1 day. He has a history of schizophrenia and prior neuroleptic malignant syndrome (NMS) from haloperidol. He has normal vital signs, a normal mental status, and normal muscle tone. He is given IV fluids but continues to vomit. What next intervention is appropriate?

A. Chlorpromazine
B. Promethazine
C. Metoclopramide
D. Ondansetron

17. A 42-year-old male presents with mild confusion, fever, diaphoresis, tachycardia, hypertension, dilated pupils, anxiety, and diarrhea. He demonstrates hyperreflexia and involuntary muscle spasms but does not have generalized muscular rigidity. His medication list, presumed to be current, includes paroxetine, risperidone, metoclopramide, and zolmitriptan. What is the most likely diagnosis?

A. Panic disorder
B. NMS
C. Anticholinergic delirium
D. Serotonin syndrome

18. A 77-year-old male with known bipolar 1 disorder presents with acute pneumonia. He is bewildered, disoriented, inattentive, unaware of his surroundings, disorganized in his thinking, and visually hallucinating. His family indicates that, before the past few days, he'd been "mentally sharp." What is the most likely diagnoses?

A. Delirium
B. Bipolar 1 disorder, current episode manic, with psychotic features
C. Psychotic disorder secondary to another medical condition
D. Major neurocognitive disorder (dementia) of rapid onset

19. A friendly 64-year-old man with a complicated medical history presents after a ground-level fall from his wheelchair where he struck and superficially lacerated his left cheek. Neurologic examination is overall normal, although the patient and family give a history consistent with mild to moderate neurologic decline. Labs demonstrate poor glycemic and hypertensive control. When asked about his medication adherence, the patient states that he takes his medications whenever his son provides them. His son seems somewhat uninterested, distracted, and unhappy. What is the most likely cause of the escalating health problems?

A. Normal aging
B. Alzheimer's disease
C. Pseudodementia
D. Elder abuse

20. Despite being divorced, a Hispanic couple in their early 60s presents after the ex-wife accidentally tripped and fell down a flight of stairs. Although no fractures are seen on radiographs of her extremities, she does admit to hitting her head and has bruising on the neck and shoulders. Her ex-husband, who is standing throughout the interaction, laughs, saying that they both might have had one too many glasses of Chardonnay. When you recommend a head CT, he waves it away and says, "she just had a little tumble is all." During the interaction she is sitting studiously on the exam table with her purse in her lap. When you ask her what she would like to do, she agrees that she is fine. When you ask to

speak to her alone, he becomes visibly irritated and says, "let's go, I can't afford any more expensive tests." What should we be most concerned about?

A. Domestic violence
B. Alcohol use disorder
C. Dementia
D. Major depressive disorder

21. A 24-year-old male with no past medical history is involved in a motor vehicle collision. He has a Glasgow Coma Scale score of 5 with agonal respirations. He is successfully endotracheally intubated using etomidate and succinylcholine with rapid sequence intubation. Fifteen minutes after the intubation, he begins to develop elevated end-tidal CO_2 readings and hyperthermia. Muscle rigidity is noted, including neck stiffness, despite the patient being on vecuronium. A chest radiograph confirms placement of the tube, and no infiltrate is seen. What intervention should be initiated next?

A. Piperacillin-tazobactam
B. Rocuronium
C. Bromocriptine
D. Dantrolene

22. A 34-year-old male is brought into the ED for flushing and vomiting. He has alcoholism as is being treated with disulfiram, and he admits to recent ingestion of ethanol. He subsequently develops hypotension and confusion. Accumulation of what toxin is responsible for this reaction?

A. Ethanol
B. Disulfiram
C. Acetaldehyde
D. Acetic acid

23. A retirement-age man presents to the ED with his adult daughter mildly intoxicated and having, according to her, made threats to kill himself. Although not disruptive, he refuses to cooperate with the interview and says that everything is fine. His very cooperative and professional daughter explains that since retiring from the police force 6 months prior, he has been more sullen, irritable, and isolated, drinking more, and struggling with increasing insomnia and chronic pain. She lets you know that he has told her on several occasions that he intends to kill himself with his service revolver on the anniversary of her mother's death, which is less than a week away. Regarding risk assessment, what is the most important factor here?

A. Insomnia
B. His uncooperative behavior

C. His intoxication
D. The collateral information from his daughter

24. An otherwise healthy patient in his mid-20s presents tremulous, tachycardic, hypertensive, agitated, and confused. This is one of a dozen similar presentations of this patient in the past year. He is known to have a history of alcohol withdrawal seizures on several occasions and delirium tremens on at least one occasion in the past. His last drink was more than 12 hours ago. What is the best initial medication for this patient?

A. Lorazepam
B. Either diazepam or chlordiazepoxide
C. Haloperidol
D. Olanzapine

25. A 32-year-old female who speaks Spanish and does not speak English presents to the ED with seizure-like activity 2 days after the death of her sister. Family states that this has happened for many years during stressful times but that she and her mother, who also suffers fits, have never been seen by a doctor for the symptoms. On history taking, the patient reports no other risk factors for seizure disorder or systemic disease. The patient has an electroencephalogram (EEG), which is read as normal. What is the next step in care?

A. Discharge with outpatient neurology referral
B. Start levetiracetam 500 mg twice daily
C. Discharge with outpatient psychiatry referral
D. Start duloxetine 30 mg

26. A 19-year-old female arrives by private vehicle complaining of sudden onset of headache, nausea, and vomiting. She has a HR of 125 bpm, BP 90/50 mm Hg, oral temperature 37.6° C, RR 20 breaths/min, and oxygen saturation 100%. On exam, she is in distress and has whole-body flushing. On further questioning she admits to receiving an IM antibiotic today to treat a "vaginal infection." Her current symptoms started at a restaurant just before arrival, where she consumed cheese and wine. What medication is responsible for her symptoms?

A. Ceftriaxone
B. Metronidazole
C. Doxycycline
D. Niacin

27. A 34-year-old male presents with acute onset of difficulty talking and swallowing. He has no chronic medical problems but yesterday was diagnosed with gastroenteritis and started on metoclopramide and sucralfate. His vital signs are HR 110 bpm, BP 135/85 mm Hg,

temperature 37.6° C, RR 16 breaths/min, and oxygen saturation 98%. His physical exam is notable for a protruding, nonswollen tongue. His skin exam is normal. CT of his head and face is normal with no swelling seen. What is the cause of this patient's condition?

    A. Degranulation of mast cells
    B. Blockade of dopamine receptors
    C. Inhibition of muscarinic acetylcholine receptors
    D. Histamine-mediated vasodilation

28. A 35-year-old man presents to the ED after having a "panic attack" on his way to work that morning. He has presented several times in the past several months for shortness of breath, insomnia, anxiety, and lower back pain. According to shared notes from primary care, the patient carries a diagnosis of major depressive disorder, recurrent, moderate, with anxious distress. He has been written for a variety of medications for his symptoms, but he discontinues them all for different reasons, including stomach upset, sexual side effects, and sedation. The patient feels that only 1 mg of alprazolam three times daily is effective for his symptoms. What is the best next step in treatment?

    A. Administer the patient a single alprazolam and discharge him
    B. Administer him nothing and refer him back to his primary care provider
    C. Write him a prescription for 10 tablets of clonazepam 1 mg and discharge him
    D. Provide him referrals for substance abuse treatment

29. A steadily employed and healthy 32-year-old woman who carries a diagnosis of bipolar disorder presents with her fiancé. In the exam room she is pacing, looking around the room distractedly, and biting her nails. When you ask her to sit down, she does so but immediately begins quickly and loudly explaining that this is just a marital issue and that she wants to go home. Her fiancé adds that she has not been taking her lamotrigine for the past 6 months, and for the past 5 days she has been sleeping less and less and has been picking fights with him over small things. What is the next step?

    A. Have her held and recommend admission to inpatient psychiatry
    B. Initiate either divalproex, lithium, or a second-generation antipsychotic medication
    C. Discharge her home into the care of her husband with outpatient psychiatry follow-up
    D. Order laboratory workup including complete blood count and thyroid-stimulating hormone

30. A 24-year-male presents to the ED complaining of vision problems. He has a history of schizophrenia and is being treated with fluphenazine. He has a HR of 125 bpm, BP 150/95 mm Hg, temperature 37.7° C, RR 20 breaths/min, and oxygen saturation 96%. On exam, he is noted to be in distress, and he has a fixed, upward, and lateral posture of both eyes. His pupils are reactive. He has no other neurologic deficits. CT of his head is normal. What treatment should be initiated?

    A. Dantrolene
    B. Droperidol
    C. Ceftriaxone plus vancomycin
    D. Diphenhydramine

31. Polysubstance abuse is common in the ED. Significantly higher rates of ED admissions and deaths are seen with opioids that are concurrently abused with which drug?

    A. Cocaine
    B. Methamphetamine
    C. Benzodiazepines
    D. Barbiturates

32. A well-groomed 42-year-old male presents on a psychiatric hold after repeatedly calling police about his next-door neighbors being terrorists. Records indicated that he made similar statements several years prior while being treated for mild abrasions from a motor vehicle collision. "I know it was foreigners that did this," he was quoted saying at that time, "they know that I know about them." On both occasions his urine toxicology was negative for any substances of abuse. Despite these ongoing beliefs, the patient is organized in his thought process, denies ever experiencing auditory or visual hallucinations, and is moving and communicating without difficulty. He states that he works full time, pays his taxes, and owns his own home. What is the most likely diagnosis?

    A. Schizophrenia, paranoid type
    B. Paranoid personality type
    C. Delirium, chronic
    D. Delusional disorder, persecutory type

33. Substance abuse can result in rare and unusual pathology. Which substance of abuse has been associated with anthrax?

    A. Heroin
    B. Cocaine
    C. Methamphetamine
    D. Marijuana

34. Police escort a 19-year-old man into the ED after he assaulted another man. He is agitated and diaphoretic and has broadly dilated pupils. The patient admits to recent methamphetamine use. His electrocardiogram (EKG) shows sinus tachycardia. The patient is rude, disruptive, and loud. He makes no attempt to leave or to assault staff and is found to be cognitively intact with no evidence of confusion or psychosis. What would be best initial treatment?

    A. Lorazepam 2 mg PO or IM
    B. PO haloperidol 10 mg
    C. IM haloperidol 5 mg, lorazepam 2 mg, and diphenhydramine 50 mg
    D. IM olanzapine 5 mg

35. An unconscious 15-year-old female is brought in by ambulance after being found down clutching an empty bottle of vodka. After routine vital signs, labs, and physical exam are performed, it appears the young woman is in no acute medical danger. After sleeping most of the night, she awakes tearful, remorseful, and deeply apologetic to her supportive family and the medical team. She is intelligent, reasonable, and emotionally responsive during conversation. She has no previous history of depression, anxiety, substance abuse, or self-harm and is an excellent student and involved in multiple sports. What is the next step in treatment?

    A. Recommend admitting to inpatient psychiatry
    B. Start fluoxetine 10 mg and have her follow up with primary care in 2 weeks
    C. Refer to outpatient mental health for individual or family therapy
    D. Refer to a school counselor to help decrease her workload

36. An otherwise healthy 27-year-old woman with frequent headaches presents to the ED with 10/10 headache pain and nausea, vomiting, and light sensitivity. This is her sixth presentation in the past month for similar symptoms. As on previous occasions, she is absolutely convinced that she is suffering a "brain bleed" and is literally begging for a CT study. She has a positive family history of migraine, and her imaging studies have been negative in the past few visits. What are the most likely diagnosis and the next step?

    A. Migraine; paired prophylactic treatment with rescue medication
    B. Somatic symptom disorder with prominent pain; referral back to primary care
    C. Acute cerebrovascular accident (CVA); stat CT and/or magnetic resonance imaging
    D. Illness anxiety disorder (hypochondriasis); outpatient psychiatry referral

37. A moderately obese 46-year-old woman with diabetes, hypertension, and fibromyalgia presents to the ED requesting opioids after a flair in her pain symptoms. Historically she had been managed on duloxetine and gabapentin but decided that she would discontinue them because of sedation and stomach upset. She feels that the most effective treatment for her was when she was managed on every-6-hour opioids and would like to return to that regimen. What recommendation should you give her?

    A. Restart opioids as the most potent treatment
    B. Restart the previous duloxetine and gabapentin regimen
    C. Refer to psychotherapy to help cope with the chronic pain
    D. Refer to physical therapy and do not refill her opioids

ANSWERS

1. ANSWER: D

This patient is on a selective serotonin reuptake inhibitor (citalopram) and was started on a drug that has serotonergic features (linezolid), therefore raising the concern for serotonin syndrome.

Serotonin syndrome is an acute-onset triad of neuromuscular dysfunction (tremor, hyperreflexia, clonus), central nervous system dysfunction, and autonomic dysfunction (tachycardia, hyperthermia). The most validated and widely used diagnostic decision rule for diagnosing serotonin syndrome is the Hunter Serotonin Toxicity Criteria, and spontaneous clonus is considered pathognomonic for serotonin syndrome.

Hyperthermia is a nonspecific finding. Xanthopsia ("yellow vision") is classically seen with digoxin poisoning. Torticollis is dystonic reaction that can be caused by dopaminergic drugs, not serotonergic drugs.

Test-taking tip: In scenario questions like this, chronology is very important. Discovering what preceded the onset of symptoms, in this case the use of linezolid, can help you determine the correct answer.

2. ANSWER: A

It is estimated that more than 1 million adults 65 years or older have a substance abuse problem. Approximately 90% of those adults abuse ethanol, resulting in more than 100,000 ED visits per year. Older adults do also use heroin, cocaine, and marijuana but at much lower rates than ethanol.

Test-taking tip: On board questions, it is important to remember that "common things are common."

3. ANSWER: A

The patient is demonstrating catatonia. Regardless of the etiology, IV lorazepam "challenge" is the gold standard for both confirmation of diagnosis and acute symptomatic alleviation. This "motor" disorder is treated by decreasing the dominant glutamatergic tone by increasing γ-aminobutyric acid (GABA).

High-potency first-generation antipsychotics, although helpful for psychosis and agitation, are more likely to worsen catatonia.

Lower potency or second-generation antipsychotics, although safer and still helpful for psychosis and agitation, are also more likely to worsen catatonia than to improve it.

IV valproic acid would be a treatment for acute seizure activity, and although likely not harmful in catatonia, it is not likely to be the most effective choice of treatment.

Test-taking tip: Try to identify the diagnosis *or* the underlying mechanism; understanding either leads directly to the specific antidote.

4. ANSWER: C

This patient was on a monoamine oxidase inhibitor and took a serotonergic drug (cocaine), and the patient now has clinical findings consistent with serotonin syndrome. Treatment for serotonin syndrome is based on cessation of the offending agents and supportive care. Cooling procedures and benzodiazepines, such as lorazepam, are first line in controlling the psychomotor agitation and preventing complications such as rhabdomyolysis.

Dantrolene is the treatment for malignant hyperthermia (MH) and would not be first-line treatment for serotonin syndrome. Bromocriptine is a potential treatment of NMS. Fentanyl has serotonergic properties and should not be given in this case.

Test-taking tip: Buzzwords, in this case "clonus," should be appreciated and indicate serotonin syndrome, so this question is asking about the treatment of serotonin syndrome.

5. ANSWER: B

Self-image and body weight are common struggles for teens. However, malnutrition and syncope are not. Failure to maintain weight and other physical markers of eating disorder require further screening.

Anorexia nervosa is an eating disorder characterized by excessively low body weight, which we see here. It also includes either restriction of calories or purging behavior, which is demonstrated here by the low BMI, dehydration, and malnutrition. Bradycardia and lanugo are symptoms of chronic and serious low body weight. What is lacking is the patient admitting to the restricting/purging behaviors or to problems with body image. Unfortunately, many patients defend their illness by denial or outright lying when confronted.

Binge-eating disorder is the most common eating disorder and is characterized by frequent episodes of consuming excessive amounts of food, over a short period of time, with a feeling of loss of control over these behaviors. Here we have abnormally low body weight, which would not be seen in an uncompensated disease of consumption.

Bulimia nervosa includes the binges of binge-eating disorder and the restriction or compensation of anorexia nervosa. Patients with bulimia by definition do not have abnormally low BMI, although at different stages of illness, patients can move between different eating disorder diagnoses.

Test-taking tip: Always pay close attention to rare or unexpected physical signs or symptoms that can be pathognomonic for certain illnesses. In this case, lanugo is pathognomonic for severe anorexia.

6. ANSWER: B

This patient has mild to moderate serotonin syndrome. While first-line treatment is benzodiazepines, cyproheptadine, an antihistamine with serotonin antagonism, can be considered as a treatment for mild to moderate cases.

Rocuronium is a nondepolarizing paralytic that could be used to treat the muscle rigidity seen in severe NMS. Dantrolene is the treatment for MH. Meperidine is an opioid with serotonergic properties and would be contraindicated in this patient.

Test-taking tip: It is common for board review questions to assume you know the initial intervention for a disease state and to then ask what the second or "next" intervention should be. Benzodiazepine would be first line and cyproheptadine would be the next treatment for serotonin syndrome.

7. ANSWER: B

Although medication side effects are common in children treated with stimulants, fractures and bruises are not among them. Most common would be decreased appetite, tremor, and insomnia.

Child abuse should be considered here considering the constellation of symptoms, including a pattern of frequent serious injuries, abnormal interpersonal family behaviors, and unexplained bruises and injuries. Parental diversion of stimulant medication can sometimes be seen and should also be considered as a factor. It should be noted that children with ADHD or other mental or physical health problems are more likely to be victims of abuse. Always attempt to speak to the patient alone when abuse is a possibility. Call child protective services immediately if you suspect abuse.

Children with ADHD are often drawn to sports and risk-taking and thus can have more frequent injuries than their peers. In this case, the number and severity of the injuries seem potentially excessive. Also, the abnormalities in the family dynamic may signal more serious problems at home than a treated patient with ADHD would warrant.

Normal childhood behavior related to sports and injuries also seems unlikely in this case. Children certainly get injured in the course of activities, but usually not to this extent.

Test-taking tip: Always look at relationships between family members in the exam room. Who is talking for the patient, how are they doing it, and how the patient responds are all useful pieces of clinical information. If something feels wrong, it probably is.

8. ANSWER: C

Schizophrenia, or a mood disorder, is unlikely because of the lack of either history or current symptoms in a 45-year-old.

Although either infection or toxic effects of antibiotics can lead to delirium including hallucinations, we are not seeing that changes in sensorium that would also be necessary.

Alcohol-induced hallucinosis involves the presence of hallucinations in a patient with a history of heavy alcohol use. It more commonly occurs during a period of cutting back on alcohol and is not usually accompanied by significant autonomic symptoms of withdrawal or the global cognitive impairment of delirium tremens.

Malingering is a diagnosis both of exclusion and evidence. In this case, there is a history of alcohol use, and no evidence of secondary gain was given to demonstrate a reason for exaggerating or manufacturing the symptoms.

Test-taking tip: Know the scope of substance-induced psychiatric disorders because continued exposures to toxic substances such as alcohol or stimulants will often accumulate over time.

9. ANSWER: A

Hopelessness has a particularly strong association with suicide, making a denial of suicidal intent, while possibly sincere, less helpful or convincing.

Anxiety symptoms or disorders convey additional risk for suicide.

Antidepressants only rarely induce or exacerbate suicidal ideation, and this has primarily been seen in transitional-age youths during early treatment.

Low energy, although an important constitutional symptom of depression, is not a particularly dangerous symptom in regard to acute suicidality.

Test-taking tip: Consider the most logical answer, even if one is not familiar with the topic.

10. ANSWER: A

Tramadol is a unique opioid that appears to have serotonergic properties and in the presence of another serotonergic drug, such as fluoxetine, may precipitate serotonin syndrome.

The other choices are not considered serotonergic drugs and would not be expected to interact with this patient's medications.

Test-taking tip: Being familiar with the indications and contraindications for commonly prescribed medications such as acetaminophen or ibuprofen can allow you to rule them out as possible answers when they are used as foils.

11. ANSWER: C

This patient has NMS, which is a poorly understood disease characterized by severe altered mental status, autonomic dysfunction, and muscle rigidity.

It is caused by antidopamine drugs, typically antipsychotics, and can manifest after patients have been on the drug for months or years. Haloperidol is the most commonly implicated drug in causing NMS. NMS has an insidious onset over days to weeks. It classically causes lead-pipe rigidity and is *not* associated with hyperreflexia or clonus. Though there is no diagnostic test for NMS, an elevated serum creatinine kinase is almost always present and considered a key diagnostic criterion.

The treatment is cessation of the offending agent with sedation and paralysis in severe cases. Bromocriptine may be of benefit. Cyproheptadine is a treatment for serotonin syndrome and has no role in the management of NMS.

Test-taking tip: Be aware of diseases and syndromes that are often grouped and tested together, in this case the "hyperthermic" toxidromes—serotonin syndrome and NMS.

12. ANSWER: B

This patient has the classic findings of severe NMS. Though NMS is more commonly associated with typical antipsychotics such as haloperidol, it can be seen with atypical antipsychotics like quetiapine as well. Treatment of NMS is based on stopping the offending agents and aggressive supportive care.

In severe cases like this one, cooling measures should be rapidly initiated, and neuromuscular paralysis with endotracheal intubation may be life-saving to treat the muscle rigidity driving the hyperthermia and prevent complications such as rhabdomyolysis and acute renal failure.

Lithium has no role in the treatment of acute NMS, and there are case reports associating it with causing NMS. Haloperidol would be contraindicated because it is the most common cause of NMS. Dantrolene is the first-line treatment for MH, and while it has been used to treat NMS, initiation of muscle paralysis is more critical in this patient.

Test-taking tip: Pay special attention to the term "most" as a qualifier because it may indicate that at least two of the answers may be correct but one is more correct for the situation presented in the stem.

13. ANSWER: D

Telling the patient there is "nothing wrong" is likely not going to reassure the patient. She is clearly experiencing a host of different physical complaints and is concerned about them. This is likely to frustrate the patient and simply send her to another institution.

Telling the patient not to worry is likely futile because the patient is clearly suffering from "worry" more than anything else. What this tells the patient is that you (the doctor) are not worried, which the patient may interpret as you not taking her seriously.

The quintessential "it is all in your head" explanation is not only unhelpful and insulting but also incorrect. The patient is truly experiencing physical discomfort, even if there is nothing primarily wrong with the areas or organs in question.

It is advisable to validate her symptoms as real and to indicate that stress etiologies are very common. Education on the body-mind connection can be very helpful if done carefully: physical stress enhances mental stress, which in turn enhances the physical stress. In addition to the cornerstone recommendation of consistent primary care follow-up, a supportive approach may increase the likelihood of her eventually meeting with a mental health professional.

Test-taking tip: Professionalism in difficult doctor-patient communications often requires a balance of the good with the bad; be honest but also be kind. Remember that rapport-building is important always, but even more so when mental health is concerned.

14. ANSWER: C

Anorexia nervosa is an eating disorder characterized by excessively low body weight, which we do not see here. It also includes either restriction of calories or excessive attempts to lose weight, which we might see here with daily exercising and focus on diet. Also required would be the perception of obesity no matter how low the BMI dropped. Lack of menses is no longer considered one of the criteria for this diagnosis.

Binge-eating disorder is the most common eating disorder and is characterized by frequent episodes of consuming excessive amounts of food, over a short period of time, with a feeling of loss of control over these behaviors. We have no indication of binges here. No body image distortions are necessary.

Bulimia nervosa includes the binges of binge-eating disorder and the restriction or compensation of anorexia nervosa. The eroded enamel and metabolic alkalosis indicate likely long-term vomiting. Patients with bulimia often maintain a BMI that is normal or slightly above normal. These patients also have a body focus that is negative and spend significant amounts of time addressing diet and/or exercise. Use of laxatives (with metabolic acidosis) or excessive exercise (with musculoskeletal injuries) are other presentations that can commonly be seen.

Factitious disorder is a conscious exaggeration or creation of symptoms in order to have emotional needs of caregiving met. Although it is possible to have an eating disorder and a factitious disorder, we have no evidence of the latter. This patient appears to be presenting because of the real medical consequences of her self-induced vomiting.

Test-taking tip: When a symptom that is pathognomonic for a particular condition is present, use the rest of the information in the question to confirm what you are already suspecting.

15. ANSWER: A

Though normally associated with antidopaminergic drugs such as antipsychotics, NMS can be precipitated by the withdrawal of dopaminergic medications, particularly in patients with Parkinson's disease (Table 14.1). The management is similar to antipsychotic-induced NMS and includes paralysis and cooling measures but also should include the restarting of the dopaminergic drug. In this case this patients' levodopa should be restarted.

Cyproheptadine is a potential treatment for serotonin syndrome, not NMS. Haloperidol would be contraindicated because of its antidopaminergic properties. Benztropine is a treatment option for acute dystonic reactions (ADRs).

Test-taking tip: In this question, the clues that this is NMS and not serotonin syndrome are the sudden stopping of levodopa before the onset of symptoms and that he is febrile and rigid. If the authors wanted you to think serotonin syndrome, they would have mentioned clonus.

16. ANSWER: D

One of the risk factors for developing NMS is a prior history of NMS. Because NMS is associated with antidopaminergic drugs, it is important to avoid exposing these patients to such drugs. Chlorpromazine, promethazine, and metoclopramide are all potent antidopaminergic drugs and all associated with causing NMS. Ondansetron is a selective serotonin antagonist and not associated with causing NMS.

Test-taking tip: Often the correct answer can be obtained by determining how the answers are similar or dissimilar compared with each other. In this case, three of the four answers act via dopamine, while ondansetron does not.

17. ANSWER: D

Although a panic attack can include physical symptoms such as anxiety, diaphoresis, and tachycardia, symptoms of marked confusion, hypertension, dilated pupils, and diarrhea would be much less likely. Hyperreflexia and involuntary muscle spasms would be even less likely.

Table 14.1 COMPARISONS ON KEY FEATURES OF NEUROLEPTIC MALIGNANT SYNDROME, SEROTONIN SYNDROME AND MALIGNANT HYPERTHERMIA

SYNDROME	PHYSICAL EXAM FINDINGS	TREATMENT	MEDICATION TRIGGERS
Neuroleptic malignant syndrome	Febrile Rigid (lead-pipe rigidity)	Paralysis and cooling	Antipsychotics Withdrawal of dopaminergic drugs
Serotonin syndrome	Febrile Clonus	Benzodiazepine Cyproheptadine	Selective serotonin reuptake inhibitors, tramadol, monoamine oxidase inhibitors, cocaine
Malignant hyperthermia	Febrile Muscle rigidity	Dantrolene	Inhaled anesthetics

Dopamine-blocking agents, such as risperidone and metoclopramide, can potentially cause NMS. Although this would include autonomic instability, the motor symptoms of NMS are characteristically an increase in muscular tone, sometimes appearing as lead-pipe rigidity, and a corresponding decrease in reflexes.

An anticholinergic delirium would be characterized by a confessional state associated with urinary retention, constipation, and dry skin, eyes, and mucous membranes.

Serotonin syndrome is usually characterized by muscle spasms, clonus, and hyperreflexia in the presence of multiple, or high-dose, serotonergic agents such as paroxetine and zolmitriptan. Antihistamines and tricyclic antidepressants are other common offenders. Serotonin syndrome can be seen as a trio of "fast" events (rapid onset, increased reflexes, and rapid recovery), whereas NMS can be seen as three "slow" events (slower onset, decreased reflexes, and a slower recovery).

Test-taking tip: In a case of distinguishing between closely related toxidromes, look for different "directions" in symptoms (increased or decreased reflexes) to decide between them.

18. ANSWER: A

An acute confusional state with disturbance of attention and awareness in particular is in keeping with delirium. The temporal correlation of these signs with an infectious illness is further confirmatory. Psychotic symptoms, in this case visual hallucinations, are common in delirium and would not warrant an additional diagnosis.

A manic episode often includes significant distractibility but not a severe global cognitive impairment. Typical features would include an elevated or irritable mood, rapid speech, flight of ideas, and an increase in goal-directed behaviors.

Psychotic disorder secondary to another medical condition could include hallucinations but would not include major disruption of the sensorium.

Major neurocognitive disorder (dementia) is usually characterized by slow or stepwise onset and rarely includes major disruption of the sensorium until advanced stages. Hallucinations, although sometimes present early in Lewy body dementia, usually present much later in the course of the dementing process.

Test-taking tip: The presence of one illness (a primary psychiatric disorder such as schizophrenia or bipolar disorder) does not preclude the development of another (delirium). In a patient older than 65 years with sudden changes to sensorium, look first to acute medical illness (CVA or delirium) before attributing changes to those that are usually more insidious.

19. ANSWER: D

Although possibly due to health problems, normal aging does not present with dementia, loss of ambulation, and the inability to manage one's own medication. Blood sugar and pressure should also be manageable medical conditions in most circumstances.

Although there are several markers of possible Alzheimer's disease (cognitive and functional), this should have little direct effect on ambulation, falls, hypertension, or diabetes.

Major depressive disorder in older adults, or pseudodementia, is a very common and disabling condition. Other than possible cognitive symptoms, however, we have no indication of depression in this case. We would want to further investigate by using a validated screening tool like the Patient Health Questionnaire (PHQ-9), Depression in the Medically Ill (DMI), or Geriatric Depression Scale (GDS).

We would be concerned about neglect or abuse here because of the clear dependence of the patient on his family for help. Presuming the patient is cooperating with care, proper medication administration and supervision should prevent escalating markers of poor health and falls. Patients with cognitive decline and mobility issues are much more likely to be victims of neglect and abuse. The behavior of the caregiver may imply either exhaustion, depression, or anger toward the patient. Remember a patient need not be 65 years or older in order to call adult protection services, only dependent on the care of others.

Test-taking tip: When considering between common causes of illness, consider the cause with the largest body of evidence initially presented.

20. ANSWER: A

This situation has several hallmarks of possible abuse present. There are multiple physical injuries with a possible but "superficial" cover story. There is evidence of a power differential in the relationship, with him standing, speaking for her, and refusing to leave the room. This is mirrored in her passivity and agreement with his recommendations without discussion. Other risk factors of domestic violence are isolation, low income, alcohol use, and divorce. Two risk factors not present here are young age and pregnancy.

As patients age they become less able to metabolize alcohol and less tolerant to the negative aspects, and they are more likely to be on medications that interact badly (pain medications or sleep aids). This will often lead to accidents, falls, or relational difficulties. Although alcohol use disorders are frequent and dangerous, we have little information to go on here.

Although a 60-year-old woman with alcohol use and a fall could be at risk for cognitive decline, there is no direct evidence of that in the scenario. We would need to see ongoing loss of cognitive skills and difficulties with activities of daily living.

Although the patient has several risk factors for depression, we do not clearly hear the hallmarks of either low mood or anhedonia. Although now found to be of limited helpfulness in predicting suicide, the SAD PERSONS mnemonic can also be used to help assess risk for depression. This includes **S**ex (male), **A**ge (under 20 or over 44 years), **D**epression history, **P**revious suicide attempt, **E**thanol abuse, **R**ational thought loss, **S**ocial support lacking, **O**rganized suicide plan, **N**o spouse, **S**ickness.

Test-taking tip: When you lack enough clear information to make a definitive diagnosis, look to what the obstacle to getting more information is. That, in and of itself, may be the diagnosis.

21. ANSWER: D

This patient is displaying classic findings of MH. MH is a genetic disease that can be triggered by certain medications, including succinylcholine. It manifests as a hypermetabolic state due to uncontrolled muscle contraction. The first sign is an elevated end-tidal CO_2 reading. Muscle rigidity, hyperthermia, and cardiovascular collapse rapidly follow unless treatment with dantrolene is initiated. Dantrolene is the antidote for malignant hyperthermia and blocks the uncontrolled muscle contractions.

Piperacillin-tazobactam would not be indicated because this patient's time course is not consistent with development of an infection or sepsis. Rocuronium is ineffective in MH because the muscle contraction is not driven by neurologic signals. Bromocriptine is a dopamine agonist that can be used to treat NMS but will not have a role in treating MH.

Test-taking tip: Antidotes for life-threatening conditions are high yield and commonly tested on the boards. It is recommended to memorize that dantrolene is the treatment for MH.

22. ANSWER: C

Disulfiram inhibits the enzyme acetaldehyde dehydrogenase, which normally converts acetaldehyde to acetic acid. When ethanol is ingested in the presence of disulfiram, acetaldehyde accumulates and causes nausea, vomiting, flushing, hypotension, headache, and confusion. Occasionally this reaction can be severe. Other substances can also inhibit or cause a disulfiram-like reaction with ethanol. Examples are metronidazole and certain cephalosporins. Disulfiram also inhibits the enzyme dopamine ß-hydroxylase, which

results in a depletion of norepinephrine and contributes to the hypotension.

Test-taking tip: From the question stem you know that the patient in the question in having a disulfiram reaction. This helps you eliminate choices A and B.

23. ANSWER: D

Alcohol use and a prior suicide attempt are the two most important factors in the assessment of risk for depression and suicide. Not only does an alcohol or other substance use disorder contribute to risk, but also many patients will attempt suicide while intoxicated or in withdrawal.

For more than a decade now, collateral from a spouse or blood relative has been considered equivalent to a patient admitting suicidal ideation, intent, or plan directly to a provider. If this patient's daughter presents a reasonable story including commentary about the patient telling her he intends to kill himself, how, and when, this information is sufficient to have the patient admitted immediately for psychiatric care.

Test-taking tip: When choosing between several good answers, remember to choose the one that gives the simplest, fastest, and most direct solution to the clinical problem.

24. ANSWER: A

Lorazepam as part of a Clinical Indications for Withdrawal Assessment (CIWA) protocol is very likely to be helpful. Along with oxazepam, it is not broken down by the liver and is thus safe for use in patients with possible acute or chronic liver failure. Unfortunately, with the severity of this patient's alcohol withdrawal history, it is highly unlikely that benzodiazepines alone will be adequate to see this patient safely through withdrawal. Rather than resorting to high doses of medication in hopes of staving off seizure and delirium, it would likely be best to augment with other agents at the outset.

Both diazepam (Valium) of chlordiazepoxide (Librium) have been staples of detoxication and withdrawal protocols for many years. Unfortunately, the very long half-lives of both of these medications cause problems in two areas. First, a patient with advanced liver disease can be further injured by the high doses of these medications that may be needed. Second, repeated studies have demonstrated that using long-acting benzodiazepines is no more effective than other agents and is much more likely to lead to delirium and extended hospitalization.

Although haloperidol is a staple of emergency control of agitation, it is not ideal in this situation for two reasons. First, it can lower seizure threshold and worsen arrhythmia, both which could be factors here. Second, we know the mechanism of the agitation and confusion and know that they will both subside with proper use of other medications that modulate the GABA-glutamate system.

Test-taking tip: You recognize from the question stem that the patient is in alcohol withdrawal. Benzodiazepines are the mainstay of therapy. You just need to recognize that lorazepam is a benzodiazepine.

25. ANSWER: C

Although a neurology referral is not unreasonable, at this point we have no evidence for a true seizure disorder and strong evidence for a mental health cause.

The evidence for true seizure is quite low in this case. Starting seizure prophylaxis is not totally benign in that all medications have side effects, and using them without clear, or even likely, evidence is not recommended. The use of this particular agent is additionally problematic. Levetiracetam is unique in that, of all drugs in the class, it is the most likely to worsen underlying mental health symptoms.

This is clearly not a psychiatric emergency but is very likely to ultimately be diagnosed as a conversion disorder. This condition is more likely in women 15 to 34 years old with low levels of education and with a family history. An outpatient referral for evaluation and treatment of underlying depression and anxiety is the best course of action. If the patient refuses this referral, frequent visits to primary care with subsequent use of an antidepressant is the next best option.

Although duloxetine may in fact help treat underlying mood, anxiety, and even neuropathic pain symptoms, this is not the time for initiation. The patient needs a more complete mental health workup before medications can be appropriately recommended or selected. Additionally, the patient may be distressed to be given a psychiatric medication for what she sees, at this time, as a purely physical condition.

Test-taking tip: Choices A and C are very similar answers. You can rule out choice A with the normal EEG in the question stem.

26. ANSWER: A

This patient is demonstrating the classic findings of a disulfiram-like reaction. Headache, nausea, vomiting, abdominal pain, flushing, and hypotension are common. Confusion and seizures can be seen in more severe cases. Though not always appreciated, several cephalosporins, including ceftriaxone, are associated with sometimes severe disulfiram-like reactions. Metronidazole is classically

described to cause a disulfiram-like reaction when taken with ethanol, but published literature refutes this [Visapää JP, Tillonen JS, Kaihovaara PS, Salaspuro MP. Lack of disulfiram-like reaction with metronidazole and ethanol. Ann Pharmacother. 2002 Jun;36(6):971–4]. Regardless, metronidazole is not given IM. Nitrofurantoin is occasionally reported to cause a disulfiram-like reaction but is not given IM and is not used to treat a "vaginal infection." Doxycycline is not associated with a disulfiram-like reaction. Niacin can cause flushing but does not interact with ethanol to cause a disulfiram-like reaction.

Test-taking tip: Answer choices that are incompatible with information presented in the stem can be easily ruled out as the correct answer. In this case the antibiotic was given IM, and neither metronidazole, doxycycline, nor niacin is given IM.

27. ANSWER: B

This patient has an ADR, which is thought to be caused by blockade of dopamine receptors, specifically the D2 receptors. ADRs are associated with multiple medications but most commonly are seen with antidopaminergic drugs such as antipsychotics and antiemetics. In this case, this patient was taking metoclopramide, which is a potent antidopaminergic drug and well known to cause ADR.

Onset of ADR is usually within 48 hours of starting the offending medication. There are multiple types of ADRs, including oromandibular dystonia; oculogyric crises; blepharospasm; complex cervical dystonia with a mixture of retrocollis, laterocollis, and antecollis; focal limb dystonia; Pisa syndrome; and opisthotonos. This patient had oromandibular dystonia, which is the most common presentation. It presents with tongue and mouth dysfunction resulting in speech and swallowing difficulties.

Degranulation of mast cells and histamine-mediated vasodilation would be consistent with a hypersensitivity reaction. Inhibition of muscarinic acetylcholine receptors does not cause ADR.

Test-taking tip: The stem will provide information ruling in or out a suspected disease and is not meant to mislead you. In this case, a negative CT scan makes hypersensitivity reaction unlikely.

28. ANSWER: B

Although providing a single dose of medication for symptomatic relief is not unreasonable and would be the simplest solution, it is likely not ideal. Presuming the patient has waited more than 30 minutes for care, it is unlikely that the same panic attack is still happening. Furthermore, each time the patient is given symptomatic relief in an emergency setting, it fosters the ideas both that this is a true emergency and that returning to the ED is an appropriate and useful behavior.

Panic attacks can be quite frightening and uncomfortable but are not medical emergencies. The best chronic care is usually a combination of cognitive behavioral therapy (CBT) and an antidepressant medication that also treats anxiety. Medications can almost always be managed in primary care and a referral made to outside therapy.

Writing a prescription for a short course of anxiolytics might feel like a humane and benign treatment for this patient but is likely not helpful in the long run. The patient is already under the care of a provider who presumably knows his history much better than you do. This history may include substance abuse, other sedative hypnotics, or suicidality, all for which additional prescriptions could put the patient at risk. Additionally, as stated before, this fosters recurrent use of emergency services for routine care.

Although a depressed and anxious patient seeking benzodiazepines is certainly at risk for a substance use disorder, we do not have enough information here to make that diagnosis. This, again, is a decision that should be made by a provider with a longer-term relationship with the patient. What might look like medication-seeking behavior could be an honest attempt to have symptoms treated, a misunderstanding of the patient of proper treatment techniques, or even undertreatment of his symptoms by his primary care physician.

Test-taking tip: When choosing a treatment in the emergency setting, first determine whether this situation is truly an emergency. Treating a chronic condition as an emergency can disrupt the longitudinal care and confuse provider roles.

29. ANSWER: D

Although it is highly likely that this woman is having a hypomanic or manic episode and may ultimately need hospitalization, we do not yet have clear evidence of danger to herself or others or of grave disability. Her behavior would need to be more erratic and uncooperative or the history more concerning to arrive at this conclusion with only the information provided. The simple presence of mania, or even psychosis, does not automatically indicate hospitalization. Dangerousness is required for hospitalization.

Starting any of the listed agents would be appropriate if the patient had been aggressive or if we had determined unambiguously that this was a full manic episode. Here, the patient is able to somewhat calm herself and has historically been treated with a milder medication most commonly used for bipolar 2 disorder. Need for emergency medications has not yet been demonstrated, nor have criteria for bipolar 1

been fully met. Other options could include administering a benzodiazepine or (after some discussion) restarting the previously helpful medication.

Discharging her home is likely the best decision given the information provided. In reality, a full safety assessment needs to be done. This would entail doing an abbreviated psychiatric history, including recent risk behaviors, as well as collecting a history of suicide attempts, violence, hospitalizations, and responses to past treatments. With her fiancé there to provide collateral, this assessment should be possible.

A laboratory workup would be indicated if this patient had no prior history of psychiatric illness and was presenting with these manic symptoms.

Test-taking tip: The question stem presents a very stable, questionably manic individual. You can rule out choice A because she does not meet the criteria to hold her against her will. You can also eliminate B because you would not initiate a new psychiatric drug out of the ED. So that narrows your decision down to C or D.

30. ANSWER: D

This patient has signs and symptoms of oculogyric crisis, a severe type of ADR brought on by antidopaminergic drug use, in this case fluphenazine. Antimuscarinic drugs such as diphenhydramine or benztropine are the first-line treatment choice.

Benzodiazepines can be used in refractory cases. Dantrolene is the treatment for malignant hyperthermia. Droperidol would potentially make this patient's symptoms worse because it is a potent antidopaminergic drug. Ceftriaxone plus vancomycin would be appropriate if there were concern for meningitis or other infections, but in this case the most likely diagnosis is oculogyric crisis.

Test-taking tip: The question stem points you toward the diagnosis of dystonic reaction because the patient is a psychiatric patient with eyes stuck in one position.

31. ANSWER: C

Opioid abuse and associated deaths are at epidemic levels in the United States. Studies have shown that the concurrent use of benzodiazepines and opioids is associated with significantly higher rates of ED visits, hospital admissions, and deaths [Day C. Benzodiazepines in Combination with Opioid Pain Relievers or Alcohol: Greater Risk of More Serious ED Visit Outcomes. The CBHSQ Report. Rockville (MD): Substance Abuse and Mental Health Services Administration (US); 2013–.] Studies have not demonstrated the same synergy with cocaine or methamphetamine. Though barbiturates may be expected to cause increased toxicity when taken with opioids, there is no published literature supporting this.

Test-taking tip: You can rule out choices A and B because both of those drugs are stimulants. This leaves the answer between C and D.

32. ANSWER: D

This clearly describes delusional disorder, persecutory type, with the characteristic long-standing fixed negative belief about persecution from a defined source. As the diagnosis requires, the patient is able to function overall within the limits of his societal environment despite the delusion. Other named delusional subtypes are erotomanic, grandiose, jealous, somatic, and mixed.

Schizophrenia would require not only delusions, which he has, but other symptoms, which he is not demonstrating. These include hallucinations, odd speech, odd appearance or behavior, and negative symptoms. Additionally, most patient with schizophrenia are unable to maintain stable employment to the extent that they would own their own homes.

Paranoid personality type is a possibility, but the intensity and specificity of the symptoms speak against it. Although persistent, like delusions, the symptoms of personality disorder are usually directed more broadly. This would include suspiciousness of most people, including doctors, nurses, and other groups of people.

Although certainly possible after an accident, we are given no evidence of waxing or waning mental status in either occurrence. Speaking further against delirium are the persistent false beliefs maintaining the same content over the span of many years. Delirium tends to be more sensory, most often with hallucinations, and any delusions tend to be connected to these disturbances.

Test-taking tip: You can eliminate choice A because the question stem describes a well-groomed man who owns his home and pays taxes. One would expect a schizophrenic man in crisis to be more disheveled. You can also rule out C because there is no waxing and waning of symptoms. So you can narrow it down to B and D.

33. ANSWER: A

Cocaine is often adulterated with levamisole, which can cause agranulocytosis.

Hyperemesis syndrome is a poorly understood disease associated with marijuana use. Anthrax has been described with injection heroin use. It is a very rare disease and is caused by the bacteria *Bacillus anthracis*. It usually presents with massive edema or necrotizing fasciitis–type symptoms. The mortality rate is usually about 30% to 40%. Treatment is with antibiotics and usually surgical debridement. Contaminated heroin is the most likely source of injection anthrax.

Methamphetamine use can be associated with lead poisoning due to use of lead acetate in its manufacturing.

Test-taking tip: Anthrax is an encapsulated bacterium *B. anthracis,* which forms exotoxins. Only choices A and C are drugs of abuse that are usually injected, so you can narrow the answer to one of these two.

34. ANSWER: A

Use of a benzodiazepine is indicated in this case because of agitation with autonomic excitation due to methamphetamines. The use of a sedative would likely calm the patient, making further escalation of violence less likely. Lorazepam is readily available and short-acting and can be administered by several routes.

PO haloperidol is not ideal for several reasons. The patient is agitated and may be unwilling to accept oral medications. Without co-administration with sedatives, haloperidol is neither rapid-acting nor strongly sedating. Third, possible adverse events, including seizure, arrhythmia, and dystonia, could further complicate care.

The combination of haloperidol, diphenhydramine, and lorazepam would certainly be effective but is likely not yet necessary. The patient is neither confused nor psychotic, and he has not yet escalated to a point at which forced treatment is appropriate. This would be overly aggressive treatment.

IM olanzapine is an adequate alternative, when available, to the classic IM haloperidol, lorazepam, and diphenhydramine combination. Although, as discussed previously, forced antipsychotic medications are likely not appropriate at this time. This treatment is further complicated because of the risk for altered mental status and even airway endangerment if combined with benzodiazepines.

Test-taking tip: Remember that the patient is a sympathomimetic, and lorazepam is the best drug of choice to calm these symptoms. The other three answers all contain an antipsychotic. Because the patient is not psychotic, you can eliminate all those (B, C, D) and pick the benzodiazepine.

35. ANSWER: C

It is unlikely that several days of hospitalization in a mental institution will be of benefit to this young woman, and it could be quite terrifying. All evidence is that she made an impulsive decision and was under the influence of alcohol and is unlikely to do so again in the near future. She has no indication of a serious underlying mental condition and has a supportive home environment to return to where she can be closely monitored.

If the patient demonstrated clear sings of major depressive disorder, then starting treatment would not be unreasonable. This would have allowed time for the medication to start working before she was seen by primary care, at which time medications could be refined, increased, or changed. If needed, a referral to mental health could be done at that time.

Because this patient does not appear to have a major mental health diagnosis, counseling is likely the treatment of choice. Depending on family dynamics, this might include parents or other siblings to a greater or lesser extent. Although sometimes available, psychotherapy is usually not available through primary care, and thus a referral to outpatient psychotherapy should be made immediately to save time during which symptoms could worsen.

Although reducing classwork and/or extracurricular activities may be a part of the treatment plan, active treatment is also necessary. This may be done in conjunction with psychotherapy but not instead of it.

Test-taking tip: When considering the best next step, try to assess how serious the patient is and then balance the risks and benefits in order to avoid overtreating or undertreating.

36. ANSWER: B

Although the presenting symptoms point to migraine, it seems evident that this is not all that is going on. It is highly unlikely that this has not been diagnosed and treatment recommendations made several times in the past. Although this treatment will likely be necessary, it needs to be done in conjunction with additional psychiatric treatment. The use of an antidepressant with neuropathic pain benefits (e.g., selective serotonin-norepinephrine reuptake inhibitor [SNRI] or tricyclic antidepressant [TCA]) may well be in order.

This disorder is defined by recurrent, excessive, and time-consuming concern or worry over the meaning of distressing physical symptoms. When pain is the primary complaint, the modifier "with prominent pain" is added. Although she likely does have recurrent migraine, it appears that she is not satisfied with this being

the answer. Something in her psychology has amplified this medical condition to be something much more. Underlying depression, anxiety, or personality disorder should be screened for and then treated in conjunction with the pain.

Performing yet another expensive test despite having no additional information or indication would be unnecessary. Although potentially uncomfortable, a conversation would need to be conducted with the patient clarifying the reason for not performing the CT scan and the need for outpatient care.

Illness anxiety disorder does include worry about having or developing serious medical illness, but does so in the absence of significant physical symptoms. The presence of pain, here, excludes this purely intrapsychic diagnosis.

Test-taking tip: You can exclude C (CVA) from the start because there are no neurologic deficits in the question stem. Six ED visits in 1 month should flag to you that this is likely a psychiatric condition and not something organic, so you can narrow the answer choices to B and D.

37. ANSWER: D

Although frequently requested and prescribed, opioids demonstrate limited benefits paired with substantial health and addiction risk. The overtreatment of chronic and neuropathic pain with opioids accounts for a large proportion of the current opioid crisis faced in the United States.

Although psychotherapy may be a helpful adjunct to exercise and medication treatment, it is unlikely to be effective on its own.

The best evidence for treatment of chronic pain and, in particular, fibromyalgia includes physical therapy followed by graded physical exercise. This appears to both reverse problematic deconditioning and allow for the return of normal physiologic function with a regression of the hyperalgesia that is often seen in these syndromes. Neuropathic pain agents and antidepressants often augment care.

Test-taking tip: Opioid refills for chronic pain are something most ED physicians stay away from, so you can eliminate choices A and B right from the start.

15.

RENAL AND GENITOURINARY EMERGENCIES

Michelle Storkan

1. A 29-year-old sexually active male presents to the emergency department (ED) with painful left testicular swelling getting worse over the last week. Cremasteric reflex is intact on both sides, and lifting the left testicle improves his pain slightly. What is the best treatment option for this patient's testicular pain?

    A. Doxycycline 100 mg PO twice daily for 10 days + ceftriaxone 250 mg IM once
    B. Levofloxacin 500 mg PO once daily for 7 days
    C. Surgery
    D. Manual detorsion in emergency department

2. A 67-year-old male presents with suprapubic abdominal pain. The patient states he has not been able to urinate for the past 8 hours. He has never had this problem before. He states he was feeling fine when he woke up this morning. He denies fever, chills, nausea, or vomiting. He is visibly uncomfortable. Bladder scan shows 950 mL of urine in his bladder. What is the next best step in management of this patient?

    A. Emergent urology consult
    B. Tamsulosin and reassess
    C. Suprapubic drainage of bladder
    D. Urinary catheter placement and discharge with urology follow-up as outpatient

3. A 21-year-old male presents with diffuse body aches and muscle soreness. He has been practicing twice a day for football season starting next month. Urinalysis (UA) dipstick is positive for blood, and microanalysis of UA shows no red blood cells (RBCs). Which of the following is the most life-threatening complication of this disease process?

    A. Hyponatremia
    B. Hypocalcemia
    C. Hyperkalemia
    D. Hypokalemia

4. A 72-year-old man with no significant past medical history presents with increased fatigue. The patient has had worsening symptoms over the past 1 to 2 weeks. He has also noticed some increased difficulty urinating with starting and stopping of his urine stream for the past several months. Vital signs are within normal limits. Basic lab findings are significant only for a creatinine of 3.1. The most likely cause of this patient's acute renal failure is:

    A. Postobstructive, most likely from hypertrophic prostate
    B. Ischemic injury from congestive heart failure
    C. Angiotensin-converting enzyme (ACE) inhibitor use
    D. Crystal-induced nephropathy from gout

5. A 27-year-old G1P0 female with an estimated gestational age of 16 weeks presents with lower abdominal cramping for the last 24 hours. The patient has no other associated symptoms. Vital signs are heart rate (HR) 86 bpm, blood pressure (BP) 105/75 mm Hg, respiratory rate (RR) 16 breaths/min, and oxygen saturation 99% on room air. Bedside ultrasound shows an intrauterine pregnancy (IUP) with fetal heart tones of 146 bpm. Vaginal exam is unremarkable, and UA shows leukocyte esterase 1+, white blood cells (WBCs) 5, and bacteria 2+. The patient has no associated urinary symptoms. What is the next best step in management?

    A. Discharge home with return precautions in case she develops symptoms associated with urinary tract infection
    B. Discharge home with prescription for nitrofurantoin 100 mg PO twice for 5 days should symptoms occur
    C. Nitrofurantoin 100 mg PO twice daily for 5 days to start now
    D. Ciprofloxacin 250 mg PO once daily for 3 days

6. A 30-year-old otherwise healthy female presents with flank pain and fever for the past 3 days. Review of

293

systems is otherwise negative. Vital signs are HR 105 bpm, BP 115/78 mm Hg, oxygen saturation 99% on room air, and temperature 38.5° C (101.3° F). On exam, the patient has costovertebral angle tenderness on the right. Urine pregnancy test is negative. UA is significant for positive nitrites and leukocyte esterase, WBCs 153, and moderate bacteria. HR and temperature are normalized after acetaminophen administration. What is the next best step in management?

A. Send urine culture, start PO antibiotics, and discharge with return precautions
B. Computed tomography (CT) study for renal stone
C. Discharge with return precautions for asymptomatic bacteriuria
D. Renal ultrasound

7. A 72-year-old previously healthy male presents with bright red hematuria off and on for the past couple days. Review of symptoms is otherwise negative. The patient quit smoking 10 years ago. Vital signs are stable, and physical exam is unremarkable. UA is significant only for gross hematuria, with microscopic hematuria significant for 363 RBCs per high-power field (hpf). What is the next best step in management of this patient?

A. Outpatient referral to urology within the next month
B. CT of the abdomen and pelvis for renal stone study
C. Renal ultrasound
D. Labs, CT of the abdomen and pelvis with contrast, and hospital admission

8. A 61-year-old male with a history of alcohol abuse presents with painful, swollen testicles. Vital signs are HR 105 bpm, BP 90/72 mm Hg, and temperature 37.7° C (99.9° F). On exam, both testicles are erythematous and swollen, with extreme pain on palpation and with some pain, tenderness, and firmness on the perineum as well. What is the patient's definitive management?

A. Testicular ultrasound
B. CT of the abdomen and pelvis with IV contrast
C. Labs, antibiotics, and admission to hospital
D. Emergent surgical consultation

9. A 10-year-old male presents with erythema on his penis. The patient is uncircumcised and is noted to have white discharge around the glans when the foreskin is retracted. His mother says that this is his third time having this in the past year. Previous episodes have been successfully treated with good cleaning and antifungal cream. Has had no dysuria or decreased urinary output. What is the next best step in management?

A. Urinary catheter placement
B. Fingerstick blood glucose
C. Emergent urology consult
D. Urology follow-up as outpatient

10. A 40-year-old uncircumcised male presents with a painful penis. The patient is not in any apparent distress. Genitourinary exam shows the picture in Figure 15.1. What is the next best step in management?

A. Circumcision as outpatient
B. Emergent urology consultation
C. Can be physiologic until adolescence—reassurance and follow-up as outpatient
D. Treat with betamethasone cream and follow up as outpatient

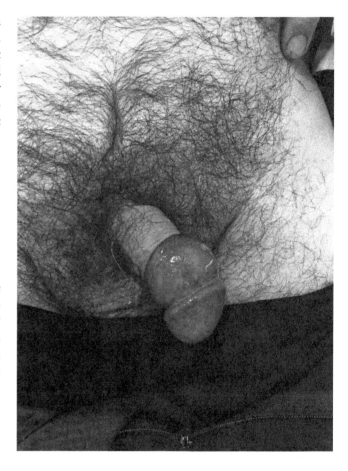

Figure 15.1 Genitourinary exam.
(Picture curtesy of Dr. Mariely Ercolano, Emergency Physician, Chile.)

11. An 8-year-old male presents after waking from sleep with acute right lower quadrant (RLQ) abdominal pain. He is in severe distress and crying. He vomited twice at home. Palpation of RLQ elicits no pain. Genitourinary exam shows a firm, right testis that appears higher than the left testis. Cremasteric reflex is intact on the left but

absent on the right. There is some relief of pain with elevation of the right testicle. Emergent ultrasound is obtained. What is the next best step in management?

A. Antibiotics and discharge
B. Emergent urology consult
C. Emergent urology consult and attempt at manual detorsion in the ED
D. CT with IV contrast

12. A 66-year-old male presents with pain during defecation and increased urinary frequency. He is afebrile, and his vital signs are otherwise stable. On exam, the patient has mild suprapubic tenderness, and rectal exam shows a boggy, tender prostate. UA is unremarkable. What is the definitive treatment?

A. Emergent urology consultation
B. Outpatient urology referral
C. IV antibiotics and admit
D. PO antibiotics for 2 to 4 weeks with primary care follow-up

13. A 3-year-old male is brought in by his mother for concern over an abdominal mass. The mother noted the mass while she was helping the boy with his sweatshirt. The child is a previously healthy male, born at full term with no significant family medical history. He has no other complaints. On exam, you palpate a mass also in the lower abdomen. What is the next best step in evaluation?

A. Deep palpation of mass to aid in diagnosis
B. Chest radiograph
C. Abdominal ultrasound
D. CT scan with contrast

14. A 2-year-old female is brought in by her mother for concern over decreased activity. The patient is still drinking liquids well but has less interest in solid foods. The mother notes that patient had a diarrheal illness a little over a week ago that has since resolved. She has noted one or two fewer wet diapers over the past 24 hours. The patient is sleeping but is easily awoken with mild stimulation, will interact, and then falls asleep again. Vital signs are HR 110 bpm, BP 90/60 mm Hg, RR 27 breaths/min, and temperature 37.2° C (99° F). No rashes are noted, and the physical exam is otherwise unremarkable. Lab results are significant for WBCs 14, hemoglobin (Hgb) 7, platelets 45, creatinine 1.8, and Na 132. What is the next best step in management?

A. Administer 10–20 mL/kg normal saline bolus, platelet transfusion, hospital admission

B. Administer 10–20 mL/kg normal saline bolus, IV antibiotics, send stool for culture, hospital admission
C. Administer 10–20 mL/kg normal saline bolus, send stool for culture, hospital admission
D. Send stool for culture, PO antibiotics, discharge with close follow-up with pediatrician

15. A 56-year-old female with past medical history of diabetes mellitus and end-stage renal disease (ESRD) on hemodialysis presents with pain in her left arm for 1 day. The patient is medically compliant and has been going to dialysis appointments as indicated. Vital signs are stable. Exam shows the patient is in mild discomfort. Left upper extremity shows the graft site where the patient gets dialysis. Distal pulses are 2+, and no palpable thrill is felt over the graft. What is the definitive treatment?

A. Heparin drip and admit for medical management
B. Antibiotics and admit for vascular consult as inpatient
C. Vascular surgery consult and possible angiography
D. Vascular surgery consult and emergent thrombectomy in the operating room

16. A 59-year-old female with past medical history of diabetes mellitus, hypertension, and chronic kidney disease has recently started hemodialysis through an arteriovenous fistula. What is the most common complication of this treatment of ESRD?

A. Hypotension
B. Air embolus
C. Hypertension
D. Dialysis disequilibrium syndrome

17. A 63-year-old male with a past medical history of ESRD on peritoneal dialysis presents with fever, chills, nausea, and vomiting. The patient is normotensive. Dialysate has been cloudy at home. Fluid analysis shows 200 leukocytes/mm³ with more than 50% neutrophils. What is the most common causative organism of this illness?

A. Fungi
B. Gram-negative bacteria
C. *Staphylococcus aureus*
D. *Staphylococcus epidermidis*

18. A 45-year-old male with a history of ESRD on hemodialysis presents with chest pain and shortness of breath. Vital signs on presentation are HR 110 bpm, BP 115/75 mm Hg, oxygen saturation 94% on room air, and RR 20 breaths/min. Electrocardiogram (EKG) shows sinus tachycardia with normal intervals and T waves.

The patient starts to complain of increased chest pain and shortness of breath along with lightheadedness. Systolic blood pressure decreases to 75 mm Hg, HR increases to 140 bpm, and the BP is not responsive to IV fluid. What is the best treatment option?

A. Heparin drip
B. Alteplase IV
C. Needle thoracostomy
D. Pericardiocentesis

19. A 75-year-old female presents 10 weeks after renal transplantation with fever and chills. The patient is not on any prophylaxis for infectious organisms. What is the most likely causative organism for infection in this patient?

A. *S. aureus*
B. Cytomegalovirus (CMV)
C. *Clostridium difficile*
D. *Streptococcus viridians*

20. A 54-year-old female presents with anuria 1 week after kidney transplantation. The patient has been taking BP medication as prescribed, as well as cyclosporine. Vital signs are HR 72 bpm, BP 205/121 mm Hg, and temperature 37.2° C (99° F). Serum creatinine is increased 20% from her last blood draw on record. Cyclosporine level is within normal limits. What is the most likely cause?

A. Renal artery thrombosis
B. Chronic rejection
C. Cyclosporine toxicity
D. Infection of urinary tract

21. A 30-year-old previously healthy, 14-week pregnant female presents with left-sided flank pain and hematuria. Vital signs are within normal limits. Microscopic analysis of UA shows RBCs 350/hpf, WBCs 250/hpf, and positive leukocyte esterase. Renal ultrasound shows hydronephrosis. What is the next best step in management?

A. Discharge with pain control and antibiotics
B. Discharge with pain control, antibiotics, and gynecology follow-up
C. Discharge with pain control, antibiotics. and urology follow-up
D. Admit with pain control, antibiotics, and urology consult

22. A 20-month-old previously healthy male is brought in by his parents for concern of testicular swelling. The parents first noted the swelling a couple of days ago when changing the patient's diapers. The swelling appears to vary in size. Urine output is within normal limits. The patient is a healthy-appearing child. Exam reveals no pain on palpation of left testicle, which is swollen compared with the right. No erythema is noted. When a penlight is placed behind the left testicle, there is illumination of the scrotum. What is the next step in management of this patient?

A. Discharge for outpatient testicular ultrasound and urology referral
B. Attempt to manually reduce in ED
C. Emergent urology consult
D. Admit for ultrasound, antibiotics, and urology consult

23. A 23-year-old previously healthy male presents with painful sustained erection for the past 4 hours. The patient is on no medications and has not taken any medications in the past 24 hours. Emergent urology consult has been called. Which of the following lab tests will be the most useful in this patient's management?

A. Complete blood count (CBC)
B. Hgb electrophoresis
C. Prothrombin time (PT)/international normalized ratio (INR), activated partial thromboplastin time (aPTT)
D. Platelets

24. A previously healthy 60-year-old male presents with acute kidney injury (AKI). He is found to have an FeNa of <1%. What is the most likely cause of this patient's kidney injury?

A. Prostatic hypertrophy
B. Recent upper respiratory infection
C. Nonsteroidal antiinflammatory drugs (NSAIDs)
D. Antibiotics

25. A 32-year-old previously healthy female presents with headache, facial swelling, and shortness of breath. The patient seems to be in mild distress. Vital signs are HR 110 bpm, BP 175/95 mm Hg, RR 20 breaths/min, and oxygen saturation 90% on room air. On exam, the patient has some periorbital swelling, clear lung sounds, and trace symmetric lower extremity edema without pain. Creatinine is within normal limits. Urinalysis shows proteinuria. Chest radiograph is clear without fluid or effusion. What is the next best test on this patient?

A. CT angiography of the chest
B. Ultrasound with Doppler of bilateral lower extremities
C. PT/INR, aPTT, platelets
D. Renal ultrasound

26. A 30-year-old male presents with penile swelling after sexual intercourse. The patient felt a painful pop and then had swelling to his penis afterward. He has no laceration on the exterior of the penis but has some painful swelling of the penis with some blood seen at the meatus. What is the definitive management?

A. Splinting of the penis
B. Surgery
C. Foley catheter placement
D. Retrograde urethrogram and, if the urethra is intact, Foley catheter placement

27. A 47-year-old female on peritoneal dialysis presents with abdominal pain. What is the minimum number of WBCs in the dialysate needed to make the diagnosis of peritonitis?

A. 5/mm^3
B. 50/mm^3
C. 100/mm^3
D. 150/mm^3

28. What is the most common cause of progressively worsening shortness of breath in a 53-year-old male on hemodialysis for ESRD?

A. Volume overload
B. Cardiac tamponade
C. Pneumothorax
D. Acute coronary syndrome

ANSWERS

1. ANSWER: A

This question is describing epididymitis. Epididymitis is inflammation of the epididymis, the long, tightly coiled tube in the scrotal sac that carries sperm. It is most often inflamed secondary to infection. In a young, sexually active male, the most common cause is a sexually transmitted infection (STI), either gonorrhea or chlamydia. Therefore, treatment is similar to that for urethritis caused by either of those two organisms (doxycycline PO for 10 days and ceftriaxone IM once). If STIs are less likely (for board purposes, this would likely be in a man aged 65 years or older with no risk factors), then the most common cause would be *Escherichia coli,* with levofloxacin being the antibiotic of choice.

Epididymitis is commonly confused with testicular torsion with a painful swollen testicle. Testicular torsion is a surgical emergency, and prompt ultrasound would help distinguish the two when in doubt. However, there are some classic clinical signs that help distinguish the two. With epididymitis, the cremasteric reflex remains intact, whereas it classically doesn't in torsion. This reflex is seen when lightly touching the inside of the thigh on the side of the swollen testicle causes the testicle to elevate slightly. Prehn's sign is also present in epididymitis, when elevating the swollen testicle will alleviate some of the pain. This is not true in torsion. Also, epididymitis usually has a more gradual onset, whereas torsion is acute.

Test-taking tip: The clinical signs and symptoms of torsion versus epididymitis may not always be clear in the ED, but for the sake of the exam, pay special attention to demographics (age) and to clues such as "sexually active" that will point you in the right direction.

2. ANSWER: D

This patient is suffering from acute urinary retention. The most common cause in this demographic (older male) is prostatic hypertrophy. Foley catheter placement and follow-up with urology within 1 week are appropriate treatment of this patient. Tamsulosin can be used in conjunction with urinary catheter placement but should not be used acutely in the ED in this way. If there is difficulty in placing the catheter, a Coudé-tipped catheter can be used to help get around the enlarged prostate, but suprapubic drainage is not the next best step, which the question asks.

Test-taking tip: Always pay attention to when the question is asking for the "next best step" or "definitive management." This is directing you to the answer choice that is literally the next best step. Although all answers may have some role in management if there are complications, only one choice points the simplest, next best step.

3. ANSWER: C

This question is describing rhabdomyolysis. UA dipstick would be positive for blood, but microanalysis would show absence of RBCs. This is because myoglobin tests positive as blood on dipstick. The deadliest complication of rhabdomyolysis is hyperkalemia; for that reason, IV fluids with potassium such as lactated Ringer's solution should be avoided. Hypocalcemia can be seen with rhabdomyolysis but is normally not considered significant.

The most common causes of rhabdomyolysis in adults are alcohol and drugs of abuse, but strenuous physical activity and heat-related illness are also common causes. Inherited metabolic disorders should be suspected in adults and children with recurrent rhabdomyolysis, especially associated with exercise intolerance.

Presenting symptoms usually are acute and include myalgias, stiffness, weakness, malaise, dark urine, and low-grade fever. Nausea, vomiting, abdominal pain, and encephalopathy can occur.

Elevated creatine kinase (CK) is the most sensitive and reliable indicator of muscle injury. Although it correlates with amount of muscle injury, it doesn't correlate with development of renal failure or other morbidity. Elevation peaks between 24 and 72 hours after onset of muscle injury.

Aggressive rehydration is the treatment of choice. The main goal is to monitor urine output with a goal of 2 mL/kg/hr. Avoid NSAIDs because of their effect on the kidneys and treat the underlying cause.

Test-taking tip: Remember to pay attention the what may sometimes seem like extraneous details in the question step. The board exam will not give information that is not necessary to understanding the clinical picture in some way. Why is it important this young man is a football player practicing twice a day? Overexertion exercise at preseason (when he may not be as well conditioned) is an important clue to the cause of rhabdomyolysis.

4. ANSWER: A

This question is describing AKI. Given this patient's age, lack of medical problems, and associated symptoms, the most likely cause is obstructive and postrenal. Prostatic hypertrophy is the most common cause of postrenal AKI. There are no findings that would suggest other causes listed. The most common cause of AKI in general is decreased kidney perfusion, caused by disorders such as congestive heart failure. ACE inhibitors and NSAIDs are the most common causes of prerenal AKI. There are no clues to this—in fact, the question stem specifically states that this patient has no known medical history. There are also no clues to suggest that this patient is also suffering from gout to explain crystal-induced nephropathy.

Test-taking tip: Remember not to overthink the question and to pay attention to the clues. The difficulty urinating and change in urine stream, along with the patient's age, are indicative of prostatic hypertrophy.

5. ANSWER: C

Asymptomatic bacteriuria treatment is recommended only in pregnant women (and in patients immediately before invasive urinary procedures). Ciprofloxacin is not recommended in pregnant woman because of the known potential to cause birth defects.

Test-taking tip: One test-taking strategy involves narrowing down the answer choices to two when you are unsure. Two answer choices are similar and recommend nitrofurantoin, so likely one is correct.

6. ANSWER: A

Acute pyelonephritis in an otherwise healthy young person can be discharged without imaging. Diagnosis of pyelonephritis is a clinical one based on costovertebral angle tenderness or flank pain with or without fever, and a positive urine culture. Frequently it can be associated with other systemic symptoms such as nausea and vomiting.

Complications of upper urinary tract infections include acute bacterial nephritis, renal abscess, and emphysematous pyelonephritis. These diagnoses are made with imaging studies, which are indicated in patients who have an inadequate or atypical response to antibiotics. Imaging should be considered in acute pyelonephritis when the patient is male, an older adult, diabetic, immunocompromised, or severely ill.

Test-taking tip: Pay attention to the answers that have the most "information" in them. Also, there are two subtly similar answers—the two imaging studies. It would be difficult for the board exam to ask you to pick between these two because both are feasible next best "imaging" steps, unless there was a relative contraindication to one, such as CT in pregnancy.

7. ANSWER: A

This is an otherwise healthy, older adult patient who is presenting with painless hematuria. This is malignancy until proved otherwise. Provided the patient doesn't have any other symptoms, such as flank pain or bladder outlet obstruction, and has stable vital signs and is able to follow up in a timely manner, this can be managed as an outpatient.

The most common kidney cancer in adults is renal cell carcinoma. It accounts for 3% of adult malignancies and 95% of cancers arising from the kidneys. It is usually clinically silent, with only 10% of patients presenting with hematuria, flank mass, and flank pain.

Test-taking tip: Pay particular attention to extra clues given in the question stem. The boards will not give you information that is not pertinent to the case. Why is it mentioned that this patient quit smoking 10 years ago? Smoking is a risk factor for malignancy in the setting of painless hematuria.

8. ANSWER: D

This question is describing Fournier's gangrene. Diabetic patients and those with a history of alcohol abuse are disproportionately affected by this disease. Mortality is high (estimates of 20%–40%), and while labs, IV antibiotics, and possible imaging are important considerations, emergent surgical consult should not be delayed in this case.

Test-taking tip: Remember to always pay attention to what the question is asking. The next "best step" or "definitive management" is a common board question, and while all the answers may have some validity in treatment, there is only one next best step.

9. ANSWER: B

Balanoposthitis is often the presenting sign of diabetes. If it is not diabetes, it can be due to poor personal hygiene, especially in a patient who has had recurrence.

Test-taking tip: The question stem is clearly describing a *Candida* infection. *Candida* infections are frequently associated with diabetes.

10. ANSWER: B

This question is asking you to know the difference between paraphimosis and phimosis. Paraphimosis is a true urologic emergency. It is the inability to reduce the proximal foreskin over the distal glans penis into its natural position. On exam, you will see a symmetric swelling of foreskin retracted behind the glans. If it remains in this position, it can result in glans edema and venous engorgement, which can then lead to arterial compromise. Paraphimosis is what is pictured in Figure 15.1.

Phimosis, on the other hand, is not an emergency as long as the patient is able to urinate. The other three answer choices are all true of phimosis but not paraphimosis.

Phimosis refers to the inability to retract the foreskin behind the glans and is benign as long as urine output is not compromised.

Test-taking tip: This is a "you know it or don't" kind of question. If you don't know it, choose an answer and move on. You can perhaps mark it for review when you are done at the end of the test. Don't, however, let these kinds of questions get you stuck and waste your time.

11. ANSWER: C

This question is showing a case of testicular torsion. Testicular torsion is a surgical emergency with a higher frequency in males up to age 18 years. Unilateral presence of a cremasteric reflex is a sensitive test for ruling out testicular torsion, although torsion can present with an intact cremasteric reflex. Often, especially in children, torsion can present as lower quadrant abdominal pain. Vomiting increases the likelihood of torsion as a diagnosis. Ultrasound image with Doppler shows a heterogeneous testicle with reduced color flow/vascularity, which is indicative of torsion. Even if manual detorsion is successful in the ED, these patients are likely to have recurrent torsion, so surgical consult is still necessary.

Test-taking tip: This question highlights the fact that you don't necessarily need to be able to interpret the image to answer the question and know that the treatment of testicular torsion is urology consult for surgery.

12. ANSWER: D

This question is describing acute prostatitis. Symptoms include low back pain; perineal, suprapubic, or genital discomfort; obstructive urinary voiding symptoms; frequency or dysuria; perineal pain with ejaculation; and fever or chills. Clinical findings are perineal tenderness, prostatic tenderness or bogginess, and rectal sphincter spasm. UA and culture are often unremarkable. Treatment is with 2 to 4 weeks of antibiotics, ideally including outpatient follow-up after 2 weeks of treatment. Prostatic massage is not necessary or indicated.

Test-taking tip: The benign presentation of this patient with normal vital signs can be used to exclude emergent consult and the need for IV antibiotics with admission.

13. ANSWER: C

This is a classic presentation of Wilms' tumor, presenting as a painless abdominal mass. It is malignant, typically in

children younger than 5 years, with good overall survival rates of more than 90%. Excessive palpation can cause tumor rupture. Chest radiograph should be obtained to evaluate for pulmonary metastases, as should CT or MRI eventually to identify extent of the disease, but the next best imaging modality in the ED is ultrasound.

Test-taking tip: There are certain disease processes that you need to know for the boards. The most important thing here is recognizing that this is Wilms' tumor. If you don't know the imaging modality of choice, try to use logic to eliminate: deep palpation is never a diagnostic modality for ED physicians. Chest radiograph for a renal tumor? Seems unlikely. CT scan versus ultrasound—a goal in pediatrics is to avoid radiation at a young age, so for most pediatric diseases, ultrasound is a reasonable first choice.

14. ANSWER: C

This question is describing hemolytic uremic syndrome (HUS). HUS is a multisystem disorder resulting in acute renal failure, thrombocytopenia, and microangiopathic hemolytic anemia. Consider the triad of anemia, high creatinine, and low platelets. There is a known association with *E. coli* O157:H7, although many cases have an obscure etiology. It often is seen in young children and follows an early, nonspecific course of respiratory illness or gastroenteritis.

A wide variety of signs and symptoms can be seen, including mild elevations in blood urea nitrogen (BUN) and creatinine with mild to moderate anemia and thrombocytopenia ranging to seizures, toxic megacolon, bloody diarrhea, hypertension, intussusception, and coma.

Platelet transfusion is not recommended, although RBC transfusion may be necessary in severe anemia. Antibiotics are generally contraindicated in pediatric diarrheal illness.

Test-taking tip: Use the clues in the question stem of an ill child with significant lab abnormalities (low Hbg, high creatinine, low platelets) to remind yourself that this is HUS.

15. ANSWER: C

This question is asking for management of a thrombosed or stenosed dialysis graft site. Complications of vascular access account for more inpatient days than any other complication of hemodialysis. Thrombosis and stenosis are the most common causes of inadequate dialysis flow and are more common in grafts than fistulas.

Vascular surgery should be consulted, but most of these cases can be treated within 24 hours either by angiographic clot removal or angioplasty. Direct injection of alteplase is also an option to be done in consult with the vascular surgeon. CT scan may be helpful to confirm thrombosis/ stenosis while waiting for consult or may be requested by the vascular surgeon.

Test-taking tip: Try to eliminate answers that don't make sense. For example, there are no clues or signs in the question stem that would indicate that antibiotics are necessary at this point.

16. ANSWER: A

Hypotension is the most common complication of hemodialysis, estimated to occur in about 50% of treatments. Air embolus is a potential complication, although not overly common. Although dialysis disequilibrium syndrome is a complication and more common in patients new to hemodialysis, it is not the most common complication. It is a syndrome that presents with nausea, vomiting, and hypertension at the end of dialysis. It can progress to seizure, coma, and death.

Test-taking tip: Hemodialysis is the removal of fluid from the body, so common sense would suggest hypotension, at least as opposed to hypertension, if unsure. Also you may not have heard of the other two options in reference to hemodialysis so they are unlikely the "most common" complications.

17. ANSWER: D

This question is asking for the most common cause of peritonitis in patients on peritoneal dialysis. *S. epidermidis* is responsible for an estimated 40% of cases. All other options are also possible, but *S. epidermidis* is the most common.

Test-taking tip: There are certain "most commons" that are important to memorize for the sake of the board exam. This is one of them.

18. ANSWER: D

Cardiac tamponade should always be considered in an unstable patient with a history of ESRD. Dialysis patients often do not present with the classic signs of cardiac tamponade. Instead, they may present with change in mental status, shortness of breath, and hypotension. Bedside ultrasound is the best modality to detect pericardial effusion.

Test-taking tip: The rapid deterioration of this patient with hypotension, not fluid responsive, along with chest pain and shortness of breath, points to either tension pneumothorax of cardiac tamponade. There is no clear suggestion of pneumothorax, and the boards will not try to trick

you on a diagnoses. The trick here is to associate ESRD with the potential complication of pericardial effusion.

19. ANSWER: B

In the 1 to 6 months after transplantation, in patients without prophylaxis or having just discontinued prophylaxis treatment, CMV infection is the most common cause of febrile illness. This is true after any transplantation, not just renal transplantation.

Test-taking tip: This is a "you know it or don't" kind of question. If you don't know it, choose an answer and move on. You can perhaps mark it for review when you are done at the end of the test. Don't, however, let these kinds of questions get you stuck and waste your time.

20. ANSWER: A

Renal artery thrombosis is a potential complication of renal transplantation, treatable by surgery. Symptoms include anuria, uncontrolled hypertension, and acute kidney failure. It can occur days to weeks after transplantation. After transplantation, acute kidney failure is defined as 20% increase in baseline creatinine, as opposed to the standard definition of 50% increase from baseline. Identifying this condition early on is important to save the graft. Chronic rejection occurs over 4 to 6 months, and increases in BP, proteinuria, and serum creatinine occur more gradually. Anuria is rare in cyclosporine toxicity, and cyclosporine levels are noted to be normal in the question stem. There are no signs that would indicate infection in this patient, although a patient on cyclosporine may be afebrile in the setting of infection.

Test-taking tip: If unsure what the question stem is alluding to, read all the possible answers. Chronic rejection after 1 week doesn't make sense. The question stem said the cyclosporine levels were normal so toxicity doesn't make sense. There are no clues in the question stem to indicate infection.

21. ANSWER: D

This patient has signs and symptoms of an infected kidney stone. Because the patient is pregnant, surgical intervention is warranted when there are hydronephrosis and signs of infection. Gynecologic consultation may also be necessary, but the most important thing to recognize here is the need for urology consult and admission.

Test-taking tip: Sometimes it can be a clue when one answer is drastically different from the others, so pay attention to those choices. In this case D is the only answer that involves admission, and that is the correct answer in this case.

22. ANSWER: A

This question stem is describing a hydrocele. A hydrocele is an accumulation of fluid around the testes and is the most common cause of painless scrotal swelling in children. The swelling is often intermittent and improved when the patient is supine. The diagnosis is confirmed by the transillumination test, which is described in this question stem. When a penlight is placed behind the affected testicle, it should illuminate like a lantern. If there was an abscess, enlarged testicle, or thickened scrotal wall, the light wouldn't penetrate. Most hydroceles reabsorb by 18 to 24 months of age. Management is described in the answer choice A: outpatient referral for urology and outpatient testicular ultrasound.

Test-taking tip: Choices B and C both describe treatment for torsion, so they can be ruled out because the question stem is not describing a torsion.

23. ANSWER: B

In a previously healthy, young male with priapism, the diagnosis of sickle cell disease should be considered. This diagnosis is made through Hgb electrophoresis.

Test-taking tip: In a young African American male with priapism, always consider sickle cell disease. This is an association to memorize.

24. ANSWER: C

Fractional excretion of sodium (FeNa) is a calculated value that helps determine whether the kidney injury is due to prerenal, intrinsic, or postrenal causes. With an FeNa of <1%, as listed in this question, it is describing prerenal causes of acute kidney failure. The most common cause is NSAID use. Other test results that could be mentioned in a question to hint at a prerenal cause of kidney injury are urine Na of <20 mEq/dL and serum BUN/creatinine ratio of >20:1. Prostatic hypertrophy is the most common cause of postrenal injury. Upper respiratory infection (i.e., streptococcal pneumonia) would be associated with glomerulonephritis, an intrinsic cause of renal injury. Antibiotics in general are not associated with kidney failure.

Test-taking tip: This question requires memorization of the meaning of FeNa (fractional excretion of sodium).

Of prerenal causes of kidney injury, NSAIDs are the most common. "Most commons" are heavily tested on the boards.

25. ANSWER: A

This question is describing nephrotic syndrome. Edema is the most common complaint. Shortness of breath and cough can often be caused by a pleural effusion. Other signs and symptoms can include nausea, vomiting, and fatigue as well as headache. Some patients describe tea-colored urine.

The main life-threatening complication of nephrotic syndrome is thromboembolic events. With a clear chest radiograph in a patient with nephrotic syndrome who is short of breath and hypoxic, pulmonary embolism should be considered. Patients with nephrotic syndrome are also at an increased risk for life-threatening infection.

Test-taking tip: Even if you don't recognize nephrotic syndrome in this patient, the patient's complaint of shortness of breath, along with tachycardia and mild hypoxia, should raise concern for pulmonary embolus.

26. ANSWER: B

This patient has a penile fracture. The classic story is pain during intercourse followed by swelling. There can sometimes be blood from the meatus. Urgent urology consult and surgery are the definitive management of this patient. Although retrograde urethrogram (RUG) and Foley placement may be used to guide treatment and surgery, this not the definitive management. Splinting and pressure dressings have led to problems with impotence and poor healing and are not part of the management.

Test-taking tip: If unsure, narrow down the answer choices to two. The last two choices are very similar, so you can use that to narrow them either in or out. Also, pay attention to the fact that the question is asking for *definitive* management, and you can rule out other choices based on that.

27. ANSWER: C

The minimum number of WBCs needed to diagnosis peritonitis is 100 WBCs per mm^3 of dialysate fluid. This, along with bacteria noted on Gram stain with 50% neutrophils, confirms the diagnosis. Peritonitis in this setting is commonly due to gram-positive organisms (*Staphylococcus* and *Streptococcus*). The treatment is intraperitoneal antibiotics (vancomycin or third-generation cephalosporin).

Test-taking tip: There are some numbers you need to memorize. The definition of peritonitis is one of them.

28. ANSWER: A

While ESRD patients are particularly susceptible to acute coronary syndrome, the most common and life-threatening cause of shortness of breath in these patient is fluid overload affecting the lungs and compromising breathing. Cardiac tamponade should be considered in ESRD patients on hemodialysis who are unstable. There is no increased risk for pneumothorax in patients on hemodialysis.

Test-taking tip: Again, pay attention to what the question is asking you—it is asking for the most common cause of progressively worsening (slow-onset) shortness of breath.

16.

THORACIC AND RESPIRATORY EMERGENCIES

Nelson Diamond, Janelle Lee, Vaishal Tolia, and Megan Tresenriter

1. A 5-year-old boy with history of asthma presents with respiratory distress. His mother notes that the patient has a runny nose and cough that started earlier today. On exam, he is tripoding with audible stridor. You give racemic epinephrine and steroids and note marked improvement of his respiratory status. The mother would now like to take the patient home because he looks a lot better. What is a reasonable observation period in the emergency department (ED) after giving racemic epinephrine?

A. 30 minutes
B. 1 hour
C. 3 hours
D. 6 hours

2. A 58-year-old male with history of chronic obstructive pulmonary disease (COPD), coronary artery disease (CAD), and hypertension presents to the ED with progressive worsening of dyspnea. On exam, the patient is tachypneic and noted to have diffuse expiratory wheezing and is saturating 86% on 2 L by nasal cannula. The rest of his vital signs are blood pressure (BP) 168/96 mm Hg, heart rate (HR) 114 bpm, respiratory rate (RR) 28 breaths/min, and temperature 37.3° C. Emergency medical services (EMS) started an albuterol treatment that was only minimally helpful. The quick bedside ultrasound is shown in Figure 16.1. Which of the following treatments would be the most appropriate?

A. Albuterol and steroids
B. Magnesium and epinephrine
C. Nitroglycerin and biphasic positive airway pressure (BiPAP)
D. Heparin

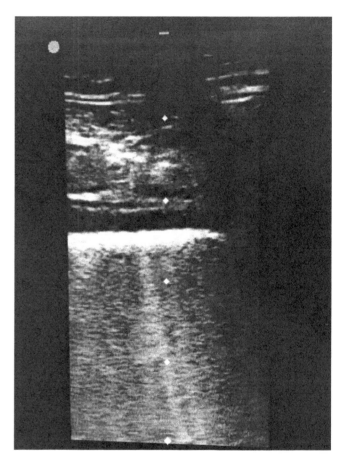

Figure 16.1 Ultrasound of the lungs.

3. The respiratory therapist calls you urgently into a patient's room, whom you've intubated for airway protection. The ventilator alarms keep going off, and you see that the patient's plateau pressures are very high.

Which of the following reasons would *not* cause high plateau pressures?

A. Pneumothorax
B. Acute respiratory distress syndrome (ARDS)
C. Bronchospasm
D. Pneumonia

4. A 36-year-old male with history of HIV presents with fever, nonproductive cough, and dyspnea for 2 weeks. He does not know his CD4 count. He feels shorter of breath with exertion. His arterial blood gases (ABGs) are as follows: pH 7.37, Pao_2 65, and Pco_2 35. His chest radiograph is shown in Figure 16.2. Besides starting Bactrim, what else should be given?

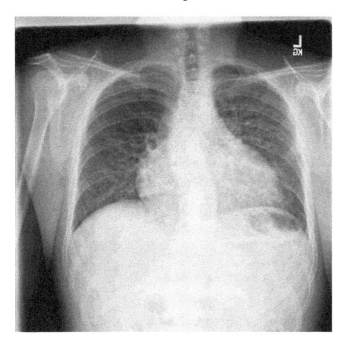

Figure 16.2 Chest radiograph.

A. Atovaquone
B. Albuterol
C. Pentamidine
D. Steroids

5. A 10-year-old girl with history of asthma presents with a severe asthma exacerbation leading to respiratory failure. After attempts with noninvasive ventilation, the patient is still not responding to therapy, so the decision is made to intubate her. Which of the following would *not* be an appropriate management strategy for her initial ventilation settings?

A. Increased expiratory/inspiratory ratio
B. Permissive hypercapnia
C. Decreased inspiratory flow rate
D. Tidal volume by ideal weight 6 mL/kg

6. A 35-year-old female presents to the ED complaining of shortness of breath, fatigue, and lightheadedness. She denies any associated chest pain. She had just been to the ED the day before for a peritonsillar abscess drainage and received some topical analgesia. She endorses less pain with swallowing and less sore throat. Her vital signs are HR 75 bpm, BP 128/74 mm Hg, RR 22 breaths/min, and oxygen saturation 85% on room air. Her oropharynx looks mildly edematous and has a patent airway. She is handling secretions and speaking full and clear sentences. Administering nasal cannula supplemental oxygen does not improve her oxygen saturations. Which of the following risk factors is *not* a contraindication to giving the treatment of choice?

A. Patient has severe renal insufficiency
B. Patient is taking citalopram
C. Patient has a history of glucose-6-phosphate dehydrogenase (G6PD) deficiency
D. Patient has a history of asthma

7. A 70-year-old male with history of end-stage renal disease (ESRD) on dialysis, diabetes mellitus (DM), congestive heart failure (CHF), and lymphoma presents with worsening dyspnea progressively over the past month. He completed his dialysis before arrival but states that dialysis only helped somewhat. He has decreased breath sounds on the right. His chest radiograph is shown in Figure 16.3. In what anatomic space is the abnormality?

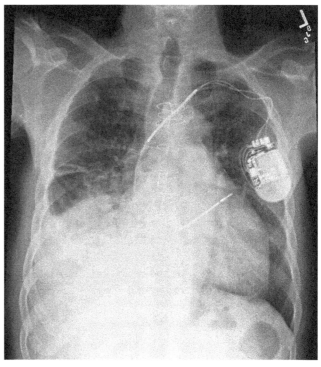

Figure 16.3 Chest radiograph.

A. In the alveoli
B. In the bronchi
C. In the interstitium
D. In the pleural space

8. A 65-year-old male with a history of pancreatic cancer presents with shortness of breath and hypoxia. His vital signs are BP 82/55 mm Hg, HR 110 bpm, RR 25 breaths/min, oxygen saturation 92%, and temperature 38.° C. Computed tomography (CT) of his chest is performed and is shown in Figure 16.4. Which of the following is *true* regarding his condition?

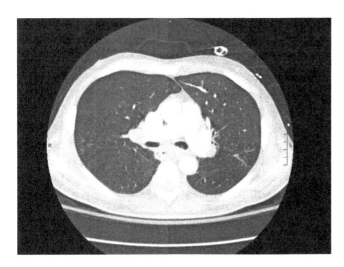

Figure 16.4 Chest computed tomography.

A. Most common electrocardiogram (EKG) abnormality is S1Q3T3
B. Most common chest radiograph abnormality is atelectasis
C. Treatment of choice in this case is heparin
D. Most common presenting sign is tachycardia

9. A 32-year-old male is transferred from a small community ED for severe pancreatitis. He has been intubated, and the paramedic notes he has been more difficult to bag. His ABG test at 60% Fio_2 reveals pH 7.35, Pao_2 90 mm Hg, and $Paco_2$ 42 mm Hg. His chest radiograph is shown in Figure 16.5. Which of the following is *true* about this condition?

A. It is classified as severe when the Pao_2/Fio_2 ratio is £200 mm Hg on positive end-expiratory pressure (PEEP) 5 mm Hg
B. Sepsis is the most common cause
C. Ventilator management includes high tidal volumes
D. It is characterized by increased lung compliance

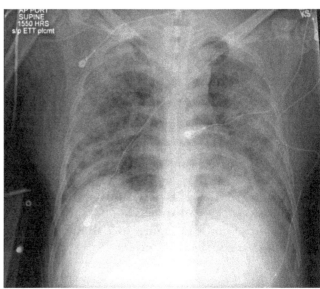

Figure 16.5 Chest radiograph.

10. A 18-year-old male from Mexico presents with cough and productive green sputum with fever for a week. He states he has had multiple lung infections since childhood. His medication list includes insulin for DM. A chest CT scan is shown in Figure 16.6. What two bacterial organisms are most likely to the trigger the exacerbation of his symptoms?

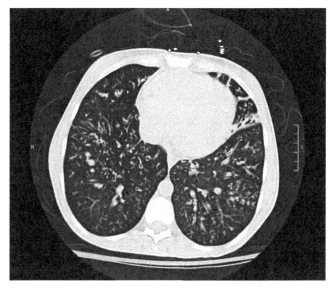

Figure 16.6 Chest computed tomography.

A. *Streptococcus pneumoniae* and *Staphylococcus aureus*
B. *Pseudomonas aeruginosa* and *S. aureus*
C. *Haemophilus influenzae* and *P. aeruginosa*
D. *S. pneumoniae* and *P. aeruginosa*

11. A 62-year-old male with a history of hypertension presents with acute shortness of breath after he received some acupuncture treatment on the left side of his torso 2 days ago. His vital signs are HR 85 bpm, BP 130/80 mm Hg, RR 23 breaths/min, and oxygen saturation 95% on room air. On exam, he has decreased breath sounds on the left. His chest radiograph is shown in Figure 16.7. What is the most appropriate next step for this patient?

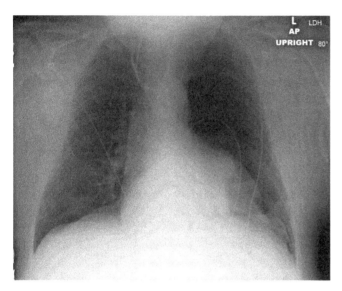

Figure 16.7 Chest radiograph.

A. Observation
B. Chemical pleurodesis
C. Needle decompression
D. Thoracostomy tube placement

12. A 4-year-old boy is brought in by his mother for a persistent cough. It started initially as a mild cough for more than 2 weeks, but his mother is concerned because the cough has worsened. She states he has abrupt spells of severe nonstop coughing, and during these spells, he has so much trouble catching his breath that he turns blue. His mother is also pregnant and concerned that he might pass the cough to her. How should you advise her?

A. His cough is not contagious. She does not need to be concerned.
B. Getting vaccinated now will protect her from infection.
C. She should be prescribed antibiotics to prevent being infected.
D. Ampicillin is the antibiotic of choice for treatment.

13. A 65-year-old male who recently had a tracheostomy 2 weeks ago is sent in from his skilled nursing facility for some mild bleeding near his tracheostomy site.

While you are examining him, you note brisk bright red bleeding around his tracheostomy site. What should you do next?

A. Obtain a chest radiograph
B. Hyperinflate his tracheostomy cuff
C. Consult pulmonology for bronchoscopy
D. Remove the tracheostomy tube

14. A 3-year-old otherwise healthy girl is brought in by ambulance for respiratory distress. Her parents explain that she was playing with her older brother in another room and suddenly the brother yelled for help because she started to forcefully cough and turned blue for 10 seconds. Here in the ED, the patient appears cyanotic, while tripoding and having stridor. What is the next best step?

A. Perform a cricothyrotomy
B. Administer racemic epinephrine
C. Perform a blind sweep of the mouth
D. Administer abdominal thrusts

15. An alcoholic male presents with cough, fevers, and rigors. His chest radiograph shows a right upper lobe consolidation with a bulging fissure. What is the most likely organism?

A. *Klebsiella pneumoniae*
B. *Legionella* species
C. *P. aeruginosa*
D. *S. aureus*

16. A 45-year-old male with a history of hypertension presents with shortness of breath and abdominal pain. He has visible angioedema with mild stridor and states that he has had several similar prior episodes. He says other family members seem to have it as well. Which of the following management steps would be indicated?

A. Give epinephrine, steroids, and antihistamines
B. Stop the offending medication
C. Cryoprecipitate
D. Administer C1-esterase inhibitor

17. A patient with a history of esophageal cancer status post–esophageal stent placement complains of shortness of breath, fatigue, cough, and fevers. A chest radiograph is performed showing infiltrates, and he is started on antibiotics for pneumonia. A bronchoscopy is performed and is shown in Figure 16.8. Which of the following antibiotics regimen would be appropriate?

A. Cefpodoxime and azithromycin
B. Vancomycin and Levaquin

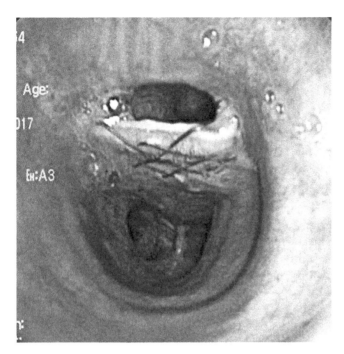

Figure 16.8 Bronchoscopy.

A. Rigid bronchoscopy
B. Intubate right main stem and place patient onto his left side
C. Interventional radiology embolization
D. Intubate patient and place patient onto his right side

C. Ampicillin-sulbactam
D. Trimethoprim-sulfamethoxazole (TMP-SMX) and levofloxacin (Levaquin)

18. A 49-year-old male with a history of lymphoma presents with blood-tinged sputum. His chest CT is shown in Figure 16.9. After returning from the scanner, he develops massive hemoptysis. What is the next best step in management?

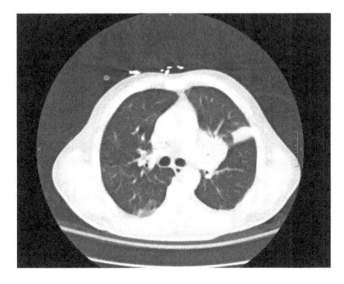

Figure 16.9 Chest computed tomography.

19. A 25-year-old female with a history of poorly controlled type 1 DM presents with severe dyspnea and chest pain acutely. She has not been compliant with her medications, so for the past 3 days, she has been vomiting frequently and experiencing abdominal pain. Her chest radiograph is shown in Figure 16.10. What is the most likely diagnosis?

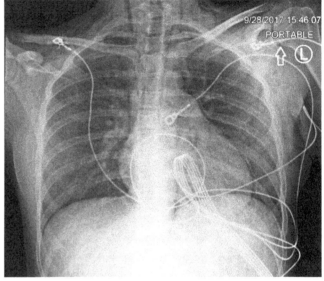

Figure 16.10 Chest radiograph.

A. Peptic ulcer perforation
B. Pneumothorax
C. Aortic dissection
D. Boerhaave's syndrome

20. A 42-year-old female with a history of allergic rhinitis and hypertension presents with complaint of a new dry cough for the past 2 weeks. She denies any rhinorrhea, productive sputum, fever or chills, abdominal pain, wheezing, shortness of breath, chest pain, or sour taste in her mouth. The cough seems to occur throughout the day. She has been complaint with her medications. She takes fluticasone and lisinopril. What is the most likely diagnosis?

A. Acute bronchitis
B. Asthma
C. Angiotensin-converting enzyme (ACE) inhibitor–induced cough
D. Gastroesophageal reflux

21. A 35-year-old previously healthy female presents with shaking chills and cough productive of rust-colored sputum for the past 24 hours accompanied by pleuritic chest pain. She denies any tobacco, alcohol, or drug use. Her vital signs are HR 115 bpm, BP 126/72 mm Hg, SpO$_2$ 97% on room air, and temperature 38.6° C. What is the most likely pathogen causing this condition?

A. *S. aureus*
B. *S. pneumoniae*
C. *P. aeruginosa*
D. *Chlamydophila pneumoniae*

22. A 65-year-old male nursing facility patient with history of stroke, hypertension, diabetes, and COPD presents to your ED for increased work of breathing and altered mental status (Glasgow Coma Scale (GCS) score of 12 from his baseline of 14). He has a G-tube, but according to family wishes, he has been advanced to liquid diet recently. He responds to painful stimuli but is unable to provide any history. Physical exam reveals skin that is hot to touch, dry mucous membranes, and coarse breath sounds bilaterally. This patient is specifically at increased risk for all of the following *except*:

A. *Mycobacterium pneumoniae*
B. *P. aeruginosa*
C. *Bacteroides* species
D. *H. influenzae*

23. A 22-year-old severely asthmatic male presents to your ED in respiratory distress. Despite maximal medical therapy and noninvasive ventilation strategies, he decompensates and requires intubation. Thirty minutes after successful rapid sequence intubation, he becomes hypotensive and hypoxic, and respiratory therapy reports that he is requiring increasing inspiratory pressures with difficulty maintaining adequate tidal volume on the ventilator. Exam reveals decreased breath sounds bilaterally and endotracheal tube (ETT) at a depth of 21 cm at the patient's incisors, where it was originally secured. What is the next step in managing this patient?

A. Withdraw the ETT 2 cm
B. Bilateral needle thoracostomies
C. Remove the patient from the ventilator circuit
D. Respiratory therapy to suction the ETT

24. A 52-year-old male with a history of daily smoking and COPD without other comorbidities presents with dry cough, dyspnea, and wheezing for the past 5 days. He has used his home albuterol with decreasing efficacy, and he has just run out. After a dose of prednisone and two 1-hour-long nebulizer treatments, his symptoms have resolved, and he is comfortable with discharge and follow-up with his primary physician. What is the most appropriate outpatient regimen?

A. Smoking cessation, oral prednisone, albuterol refill
B. Smoking cessation, oral prednisone, albuterol refill, azithromycin
C. Smoking cessation, inhaled corticosteroids, albuterol refill, azithromycin
D. Smoking cessation, IV methylprednisone, azithromycin, and admission for pulmonary function tests (PFTs)

25. A 65-year old male on 4-L home oxygen presents in respiratory distress. His eyes are open, and he follows simple commands but is unable to provide a history. He has prominent rhonchi and wheezing bilaterally with significant increased work of breathing. Chest radiograph shows hyperinflation and mild peribronchial cuffing but no infiltrate or pulmonary edema. Labs are unremarkable. Vital signs are HR 125 bpm, BP 145/86 mm Hg, RR 36 breaths/min, SpO$_2$ 85% on 2 L by nasal cannula, and temperature 37.3° C. He receives full medical therapy, and saturation improves to 100% with improved work of breathing. Thirty minutes later, nursing calls you to assess the patient, who is now obtunded and apneic, and you perform rapid sequence intubation. Which of the following most likely leads to the patient's clinical decline?

A. Inappropriate application of noninvasive positive pressure ventilation
B. Oxygen therapy that improved patient's SpO$_2$ to 100%
C. Failure to administer early antibiotics
D. Failure to obtain early ABG test

26. A 47-year-old female with wheezing and increased work of breathing is treated for COPD and admitted to the hospital after showing significant improvement with ED treatment. Her initial chest radiograph and blood tests are unremarkable. Which of the following abnormalities might be expected on repeat labs the following morning?

A. Leukocytopenia
B. Hypercalcemia
C. Hypomagnesemia
D. Hypokalemia

27. A 55-year-old male with COPD, hypertension, and diabetes reestablishes primary care after 5 years without any health care encounters when his brother dies of a heart attack. Two weeks after his first visit, he presents

to your ED with acute onset of wheezing, dyspnea, and nonproductive cough. Lab testing is unremarkable. Which of the following medications most likely triggered this exacerbation?

    A. Amlodipine
    B. Metformin
    C. Metoprolol
    D. Hydrochlorothiazide

28. A 54-year-old male presents with acute onset of shortness of breath, pleuritic chest pain, and hemoptysis 2 weeks after he began chemotherapy for testicular cancer. His vital signs are HR 125 bpm, BP 110/65 mm Hg, RR 28 breaths/min, SpO_2 93% on 2 L by nasal cannula, and temperature 37.° C. Complete blood count (CBC) and chemistry 10 panel are unremarkable, and he has a negative chest radiograph. He initially receives a 1-L normal saline bolus for tachycardia, and he later becomes hypotensive with systolic pressure in the 70s. What is the best next step in management?

    A. Another normal saline bolus, antibiotics, and immediate chest CT
    B. Central line placement for norepinephrine infusion
    C. Therapeutic anticoagulation with heparin infusion only
    D. Therapeutic anticoagulation with heparin and administration of IV thrombolytics if no contraindications

29. A 55-year-old male with AIDS is presents with productive cough, fever and chills with an infiltrate seen on chest radiograph. He is tachycardic and has a room air SpO_2 of 94%. He receives IV fluid bolus with improvement in his tachycardia and is placed on 2 L by nasal cannula. He also receives broad-spectrum antibiotics. While awaiting admission, he develops sudden onset of chest pain and on assessment exhibits jugular venous distention and tracheal deviation to the right with decreased breath sounds on the left. Which pathogen is most commonly associated with this disorder?

    A. *Pneumocystis* species
    B. *Mycobacterium avium*
    C. *S. pneumoniae*
    D. *S. aureus*

30. A 68-year-old female patient with chronic interstitial pulmonary fibrosis on chronic steroids presents to your ED with respiratory distress. Vital signs are HR 116 bpm, BP 135/85 mm Hg, RR 45 breaths/min, SpO_2 83% on room air, and temperature 36.8° C. She receives noninvasive positive pressure ventilation (NIPPV) and inhaled ß-agonist therapy with a stress dose of steroids

as well as empiric antibiotics with improvement in her respiratory rate and work of breathing. SpO_2 is now 94%. Suddenly, you are called to the room for an acute decompensation by the nurse and find the patient again hypoxic to 85% on 100% FiO_2 with increased work of breathing and complaining of right-sided chest pain. Exam reveals equal chest rise, and breath sounds are difficult to auscultate with NIPPV in place. What is the best next important step in diagnosis of this patient?

    A. Repeat EKG
    B. Repeat CBC
    C. Repeat chest radiograph
    D. Pulmonary CT angiogram

31. A 34-year-old male presents to your ED with acute sudden onset of chest pain after smoking crack cocaine. His pain is retrosternal, sharp, and nonradiating. He denies any shortness of breath, vomiting, or diaphoresis. EKG shows no ST changes. Vital signs are normal. Physical exam reveals crunching sound auscultated during systole over the precordium. He appears generally well. Which of the following is *true* of this condition?

    A. All cases require emergent esophagoscopy
    B. Cocaine and marijuana smoking are the most common risk factors
    C. Chest radiograph is the gold standard for diagnosis
    D. Cases in infants are usually benign

32. A 40-year-old African American female presents with shortness of breath, erythematous rash with tender nodules, and low-grade fever. Vital signs are as follows: HR 105 bpm, BP 120/74 mm Hg, RR 18 breaths/min, SpO_2 99% on room air, and temperature 38.2° C. Chest radiograph shows bilateral hilar adenopathy, and chemistry reveals elevated serum calcium. Which of the following is *true* of the diagnosis?

    A. HIV is commonly associated with this disease
    B. Patients require admission for urgent transbronchial biopsy
    C. If altered mental status is present, head CT is indicated emergently
    D. Extrapulmonary symptoms predominate during initial presentation

33. A 67-year-old female with known lung cancer with a large mass in the left upper lobe presents with respiratory distress. EMS reports that family called when she began to cough up large blood clots followed by bright red blood. Medics found her to have increased work of breathing, and she became increasingly obtunded with

SpO$_2$ in the 70s despite assisted respirations with bag-valve mask. She also exhibits decreased breath sounds on the left with prominent crackles. She is found to have bright, frothy blood in her posterior oropharynx but is successfully intubated with blood in the ETT and persistent hypoxia. ETT placement is confirmed with auscultation, though breath sounds remain decreased on the left as well as capnography. What is the best next step?

A. Stat chest radiograph
B. CT angiogram of chest/abdomen/pelvis to evaluate the aorta
C. Placement of a Minnesota tube for hemostasis
D. Right main stem ETT and place patient in left lateral decubitus position

34. A 63-year-old male with history of CHF presents with increased shortness of breath, cough productive of thin white sputum, dyspnea on exertion, and increasing orthopnea over the past week. He denies chest pain, fever, and chills and has not had any recent changes in medications. His EKG shows no acute ST elevations, and a chest radiograph is done and shown in Figure 16.11. If thoracentesis were performed on this patient, which of the following is most likely to be observed in the fluid?

A. Pleural fluid/serum protein ratio of 0.6
B. Pleural fluid/serum lactate dehydrogenase (LDH) ratio of 0.5
C. Pleural fluid/LDH ratio three-fourths of the normal serum value
D. Fluid white blood cell (WBC) count of 4,000/mm^3

35. A 36-year-old 18-week pregnant women presents to your ED with shortness of breath with acute onset 6 hours ago and dyspnea on exertion that is much worse than she has experienced in her pregnancy thus far. She also reports left calf pain for the past week. Her vital signs are HR 128 bpm, BP 135/86 mm Hg, RR 26 breaths/min, SpO$_2$ 92% on 4 L by nasal cannula, and temperature 37.8° C. Chest radiograph is clear, and physical exam reveals normal breath sounds and left leg swelling. Which of the following causes her hypoxia in this condition?

A. Diffusion impairment
B. Ventilation-perfusion mismatch
C. Right-to-left shunt
D. Hypoventilation

36. You are treating a patient with respiratory distress using NIPPV. The patient has a history of COPD and CHF, and the chest radiograph shows an infiltrate (Figure 16.12). The patient has mild leukocytosis. In general, which of the following is *not* a predictor of increased risk for NIPPV failure?

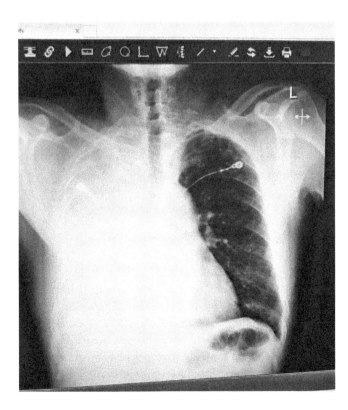

Figure 16.11 Chest radiograph.

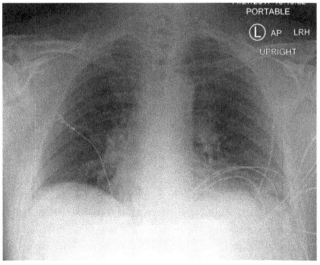

Figure 16.12 Chest radiograph.

A. Pneumonia
B. ARDS
C. Cardiogenic pulmonary edema
D. Failure to achieve PaO$_2$/FiO$_2$ ratio >150 after 1 hour of treatment

37. A 26-year-old recreational IV drug user who recently returned from travel to Southeast Asia presents with cough, fever, and hemoptysis. His vital signs are HR 118 bpm, BP 116/68 mm Hg, RR 20 breaths/min, and SpO_2 98% on room air. Chest radiograph reveals left upper lobe cavitary lesion. What is the most immediate next step in his care?

A. ABG test
B. Rapid HIV testing
C. Sputum induction for acid-fast bacillus (AFB) staining
D. Placement in respiratory isolation room

38. A previously healthy 3-month-old ex-term male is brought to the ED by his mother after an episode of irregular breathing followed by approximately 10 seconds of apnea. On exam, the child is appears well and alert. His vital signs are temperature 37.5° C, HR 126 bpm, RR 24 breaths/min, BP 84/50 mm Hg, and oxygen saturation 98% on room air. He has clear lungs and no appreciable murmur on exam. The rest of his exam is normal. The child has never had an event like this before. Additionally, there is no concerning family history. What further workup is indicated?

A. Point-of-care blood glucose
B. Viral respiratory panel
C. Admission for pulse oximetry monitoring
D. None

39. A previously healthy 9-month-old ex–31-week premature male infant is brought to the ED by his father after an episode of altered mental status. The patient's father states that the patient became "unresponsive" while feeding, characterized by decreased alertness and limp extremities. The patient returned to his baseline mental status within 1 minute of onset of symptoms. On exam, the child appears well and is playful. His vital signs are temperature 37.5° C, HR 120 bpm, RR 22 breaths/min, BP 88/54 mm Hg, and oxygen saturation 99% on room air. On exam, the patient is moving all extremities equally with normal tone, no other focal neurologic deficits are noted, and the rest of his exam is otherwise normal. The child has never had an event like this before, but the family had an infant die from sudden infant death syndrome (SIDS) several years ago. What further workup is indicated?

A. Head CT
B. Admission for workup and monitoring
C. None
D. Home cardiorespiratory monitoring

40. A 9-year-old boy with history of moderate persistent asthma is brought in by his father to the ED for difficulty breathing. The symptoms began approximately 6 hours before presentation, and the patient received three nebulized albuterol treatments before presentation. In the ED, the patient appears frightened; he is sitting up and leaning forward, and intercostal retractions are noted. His vital signs are temperature 38° C, HR 130 bpm, RR 32 breaths/min, BP 84/50 mm Hg, and oxygen saturation 92% on room air. Auscultation of the patient's chest reveals poor air movement bilaterally. The patient is started on continuous nebulized albuterol, and systemic steroids are administered. Initial ABG test shows pH 7.45, Po_2 75, Pco_2 30, HCO_3^- 18. The patient's clinical status remains unchanged after treatment. One hour later, repeat ABG test shows pH 7.5, Po_2 75, Pco_2 50, and HCO_3^- 20. Which of the following in this patient's presentation is an indication of impending respiratory failure?

A. Respiratory rate
B. Rising $Paco_2$
C. Hypoxia/hypoxemia
D. Pulsus paradoxus

41. A 4-year-old girl with history of intermittent asthma is brought in by her father to the ED for difficulty breathing. The symptoms were gradual in onset, preceded by 5 days of runny nose, watery eyes, and tactile fevers at home. In the ED, the patient is nontoxic in appearance. Her vital signs are temperature 38° C, HR 130 bpm, RR 32 breaths/min, BP 90/70 mm Hg, and oxygen saturation 88% on room air. The patient is noted to have diffuse end-expiratory wheezes on exam and mild intercostal retractions. The patient is treated for presumptive viral upper respiratory infection (URI) and reactive airway disease with acetaminophen and nebulized albuterol. The patient remains hypoxic after treatment. What is the next step in management?

A. NIPPV
B. Admission
C. Theophylline
D. Chest radiograph

42. A 16-year-old girl with no past medical history is brought into the ED by her father for cough. The patient endorses 1 week of rhinorrhea, cough, and chest tightness. She has never before been short of breath, does not smoke, and has no family history of respiratory disease. On exam, her vital signs are temperature 37.5° C, HR 90 bpm, RR 22 breaths/min, BP 125/80 mm Hg, and oxygen saturation 95% on room air. Lung auscultation

reveals scattered wheezes. Which of the following is most likely to confirm this patient's diagnosis?

    A. Chest radiograph
    B. Spirometry
    C. Rapid flu swab
    D. ABG test

43. A 7-year-old boy with no past medical history is brought to the ED by his parents for difficulty breathing. The patient developed symptoms of URI 3 days before presentation but today developed high-pitched noises with inspiration and expiration and lethargy. On exam, the patient is sitting up and leaning forward. His vital signs are as follows: temperature 39° C, HR 160 bpm, RR 34 breaths/min, BP 80/50 mm Hg, and oxygen saturation 96% on room air. The child appears ill with inspiratory and expiratory stridor. The patient was treated with nebulized racemic epinephrine with no improvement of symptoms. Which of the following organisms is most commonly implicated in development of this condition?

    A. *S. aureus*
    B. *H. influenzae*
    C. Parainfluenza virus
    D. *S. pneumoniae*

44. A 6-month-old previously healthy male infant is brought to the ED by his mother. His mother states that he has had tactile fevers, poor feeding, and copious amounts of nasal discharge for the past 3 days. Today, the patient developed labored breathing. On exam, the patient has intercostal and suprasternal retractions, temperature 37.5° C, HR 150 bpm, RR 50 breaths/min, BP 84/50 mm Hg, and oxygen saturation 88% on room air. Clear secretions are noted from the bilateral nares. Wheezing and crackles are heard on lung exam bilaterally. Four liters of supplemental oxygen by nasal cannula are applied, and the patient's oxygen saturation improves to 92%. What is the mainstay of treatment of this condition?

    A. Antibiotics
    B. Nebulized racemic epinephrine
    C. Supportive care
    D. Nebulized albuterol

45. A mother brings in her 3-year-old girl for cough and funny noises while breathing. The patient developed symptoms of "a cold" 2 days ago and now has a barking cough, which is worse at night. This evening, the patient developed high-pitched squeaking noise during inspiration. Her vital signs are temperature 37.9° C, HR 130 bpm, RR 30 breaths/min, BP 84/50 mm Hg,

and oxygen saturation 98% on room air. The patient has clear lungs on exam, mild intercostal retractions, and inspiratory stridor on exam. Which of the following therapies is indicated?

    A. Humidified oxygen
    B. Systemic steroids
    C. Inhaled ß$_2$-agonist
    D. Intubation

46. A concerned mother brings in her 5-year-old daughter to the ED for cough. Her symptoms began about 2 weeks ago with low-grade fevers and runny nose. Her runny nose has improved, but now the patient is having frequent coughing spells, sometimes so severe that they provoke vomiting immediately after. She also complains of fatigue and poor appetite. She is up to date on immunizations and has no other health problems. Her vital signs are temperature 37.8° C, HR 120 bpm, RR 24 breaths/min, BP 90/50 mm Hg, and oxygen saturation 98% on room air. Physical exam is otherwise unremarkable. The mother also has a 2-month-old male infant at home who is currently well. Polymerase chain reaction (PCR) swab tests positive for *Bordetella pertussis* the next day. Who should receive treatment, and what course of treatment should be administered?

    A. Five-year-old girl only; macrolide
    B. Five-year-old girl and 2-month-old boy; penicillin
    C. All members of household; macrolide
    D. All members of household; penicillin

47. A mother brings her 20-day-old infant boy to the ED for cough and rhinorrhea. Symptoms have been going on for 2 days. The patient reports that she received a call from her pediatrician's office that testing for pertussis came back positive today. His vital signs are temperature 37.5° C, HR 160 bpm, RR 50 breaths/min, BP 60/40 mm Hg, and oxygen saturation 98% on room air. Which of the following is the best antibiotic choice?

    A. Erythromycin
    B. Augmentin
    C. TMP-SMX
    D. Azithromycin

48. A 5-year-old male with a known history of cystic fibrosis (CF) is brought to the ED by his mother for increasing shortness of breath. Despite compliance with home therapies, symptoms have worsened in the past 3 days with increasing cough, increased sputum production, and tactile temperature at home. His vital signs are temperature 37.5° C, HR 126 bpm, RR 30 breaths/min, BP 84/50 mm Hg, and oxygen saturation 95% on room air. Coarse breath sounds and rhonchi are

heard on auscultation of the chest. Chest radiograph is similar to prior with no evidence of consolidation. Which of the following is the preferred treatment for an acute pulmonary exacerbation?

A. Ibuprofen
B. Steroids
C. Albuterol
D. Antibiotics

49. A 68-year-old man with history of CHF, COPD, ESRD on dialysis, and 60-pack-year smoking history presents with increasing dyspnea on exertion for 3 weeks. The patient also notes right-sided chest pain with deep inspiration. Review of systems also notable for weight loss and hemoptysis. On exam, his vital signs are temperature 37.5° C, HR 96 bpm, RR 22 breaths/min, BP 120/80 mm Hg, and oxygen saturation 95% on room air. Auscultation of lungs is notable for decreased breath sounds on the right. Chest radiograph is shown in Figure 16.13. Evaluation with ultrasound shows septated appearance. What is the most likely cause of the pleural effusion?

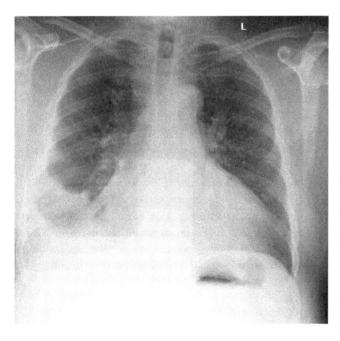

Figure 16.13 Chest radiograph.

A. Pulmonary embolism (PE)
B. Underlying malignancy
C. Heart failure
D. Pneumonia

50. A 55-year-old woman with past medical history of systolic heart failure with poor medication compliance presents to the ED with increasing dyspnea on exertion.

The patient also notes increasing swelling in bilateral lower extremities. On exam, the patient is afebrile, HR 115 bpm, RR 26 breaths/min, BP 110/50 mm Hg, and oxygen saturation 88% on room air. Chest radiograph is shown in Figure 16.14. What do you expect to find on evaluation of pleural fluid?

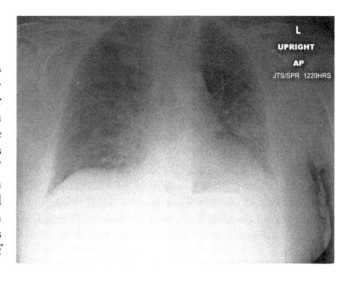

Figure 16.14 Chest radiograph.

A. Low glucose
B. High complement level
C. Ratio of pleural fluid level of LDH to serum level of LDH is greater than 0.6
D. Ratio of pleural fluid level of protein to serum level of protein is less than 0.5

51. A 36-year-old woman with no past medical history presents to ED with chest pain. The chest pain is right-sided and worse with inspiration. Her only medication is oral contraceptives. Her vital signs are temperature 37.5° C, HR 126 bpm, RR 26 breaths/min, BP 90/50 mm Hg, and oxygen saturation 91% on room air. Exam also reveals unilateral leg swelling and redness. Chest radiograph shows a small right-sided pleural effusion. Which of the following would be expected on pleural fluid analysis?

A. Low glucose
B. Low pH
C. Pleural fluid level of LDH is more than two-thirds the upper limit of the reference range for the serum level of LDH
D. Ratio of pleural fluid level of protein to serum level of protein is less than 0.5

52. A 23-year-old man without past medical history presents with cough and right-sided chest pain with breathing. He also complains of increasing shortness

of breath with activity over several days. On exam, his vital signs are temperature 37.5° C, HR 96 bpm, RR 24 breaths/min, BP 120/80 mm Hg, and oxygen saturation 96% on room air. Chest radiograph shows moderate right-sided pleural effusion. Diagnostic thoracentesis is performed and yields milky yellow fluid. Centrifugation of the fluid does not change its appearance. Analysis of the fluid is positive for chylomicrons, and no cholesterol crystals are identified. What is the most likely etiology of this condition?

A. Amyloidosis
B. Penetrating trauma
C. Malignancy
D. Pneumonia

53. A 22-year-old man with no known medical problems presents to the ED after feeling a "pop" in his chest while running. He complains of right-sided chest pain and shortness of breath. On exam, he is comfortable with no signs of respiratory distress. His vital signs are temperature 37.5° C, HR 88 bpm, RR 20 breaths/min, BP 120/80 mm Hg, and oxygen saturation 98% on room air. Absent breath sounds are noted on the right. Chest radiograph shows large pneumothorax on the right. Which of the following factors makes recurrence most likely?

A. Young age
B. Size of pneumothorax
C. Smoking tobacco products
D. Active lifestyle

54. A 17-year-old girl with no known medical problems presents to the ED for cough. The patient notes that she has been experiencing frequent, violent coughing fits for about 1 week. Her vital signs are temperature 37.5° C, HR 94 bpm, RR 20 breaths/min, BP 120/80 mm Hg, and oxygen saturation 98% on room air. Chest radiograph shows bilateral apical pneumothoraces. What is the next step in management?

A. Observation, supplemental oxygen
B. Chest CT
C. Unilateral chest tube
D. Bilateral chest tubes

55. A 55-year-old woman is brought into the ED after a motor vehicle collision. Workup is remarkable for large unilateral left-sided pneumothorax. One hour after chest tube placement, the patient becomes dyspneic and tachypneic, and she is hypoxic to 77% on room air with rales present on examination of the left lung field. Chest radiograph shows diffuse airspace opacification in the left lung field. What is the next appropriate step in management?

A. Aggressive diuresis
B. Positive pressure ventilation
C. Antibiotics
D. Replace chest tube

56. A 55-year-old man with a history of alcohol use presents to the ED complaining of one day of chest pain radiating to back, fevers, and chills. Symptoms were preceded by 2 days of nausea, vomiting, and diarrhea. The patient also complains about pain with swallowing. Vital signs are temperature 39° C, HR 135 bpm, RR 20 breaths/min, BP 100/70 mm Hg, and oxygen saturation 98% on room air. EKG and troponin are normal, and chest radiograph is unremarkable. Laboratory data are remarkable for leukocytosis to 22,000, with 15% bands. CT of the chest is obtained and shows stranding of the upper paraesophageal posterior mediastinal fat. What is the next step of management?

A. Broad-spectrum antibiotics
B. Proton pump inhibitor (PPI)
C. Flexible esophagostomy
D. CT surgery consult

57. A 35-year-old woman with history of gastro-esophageal reflux disease (GERD) and peptic ulcer disease presents to the ED complaining of sharp, substernal chest pain that is worse with deep inspiration. The patient underwent upper endoscopy yesterday without complication. Vital signs are temperature 38° C, HR 110 bpm, RR 16 breaths/min, BP 90/70 mm Hg, and oxygen saturation 98% on room air. Auscultation of the heart reveals crackles with each beat. Which of the following is most likely to reveal the diagnosis?

A. Troponin
B. EKG
C. Chest radiograph
D. CT scan

58. A 52-year-old woman is evaluated after an abdominal CT scan detected a 3-mm nodule in the right lower pulmonary lobe. The CT scan was obtained to evaluate abdominal pain, which has since completely resolved. The patient has never smoked. She works in the home and has not been exposed to potential carcinogens. She has not had a chest radiograph or other imaging procedure, except mammography. Her medical history is unremarkable, and she takes no medication. Her family history is unremarkable. The physical examination is normal. Which of the following is the required next step in the management of this patient?

A. Chest radiograph in 3 months
B. CT scan of the chest in 3 months

C. CT scan of the chest in 6 months
D. No follow-up

C. 10% to 20%
D. 25% to 50%

59. A 63-year-old man is found to have a 1.5-cm spiculated, noncalcified nodule in the right upper lobe of the lung on chest radiograph performed before elective resection of the sigmoid colon for recurrent diverticulitis. There is no lymphadenopathy or evidence of calcified lymph nodes. A chest radiograph obtained 15 years ago does not show the nodule. The patient is a lifelong nonsmoker and has no occupational risks for lung disease. Other than recurrent diverticulitis, he is healthy and takes no medication. Which of the following is the best management option for the pulmonary nodule?

A. Biopsy of the nodule
B. Positron emission tomography of the chest
C. Repeat chest radiography in 6 months
D. Spiral CT scan of the chest

60. The patient is a 58-year-old nurse who recently underwent resection of a solitary pulmonary nodule (SPN) and just moved from out of state and began a new job as a case manager in a hospital. She was completely without symptoms; her last chest radiograph was 18 years earlier and was normal. She eats sushi and, on weekends before her move, volunteered for many years at a dog shelter. Because of her age and a 42-year history of cigarette smoking, she had resection of the nodule. In the management of this patient, an infectious diseases consultation was obtained because the pathology of the nodule revealed a worm with a muscularis layer surrounded by a granulomatous reaction. She does not recall the diagnosis and is now in your ED looking for answers. The nodule was most likely due to which one of the following?

A. *Echinococcus*
B. *Anisakis*
C. *Strongyloides*
D. *Dirofilaria*

61. A 45-year-old hypochondriac male has been reading about lung cancer screening online and comes to the ED demanding a CT scan of the chest. He has no risk factors or family history and is a lifelong nonsmoker. He had a cough 3 weeks ago that has mostly resolved without any constitutional symptoms or hemoptysis, and he has no significant travel history. If CT scan screening were undertaken for the general population, what would be the likelihood of finding a malignant solitary pulmonary nodule (SPN)?

A. <5%
B. 5% to 10%

62. A 52-year-old male comes to the ED from the bronchoscopy suite after diagnostic evaluation of a 3.5-cm right pulmonary nodule noted on CT scan of the chest to evaluate for PE which was done 1 week earlier in the ED. Shortly after the procedure, the patient became immediately short of breath and felt lightheaded and started complaining of chest pain. His vital signs are BP 80/60 mm Hg, HR 122 bpm, RR 28 breathes/min, temperature 37.2° C (99° F), Sao$_2$ 94% on non-rebreather mask. Breath sounds are diminished on the right side. What is the next best step in management?

A. Needle thoracotomy
B. Chest radiograph
C. ABG test
D. Noninvasive ventilation (BiPAP)

63. A 42-year-old Caucasian man, originally from Denmark, now living in the Ohio River Valley, presents to the ED with 6 weeks of fevers and weight loss with occasional cough along with generalized weakness. A chest radiograph shows mediastinal lymphadenopathy. Laboratory findings show hypercalcemia, elevated alkaline phosphatase, and an elevated ACE level. The most likely diagnosis is:

A. Histoplasmosis
B. Pulmonary tuberculosis (TB)
C. Coccidiomycosis
D. Sarcoidosis

64. A 57-year-old African American female presents to the ED for 1 month of progressively worsening dyspnea associated with bilateral lower extremity swelling. The patient reports occasional aching and left-sided chest pain, with the most recent episode occurring 1 hour before arrival, lasting 10 minutes, and improving with rest. She denies associated nausea or diaphoresis and denies any recent travel or immobilization. She denies orthopnea and paroxysmal nocturnal dyspnea. The patient denies cardiac risk factors, recent surgeries, hospitalizations, and a personal/familial history of PE or deep venous thrombosis (DVT). Past medical history is significant for sarcoidosis (diagnosis two years prior by incidental finding on chest radiograph; asymptomatic).

Initial vital signs are BP 147/92 mm Hg, HR 101 bpm, RR 14 breaths/min, temperature 37.7° (99.8° F), and Spo$_2$ 97% on room air. Physical examination findings are as follows: cardiovascular—tachycardia, no murmurs, rubs, or gallops; pulmonary—fine bibasilar inspiratory crackles; abdominal—prominent hepatic border palpable 4 cm below the right costal margin, hepatojugular reflex present, and positive abdominal fluid wave; musculoskeletal—+3 pitting edema bilaterally.

What is the next step in the evaluation of this patient?

A. Diuresis
B. Portable chest radiograph
C. Bedside echocardiogram
D. Heparin drip

65. A 56-year-old female with stage III sarcoidosis presents to the ED with fever, chills, and flank pain with foul-smelling urine. She is being treated for progressive pulmonary sarcoidosis and was just discharged from the hospital 1 week earlier. This was her fourth admission to the hospital this year. Her initial vital signs are temperature 38.1° C (100.6° F), BP 80/50 mm Hg, HR 118 bpm, RR 22 breaths/min, and Sao$_2$ 94% on room air (same as when she was recently discharged). She denies any cough or worsening respiratory symptoms. After an appropriate fluid bolus and empiric antibiotics, her BP is 88/60 mm Hg, and she is feeling weak and light-headed. What should be the next step in management?

A. Stress dose steroids
B. Urinalysis and culture
C. Bedside echocardiogram
D. Vasopressors

66. A 33-year-old African American female, previously healthy, presents with several weeks of malaise, arthralgias, dry cough, and a nodular rash on her arms and trunk. On exam, you note she has several indurated plaques <1 cm in size over her chest, back, and arms. She also has bilateral scleral injection and a low-grade fever. She is noted to have hepatosplenomegaly. Labs show aspartate aminotransferase (AST) 35, alanine aminotransferase (ALT) 26, alkaline phosphatase 434, and total bilirubin 1.0. A chest radiograph is obtained (Figure 16.15). What is the most likely diagnosis?

A. Acute viral hepatitis
B. Cholangiocarcinoma
C. Systemic lupus erythematosus
D. Sarcoidosis

67. A 38-year-old diabetic male (last hemoglobin A1c 9.2) and sarcoidosis with recent reduction in PFTs currently on steroid taper presents with tachypnea and generalized fatigue. He has had frequent urination and muscle aches. He has been compliant with his insulin, but fluid intake has been diminished over the past few

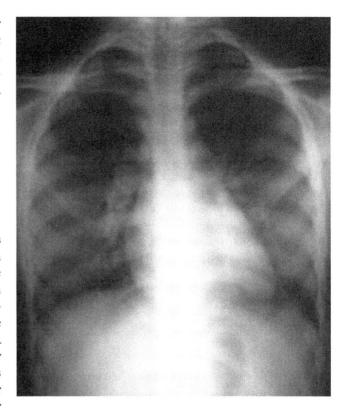

Figure 16.15 Chest radiograph.

days because of nausea. He denies fever or chest pain, but breathing is slightly worse than baseline. What is the next best step in the management of this patient?

A. IV fluid bolus
B. Point-of-care blood glucose
C. IV steroids
D. Chest radiograph

68. A 43-year-old man with a history of hypertension well controlled on hydrochlorothiazide (HCTZ) presents to the ED with cough and fever. He has had a dry cough for several weeks, which is now worsening with dark yellow sputum. He noticed a fever of 38.2° C (100.8° F) at home as well as worsening shortness of breath. A sputum sample is obtained and sent to the lab, and he is found to have spherules containing endospores. How is he most likely to have contracted his disease?

A. Hiking in the woods in Connecticut
B. Cleaning out pigeon coops in Ohio
C. Walking trails in the Arizona desert
D. Exploring caves in the Mississippi River Valley

69. A 44-year-old male physician moved from Chicago to Palm Springs, California two years ago for a new job. He is an avid hiker and otherwise healthy. He presents

to his local ED with cough, malaise, and shortness of breath progressively worsening for 3 weeks to the point at which he cannot go up the stairs in his house without stopping. He has chest pain but only with the cough. He reports no immobilization or recent travel. Initial vital signs are temperature 37.4° C (99.4° F), BP 150/84 mm Hg, HR 112 bpm, RR 23 breaths/min, and Sao$_2$ 87% on room air. Labs are unremarkable other than a WBC count of 11.8, and chest radiograph shows right-sided infiltrate with adenopathy. HIV test is negative. He completed a course of levofloxacin during an urgent care visit 10 days ago without any improvement, and his chest radiograph is slightly worse now compared with the prior done at urgent care. In addition to admission, what medications would be indicated in the ED?

A. Steroids
B. Vancomycin
C. Oseltamivir
D. Amphotericin B

70. A 25-year-old male from Yuma, Arizona with HIV/AIDS, CD4 count of 200 when tested 3 months ago, and intermittent medication compliance presents to the ED with fever, headache, joint pain, and cough that have been worsening for several days. Labs revealed leukopenia, elevated erythrocyte sedimentation rate, and normal renal function. Chest radiograph shows diffuse reticulonodular opacities. Head CT reveals mild ventriculomegaly. Lumbar puncture shows an elevated opening pressure and protein, normal glucose, and a lymphocyte predominance with no organisms on Gram stain. His vital signs and mental status are normal. What is the next step in management for this patient?

A. Amphotericin B
B. Fluconazole
C. Steroids
D. Ceftriaxone 2 g IV + dexamethasone IV

71. A 38-year-old previously healthy male who lives in Central California and works as an archaeologic excavator in the area presents to the ED with cough and fatigue for the past 2 weeks. He has also noted a mild rash that seems to be getting better. His boss at work suggested that he get evaluated for his symptoms. He denies any significant shortness of breath or respiratory symptoms. Vital signs are temperature 37.1° C (98.8° F), RR 14 breaths/min, BP 132/82 mm Hg, HR 86 bpm, and Sao$_2$ 96% on room air. His chest radiograph shows no focal infiltrate but some mild scattered reticular opacities. Serum cocci screen was positive. Remainder of the workup was unremarkable, and the patient is texting with his wife. What are the next steps in management?

A. Discharge with supportive care
B. Oral fluconazole
C. IV amphotericin B
D. Oral azithromycin

72. A 24-year-old female G3P2 at 10 weeks' gestation with a history of HIV on HAART with CD4 count of 150 presents to the ED with fever, night sweats, and hemoptysis with associated chest pain and shortness of breath. She was diagnosed with pulmonary cocci infection 3 months ago but stopped her fluconazole after finding out she was pregnant. Vital signs are temperature 37.2° C (99° F), BP 100/60 mm Hg, RR 18 breaths/min, HR 114 bpm, and Sao$_2$ 93% on room air. Chest radiograph is revealing for hilar adenopathy, scattered infiltrates, and possible cavitary changes in the upper lung fields. TB testing is negative. The patient is started on appropriate antifungal therapy and admitted. What is the most common side effect of the treatment regimen?

A. Elevated liver function test results
B. Elevated creatinine
C. Lupus-like syndrome
D. Stevens-Johnson syndrome

73. A 33-year-old male from the Upper Peninsula of Michigan presents to the ED with fever, productive cough, and shortness of breath worsening for several weeks. He appears weak and malnourished. Initial vital signs are temperature 37.3° C (99.2° F), BP 104/60 mm Hg, HR 109 bpm, RR 18 breaths/min, and Sao$_2$ 94% on room air. He has diffuse crackles on lung exam and a rash on his right lower extremity that is violet and irregular in appearance. Chest radiograph shows reticulonodular infiltrates with calcified granulomas. He is found to be HIV positive with an absolute lymphocyte count of 200. CD4 count is pending. Sputum sample KOH is positive for broad-based budding yeast. What is the first-line therapy in management for this patient?

A. Itraconazole
B. Fluconazole
C. Amphotericin B
D. Posaconazole

74. A 45-year-old woman from central Illinois with a history of psoriatic arthritis presents to the ED with 2 weeks of cough, dyspnea, fever, and malaise. She had been treated with prednisone and methotrexate for several years and had started infliximab about 10 months before this illness. On exam, she appears fatigued and short of breath with RR 32 breaths/min and oxygen saturation 96% to 100% on 100% Fio$_2$ by non-rebreather

mask. Lungs have coarse rales bilaterally with decreased breath sounds at each base. Chest radiograph shows bilateral pulmonary infiltrates. After failure to improve on levofloxacin, she undergoes lung biopsy, which reveals narrow-based budding fungal elements. The most likely diagnosis is which of the following?

A. *Pneumocystis jirovecii* pneumonia (PJP)
B. Coccidioidomycosis
C. Cryptococcosis
D. Histoplasmosis

75. A 58-year-old male with a history of kidney transplantation 5 years earlier, COPD, and previous chronic alcohol use presents with fever, night sweats, fatigue, and a 10-pound weight loss over the past few weeks. He also has purulent sputum with scant hemoptysis, shortness of breath, and uncomfortable cough with associated chest pain. A few days before the onset of symptoms, the patient was gardening and scraped his leg on the broken side of a wooden fence. Vital signs are temperature 37.7° C (99.8° F), RR 22 breaths/min, HR 116 beats/min, BP 108/76 mm Hg, and Sao$_2$ 91% on 2 L by nasal cannula. He had a negative TB test 2 weeks ago. His exam is significant for diffuse pulmonary crackles and several nodules near the site of injury near the left ankle. Chest radiograph reveals scattered nodular findings and left upper lobe cavitation. Chest CT is performed. Gram stain of sputum is negative for bacteria. What is the most likely diagnosis?

A. TB
B. *Klebsiella pneumoniae*
C. Cytomegalovirus (CMV)
D. Pulmonary sporotrichosis

76. A 51-year-old female from Arizona with relapsed acute myeloid leukemia underwent an allogeneic stem cell transplantation. Soon after discharge from the hospital she was noted in a clinic visit to be febrile and neutropenic, with fatigue and productive cough with blood streaks. Blood cultures are sent, and skin biopsy is performed. Three days later, she presents to the ED at the insistence of her hematologist with worsening fatigue and continued fever. On exam, she has 2 × 3 cm plaque-like erythematous lesions that are nontender on her left upper arm. A biopsy of the lesions done in the clinic shows septate, branching, filamentous hyphae invading cutaneous blood vessels, and blood cultures are growing them as well. In addition, her chest radiograph reveals a streaky infiltrate in the right lower lobe. Sputum sample shows the same organism as the skin biopsy. What is the most likely pathogen?

A. Histoplasma
B. Blastomycoses
C. Coccidioides
D. *Fusarium* species

77. A 29-year-old female with a history of IV drug use and AIDS (last CD4 count was 46) presents with cough, fever, and mild respiratory distress. She was started in the ED on broad-spectrum antibiotics soon after arrival. She is tachypneic and requiring supplemental oxygen at 4 to 5 L by nasal cannula. She is tachycardic. Labs are revealing for low WBCs, elevated LDH, and a chest radiograph that shows mild bilateral airspace disease. She has a sulfa allergy and has been taking PJP prophylaxis, though she just started being compliant 3 or 4 days ago. She also has an elevated A-a gradient on ABG test. She was started on clindamycin and primaquine in addition to the broad-spectrum antibiotics. Her condition acutely worsened, and she was intubated, after which a bronchoalveolar lavage (BAL) was positive for PJP. Despite treatment of her condition, she develops refractory hypoxemia and mild perioral cyanosis with elevated lactate. What is the cause of her worsening of symptoms?

A. ARDS
B. Disseminated TB
C. Carbon monoxide poisoning
D. Methemoglobinemia

1. ANSWER: C

This patient is presenting with croup, which is commonly caused by parainfluenza virus. The treatment of croup includes supplemental humidified oxygen, steroids, and nebulized racemic epinephrine. Epinephrine should be given to patients with moderate to severe croup (stridor at rest or with significant respiratory distress). These patients should be observed for 3 to 4 hours to monitor for possible rebound stridor.

For any pediatric patient presenting with stridor or signs of upper airway obstruction, always consider foreign body aspiration in your differential. However, foreign body aspiration should not have fever, cough, or URI symptoms

Test-taking tip: You can eliminate A and D because 30 minutes is too short of an observation period and 6 hours is too long. This narrows your choices down by half.

2. ANSWER: C

In this patient with acute dyspnea and wheezing, it is important to quickly differentiate the cause of this shortness of breath. Wheezing in this patient can easily be caused by his COPD, but given his cardiac risk factors, he may also have cardiac wheezing from underlying CHF resulting in pulmonary edema. A quick and easy assessment would be to use bedside ultrasound to distinguish the two. The image in Figure 16.1 shows sonographic B lines, which also are known as comet-tail artifacts. These are hyperechoic, dynamic lines coming from the pleural line. These B-lines indicate subpleural interstitial edema. A-lines, which are horizontal lines, indicate dry interlobular septa, and a predominance of A-lines over B-lines would less likely suggest pulmonary edema. The correct treatment at this time for this patient's pulmonary edema from presumed CHF would be nitroglycerin and BiPAP.

Test-taking tip: Do not be quick to assume wheezing in an adult equates to a COPD or asthma exacerbation.

3. ANSWER: C

Plateau pressures are a marker of lung compliance. Any condition that would decrease lung compliance would cause the plateau pressures to rise. In this case, bronchospasm would not cause high plateau pressures because it does not reflect lung compliance but rather airway resistance. High airway resistance will be reflected in higher peak pressures.

Peak pressure = (flow × resistance) + plateau pressure

Any time you have a question about a patient who suddenly decompensates on a ventilator, the best management strategy is to disconnect the patient off the ventilator and troubleshoot from there.

Test-taking tip: This is a "you know it or don't" kind of question. If you don't know it, choose an answer and move on. You can perhaps mark it for review when you are done at the end of the test. Don't, however, let these kinds of questions get you stuck and waste your time.

4. ANSWER: D

This HIV patient is presenting with pneumocystis pneumonia (PCP), which often occurs when the CD4 count is £200. It is the most common opportunistic respiratory infection in AIDS. The chest radiograph shows a bilateral reticular interstitial pattern with increased markings in the perihilar regions. The approach to treatment is based on the severity of the infection. Patients with PCP will have either hypoxemia at rest or with exertion or an increase in the alveolar-arterial oxygen tension gradient. Obtaining an ABG test is helpful to determine the level of hypoxemia and guide treatment. When the PaO_2 <70 mm Hg, that is an indication to give steroids because they have been shown to decrease morbidity and mortality. The steroids are thought to decrease the inflammatory response of dying organisms when antibiotic treatment is initiated. Pentamidine and atovaquone are alternate treatments for PCP if the patient is unable to tolerate Bactrim or has G6PD deficiency, allergies, or first-trimester pregnancy.

Test-taking tip: If a test question is asking about PJP pneumonia, there will be some clue that the patient has HIV, AIDS, or AIDS-defining illness. These patients tend to be hypoxemic and have out-of-proportion dyspnea with exertion.

5. ANSWER: C

In severe asthma exacerbations, severe airflow limitation occurs as a result of bronchospasm, airway edema, and mucous plugging, so work of breathing is significantly increased. The increased airway resistance in asthma exacerbation makes it more difficult to expire the air, so longer expiratory time is required to expel all the inspired air. If inspiration occurs before all the air is expired, this leads to air trapping. If significant air trapping occurs, severe hyperinflation occurs and can cause barotrauma and worsening respiratory status. Therefore, the management strategy is to decrease minute ventilation.

Minute ventilation is equal to tidal volume × respiratory rate. You can decrease your minute ventilation by prolonging expiratory time, decreasing the respiratory rate, and decreasing the tidal volumes. By increasing the inspiratory flow rate, the time for inspiration is decreased, giving the patient more time to expire. Hence, decreasing the inspiratory flow rate would potentially increase inspiratory time, decreasing the overall expiratory/inspiratory ratio. Decreasing minute ventilation would likely cause hypercapnia, but permissive hypercapnia is an appropriate strategy if pH is maintained above 7.20 or $PaCO_2$ below 90 mm Hg.

Test-taking tip: Whenever you come across a question concerning asthma or COPD ventilator management, remember to choose strategies to increase expiration.

6. ANSWER: D

This patient has developed methemoglobinemia from overapplication of topical anesthetics. Benzocaine and Cetacaine spray are common culprits because they are oxidizing agents that convert the ferrous 2+ in hemoglobin into ferric 3+ state (met-hemoglobin), which irreversibly binds oxygen. The met-hemoglobin also affects any of the remaining ferrous ions, making its affinity to oxygen tighter and causing a left shift in the oxygen dissociation curve. Therefore, oxygen delivery to the tissues is impaired, and cyanosis ensues. An important diagnostic clue that the patient has methemoglobinemia is that the cyanosis isn't corrected by oxygen. The treatment of choice for methemoglobinemia should be methylene blue, but it requires NADPH to help reduce the methemoglobin. If given to patients with G6PD, it can induce an acute hemolytic reaction and possibly increase the amount of methemoglobin. Methylene blue is a monoamine oxidase inhibitor, so patients taking selective serotonin reuptake inhibitors (SSRIs), such as citalopram, are at risk for developing serotonin syndrome. Methylene blue should not be given to patients with renal insufficiency.

Test-taking tip: If you note cyanosis that does not improve with supplemental oxygen, think of methemoglobinemia.

7. ANSWER: D

The patient has multiple risk factors for a pleural effusion given his ESRD, CHF, and lymphoma. Pleural effusions can be transudates or exudates. The radiograph shows a right pleural effusion, so the patient has a fluid collection in his pleural space. On an upright radiograph, blunting of the lateral costophrenic angle and slight elevation of the hemidiaphragm are usually seen with pleural effusions.

Typically, at least 200 to 250 mL of fluid must be present to see these findings on an upright posterior-anterior film. The layering of fluid in a pleural effusion also causes a "meniscus sign." On a lateral film, less fluid is required to blunt the posterior costophrenic sulcus. The lateral decubitus film is the most sensitive chest radiograph to pick up a pleural effusion, and a supine film is the least sensitive.

You may encounter having to interpret pleural fluid analysis to differentiate transudative versus exudative processes. A general rule of thumb is that high protein or high LDH and low glucose suggest an exudative process.

Test-taking tip: This is a "you know it or don't" kind of question. If you don't know it, choose an answer and move on. You can perhaps mark it for review when you are done at the end of the test. Don't, however, let these kinds of questions get you stuck and waste your time.

8. ANSWER: B

This patient is presenting with an unstable PE. His pancreatic cancer greatly increases his risk for developing a PE. His CT scan shows a filling defect in his main pulmonary arteries—a saddle embolus. He has a massive PE with hemodynamic instability given his hypotension. EKG is a poor tool for diagnosing PE. The EKG is useful in ruling out diagnoses other than PE. Signs of right heart strain can be present on EKG, and the S1Q3T3 classic finding is neither sensitive nor specific for PE and is relatively uncommon. Nonspecific ST/T wave changes and tachycardia are more commonly seen on EKG.

The chest radiograph is also a poor tool for diagnosing PE. The chest radiograph still tends to be abnormal in PE; atelectasis is the most common abnormality. The rare radiograph findings, such as Hampton's hump (wedge-shaped opacity) and Westermark's sign (filling defect in distal pulmonary vessels in a segmental distribution), would raise suspicion for PE. The treatment of choice in this case would be thrombolytic therapy because this is considered unstable. If the patient had a normal blood pressure, then heparin would be indicated. The most common presenting symptom in PE is dyspnea followed by chest pain. The most common presenting sign is tachypnea followed by leg swelling.

In real life, PE can present in patients without any obvious risk factors. However, on examination, the patient typically will carry risk factors for PE. Remember to think of Virchow's triad—stasis, hypercoagulability, and venous injury.

Test-taking tip: You can eliminate A and C because you know this is an unstable PE with those unstable vital signs. Therefore, more aggressive treatment than heparin is needed, and EKGs are really nonspecific.

9. ANSWER: B

The clinical scenario is describing ARDS. ARDS is an inflammatory response of the lungs to some insult, which results in diffuse alveolar injury. This results in increased fluids leaking into the interstitial spaces and alveoli, with damage to lung surfactant, leading to impaired gas exchange, pulmonary hypertension, and decreased lung compliance. This syndrome can affect all ages and is associated with high morbidity and mortality. It is considered severe when the PaO_2/FiO_2 ratio is £100 mm Hg on positive end-expiratory pressure (PEEP) of 5 mm Hg or more. There are many causes that can trigger ARDS, with sepsis being the number one cause. Other common causes include severe trauma, aspiration pneumonia, pancreatitis, massive transfusion, drug overdose, transfusion-related acute lung injury (TRALI), near drowning, and burns. On chest radiograph, you will see bilateral patchy infiltrates. With ventilator management, low tidal volumes of 4 to 8 mL/kg have been shown to improve outcomes.

Test-taking tip: ARDS is a commonly tested topic, and many questions are related to the pathophysiology. Remember low tidal volumes and higher PEEP for ventilator management. Decreased PaO_2/FiO_2 ratios are a hallmark as well.

10. ANSWER: B

The patient in this case has an acute exacerbation of CF. His CT scan shows bronchiectasis, which is a feature of CF. Patients with CF are chronically colonized with bacteria in their lungs, and the approach to treating acute exacerbations mandates one to presume a bacterial pulmonary infection is at play and to give antibiotics (grade 1C recommendations). In addition, it is thought that the bacterial infections are not caused by new strains of bacteria that the patient has not had before. Therefore, it is important to also base treatment on the patient's respiratory secretions to target the antibiotics. Typically, one or two antibiotics are always given to treat for presumed *Pseudomonas* infection and add or broaden coverage if there are some other concerning organisms in the respiratory cultures. Generally, the two most common bacterial organisms in CF in patients older than 10 years are *Pseudomonas* and methicillin-sensitive *S. aureus* (MSSA).

Test-taking tip: CF patients classically will have *Pseudomonas* infections—so remember to choose antibiotics with *Pseudomonas* coverage. Think about the diagnosis of CF if you get a young patient with either multiple lung infections, recurrent pancreatitis, or concurrent diabetes.

11. ANSWER: D

The patient presents here with a complete left-sided pneumothorax without signs of tension pneumothorax. This patient has an iatrogenic pneumothorax without any known risk factors for secondary causes of pneumothorax. Simply observing the patient without any procedural intervention would be inappropriate given the size of the pneumothorax and the patient's symptoms. Observation is indicated if the pneumothorax is very small (<1 cm) and has a high likelihood of resolving on its own (i.e., primary spontaneous pneumothorax [PSP]). Catheter aspiration can be used in a small simple pneumothorax. Needle decompression would be indicated if the patient had a tension pneumothorax, but he is hemodynamically stable. Furthermore, needle decompression would necessitate thoracostomy tube placement afterward. Chemical pleurodesis is indicated for persistent air leak or refractory pneumothorax.

Clues of hemodynamic instability with a tension pneumothorax that would need needle decompression emergently would be elevated jugular venous distention, hypotension, tachycardia, and tracheal deviation.

Test-taking tip: You can eliminate A and B because the pneumothorax is too big to just observe and it hasn't been there long enough to need a pleurodesis.

12. ANSWER: C

Pertussis infection (whooping cough) is a very contagious respiratory illness. The infection has three phases and lasts about 3 months. It is also known as the "100-day cough." After an incubation stage of about 7 to 10 days, the catarrhal phase (lasts 1–2 weeks) is characterized by nonspecific upper respiratory symptoms with dry cough that begins in the latter part of this phase. Because the symptoms are vague during this phase, it is rarely diagnosed in the early phase. The paroxysmal phase is characterized by the onset of the classic whooping cough. The whooping cough consists of severe, vigorous coughing fits followed by a loud inspiratory whoop when the patient tries to catch his or her breath. It is frequently associated with severe posttussive emesis. The convalescent phase is characterized by a decreased frequency and severity of the cough. The infection is most contagious during the catarrhal phase. Antibiotic treatment reduces the spread of the infection to others and makes the infection less contagious for about 5 days after starting treatment. Antibiotic treatment can also lessen duration of symptoms if given in the catarrhal phase but generally does not shorten symptoms in the paroxysmal or convalescent stages.

Treatment in patients typically can reduce symptoms if started within the first 3 weeks and can be considered after

3 to 6 weeks of illness to decrease transmission rate. The typical treatment of choice is macrolides—usually erythromycin. Postexposure prophylaxis is generally recommended in close household contacts and patients who are at high risk for severe or complicated pertussis even if they are already fully immunized. The mother is both a household contact and at high risk given that she is pregnant, so she should be prescribed antibiotics.

Test-taking tip: Pertussis is often missed early on but is most easily identified in the paroxysmal phase—look for clues of whooping cough, such as severe post-tussive emesis or severe coughing fits or a loud inspiratory whoop. Treatment could include macrolide antibiotics and otherwise supportive care.

13. ANSWER: B

This patient has developed a rare but life-threatening complication of tracheostomy tube placement called a tracheoinnominate fistula (TIF). This typically occurs within 3 weeks of tube placement and is usually a complication of pressure necrosis from an overinflated cuff, a low-seated tracheotomy, poor neck positioning, or prolonged endotracheal intubation. The innominate artery crosses the trachea. Patients with TIF sometimes first present with a "sentinel bleed"—a small bleed followed by the big bleed. Airway management is critical by controlling the bleeding because the patient will die from asphyxiation from the bleeding. Hyperinflating the cuff often can tamponade the innominate artery and allow time for surgical and ear-nose-throat (ENT) specialists to prepare for definitive operative management. If the patient continues to bleed with the cuff overinflated, application of direct digital pressure within the tracheostomy site or intubation from above can be performed.

TIFs should be at the top of the differential when a patient with a tracheostomy tube presents with bleeding. Otherwise, more common complications from tracheostomy include obstruction, tracheal stenosis, and pneumothorax.

Test-taking tip: You can eliminate D because removal of a fresh trach is always contraindicated because you can easily lose the track.

14. ANSWER: D

Immediate airway management is indicated in this patient because she has signs of an airway emergency given her cyanosis, stridor, and tripoding. She has aspirated a foreign body. To promote expulsion of the foreign body occluding her airway, the Heimlich maneuver should be performed in children older than 1 year or back blows in infants. If the abdominal thrusts do not expulse the object and the patient is still in respiratory distress, intubation is indicated. It is possible that intubation may push the obstructing object distally. If the object prevents intubation, then a surgical airway should be created. If the patient had presented with more mild signs and symptoms, then a workup could have been initiated, starting with a thorough history, physical exam, and neck and chest radiographs, including decubitus films. Most swallowed foreign objects are radiolucent, so a negative radiograph does not rule out foreign body aspiration. If imaging is negative but there is still moderate suspicion for a foreign body, then a rigid bronchoscopy should be performed. Performing a blind sweep of the mouth is dangerous because it can worsen airway obstruction if the object is pushed deeper into the oropharynx.

Test-taking tip: Suspect foreign body aspiration in all questions regarding children with choking, stridor, wheezing, or a new cough.

15. ANSWER: A

K. pneumoniae is a gram-negative aerobic bacterium that tends to affect impaired hosts, such as alcoholic, diabetic, COPD, and older adult patients. Patients with this infection can have classic "currant jelly" sputum. The infection can be severe and frequently results in complications such as lung abscesses, empyema, and bacteremia. On chest radiographs, a bulging fissure below an upper lobar consolidation is often seen.

Legionella pneumonia tends to be outbreak related. It is often transmitted through the water supply or inhalation of aerosols, such as mist machines, showers, and air-conditioning systems. *Legionella* can often involve gastrointestinal (GI) symptoms, bradycardia, and hyponatremia. The chest radiograph often shows hilar adenopathy, patchy infiltrate, and pleural effusions.

S. aureus pneumonia, including methicillin-resistant *S. aureus* (MRSA) pneumonia, incidence is climbing. It tends to follow influenza and causes a superinfection with high morbidity and mortality.

P. aeruginosa pneumonia tends to afflict inpatients, immunocompromised patients, intubated patients, and nursing home residents. It causes severe infections and has high mortality. Acutely, *P. aeruginosa* pneumonia usually is associated with purulent sputum, dyspnea, fever, chills, confusion, and severe systemic toxicity.

Test-taking tip: Keywords such as alcoholic and pneumonia should trigger the thought of *Klebsiella*. *S. pneumoniae* is still the most common cause of pneumonia in all ages.

16. ANSWER: D

This patient is presenting with hereditary angioedema (HAE). It is an autosomal dominant disorder. These patients have recurrent episodes of angioedema. The most common defect is dysfunction or deficiency in the C1-esterase inhibitor. Attacks can be laryngeal, GI, or cutaneous, but laryngeal attacks tend to be rarer. When there is a deficiency of C1-esterase inhibitor, excessive production of bradykinin occurs, leading to increased vascular permeability and angioedema. The treatment of choice involves replacing C1-esterase inhibitor or blocking production of bradykinin. First-line therapies include plasma-derived C1 inhibitor concentrate or recombinant C1 inhibitor, icatibant (bradykinin receptor antagonist), and kallikrein inhibitor (blocks production of bradykinin). Because these therapies take several hours to work, airway management is still the priority. If stridor and other signs of imminent airway obstruction are present, securing the airway should be the most important management step. Epinephrine, steroids, and antihistamines have not been shown to be effective. This patient's presentation also can mimic ACE inhibitor–induced angioedema, but given the positive family history and prior episodes, this is HAE. For ACE inhibitor angioedema, the offending agent needs to be stopped immediately and never to be taken again. Cryoprecipitate does not contain C1-esterase inhibitor, so it would not be indicated treatment. Fresh frozen plasma has been used as a second-line treatment for HAE.

Test-taking tip: With patients presenting with angioedema, airway management is the most important management step. Recall that the most common causes of angioedema are anaphylaxis and bradykinin-induced angioedema.

17. ANSWER: C

This patient has a tracheoesophageal fistula seen on bronchoscopy. This is a complication from the esophageal stent eroding into the trachea. The fistula puts him at high risk for aspiration pneumonia. Therefore, the appropriate antibiotic regimen needs to cover both anaerobes and gram-negative organisms. Of the regimen choices, ampicillin-sulbactam would provide adequate coverage for both. Ampicillin is a ß-lactam antibiotic, and sulbactam is a bacterial ß-lactamase inhibitor. This combination covers most gram-positive, gram-negative, and anaerobic bacteria. Cefpodoxime is a third-generation cephalosporin. It covers gram-positive and gram-negative organisms, but it specifically does not cover anaerobes or *Pseudomonas*. Azithromycin covers atypical bacteria. The combination of cefpodoxime and azithromycin would not provide adequate anaerobic coverage. Vancomycin covers MRSA, and

Levaquin covers gram-negative and atypical organisms, but this combination also lacks anaerobic coverage. Bactrim and Levaquin similarly would not have adequate anaerobic coverage.

Test-taking tip: Aspiration pneumonia occurs more frequently in alcoholic, seizure, and stroke patients and in patients with neuromuscular diseases. Right lower lobe is the most common location of pneumonia if a patient is upright or sitting, but any lobe can be affected if the patient is supine.

18. ANSWER: B

Although there is no consensus on a definition of hemoptysis, generally >600 mL in 24 hours is considered massive. With the management of massive hemoptysis, the priority is airway control. Patients die of asphyxiation from bleeding into their airway and not from exsanguination. In this case, localizing the source of bleeding and rotating the patient so that the bleeding side is down to avoid aspiration into the other lung while performing main stem intubation of the nonbleeding lung will secure the airway. If possible, use a large-bore ETT (size 8) to allow for rigid bronchoscopy. Given the patient's CT shows an invasive left-sided infection, place the patient onto his left side.

The most common cause of hemoptysis in the United States is bronchitis, and the most common cause in the world is TP. Consider the possibility of GI bleeding as the source of hemoptysis.

Test-taking tip: Always approach cases of hemoptysis by focusing on airway, breathing, and circulation management. You can eliminate A and C because they are not airway focused. That narrows your options down by two.

19. ANSWER: D

The diagnosis of Boerhaave's syndrome should be suspected in this patient with chest pain after multiple episodes of vomiting. She has pneumomediastinum on chest radiograph (Figure 16.10). The increased intrathoracic pressures from retching caused rupture of her esophagus, leading to free air dissecting into her mediastinum. The radiograph is supportive of the diagnosis, but performing a water-soluble contrast esophagram or CT scan can establish the diagnosis. These patients should be admitted to the intensive care unit (ICU) for monitoring because they can decompensate quickly. These patients should be kept NPO and be given IV fluids and started on broad-spectrum antibiotics, and a surgical consult should be made.

Test-taking tip: When confronted with a "what is the most likely diagnosis" question, consider the pertinent information/clues given in the question stem and use the answer choices to guide your thought process. The information given is generally trying to guide you to the right answer and not to trick you.

Test-taking tip: "Most common cause" questions are typical, and memorizing most common pathogens or most common causes that you encounter in your test study always has high yield.

20. ANSWER: C

ACE inhibitor–induced cough is frequently seen in patients taking ACE inhibitors such as lisinopril. The onset of this nonproductive cough usually starts within 1 week of starting therapy but can be delayed up to 6 months. It generally should not be associated with wheezing or shortness of breath. Stopping the medication should resolve the symptoms in a few days. Switching to a different ACE inhibitor usually does not resolve the cough. The other answers are less likely given the other negative review of symptoms. Cough associated with asthma tends to be worse at night and associated with other signs such as wheezing. Postnasal drip, GERD, and asthma are the most common causes of cough.

Test-taking tip: Always pay attention to medications listed in the question stem; with lisinopril listed, C is the most likely diagnosis.

21. ANSWER: B

S. pneumoniae remains the most common bacterial pathogen causing community-acquired pneumonia. The classic presentation is a cough productive of rust-colored sputum, sudden onset of shaking chills, and pleuritic chest pain; however, these patients can present with a wide variety of presentations—some with a more insidious onset.

S. aureus was found to be the second most common pathogen in some studies of hospitalized ED patients. They typically present with a higher degree of illness severity and can have cavitary lesions on chest radiograph suggestive of necrotizing pneumonia. There are several factors, including IV drug use, that place a patient at higher risk, which are not present here.

P. aeruginosa is an uncommon cause of community-acquired pneumonia and is more commonly found in patients with underlying lung disease such as bronchiectasis from CF or in patients who have been hospitalized, receive regular dialysis, or have resided in a nursing care facility in the past 90 days. Choose an antibiotic regimen that covers *Pseudomonas* in these patients.

C. pneumoniae is a common atypical pneumonia pathogen in young adults; however, it classically presents with a self-limited respiratory illness in these patients. Older adult patients can present with radiographically evident pneumonia, which may require hospitalization.

22. ANSWER: A

Mycoplasma is a relatively common cause of atypical pneumonia. Classically seen in adult patients who are healthy and younger than 40 years, this disease causes a mild respiratory illness with extrapulmonary features, most commonly a rash with diverse presentations. Although it is a common misconception that atypical pneumonias do not present in older adults, this patient is not at increased risk for this pathogen.

Pseudomonas is associated with health care encounters, including dialysis, inpatient hospitalization, and skilled nursing care facilities. This patient has increased risk for pseudomonal pneumonia and should be covered appropriately with antipseudomonal antibiotics such as piperacillin-tazobactam or cefepime in any antibacterial regimen for pneumonia.

Bacteroides is an anaerobic infection that can cause lower respiratory tract infections. It should be considered in any patient with aspiration risk as well as other anaerobes, such as *Peptostreptococcus, Fusobacterium,* and *Prevotella.* This patient's stroke puts him at risk for aspiration.

H. influenzae has become much less common in young immunized patients thanks to the advent of vaccines; however, older adult patients, especially those with chronic diseases such as COPD, malignancy, diabetes, alcoholism, or malnutrition, are at an increased risk.

Test-taking tip: Elderly patients can have a number of co-morbidities that put them at risk for a variety of diseases. Know these common associations in order to identify possible diseases both on tests and clinically.

23. ANSWER: C

A helpful mnemonic to remember is the "DOPES" mnemonic for postintubation respiratory distress. This helps you to quickly recall immediate life threats for a patient who is intubated and becomes hypoxic:

Displacement of the ETT
Obstruction of the ETT
Pneumothorax
Equipment failure (ventilator)
Stacked breaths (in patients with bronchospasm)

Intubating an asthmatic patient should be a last resort because it is difficult to match the patient's physiologic respirations while on positive pressure ventilation. The phenomenon of breath stacking or auto-peeping occurs when the patient's airway obstruction does not allow for full expiratory phase and intrathoracic pressures increase, causing decreased ventilation as well as decreased venous return that can lead to cardiac arrest. This can be prevented by setting the ventilator to rapid inspiratory phase with a decreased respiratory rate and long expiratory phase. If a patient exhibits breath stacking, immediately remove the patient from the ventilator and allow a long expiration to release the stacked breaths.

Although displacement can cause postintubation hypoxia, this patient's tube is not displaced.

While possible, bilateral tension pneumothoraxes are unlikely. Patients with COPD and emphysematous lungs are at risk for rupturing a bleb and causing pneumothorax, but this is less likely in a young asthma patient. Rapid recognition and treatment of tension pneumothorax in a patient on positive pressure ventilation is critically important, but this patient has a more likely diagnosis.

Obstruction of the ETT is a possibility in any intubated patient, and suctioning can help if a patient becomes hypoxic, but this patient needs more immediate therapy to prevent cardiac arrest.

Test-taking tip: Recognize and apply your knowledge of immediate life threats in an intubated patient. You may have only seconds to act in these patients. The DOPES mnemonic is a helpful tool to quickly remember the differential diagnosis.

24. ANSWER: A

While you should have a low threshold for starting antibiotics in COPD patients because of the high incidence of respiratory infection as an inciting factor, bacterial resistance is an ongoing concern in the practice of medicine. Antibiotic therapy has been shown to be effective only in COPD exacerbations with increased volume or purulence of sputum or in moderate to severe exacerbations requiring admission. This patient does not require antibiotics and can be discharged to see his primary physician with steroids and continued albuterol inhaler use as needed.

While this patient may benefit from inhaled corticosteroids, these are used as a preventative measure in patients who repeatedly require emergency treatment or admission for their COPD. If a patient requires inhaled corticosteroids and does not have adequate follow-up, these may be prescribed by an emergency physician for prevention of future exacerbations, but their use in acute exacerbations has not been established, and outpatient therapy should consist of a short burst of oral steroids.

This patient has a mild COPD exacerbation and improved clinically with emergency therapies so does not require admission. PFTs can be performed as an outpatient and can guide long-term management. Clinical course should be used to determine disposition in COPD patients.

Test-taking tip: Know the indication for antibiotics in a variety of conditions. Do not give empiric antibiotics when they are not indicated.

25. ANSWER: B

This patient has a severe exacerbation of COPD with hypoxia, respiratory distress, and wheezing with a clear chest radiograph. He requires maximal therapy that should include NIPPV, supplemental oxygen, IV steroids if he is unable to swallow because of distress, and inhaled ß-agonist therapy. Oxygen *should not* be withheld in a patient with severe COPD, but any patient with chronic CO_2 retention from lung disease should have a target oxygen of 90% to 92% because their respiratory drive may be dependent on hypoxia rather than hypercarbia, as in a physiologically normal patient. Discuss with your respiratory therapist to quickly titrate oxygen down with a goal of 90% to 92% to prevent apnea. If it occurs in this setting, you may need to provide ventilator support with intubation.

Although this patient may be slightly altered and cannot talk to you, studies have shown that NIPPV is safe in altered patients who are arousable and able to follow simple commands. NIPPV is appropriate in this patient and is an important feature of his care. However, NIPPV is contraindicated for patients who cannot follow simple commands because of aspiration risk.

Although antibiotics provide some benefit in caring for severe COPD exacerbations, they are not part of the most immediate care in this case and are unlikely to have influenced this patient's decline.

An ABG test can provide helpful clinical information and should be repeated serially, but emergency management based on clinical assessment of work of breathing and oxygen saturation is adequate in the acute phase, especially when obtaining an ABG test may be difficult for logistic reasons.

Test-taking tip: This is a question for which multiple answers could be right, but you are looking for the best answer. Note words like "early" in options C and D that clue you into the idea that while antibiotics and ABG testing may be important in this patient, they are not the *most* important.

26. ANSWER: D

ß-Agonists such as albuterol can cause hypokalemia, and they can be used as an adjunctive therapy for patients with critical hyperkalemia. Keep in mind that ß-agonists act by driving potassium into the cells and do not decrease total body potassium. Additionally, this effect is rarely clinically relevant.

Leukocytosis is a side effect of steroid therapy used in COPD. Leukocytopenia is not associated with steroid use or any other COPD therapy.

While there are multiple disease processes that can cause respiratory illness and could exacerbate COPD, such as malignancy or granulomatous disease, this would not be likely to occur overnight, and with initial labs that are normal, hypercalcemia should not occur on repeat testing.

Magnesium sulfate is used in some cases of severe COPD exacerbations, though its efficacy is controversial. Use of magnesium should cause *hyper*magnesemia, not *hypo*magnesemia.

Test-taking tip: Know the side effects and contraindications to common therapies used in the ED.

27. ANSWER: C

Patients who have COPD or asthma and are prone to bronchospasm should avoid taking ß-antagonists such as metoprolol or labetalol because these medications can trigger exacerbations of their chronic disease. Metoprolol is a common medication for hypertension and for rate control in atrial fibrillation, both of which are common in COPD patients. This patient has had no exacerbations in 5 years, and this visit can be very well explained by medication changes.

Amlodipine is a calcium channel blocker that is an effective antihypertensive and a good alternative to ß-blockers in a patient with COPD and should not trigger acute exacerbations.

Metformin classically causes lactic acidosis in patients with renal insufficiency but should not affect COPD. In the presence of normal labs including creatinine, metformin should be safe in this patient as an antihyperglycemic medication.

Hydrochlorothiazide is a first-line treatment for hypertension and does not cause bronchospasm. It is also a good alternative to metoprolol in this scenario.

Test-taking tip: Always consider medications, especially new ones, both in real practice and when provided on a testing stem. Polypharmacy causing medication interactions is a commonly overlooked phenomenon in emergency medicine.

28. ANSWER: D

This patient has a PE. Diagnosis can be difficult because many symptoms can overlap; however, this patient has hypoxia and tachycardia in the setting of malignancy and is undergoing active chemotherapy, and PE should be the leading suspected diagnosis. Given his hypotension, he now has a massive PE, which is defined as PE with hemodynamic instability. Benefit of thrombolytic therapy is established and should be administered in the absence of contraindications. While heparin is indicated to prevent further propagation of the clot burden, this patient is in extremis and requires more aggressive therapy.

Hemodynamic instability in PE can be due to overload of the right ventricle and cardiovascular collapse. Increasing preload to an already-strained right ventricle can hasten this collapse, and excessive IV fluid resuscitation should be avoided. While a CT is indicated in this patient, he is unstable for CT and should be stabilized first.

While vasopressors such as norepinephrine may be needed, this patient requires correction of his underlying pathophysiology with thrombolytics. He may require vasopressor therapy if thrombolytics are ineffective.

Test-taking tip: Consider PE. This is a common and life-threatening disease and requires your attention. Know the difference between massive and submassive PE and indications for thrombolytic administration.

29. ANSWER: A

Pneumocystis is an opportunistic infection in AIDS patients and is also an increasingly common cause of secondary pneumothorax. Infection with *Pneumocystis* species can cause an advanced inflammatory response with subsequent rupture of necrotic lung tissue leading to pneumothorax. This patient has a tension pneumothorax and should have intervention performed before chest radiograph.

Mycobacterium avium-intracellulare is also an opportunistic infection associated with HIV/AIDS, but it does not commonly cause pneumothorax.

S. pneumoniae is the most common bacterial pathogen in adult patients with pneumonia, including HIV patients. Antibiotic regimens for HIV patients should always cover *S. pneumoniae* in addition to opportunistic pathogens as appropriate; however, this bacteria species does not commonly cause pneumothorax.

S. aureus causes a severe pneumonia that usually requires hospitalization and even ICU care. It is common in IV drug users or immunocompromised patients with MRSA colonization, but it is not associated with significant risk for pneumothorax.

Test-taking tip: Know the common associations between disease-causing pathogens and specific features of disease. Be aware of the opportunistic infections common to HIV/AIDS patients because these are common testing topics.

30. ANSWER: C

Be aware of patients with chronic lung disease who decompensate acutely and keep pneumothorax at the top of your differential. Secondary pneumothorax is more common in patients with underlying disease, and the risk is increased by positive pressure ventilation. This patient does not show signs of tension pneumothorax, but remember that patients with chronic lung disease can decompensate severely with only a small pneumothorax. Chest radiograph should be the first initial step in evaluating for pneumothorax. You could also consider bedside ultrasound as a rapid tool for diagnosing pneumothorax.

Consideration of cardiac ischemia or new arrhythmia as a cause of acute decompensation in a critically ill patient is important. However, this patient has a presentation more concerning for acute respiratory illness due to pneumothorax. EKG is an important adjunctive diagnostic tool, but it is not the first line in this case.

Repeat CBC is unlikely to provide helpful information. Even massive hemorrhage would be unlikely to cause respiratory distress from anemia and would not account for hypoxia. Leukocytosis may be present but is a nonspecific finding and would likely have minimal to no change from initial testing.

PE can cause acute decompensation with hypoxia, shortness of breath, and chest pain. In this patient with chronic lung disease on positive pressure ventilation, pneumothorax is more likely and more immediately life-threatening and should be excluded before sending this patient to the CT scanner.

Test-taking tip: When evaluating a patient with an acute decompensation in your ED, consider the underlying disease process as well as any therapies the patient receives to help you consider most likely cause and next steps.

31. ANSWER: B

This patient has spontaneous pneumomediastinum likely related to cocaine smoking, which is the most common precipitating factor. It occurs when a sudden rise in intra-alveolar pressure causes alveolar rupture and dissection of air into the mediastinum. Read on regarding concerning or emergent cases of spontaneous pneumomediastinum, but this is usually a benign entity, and patients can be admitted for 24 hours for monitoring or, in cases in which follow-up is secure and the patient is well-appearing, may even be discharged from the ED.

Esophagoscopy is indicated in any cases in which esophageal rupture, which is an emergent condition, is suspected. These patients can become very sick, and high suspicion should be maintained if any risks for esophageal rupture are present, such as recurrent vomiting or retching or recent esophageal instrumentation (e.g., surgery or endoscopy). If esophageal rupture is diagnosed, consult thoracic surgery and give broad-spectrum antibiotics immediately.

Chest radiograph is not sensitive for pneumomediastinum. Positive findings include thin lucency surrounding the heart/mediastinum border, subcutaneous air, and air seen on lateral neck radiograph, but all these findings are rare. CT of the chest is the gold standard.

Pneumomediastinum, while benign in adults, is a very serious condition in infants, who can have cardiovascular collapse as a result. Consult surgery immediately and admit these patients.

Test-taking tip: Recognize words like "all" and "usually" as triggers to rule out answers in a multiple-choice question. They are frequently (though not always) clues that an answer is overgeneralized and incorrect.

32. ANSWER: C

This patient's presentation is suspicious for sarcoidosis. It is four times more prevalent in African Americans than in the Caucasian population and is theorized to be linked to environmental factors. There is no classic presentation for sarcoidosis because it can present in a variety of ways, but a patient with bilateral hilar adenopathy, pulmonary symptoms, and hypercalcemia should trigger consideration of this disease. Neurosarcoidosis has a 10% mortality rate, and steroids are indicated. Head CT should be obtained to identify lesions, and therapy can be tailored in conjunction with consultants.

HIV is rarely a concomitant diagnosis with sarcoidosis, though a few cases have been described. It is important to consider HIV in any young or middle-aged patient with bilateral hilar adenopathy and test for it, especially while awaiting a definitive diagnosis of sarcoidosis, but the two rarely coincide.

Transbronchial biopsy is considered the gold standard for diagnosis of sarcoidosis; however, patients do not require admission solely for the purpose of diagnosis. This can be done as an outpatient as long as the patient's other symptoms, including cardiopulmonary and extrapulmonary, do not require admission.

Extrapulmonary symptoms make up only about 10% of sarcoidosis cases. Pulmonary symptoms are much more common.

Test-taking tip: If you didn't know this one, study up on some basic patterns for rare diseases such as sarcoidosis. You can make a small flashcard and hit the highlights. It might not be efficient to spend a lot of time memorizing the whole chapter, but knowing some key bullet points on classic presentations of many rare diseases can have a high yield.

33. ANSWER: D

This patient presents with massive hemoptysis in the setting of known lung cancer on the left. Hemoptysis in these cases usually results from vascular erosion into a high-pressure bronchial artery. These patients have high mortality, which is rarely due to exsanguination but more commonly secondary to hypoxia caused by filling of the alveolar spaces with blood. Containing the bleeding to the affected lung is paramount. Ideally, intubate these patients with a large, eight-lumen ETT, or even a double-lumen ETT if available, in order to facilitate bronchoscopy and control of the bleeding if possible. In a pinch, especially if the side of the bleeding is known, selective placement of the tube in the right or left main stem can help contain hemorrhage. Normal anatomy favors the right main stem. Bronchoscopic guidance may be required to direct the ETT into the left main stem. Placing the patient in a lateral decubitus position puts the affected lung in a dependent position to limit spread of blood.

Chest radiograph should be performed to confirm the diagnosis and is helpful in an undifferentiated case or if tube placement is in question but should not delay immediate action in this patient who remains hypoxic and unstable.

Alternative causes of massive hemorrhage should be considered. such as bronchiectasis, TP or other infectious processes, and aortic dissection with erosion into vascular structures. CT can be obtained to rule out aortic pathology, but this patient is unstable and has a more likely diagnosis.

Minnesota tube is a device to control large-volume GI bleeding and acts to tamponade bleeding with balloons placed in the stomach and esophagus. Massive hemoptysis can be difficult to differentiate from massive GI bleeding. Usually hemoptysis appears frothy and bright red, whereas GI bleeding is more typically dark and may contain food particles.

Test-taking tip: When a patient is unstable or in critical condition, don't be afraid to choose an intervention first when indicated before obtaining diagnostic studies.

34. ANSWER: B

This patient has clinical and radiographic signs of CHF, which should give him a transudative pleural effusion as opposed to an exudative pleural effusion. Light's criteria are widely accepted as an instrument to differentiate exudate and transudate pleural effusions. The pleural fluid (PF) is exudative if any of the following is present:

PF/serum protein ratio >0.5
PF/serum LDH ratio >0.6

Pleural fluid LDH more than two-thirds the normal serum value for your specific lab assay

Although not specifically parts of Light's criteria, other markers of exudative fluid are:

PF cholesterol >45 mg/dL
PF protein >2.9 g/dL
Glucose <50 mg/dL
WBC >1,000/mm^3

Test-taking tip: Light's criteria are a formula worth committing to memory immediately before standardized testing just in case. They are easy to look up in everyday practice but can be used for testing. Don't worry about other markers of exudate, they are included here for your education but are less likely to be tested.

35. ANSWER: B

This patient has a PE. PE has increased risk in pregnancy, and clinical signs of DVT make the diagnosis increasingly likely. PE causes a ventilation-perfusion mismatch because blood does not perfuse lung tissue that is well oxygenated because of the embolus obstructing pulmonary blood flow.

Diffusion impairment occurs in cases in which there is interstitial fluid, edema, or blood causing decreased diffusion of gases across alveolar membranes. This can occur in pulmonary edema, pneumonia, or a myriad of other inflammatory conditions that inhibit movement of gases in lung parenchyma. This does not classically occur in PE.

Right-left shunting is usually due to a cardiac lesion in which deoxygenated blood is allowed to flow directly from the right heart to the left heart and bypasses pulmonary circulation. This type of lesion will exhibit hypoxia that does not respond to supplemental oxygenation.

Hypoventilation can be due to altered mental status, medications, or illicit drugs that affect respiratory drive secondary to obesity or mechanical limitation of ventilation, among other causes. This patient is hyperventilating, and although she may have some limitation on her diaphragm movement because of pregnancy, she is experiencing an acute change, likely due to a PE.

Test-taking tip: Recognize classic signs of PE. In answering questions with basic science or physiologic answers, reason out what you know about the disease process and use logic to find your answer. If the correct answer isn't immediately apparent, this is a good question to star or mark and come back to at the end of the test if you have a little time to think it over.

36. ANSWER: C

There is a growing body of literature supporting use of NIPPV in a variety of conditions, including asthma, cardiogenic pulmonary edema, pneumonia, neuromuscular disease, trauma and burns, upper airway obstruction, postextubation respiratory distress, and obesity hypoventilation syndrome. Cardiogenic pulmonary edema in particular is a disease process that is particularly responsive to NIPPV, and it should be a mainstay in caring for patients with CHF exacerbations.

Although pneumonia and respiratory distress are an indication for NIPPV, studies have shown that the presence of pneumonia increases the risk for failure of NIPPV. Monitor these patients carefully.

Acute respiratory distress and failure to achieve Pao_2/Fio_2 ratio >150 after 1 hour of treatment are also both conditions that increase the failure rate of NIPPV. Consider serial blood gases to monitor your patient's progress.

Test-taking tip: NIPPV and BiPAP are great but be aware of their shortcomings.

37. ANSWER: D

This patient has a cavitary lesion seen on chest radiograph in the presence of TB risk factors including IV drug use and travel to an endemic area. The most important immediate step in caring for this patient is negative pressure respiratory isolation until pulmonary TB can be ruled out. Other diseases that can cause cavitary lesions include endemic disease such as coccidiomycosis or necrotizing pneumonia, which will usually present in a patient who is critically ill with sepsis: start empiric therapy for pneumonia while working to rule out TB.

ABG testing can provide helpful information, especially for a patient who is in respiratory distress. This patient appears very stable, however, and can be deferred at this time because it is uncomfortable for the patient and is unlikely to provide immediately helpful clinical data.

HIV should always be considered in cases of TB. Furthermore, patients with HIV can often present with an atypical or even negative chest radiograph when infected with active pulmonary TB without the classic finding of cavitary lesion. Always ask about HIV risk factors and have a low threshold to send for rapid testing. This should not delay moving a patient to respiratory isolation because failure to isolate HIV patients with unrecognized TB is a common cause of nosocomial TB outbreaks in hospitals.

Sputum induction for AFB staining should occur as soon as feasibly possible but is not a critical action that supersedes placing a patient in respiratory isolation. In fact, sputum induction should be conducted in an isolation room so that respiratory particles are not spread to other patients or care providers.

Test-taking tip: Often on a standardized test, you will be asked to pick between answers that you would usually perform concurrently in the real world. In these scenarios, try to think of the big picture while reading the question stem. This is a patient who is stable (you probably don't need the ABG) and has a highly contagious disease (isolation is important) and will get empiric testing while awaiting diagnostics that are necessary but not immediately important.

38. ANSWER: D

The case describes a BRUE (brief resolved unexplained event). The term BRUE is defined as an event occurring in an infant younger than 1 year in whom the observer reports a sudden, brief, and now resolved episode of one or more of the following events that cannot be attributed to another identifiable medical condition (e.g., fever, URI) on history or exam: (1) central cyanosis or pallor; (2) absent, decreased, or irregular breathing; (3) marked change in tone (hypertonia or hypotonia); and (4) altered level of responsiveness. After a BRUE is identified, patients may be classified as low risk or high risk.

A patient is considered low risk if the following criteria are met: (1) age >60 days; (2) prematurity: gestational age ≥32 weeks and postconceptional age ≥45 weeks; (3) first BRUE (no previous BRUE ever and not occurring in clusters); (4) duration of event <1 minute; (5) no cardiopulmonary resuscitation (CPR) required by trained medical provider; (6) no concerning historical features; (7) no concerning physical examination findings. Low-risk infants such as the one described in the vignette need no further invasive testing or monitoring in the hospital or at home.

The American Academy of Pediatrics (AAP) guidelines provide strong recommendations for education of the caregiver regarding BRUE, follow-up precautions, and resources for CPR training. The provider may also elect to test for pertussis or perform an EKG if clinically warranted, but other workup is not recommended. If the event violates any of the low-risk criteria, then the patient is considered high risk for a recurrent event or underlying undiagnosed serious condition. High-risk infants fall outside the guidelines of the AAP BRUE evaluation and should be managed according to specific concerns identified on evaluation in the ED.

In 2016, the AAP replaced the term ALTE (apparent life-threatening event) with the term BRUE. Color change under BRUE definitions involves cyanosis or pallor of the face or trunk and excludes acrocyanosis or perioral cyanosis. ALTE criteria included any color change, but this has been modified and removed from BRUE criteria because redness is common in healthy infants.

39. ANSWER: B

The event described by the patient's father is consistent with BRUE, but there are several other features of the patient's history that are concerning and disqualify him from the low-risk category, thus requiring further workup. First, the patient is an ex-preemie. Second, there is a family history of SIDS. Given the concerning history, the patient should be admitted for further workup as indicated by the inpatient pediatric team. Typical workup includes EKG, basic laboratory studies, and cardiorespiratory monitoring. Genetic testing for rare diseases may be indicated if there is a strong family history. Choice A is incorrect because there is no evidence of head trauma on history or exam and no focal neurologic deficits at the time of evaluation. The AAP no longer recommends home cardiorespiratory monitoring for any type of BRUE evaluation, making D incorrect.

Keep in mind the criteria for "ruling-in" a low-risk BRUE. If the patient violates any of these criteria, he may not be considered low risk, and further workup is indicated. A patient is considered low risk if the following criteria are met: (1) age >60 days; (2) prematurity: gestational age ≥32 weeks and postconceptional age ≥45 weeks; (3) first BRUE (no previous BRUE ever and not occurring in clusters); (4) duration of event <1 minute; (5) no CPR required by trained medical provider; (6) no concerning historical features; (7) no concerning physical examination findings.

Test-taking tip: Choice A is incorrect because there is no evidence of head trauma on history or exam and no focal neurologic deficits at the time of evaluation. The AAP no longer recommends home cardiorespiratory monitoring for any type of BRUE evaluation, making D incorrect.

40. ANSWER: B

Status asthmaticus is defined as progressively worsening bronchospasm, unresponsive to standard therapy. Serial ABG tests may be useful in determining the next appropriate intervention and level of care. Although initial $PaCO_2$ may be normal or slightly below normal, normalizing $PaCO_2$ in the context of worsening clinical status is a sign of impending respiratory failure. Note that most patients also are found to have a metabolic acidosis, likely due to buildup of lactic acid. IV hydration with fluids and electrolyte repletion are important components of management of asthma exacerbations.

All of the answer choices are signs of respiratory distress, but rising $PaCO_2$ is the most concerning for impending respiratory failure, necessitating quick and expedient action.

Test-taking tip: This is a "you know it or don't" kind of question. If you don't know it, choose an answer and move on. You can perhaps mark it for review when you are done at the end of the test. Don't, however, let these kinds of questions get you stuck and waste your time.

41. ANSWER: D

The patient presents with apparent asthma exacerbation in the context of URI. However, the patient does not improve as expected after adequate treatment and remains hypoxic. Chest radiograph is not routinely obtained in patients with apparent simple asthma exacerbations, but it may be useful in cases in which the cause of wheezing or hypoxia is unclear to evaluate for conditions such as CHF, foreign body aspiration and other causes of hypoxia such as pneumonia and fever not explained by viral URI symptoms, life-threatening asthma exacerbations, and other concerning signs or symptoms such as chest pain or absence of breath sounds.

Test-taking tip: Consider chest radiograph in asthmatic patients who do not improve as expected after treatment and who have persistent hypoxia or fever.

42. ANSWER: B

Spirometry is most likely to be abnormal in this patient with URI and wheezing. In a patient with reactive airway disease, spirometry will show FEV_1 (forced vital capacity in the first 1 second of expiration) to be below the predicted value for age- and gender-matched controls. A trial of bronchodilators should be given to this patient for symptomatic improvement.

Test-taking tip: Any of the answer choices may be abnormal in this patient, but spirometry is both most likely to be abnormal and most likely to elucidate the specific cause of the patient's symptoms.

43. ANSWER: A

The patient in the vignette has bacterial tracheitis, a rare cause of infectious upper airway obstruction in children. Most cases present in children younger than 8 years and are preceded by URI symptoms. URI is thought to predispose to the condition by breaking the mucosal barrier of the trachea, making hosts susceptible to bacterial infection. The most common pathogen implicated is *S. aureus*. However, *S. pneumoniae*, group A β-hemolytic *Streptococcus, H. influenzae, M. catarrhalis,* anaerobic bacteria, and viruses have been documented as well. Treatment is with early broad-spectrum antibiotics directed against gram-positive cocci, gram-negative cocci, and anaerobes. Up to 75% of patients will require intubation for airway protection. Diagnosis is confirmed by purulent secretions, inflammation of the trachea, and subglottic narrowing with normal appearance of the epiglottis on direct laryngoscopy or bronchoscopy.

The differential diagnosis for stridor includes croup, peritonsillar abscess, retropharyngeal abscess, bacterial tracheitis, external/internal compression of the upper airway by a mass or vascular rings and slings, foreign body aspiration, angioedema, and anaphylaxis.

Test-taking tip: This is a "you know it or don't" kind of question. If you don't know it, choose an answer and move on. You can perhaps mark it for review when you are done at the end of the test. Don't, however, let these kinds of questions get you stuck and waste your time.

44. ANSWER: C

Respiratory syncytial virus (RSV) is the most common pathogen causing bronchiolitis. RSV can manifest with a variety of symptoms in any age group, but it primarily causes lower respiratory tract infection when it infects children aged 6 weeks to 2 years. There are no proven directed therapies or preventive therapies for the virus. Supportive care, including supplemental oxygen, IV hydration, and suctioning of secretions, is the mainstay of treatment. RSV infections peak in the winter months and usually peak on day 3 of illness.

Test-taking tip: You can eliminate B because there is no mention of croup with a barking cough.

45. ANSWER: B

Laryngotracheobronchitis, or croup, is most commonly caused by parainfluenza virus and is characterized by subglottic narrowing and dynamic upper airway obstruction causing a pathognomonic "barking cough" and inspiratory stridor. Croup is most often seen in children aged 6 months to 4 years, with incidence peaking in 1- to 2-year-olds. Treatment is with systemic steroids. Racemic epinephrine may be used in severe cases to rapidly improve symptoms, but it has not been shown to reduce the need for ETT or tracheotomy. Its effect is transient, lasting 2 to 3 hours, and children should be observed up until 6 hours after administration to monitor for rebound worsening of airway obstruction. Humidified oxygen may also be used to improve symptoms.

Expand your differential diagnosis for stridor in the following cases: infants younger than 4 months, patients with inspiratory and expiratory stridor, and patients with long-standing stridor.

Test-taking tip: You can eliminate C and D because these are not usual treatments for croup.

46. ANSWER: C

According to Centers for Disease Control and Prevention (CDC) guidelines, postexposure antimicrobial prophylaxis (PEP) should be administered to persons at high risk for developing severe pertussis disease and those in close contact with exposures. Specifically, the CDC recommends (1) administration of PEP to all household contacts of a pertussis case within 21 days of onset of cough in the index patient and (2) administration of PEP to persons at high risk for developing severe illness or those with close contact to persons who may develop severe illness. Persons at high risk include infants, women in their third trimester of pregnancy, and persons with preexisting health conditions that may be worsened by pertussis infection such as immunocompromised individuals or those with baseline compromised respiratory status. Some examples of persons in close contact to individuals at high risk include health care workers in child care settings, neonatal ICUs, and maternity wards. Macrolide antibiotics are the treatment for the disease and PEP. Azithromycin is preferred in infants younger than 1 month because of decreased risk for causing infantile hypertrophic pyloric stenosis (IHPS) compared with other macrolides.

Pertussis can lead to severe disease in infants younger than 1 year. About half of infants younger than 1 year will require hospitalization for treatment, and up to 23% will develop pneumonia. Infants often present with apnea instead of cough

Test-taking tip: This is a "you know it or don't" kind of question. If you don't know it, choose an answer and move on. You can perhaps mark it for review when you are done at the end of the test. Don't, however, let these kinds of questions get you stuck and waste your time.

47. ANSWER: D

The antibiotic of choice in infants younger than 1 month for both treatment and postexposure prophylaxis of *B. pertussis* infection is azithromycin. Erythromycin has been associated with IHPS. TMP-SMX is contraindicated in infants younger than 2 months because of the risk for kernicterus, but it may be used as alternative therapy to macrolide antibiotics in all persons older than 2 months. Of note, the US Food and Drug Administration (FDA) issued a warning after azithromycin had been associated with fatal arrhythmias. Thus, azithromycin should be avoided in all patients who have known cardiovascular disease, including prolongation of the QT interval, a history of torsades de pointes, congenital long QT syndrome, bradyarrhythmias, or uncompensated heart failure; patients on drugs known to prolong the QT interval; patients with ongoing proarrhythmic conditions, such as uncorrected hypokalemia or hypomagnesemia or clinically significant bradycardia; and patients receiving class IA (quinidine, procainamide) or class III (dofetilide, amiodarone, sotalol) antiarrhythmic agents. If azithromycin is contraindicated, infants should be treated with another macrolide and monitored closely for signs of IHPS. The risks of not treating pertussis outweigh the risks for developing IHPS.

Infants with a diagnosis of pertussis should be hospitalized given the high risk for mortality and complications associated with the disease in this age group.

Test-taking tip: This is a "you know it or don't" kind of question. If you don't know it, choose an answer and move on. You can perhaps mark it for review when you are done at the end of the test. Don't, however, let these kinds of questions get you stuck and waste your time.

with a careful history and physical exam, chest radiograph, and analysis of pleural fluid in appropriate circumstances. Consider pleural fluid aspiration for unilateral effusions without clear transudative etiology, bilateral pleural effusions that do not resolve with directed therapy, or symptom relief. Based on this patient's presentation, underlying malignancy is the most likely cause given unilateral effusion, weight loss, hemoptysis, and significant smoking history. Septated pleural effusions are most commonly seen in malignant pleural infections. Given that this patient is afebrile, parapneumonic effusion is less likely. PE is less likely but should also be considered. Heart failure is the most common cause of pleural effusion but typically causes symmetric, bilateral effusions. Pleural aspiration is the next appropriate step in the workup. When aspiration is performed, the sample should be sent for analysis of the following: protein, lactate dehydrogenase, Gram stain, cytology, and microbiologic culture. Additionally, it is important to note that chest CT with contrast should be performed before complete drainage of the effusion because this produces better images.

Test-taking tip: Septated effusions are most often caused by effusions associated with malignancy, and you can eliminate A and D because PE and pneumonia rarely cause pulmonary effusions.

48. ANSWER: D

Antibiotics are the mainstay of treatment in an acute pulmonary exacerbation in a patient with CF. Antibiotics are directed against the most common pathogens, typically *Pseudomonas* and *Staphylococcus*. Usually the patient is treated with two antipseudomonal antimicrobials, but this may vary depending on previous culture data, severity of symptoms, and specialist preference. Nonsteroidal antiinflammatory drugs, systemic or inhaled steroids, and inhaled ß$_2$-agonists have not been shown to improve outcomes. Given the complex multisystem involvement of CF as well as the complex medical therapies and psychosocial stressors, patients do best when managed at specialty centers with experts in pediatric CF. Specific treatment should be discussed with the patient's specialist if at all possible. Typical findings on chest radiograph for CF are bronchiectasis, hyperinflation, bullae, and pulmonary arterial enlargement.

Test-taking tip: You can eliminate A and B because the patient has no wheezing and ibuprofen will not help the patient's shortness of breath.

49. ANSWER: B

The chest radiograph in Figure 16.13 shows a right-sided pleural effusion. The causes of pulmonary effusions are diverse, and the differential diagnosis is broad. Diagnosis begins

50. ANSWER: D

The chest radiograph shows bilateral pulmonary edema, bilateral pleural effusions, and cardiomegaly.

The most common cause of bilateral pleural effusions is CHF. Based on the patient's history and exam, she appears to be having an acute heart failure exacerbation, and most likely her pleural effusions are caused by this. In cases of symmetric, bilateral pleural effusions when the clinical picture indicates cardiac, liver, or renal failure, the patient may be treated presumptively without diagnostic thoracentesis. If symptoms fail to improve as expected after several days of appropriate therapy, then guidelines recommend pleural aspiration for further workup and diagnosis. CHF causes transudative pleural effusions.

Fluid is an exudate if one or more of the following criteria are met:

1. Ratio of pleural fluid level of lactate LDH to serum level of LDH is greater than 0.6
2. Pleural fluid level of LDH is more than two-thirds the upper limit of the reference range for the serum level of LDH
3. Ratio of pleural fluid level of protein to serum level of protein is greater than 0.5

Transudative effusions are caused by imbalance in the hydrostatic and oncotic pressures, forcing protein-poor fluids into the pleural space. In contrast, exudates are typically caused by inflammatory process that allow protein-rich fluids to seep through leaky capillaries into the pleural space. Increased concentrations of LDH, protein, and lipids are seen in patients who have been treated with diuretics and may result in misclassification of many transudative effusions as exudative effusions. The most common causes of pleural effusions are CHF, parapneumonic, and malignancy.

Test-taking tip: This is a "you know it or don't" kind of question. If you don't know it, choose an answer and move on. You can perhaps mark it for review when you are done at the end of the test. Don't, however, let these kinds of questions get you stuck and waste your time.

51. ANSWER: C

The patient in the vignette has a PE. Up to 48% of patients presenting with PE will have a pleural effusion, though 90% are small. They are most often unilateral but may also be bilateral or occur on the contralateral side. Effusions associated with PE are always exudates. This is likely because the ischemia to the lung parenchyma results in release of cytokines, which cause inflammation and lead to capillary leakage.

Fluid is an exudate if one or more of the following criteria are met:

1. Ratio of pleural fluid level of LDH to serum level of LDH is greater than 0.6
2. Pleural fluid level of LDH is more than two-thirds the upper limit of the reference range for the serum level of LDH
3. Ratio of pleural fluid level of protein to serum level of protein is greater than 0.5

Test-taking tip: The question stem describes a person with a PE. It's important to know that pleural effusions associated with PE are always exudates, and it's important to know the criteria that distinguish exudative effusions from transudative effusions.

52. ANSWER: B

The main differential diagnosis for milky-white or yellow pleural fluid includes chylothorax, pseudochylothorax, and empyema. Chylothorax most often occurs when the thoracic duct is damaged, either by direct violation or compression. Thoracic trauma is the leading cause of chylothorax. Iatrogenic damage during surgery is another leading cause. Other causes include cancer, childbirth,

dislocation of the spine, sarcoidosis, amyloidosis, TP, and primary diseases of the lymph vessels. Chylothorax may also be caused by transdiaphragmatic movement of chylous ascites. Pseudochylothorax is caused by accumulation of cholesterol crystals in the pleural fluid, typically by conditions causing chronic inflammation of the pleura, and is characterized by markedly thickened pleura. Chylothorax and pseudochylothorax will appear the same after centrifugation; thus, the fluid should be sent for lipid analysis, including cholesterol crystals, chylomicrons, and triglycerides. High triglycerides, low cholesterol, and presence of chylomicrons are characteristic of chylothorax, whereas high cholesterol, presence of cholesterol crystals, and absence of chylomicrons are typical of pseudochylothorax. Finally, empyema may occasionally mimic the findings of chylothorax. In the case of empyema, the patient would also likely have infectious symptoms. Centrifugation of the empyema fluid would yield a clear supernatant layer above the layer of cellular matter causing the opacity.

Test-taking tip: The leading cause of chylothorax is trauma, either natural or iatrogenic.

53. ANSWER: C

The patient in the vignette has a PSP. Risk factors for the development of PSP include smoking and tall height. There is no relationship between activity and development of PSP, and they are just as likely to occur at rest as they are with activity. Risk for recurrence of PSP after a first episode exceeds 50% in some studies, with risk factors identified as age >60 years, tall height, and smoking. Patients should be counseled regarding smoking cessation.

Smoking tobacco is an important modifiable risk factor in the development and progression of many health conditions.

Test-taking tip: You can eliminate D because active lifestyle is never a bad thing.

54. ANSWER: D

Bilateral PSPs are a rare occurrence. The management of pneumothoraces is determined by both the radiographic size and patient's clinical status. In unilateral spontaneous pneumothorax, invasive intervention may be deferred if the pneumothorax is small and the patient is asymptomatic. Active intervention (e.g., with chest tube, Heimlich valve, needle aspiration) is recommended in large pneumothoraces and those of any size causing breathlessness. Bilateral PSPs, however, always require active intervention because they have the potential to deteriorate rapidly and cause life-threatening events such as tension-type physiology. Thus, chest tube insertion should not be delayed for further workup.

According to the American College of Chest Physicians, the size of a pneumothorax is determined by the distance from the lung apex to the ipsilateral thoracic cupola at the parietal surface as determined by an upright standard radiograph. A small pneumothorax measures <3 cm from apex to cupola, and a large pneumothorax measures ≥3 cm from apex to cupola.

Test-taking tip: This is an action patient, so any answer that is not an acute intervention can be excluded. Therefore, you can eliminate A and B easily.

55. ANSWER: B

This case describes re-expansion pulmonary edema, a rare complication of chest drainage for pneumothorax. Symptoms typically present within hours of lung re-expansion and are characterized by dyspnea, tachypnea, and hypoxia. Rapid clinical and radiologic assessment of patients is necessary. In this case, unilateral opacification of the left lung is suggestive of alveolar edema. Treatment is primarily supportive with oxygen and positive pressure ventilation (noninvasive measures may be tried first). Physiologic shunting may be reduced by positioning patient in the lateral decubitus position on the affected side. Intrapulmonary shunting is the primary cause of the patient's hypoxia, and care must be taken to ensure adequate intravascular volume. Thus, diuresis is contraindicated in these situations.

Risk factors for re-expansion pulmonary edema include younger age, longer existing pneumothorax, and swift drainage of large amounts of fluids or air.

Test-taking tip: When thinking about "next best steps" in management of patients, it is often about treating the suspected underlying cause of their disease with an agent or action that works quickly.

56. ANSWER: A

Broad-spectrum antibiotics are the initial step in management of mediastinitis. Mediastinitis is a rare complication of esophageal perforation and is most commonly seen in alcoholics and men. Perforation of the esophagus allows gastric contents and normal flora of the esophagus to spread into the surrounding tissue, resulting in inflammation and infection. If untreated, mortality approaches 100%. High index of suspicion is required in a septic-appearing patient with chest pain. Blood cultures, fluid resuscitation, IV PPI, and NPO are all important parts of management. CT surgery should be consulted for possible surgical intervention.

Test-taking tip: This is an ill, septic patient. Only choice A addresses the underlying infection.

57. ANSWER: D

CT scan is the best test in diagnosing acute mediastinitis. CT findings include extraluminal air, extravasation of ingested contrast into the extraluminal space, widening of the mediastinum, and mediastinal air-fluid levels. Chest radiograph may show widened mediastinum or air-fluid levels, but it is not possible on the basis of chest radiography alone to precisely characterize mediastinal infection and mediastinal abscess. CT is useful for assessing the extent of mediastinal infection.

Have a high index of suspicion for esophageal perforation and acute mediastinitis in a patient who has recently undergone upper endoscopy, intubation, or open cardiac surgery.

Test-taking tip: You can eliminate choices A and B because this patient is presenting septic after a recent esophagogastroduodenoscopy, and troponin and EKG do not help identify the source of infections.

58. ANSWER: D

Fleischner Society guidelines have been updated in 2017 to reflect the accumulating data on the malignancy risk of incidental pulmonary nodules and growth rates of lung cancer. Important changes include guidance on identifying benign nodules with minimal follow-up imaging. For patients with a solid or subsolid (ground-glass or part-solid) SPN measuring <6 mm, follow-up CT is optional but no longer required. An SPN that is solid and unchanged on serial CT over a 2-year period, or subsolid and unchanged over a 5-year period, is likely benign and does not need further diagnostic evaluation.

Test-taking tip: Know the latest guidelines for imaging and management of an SPN, as well as the patient risk factors and size of the lesion.

59. ANSWER: A

SPNs need to be assessed for their risk for malignancy by patient characteristics, symptoms, or features of the nodule. Both the size of the nodule and its appearance would be concerning for malignancy, and thus biopsy should be the next plan and best management option for this patient.

Test-taking tip: In answer choices there are three imaging modalities and one surgical. Thus, the answer is likely to be the one that is different from the others. Also, be sure to read the stem, which says, "management option," not necessarily the next step in the workup.

60. ANSWER: D

Dirofilaria, the dog heartworm, may present as a solitary nodule in humans. The larval forms of the worm that are transmitted to humans from dogs by mosquito bites wind up in the right heart. In humans, however, they cannot develop into mature worms; the larvae die and are embolized to the lung, inducing a granulomatous reaction. Typically the diagnosis is made when a nodule is resected and the worm is seen.

Echinococcus may cause asymptomatic lung infection but typically produces cystic disease.

Anisakis is a roundworm that can cause human GI illness after ingestion of raw fish such as sushi, but would not cause a pulmonary nodule.

Cysts and tachyzoites of *Toxoplasma* do not resemble worms and have no muscularis structures.

Strongyloides larvae migrate through the lung and may cause a diffuse infiltrate in the hyperinfection syndrome but do not form solitary nodules in the lung.

Test-taking tip: Know uncommon causes of SPNs, especially infectious causes because they are a test writer's favorite.

61. ANSWER: A

Screening studies of smokers who are at high risk for malignancy suggest that the vast majority of nodules identified on CT are benign. As an example, in the Pan-Canadian Early Detection of Lung Cancer and the British Columbia Cancer Agency studies, among the 12,029 nodules found, only 144 (1%) were malignant.

Test-taking tip: The key word in this question stem is "general population." In this case, the prevalence in the general population is low, and thus it would be inappropriate to invoke such a high-cost screening test in an overall low-prevalence disease (malignant SPNs).

62. ANSWER: A

The patient likely had a transthoracic needle biopsy (TTNB) as part of the workup for the concerning SPN and now has a tension pneumothorax with hemodynamic compromise. TTNB is performed by passing a needle through the chest wall into the target nodule, usually under CT guidance. The

needle frequently traverses pleura and lung to either aspirate or excise tissue for biopsy, and pneumothorax rates range from 10% to 60% depending on the location of the nodule being sampled. Typically, the diagnostic yield of TTNB is >88% for benign and malignant nodules, but this is dependent on the location and characteristics of the nodule.

Test-taking tip: This is an action patient, so any answer that is not an acute intervention can be excluded.

63. ANSWER: D

Sarcoidosis is a systemic granulomatous disease that is characterized by noncaseating granulomas that may affect multiple organ systems. The condition occurs mainly in people ages 20 to 40 years and is most common in Northern Europeans and African Americans. Symptoms are variable, and the etiology is unknown. Fever, weight loss, arthralgias, and erythema nodosum (more commonly seen in Europeans) are the usual initial presenting symptoms. Cough and dyspnea may be minimal or absent. Other manifestations include mediastinal lymphadenopathy seen on chest radiograph (hallmark finding in 90% of cases), hepatic granulomas, granulomatous uveitis, polyarthritis, cardiac symptoms (including angina, CHF, and conduction abnormalities), cranial nerve palsies, and diabetes insipidus. Laboratory findings include leukopenia, hypercalcemia, hypercalciuria, and hypergammaglobulinemia (particularly in African American patients). Other abnormalities include elevated uric acid (not usually associated with gout), elevated alkaline phosphatase, elevated γ-glutamyl transpeptidase, elevated levels of ACE, and PFTs showing restriction and impaired diffusing capacity. Diagnosis can be made with biopsy of peripheral lesions or fiberoptic bronchoscopy for central pulmonary lesions. Whole-body gallium scans can be used to show useful sites for biopsy and, in some cases, to follow disease progression. Serial PFTs are important for assessing disease progression and guiding treatment. The prognosis depends on the severity of the disease. Spontaneous improvement is common; however, significant disability can occur with multiorgan involvement. Pulmonary fibrosis is the leading cause of death. Treatment for symptomatic patients consists of corticosteroids, methotrexate, and other immunosuppressive medications if steroid therapy is not helpful.

Test-taking tip: Caucasians of Northern European descent are also at risk for sarcoidosis, not just African Americans.

64. ANSWER: C

Complications of sarcoidosis involve a multitude of cardiac abnormalities, including aneurysms, pulmonary hypertension leading to CHF, pericardial effusion, and acute valvular regurgitation from papillary muscle rupture due to granulomatous infiltration. A bedside echocardiogram (after an EKG) should be the next step in the evaluation of this patient because many of the life-threatening etiologies related to sarcoidosis can be identified.

Test-taking tip: Always prioritize the life-threatening conditions. Echocardiogram is the safest, cheapest, fastest, and most useful next step.

65. ANSWER: A

This patient has had a number of flares of sarcoidosis and disease progression as noted by her multiple and recent admissions for the same over the past year. She is undoubtedly on steroids and likely long-term steroids. Because of this, because she presents with severe sepsis from likely pyelonephritis, the next step in her management should be empiric stress dose steroids, which are often forgotten in patients who receive long-term steroids. For sarcoidosis, initial therapy with steroids can last 4 to 6 weeks, and patients who have multiple flares and/or progression of disease can be on steroids for much longer, as in the case of this patient. Many patients end up on steroids for more than 1 year.

Test-taking tip: Know the treatment of sarcoidosis with steroids and the risk for adrenal suppression.

66. ANSWER: D

While an isolated elevation in alkaline phosphatase can be seen with malignancy, infection, granulomatous inflammation, or drug toxicity, the presence of bilateral hilar lymphadenopathy makes sarcoidosis the most likely diagnosis. The patient has a form of acute sarcoidosis called Lofgren's syndrome, and the rash likely represents erythema nodosum. In this clinical context, none of the other conditions is likely, particularly with the associated isolated alkaline phosphatase elevation.

Test-taking tip: Put all the findings together and know the pathognomonic chest radiograph for sarcoidosis.

67. ANSWER: B

Steroids are the mainstay of treatment for sarcoidosis. The prognosis is difficult to determine, but patients who are deteriorating from baseline, such as having a decrease in PFTs, should be initiated on steroids. This patient has underlying, poorly controlled diabetes as indicated by the A1C. He is at risk for complications from hyperglycemia,

and there is a risk he is currently presenting with diabetic ketoacidosis (DKA). Thus, the next best step would be to find out what the glucose is and likely then start IV fluids if there is no contraindication. Steroids would be the wrong choice because there is no evidence of an acute sarcoidosis complication at present. The other choices would be appropriate after the glucose is known and therapy can be initiated.

Test-taking tip: In someone with diabetes and systemic illness, it is rare that any other test before a point-of-care blood glucose is the right answer.

68. ANSWER: C

This patient's clinical presentation and biopsy showing spherules containing endospores is consistent with *Coccidioides immitis* infection, which is endemic in the southwestern United States.

C. immitis is one of the four "systemic" mycoses along with *Histoplasma capsulatum*, *Blastomyces dermatitidis*, and *Paracoccidioides brasiliensis*. All four cause a mild pneumonia in immunocompetent patients and can cause disseminated disease in the immunocompromised. As seen on biopsy, *Coccidioides* is a spherule in tissue, differentiating it from the other systemic mycoses, which assume a yeast form in tissue.

Coccidioides is most commonly found in the southwestern United States, including Arizona.

Lyme disease, a tick-borne illness that presents with the classic target-shaped erythema migrans rash as well as fever and arthritis, is endemic to the northeastern United States.

H. capsulatum is a systemic mycosis endemic to Ohio and the Mississippi River Valley. It is commonly found in bird and bat droppings.

Cryptococcus is another systemic mycosis that can cause pneumonia and is commonly found in soil contaminated with pigeon droppings.

Test-taking tip: Though we often don't need to know the microscopic appearance of organisms, *cocci* have a distinct appearance that differentiates them among other endemic pathogens.

69. ANSWER: D

Based on the available information and the fact that this individual recently moved to an area endemic for coccidioidomycosis, it is reasonable to consider the infiltrates and his presentation to be related to severe coccidioidomycosis infection with possible fungemia. This is especially concerning given the lack of response to an antimicrobial agent that would have treated a typical community-acquired pneumonia. Mild disease with suspected or proven cocci infection in the immunocompetent host rarely requires treatment with an azole antifungal. Patients with severe disease or those who are immunocompromised can be treated with amphotericin B initially and then switched to oral azole therapy. There is no indication for steroids, antivirals, or other antibiotics in this case.

Test-taking tip: More antibiotics are rarely the correct answer, and two of the choices are antivirals. The stem of the question mentions geographic region, which is almost always a key in the answer to a board question.

70. ANSWER: B

This patient has cocci meningitis at risk for disease progression and will need lifelong antifungal therapy. He also needs admission for serial lumbar punctures to decrease intracranial pressure. The medication that should be used for this is fluconazole. The patient is not displaying signs of serious infection, and thus you would hold off at present on using amphotericin B given its poor side-effect profile. There is no indication for steroids or antibiotics at present.

Test-taking tip: Know standard therapies for treatment of coccidioidomycosis. Severe disease is treated with amphotericin B from the start.

71. ANSWER: A

Antifungal therapy is not needed for healthy patients without evidence of extensive coccidioidal infection or risk factors for more serious infection such as an immunocompromised state because most patients resolve their infection without treatment. This patient does not have prolonged fatigue or night sweats and does not appear sick based on vital signs and exam. Because he is immunocompetent with mild symptoms, supportive care is all that is required. There is no role for antifungals or antibiotics to treat mild pulmonary cocci infections.

Test-taking tip: In a relatively healthy person with mild disease and no risk factors, cocci are usually self-limited and do not require antifungal therapy.

72. ANSWER: B

This AIDS patient has a complication of long-standing pulmonary cocci infection (not appropriately treated) known as fibrocavitary pneumonia. To complicate matters, she is also pregnant. Thus, for at least the first trimester, she will need to be treated with amphotericin B because of the teratogenicity of azoles. Patients on ampho B, even the liposomal formulation, are at risk for acute kidney injury along with hypokalemia. It is important for the ED team to get a baseline creatinine before initiating therapy and to continue monitoring kidney function for the duration that the patient is on amphotericin B. Once she is out of the first trimester, she can be switched to azoles. The other complications are not common adverse drug reactions to amphotericin B. This is why it is often referred to in the colloquial sense as "ampho-terrible"!

Test-taking tip: Know common side effects of the antifungal drug class. They are not used often in the ED but have a role in therapy, and we need to know the reasons for dosing adjustments, the drug-drug interactions, and common adverse effects.

73. ANSWER: A

Patients with mild to moderate disease without central nervous system involvement should initially be started on itraconazole because of its better absorption and antifungal activity and fewer side effects when used for non–life-threatening blastomycosis. This patient, who is chronically ill from newly diagnosed AIDS and has calcifications on chest radiograph from prior blastomycosis exposure, is presenting with more significant disease in the setting of immunosuppression from AIDS. It is rare in the ED to have a CD4 count result available, but the absolute lymphocyte count (ALC) can be a good surrogate for the CD4 count. At the current ALC, the patient is definitely in the <200 category. Fluconazole is a mainstay in many other pulmonary fungal infections but is not as effective in pulmonary blastomycosis.

Test-taking tip: Knowing the morphologic appearance of blastomycosis is the key to this question.

74. ANSWER: D

The patient has disseminated histoplasmosis in the setting of tumor necrosis factor (TNF) inhibitor (infliximab) use. Her blood cultures and BAL cultures grew *H. capsulatum*. She was treated with amphotericin B and gradually improved. She was discharged on a prolonged course of oral itraconazole. Histoplasmosis, the most prevalent endemic mycosis in the United States, has been reported in patients treated with TNF blockers. The morphology of the organism in the pathologic specimen is one of the keys to distinguishing between the potential diagnoses. The aspirate shows the typical narrow-based budding morphology of *Histoplasma*. By contrast, *Blastomyces* typically has broad-based budding and is larger than *Histoplasma*. *Coccidioides* usually appears as a large spherule. *Cryptococcus* has a surrounding capsule. Although PJP has been reported in the setting of TNF antagonist use, the histologic appearance of the organism's trophozoites and cysts is distinct from that of the morphology of *Histoplasma*. An increased risk for serious infection has been observed among patients treated with TNF inhibitors. These infections include: mycobacterial—TB, nontuberculous *Mycobacteria*; bacterial—listeriosis, nocardiosis; viral—hepatitis B vaccine reactivation, possibly zoster (with TNF monoclonal antibody); fungal—PJP, *Histoplasma*, *Coccidioides*, *Cryptococcus*, *Aspergillus*, and *Candida*.

75. ANSWER: D

This patient is immunocompromised because of his kidney transplantation and is taking immunosuppression drugs; he presents after receiving a wound in the garden and developing pulmonary symptoms. Though this could be bacterial pneumonia or TB, the exposure and nodules near the site of injury make sporotrichosis the most likely cause of his symptoms. Influenza and CMV rarely would have a cavitary lesion.

Test-taking tip: Think about what is going on in that garden. Sporothrix is a soil organism, typically associated with rose bush thorns, but it can occur in any activity that involves soil through the skin. Pulmonary sporotrichosis occurs primarily in the immunocompromised host.

76. ANSWER: D

Disseminated *Fusarium* infection is a rare but serious infection in neutropenic fever patients. In the ED, we need to be aware of the complications of neutropenia as well as stem cell transplantation. The *Fusarium* fungus is known to cause skin lesions but more extensive in the immunocompromised host with the possibility of becoming disseminated. *Fusarium* is often resistant to antifungal therapy. The pathologic appearance of the other organisms is very different.

Test-taking tip: For fungal infection, knowing the morphology can be very helpful in distinguishing the infection. Also, know the situations in which patients can get invasive fungal infections.

77. ANSWER: D

Common causes of acquired methemoglobinemia include a whole host of drugs in the hospital setting. The patient was at risk from her dapsone prophylaxis as well as now being initiated on primaquine. This is important in the ICU setting because this patient is already quite ill and the methemoglobinemia is causing multiorgan failure. Methylene blue is the treatment modality of choice based on methemoglobin levels but would likely be used in this case because this patient is critically ill. Mild cyanosis is characteristic, and the decreasing oxygen delivery to tissues is due to increased oxygen and hemoglobin affinity and shifting of the dissociation curve to the left.

Test-taking tip: Remember the common causes of acquired methemoglobinemia and the way it typically presents in the hospital setting.

17.

TOXICOLOGIC EMERGENCIES

Michael A. Darracq and Danielle Holtz

1. A group of teenagers are at a party. In addition to drinking alcohol, they consume a tea brewed from a plant that they were told would cause hallucinations. Several of the teens present to the emergency department (ED), confused but not violent, tachycardic, with dry flushed skin and dilated pupils. Which of the following plants is the most likely culprit?

A. Jimson weed
B. Death cap mushroom
C. Water hemlock
D. Dumb cane

2. A 17-year-old male is started on phenytoin for seizures. Two weeks later, he develops rash, malaise, sore throat, and right upper quadrant abdominal pain. On exam, he has a diffuse maculopapular rash, facial swelling, pharyngitis, and tender cervical lymphadenopathy. Laboratory evaluation reveals elevation in aspartate aminotransferase (AST), alanine aminotransferase (ALT), total bilirubin, and creatinine, as well as hematuria. Eosinophils are noted on peripheral smear. What is the most likely etiology of this presentation?

A. Streptococcal pharyngitis
B. Drug rash with eosinophilia and systemic symptoms (DRESS)
C. Viral syndrome
D. Anaphylaxis

3. An ambulance crew is en route to your facility following an explosion at a local water treatment plant. There are several victims who have been exposed to chlorine gas. Which of the following is the most appropriate method of decontamination for the victims?

A. No decontamination is necessary, removal from the area of exposure is sufficient
B. Copious soap and water
C. Copious water alone

D. A shower of diluted household bleach in water (1:10 dilution)

4. A 17-year-old girl is brought to the ED by ambulance after being found unresponsive in her bedroom. An empty bottle of her grandmother's amitriptyline was next to her on the floor when emergency medical services (EMS) arrived. Enroute to the hospital, she had a tonic-clonic seizure. Which pharmacologic effect of this medication is most responsible for the electrocardiogram (EKG) changes seen in Figure 17.1, as well as the seizure?

A. α-Adrenergic receptor antagonism
B. Antihistamine effects
C. GABA-A receptor antagonism
D. Sodium channel blockade

5. A 16-year-old Boy Scout is hiking with his troop near a stream. He attended a wilderness survival course and feels fairly confident about his ability to identify edible wild plants. He eats the root of a plant that he believes to be a wild carrot. Shortly thereafter, he develops nausea, vomiting, and abdominal pain, followed by seizures. Which of the following plants did he most likely consume?

A. Peyote
B. Pokeweed
C. Water hemlock
D. Dumb cane

6. A 26-year-old female presents following a suicide attempt by medication ingestion. She is not forthcoming with what she took or the exact time of the ingestion. She has bipolar disorder, and her medication list includes valproic acid. She gets progressively more somnolent and minimally responsive to stimuli during the history and physical exam. Serum acetaminophen and salicylate levels are undetectable. A serum valproic acid

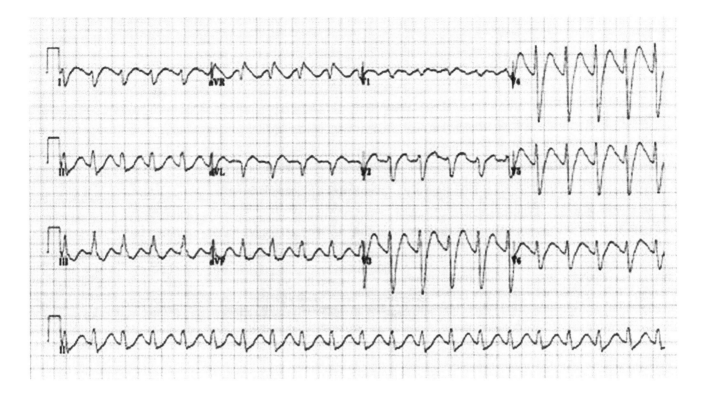

Figure 17.1 Electrocardiogram.

level is 700 mg/L (therapeutic: 50–120 mg/L). Which of the following is most appropriate next step in management of this patient?

A. Admission for valproic acid toxicity without further valproic acid levels because she is already manifesting signs of toxicity
B. Placement of vascular hemodialysis catheter and consultation with nephrology
C. Administration of activated charcoal and whole bowel irrigation
D. Medical clearance for psychiatric evaluation

7. A 19-year-old female presents to the ED with a depressed level of consciousness. She has a history of IV heroin abuse. On presentation, she has pinpoint pupils, a respiratory rate (RR) of 10 breaths/min, heart rate (HR) of 55 bpm, blood pressure (BP) of 100/60 mm Hg, and pulse oximetry of 92%. If a blood gas were obtained, which of the following would be most consistent with this presentation?

A. pH 7.20, P_{CO_2} 60, HCO_3 24
B. pH 7.20, P_{CO_2} 35, HCO_3 18
C. pH 7.50, P_{CO_2} 30, HCO_3 24
D. pH 7.50, P_{CO_2} 40, HCO_3 30

8. A 74-year-old woman presents to the ED with complaint of generalized weakness. Labs reveal sodium 137, potassium 2.7, chloride 107, bicarbonate 20, blood urea nitrogen (BUN) 22, creatinine 1.1, and glucose 124. Arterial pH is 7.30, and urine pH is 7.50. Which of the following is the most likely cause of the patient's presentation?

A. Salicylate toxicity
B. Renal tubular acidosis
C. Loop diuretics
D. Methanol toxicity

9. A 17-year-old male presents from home with ataxia, dysarthria, and nystagmus. He became despondent and took several handfuls of his anticonvulsant in an apparent suicide attempt. His EKG is shown in Figure 17.2. What is the next step in management?

A. Overdrive pacing
B. Multiple-dose activated charcoal (MDAC)
C. Sodium bicarbonate
D. Magnesium

10. A 36-year-old female presents after a terrorist attack with a chemical weapon in a nearby subway station. She presents with diaphoresis, pinpoint pupils, diarrhea, and vomiting. Her HR is 45 bpm and RR is 27 breaths/min. On physical examination, rales and rhonchi are heard in all lung fields. Which of the following agents was most likely used in the attack?

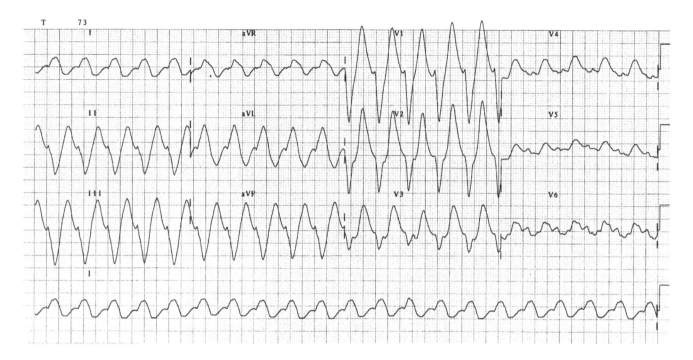

Figure 17.2 Electrocardiogram.

A. Organophosphate nerve agent
B. Hydrogen cyanide
C. Chlorine gas
D. Sulfur mustard

11. A 32-year-old male is hiking through thick brush along a lakeshore in Florida when he steps on the snake that has red bands touching smaller bands of yellow (Figure 17.3). The snake bites him in the lower leg. What symptoms may this patient experience as a result of this bite?

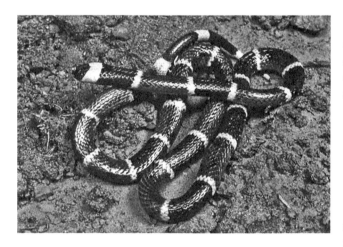

Figure 17.3 Snake.

A. None given that this a nonvenomous kingsnake
B. Marked local swelling and ecchymosis at the bite site without systemic effects

C. Dyspnea, diplopia, muscle weakness, and seizures
D. Severe pain

12. A 43-year-old male with a history of alcohol abuse presents to the ED with a depressed level of consciousness. He was found in the garage with an empty bottle next to him that was not labeled. He is somnolent but arousable. He reports epigastric pain, generalized weakness, and blurred vision. There are no external signs of trauma, and he is moving all extremities. Vital signs are normal. Laboratory studies show Na 140 mEq/L, Cl 100 mEq/L, K 4.2 mEq/L, bicarbonate 14 mEq/L, BUN 20 mg/dL, creatinine 0.9 mg/dL, glucose 120 mg/dL, and serum osmolality 305 mOsm/kg. A urine drug screen is negative for illicit substances, and there is no ethanol detected in the serum. Which of the following substances did this patient likely ingest?

A. Aspirin
B. Methanol
C. Heroin
D. Metformin

13. A 3-year-old boy presents to the ED after ingesting a small volume of gasoline from a gas can in the garage of his home approximately 30 minutes ago. He appears well and is asymptomatic with normal vital signs. His abdomen is soft and nontender. His lungs are clear to auscultation bilaterally. Which of the following is the most appropriate management of this patient?

A. Discharge home now
B. Admit for 24-hour observation
C. Gastric lavage
D. Observe for 6 hours and obtain chest radiograph at that time

14. A 26-year-old male presents to the ED with a depressed level of consciousness. He is somnolent but briefly opens his eyes to sternal rub. His pupils are 2 mm and minimally reactive bilaterally. Vital signs are BP 90/60 mm Hg, HR 56 bpm, RR 10 breaths/min, and oxygen saturation 98% on room air. His EKG shows sinus bradycardia with a QTc of 505. Which of the following is most likely responsible for his current condition?

A. Heroin
B. Diltiazem
C. Alprazolam
D. Methadone

15. A 16-year-old female presents to the ED on a psychiatric hold after a suicide attempt by ingestion. Her boyfriend broke up with her today, and she reports taking an unknown quantity of acetaminophen 3 hours ago because she "cannot live without him." She denies ingesting any other substances. She is well-appearing and asymptomatic. Her vital signs and EKG are normal. Pregnancy test is negative, chemistry panel is unremarkable, and her acetaminophen level is zero. Which of the following is the next step in management?

A. Repeat acetaminophen level in 1 hour (4 hours postingestion)
B. Administer *N*-acetylcysteine
C. Give activated charcoal
D. Medically clear for psychiatric evaluation

16. Which of the following alcohols is correctly paired with its toxic metabolite?

A. Methanol—formaldehyde
B. Ethylene glycol—oxalic acid
C. Isopropanol—propylene glycol
D. Ethanol—acetic acid

17. A 4-year-old boy is brought into the ED by his mother after he ingested an unknown quantity of her iron pills approximately 15 minutes ago. She was in the kitchen making dinner when she realized that he had wandered out of the living room. She found him in the bathroom with the bottle that had previously been full and was now nearly empty. He is currently asymptomatic and well-appearing with normal vital signs. A plain film of the abdomen reveals a large number of radiopaque

tablets in the stomach. Which of the following is the most appropriate next step in management?

A. Observation for 6 hours, discharge home if asymptomatic
B. Activated charcoal
C. Gastric lavage
D. Whole bowel irrigation

18. A 32-year-old female is the victim of a house fire. She is found on the floor inside the burning home. She does not have any noticeable burns but does have soot around her nose and mouth. She briefly responds to sternal rub by opening her eyes and moving all extremities but is quite somnolent and confused. Her vital signs include BP 90/50 mm Hg, HR 130 bpm, SpO_2 98% on non-rebreather mask, and RR 24 breath/min. Laboratory studies reveal sodium 140 mEq/L, potassium 4.5 mEq/L, chloride 100 mEq/L, bicarbonate 12 mEq/L, BUN 18 mg/dL, creatinine 0.9 mg/dL, lactate 12 mmol/L, and carboxyhemoglobin 10%, and human chorionic gonadotropin (hCG) negative. Which of the following treatments is most likely to provide the greatest benefit to this patient?

A. Hydroxocobalamin
B. Hyperbaric oxygen
C. Sodium bicarbonate
D. Hemodialysis

19. A 27-year-old male presents to the ED for nausea, vomiting, and diarrhea. He thinks he may have food poisoning from fish that he ate for dinner a few hours ago. He also reports headache, myalgias, and painful tingling in his hands. He is particularly disturbed by the sensory changes in his hands, endorsing burning pain when he picked up a glass of ice water. His BP is 88/50 mm Hg and HR is 54 bpm. Which of the following is the most likely cause of his presentation?

A. Scombroid
B. Ciguatera
C. Tetrodotoxin
D. *Vibrio parahaemolyticus*

20. A 6-month-old female is brought in by ambulance for lethargy. Her parents report that she has had a cough, and they have been giving her a cough suppressant they purchased at a natural food store. She has also been constipated and not feeding well. On exam, she is afebrile, tachycardic, and lethargic. She has poor tone and head control. She is not handling her oral secretions well and is intubated for airway protection. Chest radiograph shows the endotracheal tube in good position and is otherwise unremarkable. All initial laboratory results, including a urinalysis and lumbar puncture, are normal. Which of the following is the definitive treatment for her condition?

A. Supportive care alone
B. IV antibiotics
C. Dialysis
D. IV botulism immune globulin

21. A 70-year-old female presents to the ED for confusion, lethargy, and diaphoresis. Per EMS, her blood sugar on scene was 35. She was given D50 en route with improvement in her mental status. She is now feeling well and is without complaint. She reports taking "some pills" for her diabetes, but she does not know the names of her medications. She denies using any form of insulin. Chemistry panel is unremarkable other than a blood sugar of 205. You decide to feed her and observe her in the ED. A few hours later, her nurse reports that the patient is confused again. Her repeat blood sugar is 43. Which of the following is the correct management for this patient?

A. Administer D50 and octreotide
B. Administer D50 and glucagon
C. Activated charcoal
D. Emergent dialysis

22. Which of the following antidepressants is most likely to cause QRS prolongation and convulsions in overdose?

A. Fluoxetine
B. Sertraline
C. Trazodone
D. Venlafaxine

23. A 78-year-old male with history of coronary artery disease, congestive heart failure, hypertension, and dementia presents to the ED with generalized weakness, nausea and vomiting, and worsening confusion. At baseline, he is intermittently confused per family, but he insists on being independent. His vital signs include BP 110/70 mm Hg, HR 52 bpm, RR 18 breaths/min, oxygen saturation of 97% on room air, and temperature 37.2° C. His home medications include metoprolol, furosemide, digoxin, aspirin, lisinopril, and simvastatin. He is somnolent but arousable and is oriented to person and place only. His complete blood count (CBC) is normal. His chemistry panel is remarkable for a potassium of 6.5 mEq/L, BUN of 38 mg/dL, and creatinine of 3.1 mg/dL. He does not have any known renal insufficiency at baseline. His serum digoxin level is 3.2 ng/dL. Which of the following is the next best step in the management of this patient?

A. Insulin, D50, and sodium bicarbonate
B. Digoxin-specific antibody fragments
C. Activated charcoal
D. Hemodialysis

24. A 41-year-old male with a history of diabetes and hypertension presents to the ED with lethargy. His pupils are pinpoint. His BP is 96/48 mm Hg and HR is 56 bpm. His RR is 8 breaths/min, and respirations are shallow. He has no known history of substance abuse. Which of the following in overdose may be the cause of the patient's condition?

A. Cocaine
B. Clonidine
C. Amitriptyline
D. Metformin

25. A 21-year-old male presents to the ED with a depressed level of consciousness. Per EMS, he was picked up at a nightclub after a friend found him unresponsive in the bathroom. There was vomit next to him on the floor, and he was incontinent of urine. Vital signs include RR 8 breaths/min, HR 56 bpm, BP 120/80 mm Hg, and temperature 37.5° C. His Glasgow Coma Scale (GCS) score is 7. Naloxone is given with no response. He is intubated for airway protection. While his workup is in progress, he suddenly wakes up approximately 2 hours after arrival to ED. He is following commands, passes a spontaneous breathing trial, and is extubated. He reports using a drug at the club to experience euphoria, but he is unsure what it was. He now feels fine and is asking to go home. Which of the following did he most likely use?

A. Oxycodone
B. MDMA
C. γ-Hydroxybutyrate (GHB)
D. Salvia

26. A 18-year-female presents to the ED on a psychiatric hold after a suicide attempt. She reports ingesting "most of the bottle" of sustained-release lithium less than an hour ago. She is withdrawn and not willing to participate with any further history but otherwise appears well. Her vital signs are normal. Which of the following treatments should be initiated?

A. Activated charcoal
B. Hemodialysis
C. Observation alone
D. Whole bowel irrigation

27. You are called to the bedside of a 33-year-old male who had just undergone bedside incision and drainage

of a peritonsillar abscess less than 1 hour prior by your colleague who has now gone home. The nurse was about to discharge the patient when she noted perioral cyanosis. The patient also reports generalized weakness and headache. He denies shortness of breath or chest pain. Vital signs include BP 118/76 mm Hg, HR 112 bpm, RR 22 breaths/min, and oxygen saturation 85% on room air. There is no stridor, and his airway appears widely patent. His lungs are clear to auscultation, and his heart rhythm is regular without murmur. He has no peripheral edema. You administer supplemental oxygen with no improvement. The nurse places an IV line and notes that the patient's blood appears brown. An arterial blood gas is drawn, and the PaO_2 is normal. Which of the following treatments is most likely to resolve his cyanosis and symptoms?

A. Methylene blue
B. Hyperbaric oxygen
C. Positive pressure ventilation
D. Hydroxocobalamin

28. A 53-year-old male is brought in by ambulance from a psychiatric facility for fever and altered mental status. He has a history of schizophrenia that is refractory to medications. His current medication list includes clozapine, risperidone, and lorazepam. He was noted by staff to be lethargic this morning. Vital signs include BP 172/98 mm Hg, HR 124 bpm, RR 24 breaths/min, oxygen saturation 97% on room air, and temperature 39° C. He is noted to be rigid, but there is no myoclonus. Which treatment is most appropriate?

A. Diphenhydramine
B. Supportive care
C. Cyproheptadine
D. Acetaminophen

29. A 57-year-old male with history of hypertension, chronic kidney disease, depression, alcohol abuse, and gout is sent to the ED by his primary care doctor for generalized weakness and severe anemia. His hemoglobin was noted to be 6.2 g/dL on the outpatient labs. The repeat CBC in the ED shows white blood cells (WBCs) $3.2 \times 10^3/\mu L$, hemoglobin 6.1 g/dL, and platelets $65 \times 10^3/\mu L$. Chemistry panel shows Na 135 mEq/L, Cl 105 mEq/L, K 4.2 mEq/L, bicarbonate 20 mEq/L, BUN 32 mg/dL, creatinine 1.9 mg/dL, and glucose 105 mg/dL. On exam, he is noted to have proximal muscle weakness and numbness in his hands and feet. Which of the following is the likely etiology of his presentation?

A. Clozapine toxicity
B. Colchicine toxicity

C. Botulism
D. Lisinopril toxicity

30. A 2-year-old boy presents to the ED after drinking drain cleaner that contained sodium hydroxide. He is stridulous, coughing, drooling, and vomiting. Burns are noted on his lips, and there is significant edema of the oropharynx. He has increased work of breathing. He is intubated for airway protection. Which of the following is the most appropriate next step in management?

A. Neutralize the sodium hydroxide with citric acid to prevent further tissue damage
B. Administer activated charcoal
C. Perform gastric lavage
D. Consult gastroenterology for possible endoscopy

31. A 29-year-old female presents to the ED after a seizure. She had a witnessed generalized tonic-clonic seizure that lasted approximately 2 minutes and is now in a postictal state. She recently had knee surgery but has been recovering well and is otherwise healthy. She has never had a seizure, but her sister has epilepsy. Which of the following most likely contributed to her seizure?

A. Acetaminophen
B. Ibuprofen
C. Tramadol
D. Hydrocodone

32. A 53-year-old female artist presents to the ED with a painful lesion to her left lower leg. She was working with a glass etcher approximately 12 hours ago when she accidentally spilled it on her leg. She wiped it off with a rag, and initially noted some mild pain ,which has been progressively worse. The affected area is now swollen and erythematous with an ulcerated lesion in the center. She is in excruciating pain. In addition to pain control, which of the following is the best initial treatment for this patient's condition?

A. Broad-spectrum antibiotics
B. Surgical debridement
C. Calcium gluconate
D. Bacitracin and petrolatum-impregnated gauze dressing

33. A 42-year-old woman presents to the ED from her job at a commercial farm with a chief complaint of generalized weakness. She is actively vomiting and defecating and is in respiratory distress. Physical exam reveals diaphoresis, bradycardia, hypotension, diffuse wheezing and rhonchi, pinpoint pupils, and muscle fasciculations. You are concerned for organophosphate exposure and plan to give atropine. Which of the

following would you expect to persist despite administration of atropine?

A. Pinpoint pupils
B. Wheezing and rhonchi
C. Muscle weakness
D. Diaphoresis

34. A 67-year-old female is sent to the ED by her primary care doctor for an international normalized ratio (INR) of 10.2 noted on routine labs. The patient has a history of a mechanical valve replacement and is anticoagulated with warfarin. She currently has no complaints and denies any known sources of bleeding. Her hemoglobin and vital signs are normal. What is the best course of action in this case?

A. Withhold warfarin, administer vitamin K
B. Withhold warfarin, administer prothrombin complex concentrate (PCC)
C. Withhold warfarin, administer fresh frozen plasma (FFP)
D. Withhold warfarin, no other intervention indicated

35. A 3-year-old female is brought in by ambulance for seizure. She was given multiple doses of benzodiazepine en route but continues to seize. The patient's mother is an herbalist, and there are many potential toxins in the home. Which of the following did she most likely ingest?

A. Nutmeg
B. Camphor oil
C. Oil of wintergreen
D. Tea tree oil

36. A 38-year-old male presents to the ED for medical clearance for jail. He is agitated and making nonsensical statements. He appears to be responding to internal stimuli. Vertical nystagmus is noted. Which of the following drugs did he most likely use before he was taken into custody by the police?

A. Cocaine
B. Methamphetamine
C. Lysergic acid diethylamide (LSD)
D. Phencyclidine (PCP)

37. A 32-year-old female presents to the ED after being stung by a Portuguese man-of-war while snorkeling off the coast of Florida. Which of the following treatments should be initiated?

A. Tap water irrigation
B. Salt water irrigation

C. Cold water immersion
D. Acetic acid irrigation

38. A 45-year-old female presents to the ED with necrosis to the tip of her nose and both of her pinnae. She has no known medical problems. She smokes a pack of cigarettes daily and uses cocaine. Exposure to which of the following is the most likely cause of her current presentation?

A. Lead
B. Mercury
C. Boric acid
D. Levamisole

39. A 50-year-old male presents to the ED with a large laceration to his left arm after an alleged assault with a knife. After a thorough examination, it is determined that there is no significant underlying injury, and you plan to close the laceration at the bedside with sutures. The patient's chart indicates that he has had an anaphylactic reaction to tetracaine in the past. Which of the following local anesthetics would be the safest option in this patient?

A. Bupivacaine
B. Procaine
C. Benzocaine
D. Chloroprocaine

40. A 30-year-old male with a history of substance abuse presents to the ED with intermittent episodes of painful muscle spasms. He is lying on the bed with an arched back, rigid extremities, and facial grimacing, but he is awake and alert. Which of the following is most likely responsible for these findings?

A. Serotonin syndrome
B. Neuroleptic malignant syndrome (NMS)
C. Strychnine poisoning
D. Alcohol withdrawal seizure

41. A 26-year-old female field worker in California presents to the ED with sudden onset of severe pain in her left arm that occurred while she was at work. Shortly thereafter, she developed diffuse abdominal pain, nausea, vomiting, and headache. On exam, she is tachycardic, hypertensive, and diaphoretic. Her abdomen is rigid. You note a small area of erythema on the left upper extremity. What is the most likely outcome of this patient's condition?

A. Necrosis of the left upper extremity in the area of erythema
B. Death

C. Recovery without sequelae

D. Compartment syndrome of the left upper extremity requiring fasciotomy

42. A 3-year-old female presents from home with very concerned parents. She is sleepy but arousable. She was found in the garage drinking from an unlabeled mason jar and has a faint blue color around her lips. Her initial vital signs are age appropriate. The compound that she drank is pictured in Figure 17.4. Her CBC is normal, her chemistry panel reveals sodium 137 mmol/L, potassium 3.7 mmol/L, chloride 110 mmol/L, bicarbonate 21 mmol/L, BUN 7 mg/dL, and glucose 132 mg/dL. Her serum osmolality is measured at 355. What is the most likely substance that she ingested?

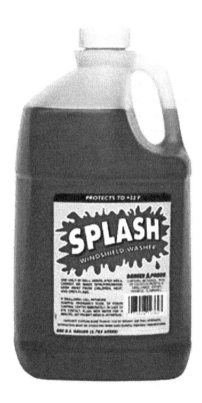

Figure 17.4 Windshield washer fluid.

A. Methanol

B. Ethylene glycol

C. Isopropyl alcohol

D. Propylene glycol

43. A 72-year-old male presents to your rural ED complaining of blurred vision. He states his vision looks like a "snowstorm" or a "television with static." In questioning, he reports that he frequently drinks "homemade" alcohol. What is the underlying mechanism for his visual disturbance?

A. Lead toxicity

B. Formic acid–mediated destruction of retinal cells

C. Direct ocular exposure to methanol

D. Lactic acidosis

44. Your next door neighbor knows that you are an emergency medicine provider and wants your opinion about a plant that is in her backyard. She has been told that it is a poisonous plant and is wondering whether she needs to remove it because her toddler is just beginning to walk. The plant in question is shown in Figure 17.5. What is the most appropriate response to her question?

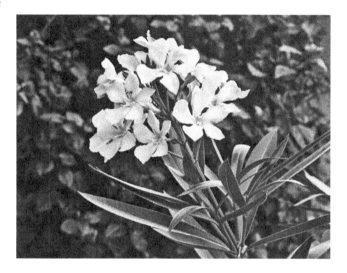

Figure 17.5 Plant.

A. No need to worry because the plant is nontoxic

B. The plant is toxic, but pediatric ingestions rarely result in serious clinical symptoms, therefore removal is not necessary

C. The plant should be removed immediately because deaths and serious toxicity result from ingestions

D. All botanicals have the potential to cause toxicity and should therefore be removed

45. A 17-year-old female presents to the ED with abdominal discomfort, nausea, and vomiting. She is tearful and reports that her boyfriend just broke up with her. She is alert, awake, oriented to person, place, and time, but she repeatedly asks you to repeat your questions and speak louder. Her vital signs include HR 120 bpm, BP 135/80 mm Hg, RR 22 breaths/min, and temperature 37.8° C. Laboratory studies reveal sodium 140, chloride 100, bicarbonate 18, BUN 20, creatinine 1.5, and glucose 100. A blood gas is obtained that reveals pH 7.50, P_{CO_2} 25, and bicarbonate 19. Which of the following is the likely cause of her acid-base disturbance?

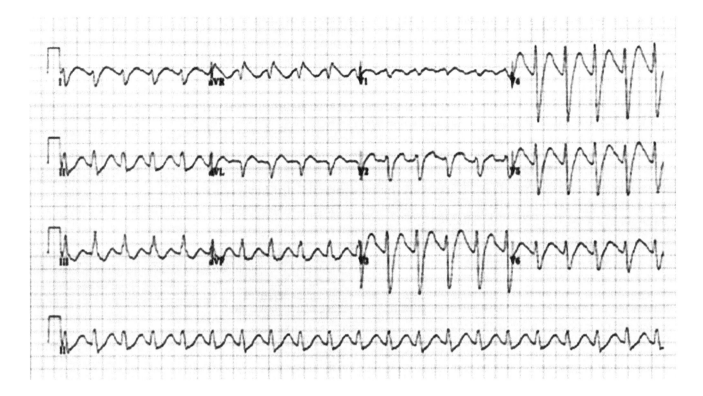

Figure 17.6 Electrocardiogram.

A. Salicylate ingestion
B. Methanol ingestion
C. Diabetic ketoacidosis
D. Excessive vomiting

46. A 23-year-old male is intubated following an intentional overdose of amitriptyline. An EKG is obtained and is shown in Figure 17.6. Which of the following is the most appropriate medication to administer?

A. Calcium gluconate
B. Magnesium sulfate
C. Potassium chloride
D. Sodium bicarbonate

47. Which of the following is the most appropriate to treat convulsions associated with a tricyclic antidepressant (TCA) overdose?

A. Flumazenil
B. Lorazepam

C. Physostigmine
D. Sodium bicarbonate

48. A 33-year-old female with history of depression presents to the ED with seizures. Per EMS, she has been having generalized tonic-clonic seizure activity for 30 minutes despite 4 mg of IV lorazepam en route. She is given an additional 4 mg of IV lorazepam in the ED without resolution of seizures. Phenytoin and phenobarbital also fail to stop the seizing. Her blood sugar and sodium levels are normal. She is afebrile, and there are no external signs of trauma. Her roommate arrives and reports that the patient recently immigrated from Mexico. She has no known history of seizures. She has had a hard time adjusting to life in the United States away from her friends and family and has been very depressed. Which of the following medications is most likely to terminate the seizures?

A. Diazepam
B. Pyridoxine
C. Carbamazepine
D. Levetiracetam

ANSWERS

1. ANSWER: A

This clinical presentation is most consistent with an antimuscarinic (anticholinergic) toxicity. The mnemonic "hot as a hare, red as a beet, blind as a bat, dry as a bone, and mad as a hatter" is often used to remember the features of the antimuscarinic toxidrome.

Of the answer choices, only jimson weed (*Datura stramonium*) contains atropine-like alkaloids throughout the plant but concentrated in the seeds. It is not uncommon for teenagers to brew teas from this plant in an attempt to get high and hallucinate.

The other answers are not consistent with this presentation. The death cap mushroom (*Amanita muscaria*) is associated with fulminant liver failure following ingestion. Water hemlock is associated with convulsions and seizures. Dumb cane (*Dieffenbachia*) is a common household ornamental plant that causes mouth pain if ingested because of insoluble oxalate crystals that are fired into the lips and tongue.

Test-taking tip: Brush up on common toxidromes that present to the ED before the test, including anticholinergic, cholinergic, sedative-hypnotic, opioid, and stimulant.

2. ANSWER: B

This patient is experiencing the DRESS syndrome. This occurs most commonly with anticonvulsants and is thought to involve inadequate metabolism of these compounds. It results in dysfunction of multiple organ systems. The liver is the most commonly involved. Patients may also develop nephritis, pneumonitis, myocarditis, encephalitis, and thyroid abnormalities.

Streptococcal pharyngitis and a viral syndrome might explain some of the symptoms and signs described but not all of them. This patient's clinical condition is not consistent with anaphylaxis.

Test-taking tip: When faced with a question for which you don't solidly know the answer, a helpful strategy is to eliminate answer choices that are clearly wrong, such as anaphylaxis and streptococcal pharyngitis for this question.

3. ANSWER: A

Decontamination is an important step in the care of chemically exposed patients and is a preventative step to avoid exposures to hospital and prehospital staff. Substances that are exclusively gas at normal temperature and pressure such as chlorine, phosgene, and hydrogen cyanide require only the removal of patients from the source of exposure.

Only chemical weapons dispersed as liquids require decontamination in the form of showers and removal of patient clothing. In this stem, the victims have been exposed to gas only. The other answer choices would not help in the care of this patient.

Test-taking tip: Remember that gas goes away, so no decontamination is necessary.

4. ANSWER: D

The EKG demonstrates a widening of the QRS complex that occurs with sodium channel blockade caused by TCA toxicity. This is also the mechanism that causes seizures with TCA overdose.

All of the other answer choices are also effects of TCAs. α-Adrenergic receptor antagonism will result in orthostatic hypotension, not QRS prolongation or seizures. Antihistamine effects result in sedation and somnolence. GABA-A receptor antagonism would be expected to cause seizures but not QRS prolongation.

Test-taking tip: Sodium channel blockade is a very common mechanism of action for a wide variety of medications and toxins. When in doubt, guessing sodium channel blockade is a very reasonable and appropriate strategy.

5. ANSWER: C

This boy most likely ate water hemlock. This plant is often mistakenly identified as wild carrots or parsnips. All parts of the plant contain cicutoxin, but the roots have the highest concentrations. Following initial gastrointestinal symptoms, seizures are not uncommon. Mortality following ingestion is as high as 70%. The exact mechanism of toxicity is not entirely clear but is thought to be due to GABA antagonism.

Peyote is a cactus that is a known hallucinogen. Pokeweed produces a severe gastroenteritis when ingested, but it does not cause seizures. Dumb cane (*Dieffenbachia*) is a common household plant that results in mucous membrane irritation if ingested but not seizures.

Test-taking tip: This is a "you know it or don't" kind of question. If you don't know it, choose an answer and move on. You can perhaps mark it for review when you are done at the end of the test. Don't, however, let these kinds of questions get you stuck and waste your time.

6. ANSWER: B

This patient is clearly showing signs of toxicity, including a depressed level of consciousness. This is confirmed by a markedly elevated serum valproic acid concentration. Admission is warranted, but additional levels should be obtained to determine the direction of toxicity.

The most appropriate management is to place a hemodialysis catheter and consult nephrology for dialysis. At therapeutic doses, valproic acid demonstrates characteristics that do not lend themselves to hemodialysis, namely a high degree of protein binding. However, in overdose, protein binding becomes saturated, and a high degree of valproic acid is free. Valproic acid is a small molecule and has a small volume of distribution, making it amenable to dialysis.

While activated charcoal may be indicated in some valproic acid ingestions, it is contraindicated in this patient given her depressed level of consciousness. Medical clearance is ill advised because cerebral edema, seizures, and death have all been reported after valproic acid toxicity.

Test-taking tip: When faced with a question for which you don't solidly know the answer, a helpful strategy is to eliminate answer choices that are clearly wrong, such as medical clearance or administration of activated charcoal to a somnolent patient for this question.

7. ANSWER: A

This patient is presenting with an acute opioid intoxication. This is manifested by the depressed level of consciousness, constricted pupils, decreased respiratory rate, and history of IV heroin abuse. The blood gas that is correct will correspond to these physiologic changes. In particular, a decreased RR will result in an accumulation of CO_2 and a decrease in pH. This is the definition of a respiratory acidosis. The only answer choice that demonstrates a pure respiratory acidosis is pH 7.20, P_{CO_2} 60, and HCO_3 24.

Choice B is consistent with a metabolic acidosis, and both C and D represent alkalotic states.

Test-taking tip: Depressed respirations equals respiratory acidosis, allowing you to eliminate two of the answers.

8. ANSWER: B

The presence of hypokalemia, a non–anion gap acidosis, and alkaline urine suggests a renal tubular acidosis (RTA). Distal RTA (type I) refers to the inability of the urine to be acidified in the distal tubule (resulting in alkaline urine). Proximal RTA (type II) refers to the inability of the proximal renal tubule to reabsorb bicarbonate. Both of these conditions result in an acidic serum pH but a normal anion gap.

Both salicylates and methanol result in anion gap acidosis. Loop diuretics produce a metabolic alkalosis, not acidosis.

Test-taking tip: A solid understanding of how to calculate an anion gap and the things that cause an anion gap

acidosis is important for standardized tests in emergency medicine and clinical practice.

9. ANSWER: C

This patient is demonstrating QRS prolongation due to sodium channel blockade. This finding portends the potential for serious cardiac dysrhythmias and cardiovascular collapse. Sodium bicarbonate is the treatment of choice for QRS prolongation regardless of the cause.

While MDAC has been demonstrated to reduce the enterohepatic and enteroenteric recirculation of certain medications, this would not be appropriate therapy for QRS prolongation. Overdrive pacing and magnesium are both appropriate therapies for QT prolongation, not QRS prolongation.

Test-taking tip: A prolonged QRS in the setting of suspected or confirmed ingestion should be treated with sodium bicarbonate regardless of the cause.

10. ANSWER: A

There are many potential agents that can be used in a terrorist attack. Organophosphate nerve agents are among those that have been most often described or actually released. These nerve agents work by inhibiting the enzyme acetylcholinesterase, resulting in excess levels of acetylcholine and a cholinergic toxidrome. The mnemonics DUMBELS and SLUDGE have been used to describe these clinical effects. DUMBELS stands for diarrhea, urination, miosis, bradycardia, bronchorrhea, bronchospasm, emesis, lacrimation, and salivation. SLUDGE stands for salivation, lacrimation, urination, defecation, gastrointestinal motility (emesis), and eyes (miosis). Patients often die as a result of the "killer Bs," including bradycardia, bronchorrhea, and bronchospasm.

Hydrogen cyanide exposure would turn off aerobic respiration, resulting in hypoxia and acidosis. Chlorine increases alveolar capillary permeability, resulting in pulmonary edema. Sulfur mustard is a vesicant that produces blistering of mucous membranes, skin, and pulmonary tissue.

Test-taking tip: Brush up on common toxidromes that present to the ED before the test, including anticholinergic, cholinergic, sedative-hypnotic, opioid, and stimulant.

11. ANSWER: C

The snake depicted in the photo is an Eastern coral snake, a member of the Elapid family of venomous snakes. This snake may be confused with similar-appearing nonvenomous snakes, such as kingsnakes. In the coral snake, the red and yellow bands touch, whereas in nonvenomous snakes, the red and black bands touch. This can be remembered using the mnemonic "Red on yellow, kill a fellow; red on black, venom lack." Coral snake venom contains a neurotoxin that can cause all of the symptoms in choice C, in addition to dysarthria, dysphagia, and tremors. The most common cause of death is respiratory failure due to paralysis of the respiratory muscles. Choices B and D are incorrect because there tends to be only minimal pain or local injury with coral snake envenomations. These symptoms would be more common with crotalid envenomation (i.e., rattlesnake).

Test-taking tip: Brush up on common envenomations that present to the ED and their associated symptoms and treatment.

12. ANSWER: B

This patient has an anion gap metabolic acidosis (bicarbonate 14, anion gap 26) and an elevated osmole gap of 11. These findings are suggestive of methanol toxicity. Methanol is a toxic alcohol commonly found in windshield wiper fluid and many solvents. It may be ingested by alcoholics when they do not have access to ethanol. Initial signs/symptoms are similar to those of ethanol ingestion, followed by anion gap metabolic acidosis, blindness, acute renal failure, seizures, and death. In addition to supportive care, treatment is with fomepizole, which prevents the breakdown of methanol into its toxic metabolite, formic acid, by competing for the enzyme alcohol dehydrogenase.

While aspirin and metformin may produce an anion gap metabolic acidosis, they do not result in an elevated osmole gap. Heroin does not cause an anion gap metabolic acidosis or elevated osmole gap.

Test-taking tip: Visual changes in the setting of an ingestion should make you think methanol.

13. ANSWER: D

This patient ingested gasoline, which is a hydrocarbon. Hydrocarbon ingestion can cause multiple organ system dysfunction, including dysrhythmia, lethargy, ataxia, paresthesias, nausea, vomiting, abdominal pain, and hepatotoxicity. Aspiration pneumonitis is of particular concern with hydrocarbon ingestion. Most patients with clinically significant aspirations have an abnormal chest radiograph and some symptoms such as tachypnea, wheezing, retractions, or fever. However, even asymptomatic patients may develop signs of pneumonitis later. Most cases of pneumonitis will be apparent on radiograph within 6 hours. This patient therefore should not be immediately discharged but rather should have

a chest radiograph performed after 6 hours to evaluate for development of pneumonitis. He does not need to be admitted if he is asymptomatic with a normal chest radiograph at 6 hours postingestion. Gastric lavage should be avoided given that the risk for aspiration outweighs potential benefit.

Test-taking tip: A period of 6 to 8 hours of observation in asymptomatic or minimally symptomatic ingestions is a common recommendation, so if it is one of the potential answers in such a setting, it is probably the correct answer.

14. ANSWER: D

This patient most likely ingested methadone. Methadone overdose presents like opioid overdose with a depressed level of consciousness, bradypnea, hypotension, bradycardia, and pinpoint pupils, but methadone is classically associated with a prolonged QT interval, and this may help distinguish the two clinically.

Diltiazem is a nondihydropyridine calcium channel blocker that may cause hypotension and bradycardia but does not prolong the QT interval. Alprazolam is a benzodiazepine commonly abused for recreation. It may produce somnolence and hypotension but does not prolong the QT interval.

Test-taking tip: Brush up on common toxidromes that present to the ED before the test, including anticholinergic, cholinergic, sedative-hypnotic, opioid, and stimulant.

15. ANSWER: D

This patient is unlikely to have ingested a significant amount of acetaminophen given that the level was undetectable 3 hours after ingestion. For acute ingestions, an acetaminophen level should be collected at least 4 hours after ingestion to be interpreted using the Rumack-Matthew nomogram. Levels drawn before 4 hours cannot be interpreted unless they are undetectable, as in this case.

With a clinically significant ingestion, there should be some acetaminophen detected between 1 and 4 hours, and the level should be repeated after the 4-hour mark has been reached to determine whether the antidote, N-acetylcysteine, should be administered. Given that the remainder of her workup is unremarkable, this patient can be medically cleared at this point for psychiatric evaluation.

Activated charcoal can be used for acute acetaminophen ingestions if there are no contraindications but is not generally indicated if the ingestion was more than 2 hours before arrival, unless there is suspicion for ingestion of extended-release formulations.

Test-taking tip: Sometimes less is better in asymptomatic patients with normal labs, on tests and in emergency medicine practice.

16. ANSWER: B

Both ethanol and isopropanol toxicity are directly related to the parent compound rather than a metabolite. This distinguishes these alcohols (which are generally considered less toxic) from methanol and ethylene glycol. The most serious complications and toxicity result from the metabolism of these alcohols into acid-containing metabolites (Figure 17.7).

Methanol is metabolized through formaldehyde to formic acid, which is implicated as the cause of most of the toxicity resulting from methanol ingestions.

Ethylene glycol is metabolized through a number of intermediates (including glycoaldehyde) to oxalic acid. Oxalic acid is the metabolite that is the cause of most of the serious toxicity following ethylene glycol ingestion.

Ethanol is ultimately metabolized to acetic acid, but acetic acid has very limited toxicity; isopropanol is metabolized to acetone.

$$\text{(ADH)} \quad\quad \text{(ALDH)} \quad\quad \text{(folate)}$$
Methanol → Formaldehyde → Formic Acid → CO_2 + H_2O

$$\text{(ADH)} \quad\quad \text{(ALDH)}$$
Ethylene Glycol → Glycoaldehyde → Glycolic Acid → Glyoxylic Acid → Oxalic Acid

$$\text{(ADH)}$$
Isopropanol → Acetone

$$\text{(ADH)} \quad\quad \text{(ALDH)}$$
Ethanol → Acetaldehyde → Acetic Acid

(ADH) = Alcohol dehydrogenase

(ALDH) = Aldehyde dehydrogenase

Figure 17.7 Metabolism of potentially toxic alcohols.

Test-taking tip: This is a "you know it or don't" kind of question. If you don't know it, choose an answer and move on. You can perhaps mark it for review when you are done at the end of the test. Don't, however, let these kinds of questions get you stuck and waste your time.

17. ANSWER: D

Iron supplements are commonly ingested by curious children given that they are readily available and may come in containers that are not child resistant. Iron toxicity can be life-threatening, particularly in children.

There are four stages of iron toxicity. Initially there is gastrointestinal upset from direct corrosion to the gastrointestinal tract. This causes nausea, vomiting, and diarrhea, which is often bloody and may result in perforation. This is followed by a quiescent second stage. In the third stage, toxicity progresses to multisystem organ failure that may result in shock and death. If the patient survives stage three, the final stage involves scarring of the gastrointestinal tract with subsequent gastric outlet or bowel obstruction.

In patients with a known minor ingestion and those who present more than 6 hours after ingestion and remain asymptomatic, observation may be appropriate. However, patients with a significant ingestion should be treated aggressively, even if initially asymptomatic. The treatment of choice in this case is whole bowel irrigation. Activated charcoal is not effective because it does not bind metals. Gastric lavage may be indicated in ingestion of liquid formulations, but whole tablets are unlikely to be removed by lavage.

Test-taking tip: There are a number of mnemonics that describe drugs that appear on plain radiography. CHIMPS is a commonly used mnemonic: chloral hydrate, hydrocarbons, iron, metals, pesticides, and solvents.

18. ANSWER: A

This patient is exhibiting signs of both cyanide and carbon monoxide poisoning. The anion gap metabolic acidosis with a significantly elevated lactate is highly suggestive of cyanide toxicity in the setting of smoke exposure. Lactate has been used as a surrogate marker for cyanide given that cyanide levels are not readily available at most hospitals. Cyanide prevents the use of oxygen during aerobic respiration. Hydroxocobalamin is an antidote for cyanide toxicity.

The patient also has an elevated carboxyhemoglobin level, indicating exposure to carbon monoxide. This can be treated with supplemental oxygen, but hyperbaric oxygen is not necessarily indicated in this case if the patient responds to the treatment for cyanide toxicity. Indications for hyperbaric oxygen include carboxyhemoglobin >25% (or 15% in pregnant women given that fetal hemoglobin has a greater affinity for carbon monoxide), severe metabolic acidosis, loss of consciousness, and abnormal neurologic exam.

Sodium bicarbonate is not necessary in this patient because her acidosis will likely improve with proper treatment for cyanide and carbon monoxide toxicities. Dialysis is not indicated for the treatment of cyanide or carbon monoxide.

Test-taking tip: Brush up on antidotes to common poisonings that may present to the ED.

19. ANSWER: B

This patient is most likely suffering from ciguatera. This ciguatoxin is produced by dinoflagellates that are consumed by reef fish. Grouper, snapper, and barracuda are common sources. Symptoms typically occur within the first 6 hours after ingestion and include nausea, vomiting, diarrhea, paresthesias, myalgias, hypotension, bradycardia, and the pathognomonic finding of hot-cold reversal as seen in this patient.

Scombroid is also caused by consumption of fish, typically those that have not been properly refrigerated. The fish may have tasted "peppery" and results in release of histamine. This causes flushing, abdominal cramping, diarrhea, headache, tachycardia, hypotension, and respiratory distress. The treatment is with antihistamines.

Tetrodotoxin is found in puffer fish. It produces vomiting, paresthesias, weakness, hypotension, and bradycardia. It may result in flaccid paralysis and respiratory failure requiring intubation. The treatment is supportive.

V. parahaemolyticus is found in shellfish and causes bloody diarrhea and fever, but not the other symptoms this patient is experiencing.

Test-taking tip: This is a "you know it or don't" kind of question. If you don't know it, choose an answer and move on. You can perhaps mark it for review when you are done at the end of the test. Don't, however, let these kinds of questions get you stuck and waste your time.

20. ANSWER: D

This infant is suffering from botulism, likely due to exposure to honey from the natural cough suppressant. Botulism is caused by the botulin toxin that prevents release of acetylcholine at the neuromuscular junction. Infant botulism is caused by ingestion of spores with subsequent production of toxin in the gut rather than ingestion of preformed toxin. Children younger than 1 year should never consume honey because it often contains spores. Infant botulism classically presents with a "floppy baby." Infants may have hypotonia, poor head control, poor feeding, loss of reflexes, weak gag and suck, lethargy, constipation, and tachycardia. The treatment is administration of IV botulism immune globulin.

Although sepsis can present with many of the same symptoms, this child has a normal temperature and no apparent source of infection. Although dialysis may be indicated for a variety of toxic ingestions, there is no role for dialysis in botulism. Supportive care is important for this patient but will not treat the underlying cause of her disease process.

Test-taking tip: Floppy infants should make you think botulism, on standardized test and in practice.

21. ANSWER: A

This patient is likely taking a sulfonylurea for diabetes. Sulfonylureas stimulate insulin release from the pancreas; therefore, toxicity may result in recurrent severe hypoglycemia. The correct treatment for sulfonylurea toxicity with recurrent hypoglycemia despite administration of glucose is octreotide. Octreotide suppresses insulin release, thereby decreasing glucose requirements and preventing rebound hypoglycemia. Patients treated with octreotide should be admitted for close monitoring.

Glucagon is not generally used for hypoglycemia because of its slow onset. Glucagon is the treatment for ß-blocker toxicity. Although activated charcoal can be given for sulfonylurea ingestion, it is not appropriate in this patient given unknown time of ingestion and her depressed level of consciousness. Sulfonylureas are highly protein bound, and therefore dialysis is not an effective treatment. Dialysis will remove metformin in the event of toxicity, but metformin toxicity presents with lactic acidosis, not recurrent hypoglycemia.

Test-taking tip: When two answers have the same root, in this case "administer D50," one of these answers is probably the correct one.

22. ANSWER: D

Of the answer choices listed, venlafaxine is well described to cause convulsions and QRS prolongation in overdose. Venlafaxine has potent sodium channel blocking effects. The other answer choices do not have this as a pharmacologic effect.

Fluoxetine and sertraline are both selective serotonin reuptake inhibitors. Overdose is associated with somnolence and occasionally serotonin syndrome. Trazodone is a serotonin reuptake inhibitor but lacks sodium channel blockade or antimuscarinic effects common to other antidepressants such as TCAs or monoamine oxidase inhibitors. Priapism is commonly associated with trazodone in overdose.

Test-taking tip: This is a "you know it or don't" kind of question. If you don't know it, choose an answer and move on. You can perhaps mark it for review when you are done at the end of the test. Don't, however, let these kinds of questions get you stuck and waste your time.

23. ANSWER: B

This patient is exhibiting signs of acute digoxin toxicity. A serum digoxin level >2.5 ng/mL is considered toxic. Patients may report vague, nonspecific symptoms such as generalized weakness, nausea, vomiting, abdominal pain, or confusion. A classic finding not given in the question stem is xanthopsia, a phenomenon in which patients will see yellow-green halos around objects. Bradycardia is common, and a variety of dysrhythmias may occur. Digoxin inhibits the sodium-potassium adenosine triphosphatase (ATPase); thus, acute toxicity can result in severe hyperkalemia.

The use of insulin, dextrose, and sodium bicarbonate does not reduce mortality from hyperkalemia caused by digoxin. The treatment of choice is digoxin-specific antibody fragments (digoxin-Fab).

Activated charcoal may play a role in acute digoxin ingestion; however, the time of ingestion is not known for this patient. Hemodialysis is not beneficial for digoxin toxicity.

Test-taking tip: Brush up on antidotes to common poisonings that may present to the ED.

24. ANSWER: B

This patient most likely is experiencing clonidine toxicity. Clonidine toxicity may look very similar to opioid intoxication. Clonidine is a centrally acting α_2-agonist that prevents release of catecholamines. It has primarily been used as an antihypertensive; however, it also has some opioid agonist properties and can be used for opioid withdrawal. The treatment of clonidine toxicity is primarily supportive. Although response to naloxone may be variable, it should be given because it may reverse some of the effects of clonidine. Additionally, naloxone will reverse opioid toxicity if there is diagnostic uncertainty given that it may be difficult to distinguish opioid from clonidine overdose clinically.

Cocaine causes the release of catecholamines and therefore should result in the opposite effects of those seen in this patient.

Amitriptyline is a TCA. TCA toxicity has variable presentations ranging from an antimuscarinic toxidrome to severe cardiotoxicity from sodium channel blockade. Signs and symptoms may include somnolence, ataxia, confusion, dry mucous membranes, and ileus. Tachycardia is more likely than bradycardia with TCA toxicity. Classically, the EKG in TCA toxicity will show sinus tachycardia with prolonged PR, QRS, and QT intervals; however, the EKG may be normal or show other abnormalities as well.

Metformin toxicity results in lactic acidosis. While lactic acidosis may produce lethargy and hypotension, it is not generally associated with respiratory depression or pinpoint pupils.

Test-taking tip: When faced with a question for which you don't solidly know the answer, a helpful strategy is to eliminate answer choices that are clearly wrong, such as cocaine and metformin for this question.

25. ANSWER: C

This patient most likely took GHB. This drug is commonly known as the "date rape" drug, but is also abused at nightclubs and raves for its euphoric effects. It acts on GABA receptors, and its effects can be potentiated by co-ingestion of alcohol. After a period of euphoria, users may develop delirium, coma, myoclonus, seizures, urinary incontinence, vomiting, bradypnea, and bradycardia. The effects are short-lived, and classically those who require intubation are extubated a few hours later. Treatment is supportive because there is no antidote.

Oxycodone overdose may present with bradypnea and depressed level of consciousness, but there should have been some improvement with naloxone. MDMA, commonly known as Ecstasy, is another popular club/rave drug, but it presents with a sympathomimetic toxidrome. Severe hyponatremia may also occur with MDMA. Salvia is a plant in the mint family that when consumed causes altered visual perception and hallucinations, but it is unlikely to produce respiratory depression or coma.

Test-taking tip: Brush up on common toxidromes that present to the ED before the test, including anticholinergic, cholinergic, sedative-hypnotic, opioid, and stimulant.

26. ANSWER: D

Lithium toxicity may result in weakness, lethargy, ataxia, dysrhythmia, delirium, coma, or seizures. Whole bowel irrigation is the best method of gastrointestinal decontamination in acute lithium overdose for patients with a normal mental status.

Activated charcoal is ineffective because it does not bind lithium. A good mnemonic for toxins that do not bind to charcoal well is PHAILS: pesticides, hydrocarbons, alcohols, acids/alkalis, iron, lithium, lead, and solvents.

Hemodialysis may be indicated for severe toxicity such as in those with altered mental status, coma, seizures, dysrhythmias, or lithium levels >4 mEq/L in acute ingestions.

Observation alone is not safe in suspected significant lithium overdose because lithium toxicity can lead to significant morbidity and mortality if not properly treated.

Test-taking tip: This is a "you know it or don't" kind of question. If you don't know it, choose an answer and move on. You can perhaps mark it for review when you are done at the end of the test. Don't, however, let these kinds of questions get you stuck and waste your time.

27. ANSWER: A

This patient is most likely suffering from methemoglobinemia induced by the topical anesthetic spray that was used during the incision and drainage. Methemoglobin is hemoglobin with the iron moiety in the ferric (rather than the normal ferrous) form that is unable to transport oxygen. The pulse oximeter will give falsely low oxygen saturation readings, and cyanosis does not improve with supplemental oxygen. The PaO_2 should be normal. A chocolate-brown color to the blood is classically associated with methemoglobinemia, which is confirmed by an elevated methemoglobin level. There are many potential causes, including anesthetics, nitrates, and antimalarials. Among the local anesthetics, benzocaine is most commonly associated with methemoglobinemia. The antidote is methylene blue, which reduces the iron in the methemoglobin back to the ferrous state. Methylene blue is indicated in symptomatic patients or asymptomatic patients with a methemoglobin level greater than 25%.

Hyperbaric oxygen is sometimes used for carbon monoxide poisoning, which is unlikely in this patient. Positive pressure ventilation is unlikely to improve his cyanosis given that he is not in respiratory distress, and his issue is oxygenation, not ventilation. Hydroxocobalamin is indicated for the treatment of cyanide toxicity, not methemoglobinemia.

Test-taking tip: A low pulse oximetry read that does not improve with oxygen in the setting of a possible toxidrome is methemoglobinemia until proved otherwise.

28. ANSWER: B

This patient is likely experiencing NMS from his antipsychotic medications. The hallmark findings of NMS are fever, muscle rigidity, altered mental status, and autonomic instability. Patients may develop transaminitis, rhabdomyolysis, acute kidney injury, and metabolic acidosis. NMS can be fatal.

This condition does not indicate overdose because levels are generally within therapeutic range. Rather, NMS tends to occur after initiating therapy or changing the dose. Treatment is supportive, and all antipsychotics should be discontinued. Dantrolene, bromocriptine, and amantadine have all been proposed as treatments for NMS, but the evidence is lacking.

Diphenhydramine is commonly used with antipsychotics to prevent extrapyramidal symptoms; however, it does not have a role in the treatment of NMS.

Cyproheptadine is indicated for the treatment of serotonin syndrome. While serotonin syndrome shares many features with NMS, such as hyperthermia, altered mental status, and hypertonia, it can be distinguished by the presence of myoclonus and exposure to serotonergic medications.

While cooling measures should be initiated, acetaminophen is not indicated because it does not lower body temperature in NMS.

Test-taking tip: This is a "you know it or don't" kind of question. If you don't know it, choose an answer and move on. You can perhaps mark it for review when you are done at the end of the test. Don't, however, let these kinds of questions get you stuck and waste your time.

29. ANSWER: B

This presentation is consistent with chronic colchicine toxicity. This patient has a history of gout that may be treated with colchicine. He also has renal insufficiency, and potentially some degree of liver dysfunction from his alcohol abuse, both of which can increase colchicine levels, ultimately resulting in toxicity. Colchicine inhibits formation of microtubules, thereby arresting cells in mitosis. Effects of chronic toxicity include bone marrow suppression, proximal muscle weakness, and polyneuropathy. Acute toxicity may result in vomiting, bloody diarrhea, lactic acidosis, rhabdomyolysis, delirium, seizures, and death.

Clozapine may cause agranulocytosis, seizures, and pancreatitis but is not generally associated with proximal muscle weakness or neuropathy. This patient is also unlikely to be on clozapine because it is an antipsychotic, not antidepressant.

Botulism is a neuromuscular disorder that classically causes descending paralysis that affects bulbar muscles first. It does not cause sensory deficits or pancytopenia.

Lisinopril is an angiotensin-converting enzyme (ACE) inhibitor that is used to treat hypertension. The most common side effect is dry cough, but ACE inhibitors have also been associated with angioedema. They do not cause significant morbidity in overdose.

Test-taking tip: When faced with a question for which you don't solidly know the answer, a helpful strategy is to eliminate answer choices that are clearly wrong, such as lisinopril toxicity for this question.

30. ANSWER: D

This child ingested sodium hydroxide, which is an alkaline substance commonly used in drain cleaner. Alkaline ingestions produce liquefaction necrosis and therefore may result in extensive tissue damage, including esophageal and/or tracheal perforation. Alternatively, acid ingestions result in coagulation necrosis and thus are less likely to cause significant tissue injury. In patients with evidence of serious injury, such as airway compromise, significant oropharyngeal burns, or active vomiting, early consultation with a gastroenterologist for possible endoscopy is indicated. Endoscopy is the best method to assess the extent of the injury and determine the proper course of treatment. It should be done ideally within the first 12 hours to prevent iatrogenic perforation.

Attempts at neutralization will produce heat, ultimately resulting in more damage, and therefore should be avoided. Activated charcoal is contraindicated in caustic ingestions because it will prevent adequate endoscopic evaluation of the tissues, and it typically does not bind caustic agents well. Gastric lavage is unlikely to be helpful, and in general, nasogastric tubes should not be placed until endoscopy has been performed to assess the extent of the tissue damage.

Test-taking tip: This is a "you know it or don't" kind of question. If you don't know it, choose an answer and move on. You can perhaps mark it for review when you are done at the end of the test. Don't, however, let these kinds of questions get you stuck and waste your time.

31. ANSWER: C

Tramadol is an analgesic that acts at the μ-opioid receptor, although it is structurally unrelated to other opioids. Tramadol is known to lower the seizure threshold. This patient was likely prescribed this medication for postoperative pain control.

Acetaminophen, when taken in excess, may result in liver toxicity but is not typically associated with seizures. Ibuprofen overdoses are often asymptomatic or may be associated with mild gastrointestinal symptoms. Only massive ingestions of ibuprofen have been associated with seizures, and therefore this choice is less likely to be the cause of this patient's seizure.

Hydrocodone is an opioid pain medication that may be associated with lethargy and respiratory depression. While certain opioids may cause seizure when overdosed, this is rare, and seizure is not generally caused by hydrocodone.

Test-taking tip: Tramadol is the only analgesic at therapeutic doses known to cause seizures.

32. ANSWER: C

This patient was most likely exposed to hydrofluoric acid, which is commonly found in glass etcher and rust remover. When hydrofluoric acid comes in contact with skin, the fluoride ions penetrate deeply and rapidly bind calcium. This may result in extensive tissue loss, bone destruction, systemic hypocalcemia, and hypomagnesemia. Hyperkalemia may also be due to cellular destruction. Any contaminated

clothing should be removed, and the affected area should initially be irrigated to remove any residual acid solution. After decontamination, a calcium gluconate gel should be applied topically. Depending on the severity of the exposure, patients may also require IV, or even intra-arterial, calcium. Electrolyte disturbances can result in dysrhythmias that may be fatal and should therefore be corrected.

Antibiotics are not indicated. Surgical debridement may be necessary if calcium therapy fails, but this should not be the initial treatment modality. Finally, bacitracin and petrolatum-impregnated gauze are commonly used for a variety of both thermal and chemical burns, but this is not appropriate in the management of hydrofluoric acid given the extensive tissue damage and systemic effects that may occur if the highly reactive fluoride ions are not neutralized.

Test-taking tip: Calcium gluconate stands out as different form the other three answers, making it most likely the correct answer.

33. ANSWER: C

This patient is exhibiting classic signs of a cholinergic toxidrome, likely from organophosphate exposure at her job on the farm. Organophosphates inhibit the enzyme acetylcholinesterase, resulting in excess levels of acetylcholine. The antidote for this poisoning is atropine, which reverses the muscarinic but not the nicotinic effects of organophosphates. Muscle weakness is a nicotinic effect and therefore will persist after atropine administration, while the other symptoms should improve.

The mnemonics DUMBELS and SLUDGE have been used to describe the clinical effects of a cholinergic toxidrome. DUMBELS stands for diarrhea, urination, miosis, bradycardia, bronchorrhea, bronchospasm, emesis, lacrimation, and salivation. SLUDGE stands for salivation, lacrimation, urination, defecation, gastrointestinal motility (emesis), and eyes (miosis). Patients often die as a result of the "killer Bs," including bradycardia, bronchorrhea, and bronchospasm.

Test-taking tip: Brush up on common toxidromes that present to the ED before the test, including anticholinergic, cholinergic, sedative-hypnotic, opioid, and stimulant.

34. ANSWER: A

This patient has a supratherapeutic INR without any evidence of active bleeding. In patients with an INR >9 without bleeding, warfarin should be held, and the patient should be given vitamin K.

If the INR is <5 without bleeding, warfarin is held, but vitamin K is typically not indicated. There is some disagreement about how best to handle an INR between 5 and 9 without bleeding; Some providers will simply hold warfarin and monitor the INR closely, while others will give a dose of vitamin K, particularly if there is any concern that the patient may be at risk for bleeding (older adult, recent surgery, concomitant use of antiplatelet medications, liver disease).

In nonbleeding patients, PCC and FFP should not be given because of the risk for transfusion reactions and fluid overload.

Test-taking tip: Less is usually appropriate in asymptomatic patients, allowing you to eliminate answers B and C.

35. ANSWER: B

This child most likely ingested camphor oil. Camphor oil is an essential oil that stimulates the central nervous system to cause seizures that are refractory to antiepileptic medications and may result in status epilepticus. It is commonly found in over-the-counter decongestant ointments, but it is also sold as pure oil.

Nutmeg contains myristica oil, which is a hallucinogen and has amphetamine-like effects. Oil of wintergreen contains methyl salicylate and may result in salicylate toxicity. Tea tree oil ingestion may result in lethargy, confusion, and ataxia.

Test-taking tip: This is a "you know it or don't" kind of question. If you don't know it, choose an answer and move on. You can perhaps mark it for review when you are done at the end of the test. Don't, however, let these kinds of questions get you stuck and waste your time.

36. ANSWER: D

This patient is likely intoxicated with PCP. PCP is a dissociative anesthetic that is abused for recreation. It produces euphoria and hallucinations but is primarily known for causing significant agitation and violent behavior. Both vertical and horizontal nystagmus are associated with PCP intoxication.

Cocaine and methamphetamine both result in a sympathomimetic toxidrome and may be associated with hallucinations, but neither causes vertical nystagmus. LSD is a potent hallucinogen but also does not produce vertical nystagmus.

Test-taking tip: Brush up on common toxidromes that present to the ED before the test, including anticholinergic, cholinergic, sedative-hypnotic, opioid, and stimulant.

37. ANSWER: B

The Portuguese man-of-war is a jellyfish found in the Atlantic, Pacific, and Indian Oceans that is capable of delivering an excruciatingly painful sting by harpoon-like nematocysts. The initial treatment of most jellyfish stings, including the Portuguese man-of-war, involves irrigation with salt water to remove as many of the nematocysts as possible. This should be followed by warm water immersion because the toxin is heat labile.

Tap water should not be used because the hypotonic solution may cause the nematocysts to fire, resulting in worsening pain. Acetic acid is found in vinegar and is commonly used to irrigate jellyfish stings, but in general, this is not recommended, and with certain species of jellyfish, it may even worsen stinging.

Test-taking tip: Brush up on common envenomations that present to the ED and their treatment.

38. ANSWER: D

This presentation is consistent with levamisole-induced vasculitis. Levamisole is an antihelminthic agent that is often used to cut cocaine. Levamisole was pulled from the market after it was found to cause vasculitis and agranulocytosis but is still used in veterinary medicine. Exposure may result in skin necrosis that primarily involves the nose and ears. Treatment is primarily supportive, and patients should avoid further cocaine use because recurrence is likely with repeat exposure.

Lead toxicity may present with confusion, ataxia, foot or wrist drop, microcytic anemia, abdominal pain, and constipation. Manifestations of mercury toxicity vary based on the form of mercury, as well as the route and chronicity of exposure. Signs and symptoms may include tremor, ataxia, memory issues, paresthesias, visual changes, pneumonitis, gingivostomatitis, hemorrhagic gastroenteritis, and renal failure.

Boric acid is another agent commonly used to adulterate cocaine. If ingested in sufficient quantities, boric acid may cause diarrhea and vomiting with a blue-green discoloration, seizures, renal failure, and an erythematous rash that is said to look like "boiled lobster."

Test-taking tip: Brush up on common toxidromes that present to the ED before the test, including anticholinergic, cholinergic, sedative-hypnotic, opioid, and stimulant.

39. ANSWER: A

Allergies to local anesthetics are rare but occur in much higher incidence with ester-linked anesthetics than amide-linked anesthetics. Tetracaine is ester-linked, as are procaine, benzocaine, and chloroprocaine. Remember the esters have one I in their names, while the amides have two I's. Given that this patient has had a serious allergic reaction to tetracaine in the past, it would be safer to use an amide-linked anesthetic such as bupivacaine.

Test-taking tip: Ester has no I and is allergic; amide has an I and is less allergenic.

40. ANSWER: C

This patient is exhibiting signs of strychnine poisoning, including opisthotonus (muscle spasms that cause arching of the back and neck) and facial grimacing. Strychnine toxicity can look similar to tetanus. Mental status is typically normal, and patients are painfully aware of the muscle spasms. Death may be caused by respiratory arrest or renal failure from rhabdomyolysis. Strychnine is found in rodenticides and sometimes used as an adulterant in heroin.

Serotonin syndrome and NMS both result in hypertonia but are generally accompanied by altered mental status. Opisthotonus is not typical in either serotonin syndrome or NMS.

Although strychnine-induced spasms can look similar to the tonic phase of generalized seizures, they differ in that patients are alert throughout the episodes.

Test-taking tip: This is a strange presentation that should make you think of a strange diagnosis, strychnine poisoning.

41. ANSWER: C

This patient is most likely suffering from a black widow spider envenomation. The black widow is common in California, and exposures typically occur outdoors. Most bites involve the extremities. This patient's symptoms are characteristic. Muscle spasms commonly occur in the abdomen, chest, and back and may mimic a surgical abdomen.

Necrosis at the bite site is a feature of brown recluse spider envenomation but does not occur with black widow bites. In fact, the bite itself is generally minor.

While death may occur with black widow envenomations, it is uncommon, even in young children who tend to manifest more severe reactions.

Patients often have severe pain in the bitten extremity and may develop paresthesias, but compartment syndrome is unlikely.

The most likely outcome is recovery without sequelae after treatment with opioids and benzodiazepines to control pain and muscle spasms. Antivenom is generally reserved for severe envenomations unresponsive to supportive treatment because allergic reactions are common, and risks may outweigh benefits in this generally self-resolving condition.

Test-taking tip: Brush up on common envenomations that present to the ED and their treatment and outcomes.

42. ANSWER: A

The child likely drank methanol-containing windshield washer fluid. Other common sources of methanol available around the home include carburetor-cleaning fluids, model engine fuels, Sterno, shellacs, lacquers, adhesives, and inks. This case also illustrates a common route of exposure. Parents and others commonly rebottle potentially dangerous solutions into unmarked containers. Many potentially toxic alcohols look like fluids that may appeal to a child (e.g., a sports drink).

Ethylene glycol is typically green in color because of the addition of fluorescein to aid mechanics in the detection of leaks. Isopropyl alcohol and propylene glycol are both clear. Ethanol similarly is not typically blue in color.

Test-taking tip: Blue equals methanol, and green equals ethylene glycol.

43. ANSWER: B

Homemade alcohols or "moonshine" are a relatively uncommon problem in the United States, but in other parts of the world, this is a common source of toxicity.

Historically, in the United States, stills were made from automobile radiators that contained a significant amount of lead. However, lead toxicity does not typically present with visual disturbances.

Ocular exposure to methanol would not be expected to result in visual disturbances as described.

"Snowstorm" or "static" vision is often described following significant ingestion of methanol. Methanol does inhibit oxidative phosphorylation and therefore can lead to an increase in lactate, but this is not the mechanism of visual disturbances.

The underlying mechanism of visual disturbance in methanol ingestions is thought to involve predominantly the Muller cells, the principle glial cells for photoreceptors and retinal cells. These cells possess the enzymes necessary for conversion of methanol to formic acid, which can destroy retinal cells. Other central nervous system changes, including hypodensities, hemorrhages, and necrosis of the basal ganglia, may occur after significant methanol ingestion.

Test-taking tip: This is a "you know it or don't" kind of question. If you don't know it, choose an answer and move on. You can perhaps mark it for review when you are done at the end of the test. Don't, however, let these kinds of questions get you stuck and waste your time.

44. ANSWER: B

This is a picture of oleander, which is a very common shrub that is used in both home and commercial landscaping. In fact, many highway medians are lined with oleander plants. All parts of the oleander plant contain cardiac glycosides similar to digoxin. Cardiac glycosides act by inhibiting the sodium-potassium ATPase in order to increase intracellular calcium. Fortunately, the primary toxicity following acute ingestions is nausea, vomiting, abdominal pain, and diarrhea. In essence, the body self-expels the foreign substance, preventing further toxicity.

In certain parts of the world, oleander is a common method for self-harm, but these individuals will consume antiemetics concomitantly to prevent vomiting. Fortunately, pediatric ingestions of oleander leaves rarely produce serious clinical toxicity, and therefore removal of the plant is not necessary.

Test-taking tip: This is a common plant, and presentations to the ED for ingestions of it are unheard of, allowing you to eliminate C and D.

45. ANSWER: A

This patient has a classic presentation of salicylate intoxication. The patient's boyfriend just broke up with her (a common inciting event for impetuous ingestions), and she appears to have a change in hearing, tachypnea, and mildly elevated temperature. While tinnitus is most commonly described with salicylate toxicity, other changes in hearing such as rushing sensation or decreased acuity are also described. Additionally, the patient has a mixed acid-base disturbance on blood gas. Both a metabolic acidosis and respiratory alkalosis are present, and the anion gap is elevated.

The patient's normal mental status argues against methanol intoxication. With methanol, the patient would be expected to have a decreased level of consciousness by the time the acid-base disturbance develops. The normal blood sugar argues against diabetic ketoacidosis, and excessive vomiting alone should not cause the clinical presentation described.

Test-taking tip: A mixed acid-base disturbance (both a metabolic acidosis and respiratory alkalosis) is almost always salicylate toxicity in the setting of a potential ingestion.

46. ANSWER: D

Sodium bicarbonate is the most appropriate answer choice. The patient is manifesting prolongation of the QRS, a known effect of TCAs in overdose caused by sodium channel blockage. Of the answer choices listed, only sodium bicarbonate can reverse this effect.

Calcium gluconate is used in the treatment of hyperkalemia. TCAs are not anticipated to cause hyperkalemia. Magnesium sulfate is used in the treatment of torsades de pointes, which is not demonstrated in this EKG. Potassium chloride is used to treat hypokalemia. Hypokalemia manifests with a long QT interval, T wave flattening, and the development of U waves. These are not present in the EKG.

Test-taking tip: A prolonged QRS in the setting of suspected or confirmed ingestion should be treated with sodium bicarbonate regardless of the cause.

47. ANSWER: B

The most appropriate agent listed to treat seizures in TCA overdose is lorazepam.

Flumazenil is used to reverse benzodiazepine overdoses in the setting where it is known that a benzodiazepine is the only involved agent (e.g., reversal from procedural sedation).

Physostigmine is used as antidotal therapy in antimuscarinic (anticholinergic) toxicity.

Sodium bicarbonate can be used to narrow the QRS complex in TCA and other sodium channel blocking drug overdoses, but it will not treat the seizures.

Test-taking tip: Benzodiazepines are first-line therapy of most seizures, regardless of their etiology.

48. ANSWER: B

This patient is in status epilepticus that is refractory to multiple agents in a setting of possible ingestion; this should raise the concern for isoniazid ingestion. The treatment for seizures related to isoniazid ingestions is pyridoxine. Pyridoxine should be given in a dose equivalent to the suspected amount of isoniazid ingested. If the amount of ingested isoniazid is not known, 5 g of pyridoxine should be given IV over 5 to 10 minutes. Dosing should be repeated until seizure activity ceases.

Additional doses of benzodiazepines are unlikely to have any benefit in this case scenario. While carbamazepine and levetiracetam may be tried, if the seizures are in fact related to isoniazid, these are also unlikely to be effective in controlling the seizure activity.

Test-taking tip: Refractory seizures in the setting of a possible ingestion should make you think isoniazid ingestion.

18.

TRAUMA AND ORTHOPEDIC EMERGENCIES

Anjali Gupta, Jordan Harp, and Desiree Crane

1. A 65-year-old man presents after a ground-level fall. He opens his eyes to voice, localizes to sternal rub, and can tell you his name. Which of the following would you most likely expect to see on computed tomography (CT) of his head?

A. Biconvex-shaped white density
B. Crescent-shaped white density
C. White densities in the cisterns and sulci
D. A normal head CT

2. Which of the following clinical situations would warrant emergent evacuation of an acute subdural hematoma (SDH)?

A. A patient with a Glasgow Coma Scale (GCS) score of 12 with a subdural but no midline shift on CT
B. A patient who with a GCS score of 14 with a slim subdural of less than 10 mm on CT
C. A comatose patient with a GCS score drop of two points from the time of injury to hospital presentation
D. A patient taking antiplatelet medications with a subdural of less than 5 mm on CT who has a GCS score of 15

3. A 21-year-old male presents to the emergency department (ED) following a bar fight during which he is struck in the head with an unknown object. A CT scan of the brain shows a basilar skull fracture. What physical exam finding is most highly associated with this injury?

A. Periorbital ecchymosis
B. Blurry vision
C. Ecchymosis behind the ears
D. Subconjunctival hemorrhage

4. A 14-year-old female is brought in by her parents after being struck in the head by a soccer ball during a game earlier. She complains of a headache and feeling dizzy after getting hit. She denies loss of consciousness or any nausea, vomiting, or vision changes. On exam, she is acting appropriately and has no signs of trauma or any gross neurologic deficits. What is the most appropriate management for this patient?

A. Obtain a head CT
B. Consult pediatrics
C. Discharge and clear for return to sports
D. Discharge with instructions to not return to sports until further evaluation as an outpatient

5. A 9-year-old presents with the finding in Figure 18.1 after falling forward onto concrete. What is the most appropriate management of this condition?

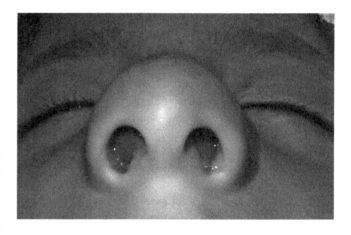

Figure 18.1 Nares.

A. Nasal packing
B. Discharge with no treatment in the ED and referral to ear-nose-throat (ENT) clinic
C. Obtain a maxillofacial CT
D. Perform incision and drainage

6. In an orbital blowout fracture, what wall is most commonly involved?

  A. Inferior
  B. Lateral
  C. Medial
  D. Superior

7. What nerve is most commonly injured in an orbital blowout fracture?

  A. Inferior orbital nerve
  B. Anterior-superior alveolar nerve
  C. Zygomatic branch of facial nerve
  D. Oculomotor nerve

8. A 40-year-old female presents after a high-speed motor vehicle collision (MVC). She was the unrestrained front seat passenger. She complains of face pain. On exam, you note that the hard palate and nose move independently of the eyes with pressure. What is the classification of this injury?

  A. Le Fort I
  B. Le Fort II
  C. Le Fort III
  D. Le Fort IV

9. A 28-year-old male presents after being assaulted. He was punched once on the left side of his face. He now reports pain over the angle of the mandible. On exam, he has small cuts on his cheek, left lip, and inside of his mouth. A panorex shows a fracture of the mandible. What is the most appropriate management of this patient?

  A. Discharge with a 2-week course of amoxicillin/ clavulanate and follow up with primary care physician
  B. Administer penicillin G IV and consult oral maxillofacial surgeon
  C. Obtain a maxillofacial CT
  D. See if patient can tolerate food and water, and if he can, discharge him with outpatient follow-up with his primary care physician

10. A 17-year-old male presents after being stabbed on the left side of the chest. His initial vital signs are blood pressure (BP) 80/50 mm Hg, heart rate (HR) 127 bpm, and respiratory rate (RR) 28 breaths/min. Physical exam reveals a young male who is alert and talking but in severe respiratory distress. Breath sounds are absent over the left hemithorax, and his trachea is deviated to the right. What is the most appropriate initial management of this patient?

  A. Chest radiograph
  B. Chest tube placement on right side

C. Needle decompression
D. Endotracheal intubation

11. A 45-year-old female presents after an MVC. She was the restrained driver of a car that hit a tree at a moderate rate of speed. She complains of chest pain. Her initial chest radiograph is negative, but a sternal fracture is diagnosed on chest CT. Vital signs are within normal limits during her ED stay. An electrocardiogram (EKG) is unchanged from prior. Her pain is controlled with oral analgesics. What is the most appropriate next step in the management of this patient?

  A. Obtain a stat EKG
  B. Admit to surgical service
  C. Discharge with outpatient follow-up
  D. Admit to telemetry

12. A 50-year-old male presents after an MVC. He was a restrained driver who was going about 55 mph when he lost control and struck the freeway median. He recalls striking his chest against the steering wheel. He complains of chest pain in his mid to left chest. His vital signs are BP 140/90 mm Hg, HR 115 bpm, and RR 18 breaths/min. The lateral view of his chest radiograph is shown in Figure 18.2. What is the next most appropriate diagnostic testing you should order on this patient?

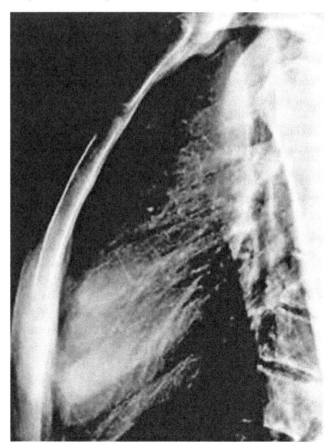

Figure 18.2 Lateral chest radiograph.

A. Cardiac CT
B. Echocardiogram
C. EKG and troponin I
D. Troponin I

13. A 52-year-old female presents after a moderate-speed MVC. She complains only of neck pain and has midline tenderness to palpation on exam. She has normal strength in both upper and lower extremities, and sensation is intact. A CT of the cervical spine is obtained that demonstrates a unilateral facet dislocation at C5 and C6. What is the most appropriate next step in management of this patient?

A. MRI cervical spine
B. Urgent neurosurgery consultation
C. Discharge with cervical collar and outpatient follow-up with neurosurgery
D. Obtain a computed tomography angiogram (CTA) of the neck

14. A fracture of which of the following would prompt the greatest suspicion for associated pulmonary injury?

A. Scapula
B. Sternum
C. Spinal transverse process
D. Clavicle

15. A 75-year-old male presents after being hit in the head with his garage door. He currently has a GCS score of 14. Exam shows an abrasion to the top of his scalp. His head CT head is shown in Figure 18.3. He takes warfarin for atrial fibrillation. His international normalized ratio (INR) is 2.7. What is the most appropriate next step in treatment?

A. PO vitamin K
B. Cryoprecipitate
C. Prothrombin complex concentrate (PCC)
D. Platelets

16. A 20-year-old female presents after being stabbed by her boyfriend in the right upper back and right chest. Initial vital signs are BP 120/75 mm Hg, HR 105 bpm, RR 18 breaths/min, and oxygen saturation 95%. She complains of some mild shortness of breath. Her initial chest radiograph is shown in Figure 18.4. What is the most appropriate treatment plan for this patient?

A. Insert a chest tube into the right pleural space
B. Perform needle decompression
C. Discharge patient with outpatient follow-up
D. Observe patient and repeat chest radiograph in 4–6 hours

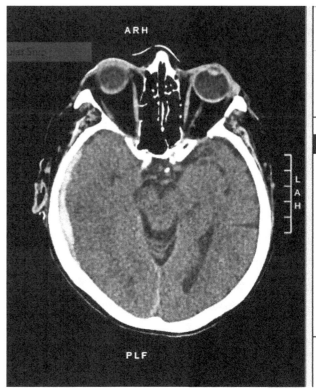

Figure 18.3 Head computed tomography.

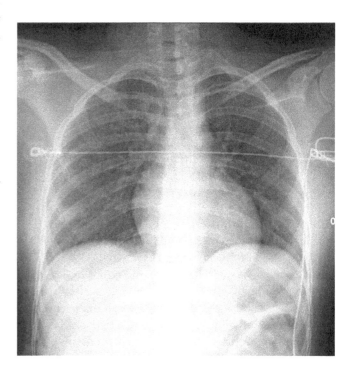

Figure 18.4 Chest radiograph.

17. In which of the following patients should an ED resuscitative thoracotomy be considered?

A. A 25-year-old male with stab wound to the chest in respiratory distress with BP 95/palp mm Hg and HR 119 bpm

B. A 46-year-old female with self-inflected gunshot wound whose initial BP was 60/palp mm Hg, now 110/60 mm Hg after 2 L of normal saline and 1 unit of packed red blood cells (pRBCs)

C. A 36-year-old male with gunshot wound to the left chest in whom cardiopulmonary resuscitation (CPR) has been ongoing for 20 minutes

D. A 20-year-male in motorcycle crash with extensive bruising over chest who becomes unresponsive on arrival to the ED

18. Which of the following patients can be cleared by the NEXUS cervical spine criteria?

A. A 47-year-old male following an MVC, who drank a pint of vodka 2 hours ago, denies any midline neck pain or tenderness to palpation and is moving all of his extremities

B. An 86-year-old female with a history of dementia who presents after a ground-level fall. She denies midline neck pain or tenderness to palpation and has normal strength but is only able to tell you her name

C. A 37-year-old male involved in an MVC who has a GCS score of 15 with no neurologic deficits but who is in distress because of pain and has a clinical left femur fracture

D. A 59-year-old male who fell down two stairs, hit his head, and suffered from a loss of consciousness. He currently has a GCS score of 15 with a contusion to his forehead but with an otherwise normal physical exam

19. A 26-year-old male presents after accidentally being shot with a 45-caliber handgun. The patient presents awake, alert, and speaking but in respiratory distress, with vital signs showing RR 28 breaths/min, oxygen saturation of 92%, and BP 135/85 mm Hg. Physical exam shows a penetrating wound to the right side of the chest that appears to be leaking air. What is the most appropriate immediate management for this patient?

A. Obtain a portable chest radiograph
B. Needle decompression of right chest
C. Apply a three-sided dressing to the chest wound
D. Endotracheal intubation

20. What is the preferred site for a tube thoracostomy for a pneumothorax?

A. Second intercostal space mid-clavicular line above the rib
B. Fifth intercostal space mid-axillary line below the rib
C. Fifth intercostal space mid-axillary line above the rib
D. Sixth intercostal space mid-axillary line above the rib

21. A 41-year-old female presents after an MVC. She was going about 65 mph when she hit another car. She was not wearing a seat belt. On presentation, vital signs are BP 95/palp mm Hg, HR 121 bpm, and oxygen saturation 94%. She is in distress and complains of chest pain and shortness of breath. Physical exam shows a round contusion on her chest. What is the most sensitive finding on chest radiography for aortic injury in this patient?

A. Widened mediastinum
B. Fracture of the first rib
C. Hemothorax
D. Scapular fracture

22. A 19-year-old female presents after getting hit in the face by a softball. She complains of severe pain and vision loss in the right eye. Physical exam demonstrates extensive swelling and ecchymosis around the right eye. Intraocular pressure (IOP) testing demonstrates a pressure of 53 mm Hg. What is the most appropriate immediate management at this time?

A. Obtain orbits CT
B. Provide analgesia and a cool compress to the eye
C. Administer acetazolamide orally
D. Perform a lateral canthotomy

23. A patient presents after being hit in the head. Physical exam shows the finding in Figure 18.5. What medication should be avoided in this patient?

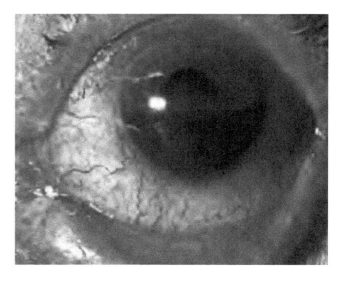

Figure 18.5 Eye.

A. Toradol
B. Morphine
C. Acetazolamide
D. Topical corticosteroids

24. A 39-year-old male presents after being assaulted with a baseball bat to the face and head. The patient currently has a GCS score of 15. He exhibits diffuse facial ecchymosis and swelling. No other findings are noted on physical exam. A maxillofacial CT is obtained that demonstrates a Le Fort III fracture. CT scans of the head and cervical spine are negative. In addition to consulting with an oral maxillofacial surgeon, which of the following is recommended at this time?

A. Chest, abdomen, and pelvis CT
B. Nasogastric tube
C. Soft tissue neck radiograph
D. CTA of the neck

25. Which of the following is considered an unstable cervical spine injury?

A. Unilateral facet dislocation
B. Clay shoveler's fracture
C. Transverse process fracture
D. Hangman's fracture

26. A 19-year-old male patient is brought in by ambulance after falling 50 feet while rock climbing. His GCS score is 8, and he was intubated on arrival to the ED for airway protection. Which of the following should be avoided in this patient?

A. Methylprednisolone
B. Mannitol
C. Levetiracetam
D. Ketamine

27. What is the most common cardiac dysrhythmia seen after traumatic brain injury (TBI)?

A. Prolonged QT interval
B. First-degree atrioventricular (AV) block
C. Supraventricular tachycardia (SVT)
D. Ventricular tachycardia

28. An 8-month-old presents after being accidentally dropped by his 10-year-old sibling onto a carpeted surface about 20 minutes before presentation. His mother reports that 1 or 2 seconds after being dropped he started crying. Other than being fussy, he is acting normally according to the mother. Physical exam shows a fussy, active infant. He has a hematoma over his forehead but

otherwise no other signs of trauma. What is the most appropriate management at this time?

A. Head CT
B. Admit to pediatric service
C. Discharge with outpatient follow-up
D. Administer Keppra for seizure prophylaxis

29. A 37-year-old female presents after an MVC. On exam, she is able to shrug her shoulders but has no motor function caudally. At what spinal cord level has this patient suffered a cord injury?

A. C5
B. C6
C. C7
D. T1

30. A 54-year-old male presents after an MVC. He was not wearing a seat belt and hit his chest on the steering wheel. He is hypotensive and tachycardic. He complains of pain in the middle of his back. You are concerned about aortic rupture. Where is the most common site of injury for this condition?

A. Ascending aorta
B. Descending thoracic aorta at the subclavian artery
C. Descending thoracic aorta at the diaphragm
D. Abdominal aorta

31. A 45-year-old female presents after an MVC. She complains of chest pain and shortness of breath. Her RR is 26 breaths/min, HR 110 bpm, and BP 115/79 mm Hg. Her chest radiograph is shown in Figure 18.6. What is the appropriate management for this patient?

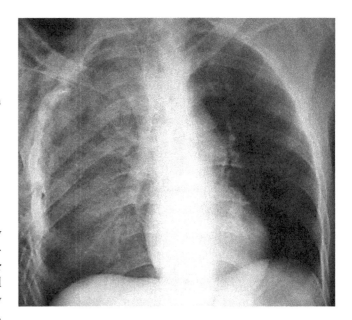

Figure 18.6 Chest radiograph.

A. Aggressive fluid resuscitation
B. Steroids
C. Positive pressure ventilation
D. Antibiotics

32. **A 33-year-old presents after an MVC. He was going about 30 miles per hour when he hit a pole. He was wearing a seat belt, and the airbags deployed. He denies loss of consciousness. He endorses chest pain. On exam, he does not exhibit any tenderness to the chest wall, sternum, scapula, or thoracic spine. His lungs are clear to auscultation bilaterally. He currently has a GCS score of 15. He has no other identifiable injuries on exam. His initial chest radiograph does not show any acute intrathoracic pathology. What is the most appropriate next step in the management of this patient?**

A. Chest CT
B. Head CT
C. Consult trauma surgery
D. Discharge with pain medication

33. **A patient presents after his car fell on him while he was working under it. He is hypotensive and tachypneic. A chest tube is placed on the right side because of a hemothorax on chest radiograph. At what amount of immediate drainage from the chest tube should an urgent operative thoracotomy be considered?**

A. 500 mL
B. 200 mL
C. 750 mL
D. 1,500 mL

34. **A 20-year-old male gets hit in the right eye by a baseball during a game. On exam, there is significant periorbital swelling, and a picture of the eye is shown in Figure 18.7. His vision is 20/30 in the left eye and 20/200 in the right. Which of the following should be avoided in this patient?**

A. Antibiotics
B. Ketamine
C. IOP measurement
D. Fluorescein

35. **A 32-year-old professional bicyclist presents to your ED after he was struck by a vehicle while on a training ride. He is tachycardic and hypotensive with some abdominal bruising. What is the initial preferred imaging?**

A. Immediate CT of the abdomen and pelvis with IV contrast
B. Kidney-ureter-bladder (KUB) study

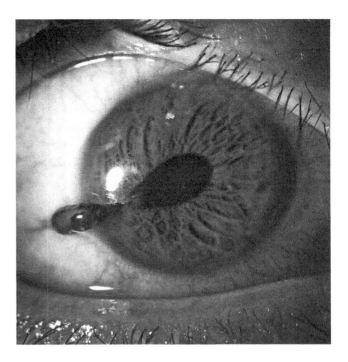

Figure 18.7 Eye.

C. Bedside ultrasound/focused assessment with sonography for trauma (FAST) exam
D. Diagnostic peritoneal lavage (DPL)

36. **Which of the following is true regarding imaging studies for assessment of injuries in blunt abdominal trauma?**

A. In hemodynamically unstable patients with a positive FAST exam, CT is recommended
B. IV, PO, and rectal contrast CT is the preferred diagnostic study for determining injuries of the bowel, diaphragm, and pancreas in blunt abdominal trauma
C. Oral contrast is not essential to the evaluation of blunt abdominal trauma
D. DPL is reliable for detecting bowel injuries and retroperitoneal injuries.

37. **A 27-year-old female was thrown from her horse and presents with complaints of abdominal pain, chest pain, and shortness of breath. Vital signs reveal HR 110 bpm, BP 148/82 mm Hg, RR 20 breaths/min, and oxygen saturation 90% on room air. On your exam, you auscultate borborygmi in the left lower pulmonary field. The chest radiograph obtained is seen in Figure 18.8. What is your diagnosis?**

A. Hiatal hernia
B. Ruptured bleb

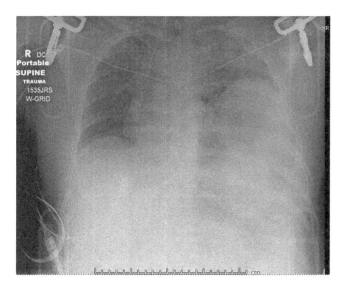

Figure 18.8 Chest radiograph.

C. Diaphragmatic injury
D. Pneumomediastinum

38. An obese 52-year-old female who was a restrained driver (lap belt only) presents to the ED after rear-ending another vehicle while traveling 50 mph. Exam reveals a "seat belt" sign. CT of spine is obtained and seen in Figure 18.9. Initial FAST exam is negative, and

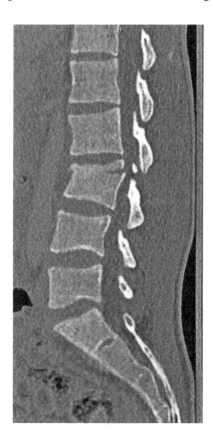

Figure 18.9 Spine computed tomography.

CT of the abdomen and pelvis is unremarkable. What is the most appropriate next step in management?

A. Admit for observation and serial abdominal exams
B. Orthopedics consult
C. Perform a DPL
D. Order magnetic resonance imaging (MRI) of the spine

39. A 19-year-old restrained driver presents after a high-speed rollover MVC. He is tachycardic and hypotensive. On exam, he is noted to have a "seat belt sign" and diffuse tenderness to palpation of his abdomen. He endorses some left shoulder pain with a normal shoulder exam. He is persistently tachycardic and hypotensive despite aggressive fluid resuscitation. Your FAST exam is inconclusive. You prepare to transfuse blood. What is the most appropriate next step?

A. Immediate IV contrast CT of abdomen and pelvis
B. Immediate surgical consultation and laparotomy
C. Re-evaluate vital signs after your patient has received the blood transfusion
D. Repeat FAST exam in 20 minutes

40. What is the most commonly injured organ with penetrating stab wounds to the abdomen?

A. Colon
B. Small bowel
C. Liver
D. Kidney

41. A 26-year-old female who is in her third trimester of pregnancy presents to your ED as a trauma patient. She was a restrained driver of a vehicle that rear-ended another vehicle at low speeds. There was no airbag deployment. Vital signs are stable. She has some mild low abdominal pain without bruising or vaginal bleeding. Chest radiograph, bedside ultrasound, and urinalysis are unremarkable. What is the most appropriate next step in this patient's management?

A. External tocodynamometric monitoring for a minimum of 4–6 hours
B. Admit for serial abdominal exams
C. Emergent obstetric/gynecologic (OB/GYN) consultation for sterile speculum exam
D. Discharge home with outpatient OB/GYN follow-up and strict return precautions

42. All of the following regarding abdominal trauma in a pregnant patient are true *except*:

A. Tetanus prophylaxis should be given for appropriate indications
B. Rho(D) immunoglobulin should be administered to all Rh-negative pregnant women with abdominal trauma
C. Pregnant patients should be kept in the semi–lateral decubitus position
D. Ultrasound is the only indicated method of imaging for trauma in pregnant patients

43. A 32-year-old pregnant female is brought to the ED by emergency medical services (EMS). She was in an altercation with her significant other and was hit and kicked in her abdomen. She is having some abdominal pain and vaginal spotting. What is the most sensitive clinical finding for placental abruption?

A. Uterine irritability
B. Fetal tachycardia
C. Loss of uterine contour
D. Vaginal bleeding

44. A 19-year-old pregnant female, estimated to be approximately 26 weeks' pregnant by fundal height, presents to your ED as a trauma patient. She was an unrestrained passenger of a vehicle that was involved in a rollover. On arrival to the ED, she becomes hypotensive and loses pulses. You start chest compressions, intubate her, and provide appropriate advanced cardiac life support (ACLS) treatment. After 4 minutes of resuscitation, she remains pulseless. What is the next most appropriate step in management?

A. Place a femoral central venous catheter
B. Perform FAST exam and ultrasound for fetal evaluation
C. Transfuse 2 units O-negative blood
D. Perform perimortem cesarean delivery

45. An 87-year-old female with a history of osteopenia presents to your ED with complaints of left hip pain after falling while getting up from the toilet. She did not hit her head or pass out. Exam reveals stable vital signs and left iliac tenderness to palpation. She is neurologically intact distally. Her radiographs are unremarkable. She has continued pain, and you astutely order a pelvic CT for further diagnostic evaluation. CT imaging is also negative. She continues to have pain and is unable to bear weight. What is the most appropriate next step in management?

A. Discharge home with pain control, crutches, and follow-up with orthopedics in 1 week
B. Admit for pain control
C. Order a pelvic MRI

D. Discharge to a skilled nursing facility for physical therapy and rehabilitation

46. A 22-year-old female presents to your ED as a trauma patient. She is hypotensive and tachycardic with an unstable pelvis. A pelvic binder is placed, and she initially responds to an IV crystalloid bolus with improvement in her blood pressure. The FAST exam is negative, and a preliminary CT scan of the abdomen and pelvis is negative for solid organ injury. On return from CT, she again becomes hypotensive. What is the most appropriate next step in management?

A. Emergent orthopedics consult and laparotomy
B. Pelvis radiograph
C. Angiography
D. Pelvic exam

47. A 72-year-old intoxicated male presents after he fell from a third-story window. He has low abdominal pain and swelling, an unstable pelvis, scrotal edema, and blood noted at the meatus. What genitourinary (GU) structure should you have a high index of suspicion of injury?

A. Urethra
B. Bladder
C. Ureter
D. Kidney

48. A previously healthy 28-year-old male presents as a walk-in to your ED after an MVC. He was a restrained driver traveling 55 mph and rear-ended another vehicle. His vital signs reveal BP 132/76 mm Hg, HR 95 bpm, RR 14 breaths/min, and oxygen saturation of 99% on room air. He has vague complaints of diffuse flank pain and abdominal pain. On your secondary exam, he has no blood at the meatus, and you proceed to place a Foley catheter with urinalysis showing 75 RBCs per high-power field (hpf). Regarding your patient's hematuria, what is the most appropriate next step in the workup?

A. Nothing, the hematuria is likely related to trauma from the Foley catheter placement
B. Order an outpatient CT cystography
C. Order an intravenous pyelogram (IVP)
D. Obtain an immediate IV contrast CT of the abdomen and pelvis

49. A 58-year-old female presents to your ED as a trauma alert after hitting her face on the bottom of a swimming pool while diving in the shallow end. Your exam reveals bilateral upper extremity weakness and numbness, but normal strength and sensation in the lower extremities. What is your clinical diagnosis?

A. Central cord syndrome
B. Anterior cord syndrome
C. Brown-Sequard syndrome
D. Transient spinal shock

50. Correctly match the neck zone and anatomic boundaries.

    A. Zone I: angle of the mandible and base of the skull
    B. Zone II: clavicles to the cricoid cartilage
    C. Zone II: cricoid cartilage to the angle of the mandible
    D. Zone III: clavicles to the cricoid cartilage

51. Correctly match the penetrating neck injury with the most likely clinical findings.

    A. Vascular injury, hoarseness
    B. Laryngotracheal injury, stridor
    C. Laryngotracheal injury, saliva draining from the wound
    D. Pharyngoesophageal injury, tracheal deviation

52. A 39-year-old male was hunting with his friends when he was accidentally shot with an arrow, which lodged into his neck. He is having some painful difficulty swallowing and has some blood in his mouth. What is the most appropriate imaging to determine the extent of his injuries?

    A. CTA
    B. Esophagram or esophagoscopy
    C. Bronchoscopy
    D. Color-flow Doppler ultrasound

53. A 62-year-old female presents to the ED for evaluation of injuries sustained in a high-speed MVC rollover. She has a GCS score of 8 and notable weakness on the left. Her head CT scan and cervical spine CT scan are negative. You are concerned about possible vertebral artery injury. What is the gold standard for diagnosis of vertebral artery injury in blunt cervical trauma?

    A. CTA
    B. MRI
    C. Duplex ultrasonography
    D. Catheter angiography

54. A 31-year-old male was dropped off at the ambulance bay. He is unconscious and is profusely bleeding from a neck wound. Which of the following statements regarding penetrating neck trauma is correct?

    A. Vascular injuries are the leading cause of death from penetrating neck trauma

B. Zone I is the most commonly injured zone of the neck
C. Management of penetrating wounds in zone II consists of color-flow Doppler ultrasonography
D. Injuries that do not violate the platysma still need imaging to evaluate for damage to vital structures

55. A 22-year-old male with history of IV heroin abuse, who is very well known at your rural ED, presents with severe hand pain after injecting heroin into his wrist vessels. Your exam reveals significant tense swelling of the hand and pain with movement. You are concerned about compartment syndrome. Which of the following is true?

    A. Normal compartment pressure is 20 mm Hg
    B. He only has pain and swelling, and therefore, you cannot diagnose compartment syndrome
    C. Compartment syndrome is a diagnosis of exclusion; you must rule out other sources of his symptoms before diagnosing compartment syndrome
    D. Hand compartment syndrome may not be associated with paresthesia

56. A right-handed male carpenter presents to the ED for evaluation of a right finger injury. He was using a skill saw just before arrival when the saw kicked back, cutting his fingers. He brings with him an amputated finger at the level of the proximal interphalangeal joint. Bleeding is controlled. You assess that this patient is a candidate for reimplantation and provide tetanus update and IV antibiotics. Which of the following is appropriate management of this amputation?

    A. Splint the stump
    B. Clamp arterial bleeders to minimize blood loss
    C. Wrap the amputated digit in gauze and then place it directly on ice
    D. Debride all wound edges

57. A 42-year-old professional house painter presents with finger pain after accidentally shooting himself with paint while checking the nozzle to a pressurized paint gun. His exam reveals a very small puncture wound to the palmar aspect of his index finger with some localized edema. The remainder of his exam is unremarkable. What is the most appropriate management of this injury?

    A. Pain medication, updated tetanus, and discharge home
    B. Radiograph, splint, and discharge home with orthopedic referral
    C. Emergent orthopedics consultation
    D. Irrigate wound and admit for observation

58. You receive an EMS call that they are en route with a 37-year-old who was working outside and involved in a gas explosion. EMS reports that the patient was hypoxic with singeing of eyebrows and nose, stridulous, and coughing up carbonaceous sputum, with severe burns to the face and torso. EMS personnel intubate the patient, and on arrival to the ED, vital signs reveal BP 110/72 mm Hg, HR 105 bpm, and oxygen saturation 92% on 100% FiO_2. You complete your primary survey and appropriately fluid-resuscitate your patient. On your secondary survey, you note circumferential, full-thickness burns to the chest and abdomen. The respiratory therapist then tells you that his peak inspiratory pressure is high at 40 mm H_2O. What is the most appropriate next step?

A. Decrease FiO_2 to 80%
B. Administer IV methylene blue
C. Perform emergent escharotomy
D. Transfer the patient for hyperbaric oxygen therapy

59. A 27-year-old, 90-kg male presents after sustaining partial-thickness circumferential burns to his bilateral lower legs after his pants caught fire. He has no inhalation injury and no other burns. Using the Parkland formula, determine the correct amount of crystalloid solution that is required in the first 8 hours.

A. 3,240 mL
B. 6,480 mL
C. 9,720 mL
D. 12,960 mL

60. Correctly match the depth of burn and initial clinical findings.

A. Superficial burn: redness with associated blistered skin
B. Superficial partial-thickness burn: blistered skin with exposed dermis that is red, moist, painful
C. Deep partial-thickness burn: blistered skin with exposed dermis that is pale, blanchable, and painful
D. Full-thickness burn: charred skin that is pale, leathery, and painful

61. A 45-year-old right-hand–dominant female presents to your ED from a nearby electronics manufacturing plant with severe finger pain after a chemical that she works with contacted her skin through a torn glove. Clinical findings are as noted in Figure 18.10. What is the correct diagnosis and initial treatment?

A. Hydrofluoric acid burn, calcium gluconate gel
B. Thermal burn, skin graft

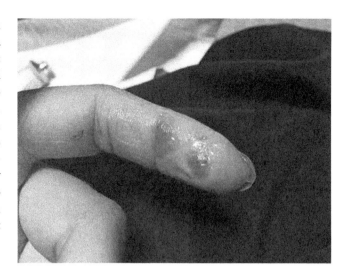

Figure 18.10 Finger.

C. Chemical burn, irrigation with normal saline
D. Phenol burn, irrigation with water

62. Which of the following substances will cause deep tissue burns?

A. Acetic acid
B. Hydrochloric acid
C. Wet cement
D. Sulfuric acid

63. What is the most common finding in cauda equina syndrome?

A. Lower extremity weakness
B. Hyporeflexia
C. Saddle anesthesia
D. Urinary retention

64. A 23-year old-male presents to the ED 1 week after sustaining an open right ankle fracture after an MVC. He underwent an open reduction and internal fixation (ORIF) to the right ankle on the day of injury. He now presents with redness, pain, and swelling to the right lower extremity. You have a high degree of suspicion that the patient has osteomyelitis. Which of the following is the most common causative organism in this scenario?

A. *Pseudomonas aeruginosa*
B. *Staphylococcus aureus*
C. *Salmonella paratyphi*
D. *Haemophilus influenzae*

65. A 25-year-old male comes to the ED after a fall off his unicycle complaining of left wrist pain. His radiograph is shown in Figure 18.11. Which of the following best describes his fracture?

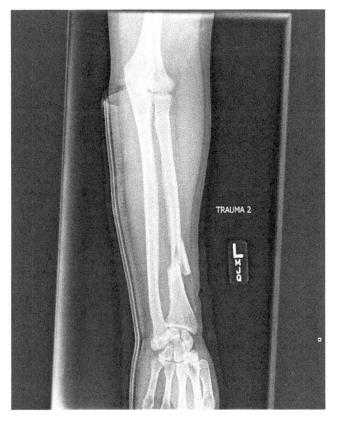

Figure 18.11 Forearm radiograph.

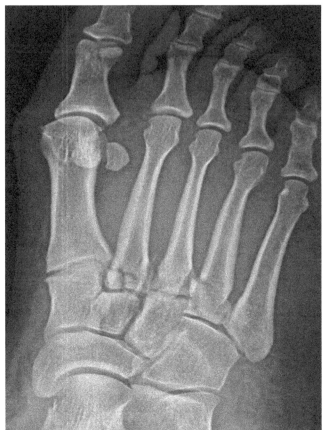

Figure 18.12 Foot radiograph.

A. Colles
B. Monteggia
C. Galeazzi
D. Smith

66. Which of the following is *not* true of the condition depicted in the radiograph shown in Figure 18.12?

A. This injury always results from a high-energy mechanism
B. Patients with this injury commonly have plantar ecchymosis
C. Patients with this injury can be sent home with outpatient orthopedics follow-up
D. This injury would be unlikely to result from an MVC

67. A 40–year-old man fell off his motorcycle and sustained the fracture pictured in Figure 18.13. Which statement is most accurate?

A. This is a Rolando fracture that requires emergent hand service consultation in the ED
B. This is a Bennett fracture, which should be placed in a thumb spica splint and discharged with immediate outpatient hand service follow-up

C. This is a Rolando fracture, which has a worse prognosis than the Bennett fracture
D. This is a Bennett fracture, which has a worse prognosis than the Rolando fracture

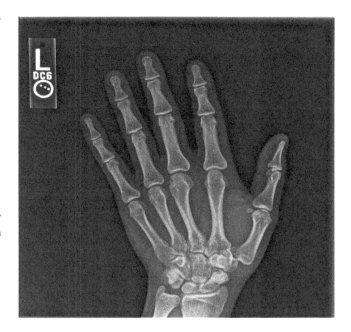

Figure 18.13 Hand radiograph.

68. All of the following are Kanavel's signs *except*:

A. Diffuse fusiform swelling
B. Finger held in slightly flexed position
C. Puncture wound over volar surface
D. Severe pain on extension

69. Which of the following is *not* true of this condition pictured in Figure 18.14?

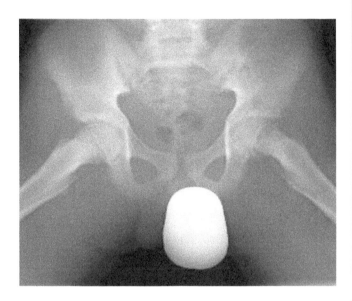

Figure 18.14 Pelvis radiograph.

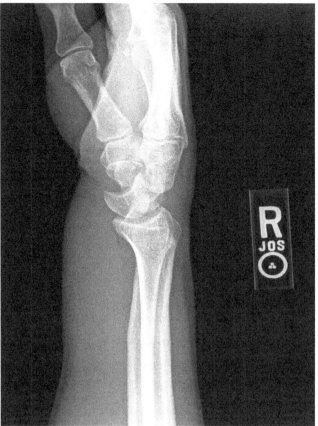

Figure 18.15 Wrist radiograph.

A. Tends to occur in young children about age
   4–8 years
B. Treatment is ORIF
C. Patients are often obese
D. Tends to occur bilaterally

70. The radiograph in Figure 18.15 shows which type of dislocation?

A. Scapholunate dissociation
B. De Quervain's dislocation
C. Lunate dislocation
D. Perilunate dislocation

71. All of the following statements are true of the condition depicted in Figure 18.16 *except*:

A. This condition is relatively uncommon
B. This may be a result of a seizure or electric shock
C. Neurovascular injuries are common
D. Associated fractures are common

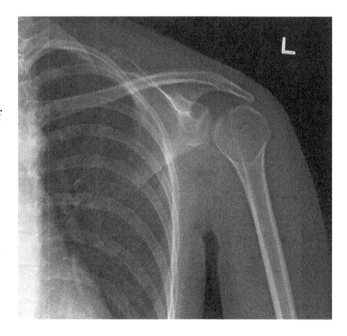

Figure 18.16 Shoulder radiograph.

72. Disruption of the extensor hood mechanism of the finger with intact lateral bands leads to which of the following?

    A. Mallet finger
    B. Boutonnière deformity
    C. Gamekeeper's thumb
    D. Volar plate injury

73. A 45-year-old man presents with knee pain after a high mechanism rollover MVC. There is no deformity, but there is laxity on both anterior and posterior drawer tests. Patient denies any other pain or injuries. Radiograph shows no acute fracture. Which of the following imaging studies would be most important in this patient's acute evaluation?

    A. MRI
    B. CT without contrast
    C. CTA
    D. Radiographs of the joints above and below the injury

74. Which of the following regarding compartment syndrome is *false*?

    A. Injury is most commonly due to a proximal tibial shaft fracture
    B. The earliest symptom is paresthesias
    C. The most commonly injured compartment is the anterior tibial compartment
    D. Compartment pressure of 40–55 mm Hg is an indication for fasciotomy

75. Which of the following is *true* of the fracture pictured in Figure 18.17?

    A. There is a low incidence of nonunion
    B. This fracture occurs at the insertion of the peroneus brevis
    C. This fracture rarely needs operative fixation
    D. The patient should be placed in a non–weight-bearing splint or cast with podiatry/orthopedic follow-up

76. Which statement is most accurate in regard to the radiograph shown in Figure 18.18?

    A. This patient's injury was likely due to inversion
    B. This is usually an isolated ankle injury
    C. This injury is due to rupture of the lateral ligament complex
    D. This may be associated with a proximal fibula fracture

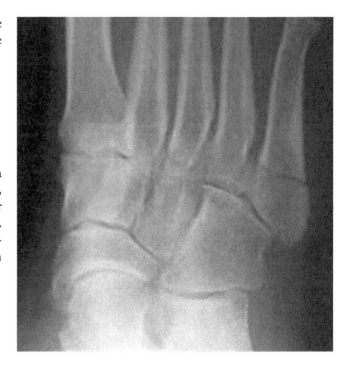

Figure 18.17 Foot radiograph.

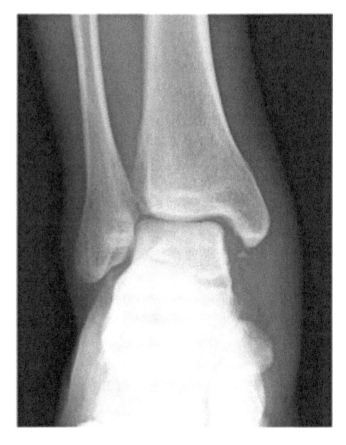

Figure 18.18 Ankle radiograph.

77. Which of the following fractures is least suspicious for nonaccidental trauma?

A. A 2-year-old with a nondisplaced spiral fracture of the distal tibial shaft
B. A 2-year-old with a bucket handle fracture
C. A 2-year-old with a metaphyseal corner fracture
D. A 1-year-old with a spiral fracture of the humerus

78. The elevated arm stress test (EAST) is used to diagnose which of the following?

A. Adhesive capsulitis
B. Rotator cuff tear
C. Impingement syndrome
D. Thoracic outlet syndrome

79. The radiograph shown in Figure 18.19 depicts which injury?

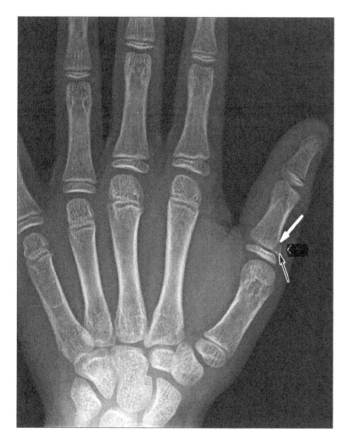

Figure 18.19 Hand radiograph.

A. Salter-Harris I
B. Salter-Harris II
C. Salter-Harris III
D. Salter-Harris IV

80. Which of the following are present in the radiograph shown in Figure 18.20?

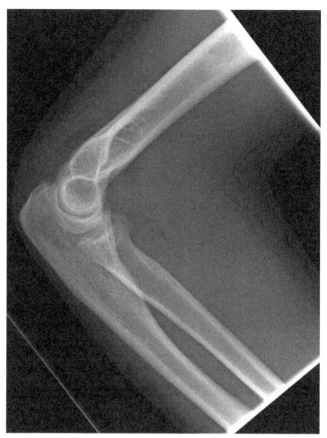

Figure 18.20 Elbow radiograph.

A. Anterior fat pad
B. Sail sign
C. Posterior fat pad
D. All of the above

81. A 45-year-old male IT professional comes in complaining of severe atraumatic pain on the thumb side of the wrist when turning door knobs or opening containers. Which of the following is associated with a diagnosis of de Quervain's tenosynovitis?

A. Tinel's sign
B. Phalen's sign
C. Finkelstein's test
D. Thompson's test

82. What is the most common cause of a painful hip in ambulatory children?

A. Septic arthritis
B. Legg-Calvé-Perthes disease

C. Slipped capital femoral epiphysis (SCFE)
D. Toxic synovitis

83. A patient presents with foot pain after tripping while hiking. What is the best way to manage this patient whose injury is depicted in the radiograph in Figure 18.21?

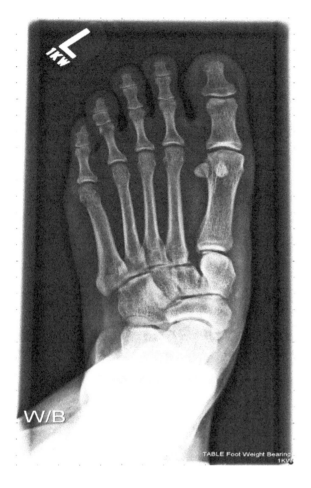

Figure 18.21 Foot radiograph.

A. Postop shoe
B. CAM boot
C. Weight-bearing cast
D. Urgent orthopedic consultation

84. Which of the following is most likely *not* a candidate for replantation?

A. A 25-year-old woman status post electric saw injury resulting in amputation of distal phalanx of the thumb
B. A 10-year-old boy who accidentally closed the car trunk on his hand, with resulting amputation of the index finger just distal to the proximal interphalangeal (PIP) joint
C. A 30-year-old man whose hand was run over by a tractor, resulting in amputation of the index finger just proximal to the distal interphalangeal (DIP) joint
D. A 50-year-old male chef whose sushi knife slipped, resulting in amputation of the index and middle fingers at the DIP

85. An 8-year-old girl fell off her bicycle and presents complaining of elbow pain. Her radiograph is shown in Figure 18.22. Which of the following *best* describes her fracture?

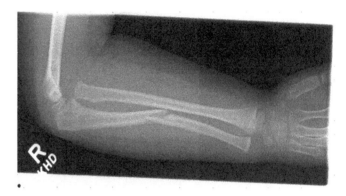

Figure 18.22 Elbow radiograph.

A. Proximal ulnar shaft fracture
B. Monteggia
C. Galeazzi
D. Nightstick fracture

86. A 25-year-old woman presents after an inversion injury of her right ankle while trail running. Which of the following is *not* an indication for radiograph?

A. She is tender along the anterior edge of distal 6 cm of the medial or lateral malleolus
B. She is unable to bear weight on the ankle
C. She is tender over the base of the fifth metatarsal
D. She has point tenderness over the navicular bone

87. A patient presents with knee pain after falling out of a tree. Which of the following is *not* true of the injury depicted in the radiograph in Figure 18.23?

A. The examiner should evaluate for compartment syndrome
B. The indication for surgery is independent of the degree of depression
C. The most common complication is post-traumatic arthritis
D. This may be associated with deep peroneal nerve injury

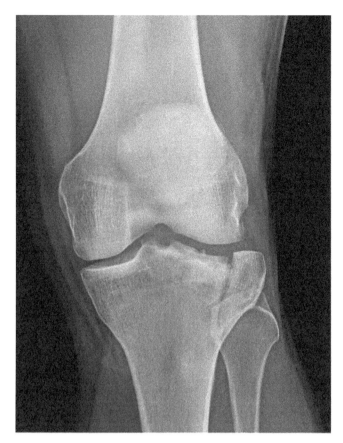

Figure 18.23 Knee radiograph.

88. Which of the following is most likely to be associated with a concomitant radial head dislocation?

A. Nightstick fracture
B. Colles fracture
C. Galeazzi fracture
D. Salter-Harris fracture

89. A 28-year-old woman comes in after falling off her mountain bike and is complaining of wrist pain. She is tender in the anatomic snuff box, but her radiograph is normal. Which of the following statements is *true*?

A. She should be placed in a thumb spica splint for 2 weeks followed by early range of motion
B. She needs a repeat radiograph in 6 weeks
C. She may develop avascular necrosis
D. This is an uncommon carpal bone injury

90. What is the most common cause of compartment syndrome in the forearm?

A. Supracondylar fracture
B. Both bone forearm fracture
C. Monteggia fracture

D. Galeazzi fracture

91. Thompson's test is positive in which of the following?

A. Patellar tendon rupture
B. Achilles tendon rupture
C. Gastrocnemius rupture
D. B and C

92. The radiograph in Figure 18.24 shows which of the following?

A. Greenstick fracture
B. Torus fracture
C. Plastic deformity
D. Salter-Harris fracture

93. Which of the following is the most important to examine in a patient with a humeral shaft fracture?

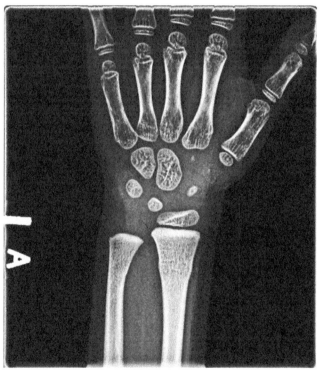

Figure 18.24 Wrist radiograph.

A. Sensation over the first dorsal webspace of the hand and thumb extension
B. Sensation over the thenar eminence and thumb opposition
C. Sensation over the pinky and ring finger and finger abduction
D. Sensation over the thenar eminence and extension of the ring and pinky fingers

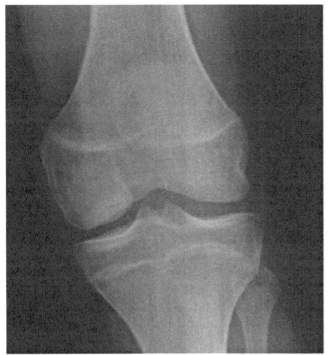 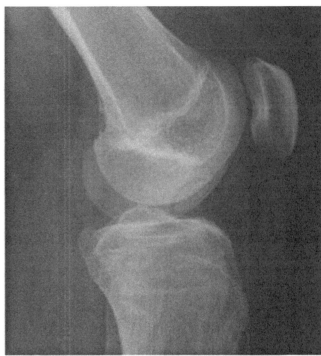

A   B

Figure 18.25 Knee radiograph.

94. Regarding the radiograph shown in Figure 18.25, which of the following is *false*?

A. This condition is common in adolescents
B. This condition most commonly occurs on the lateral femoral condyle

C. This condition may result in a locked joint due to a free-floating segment
D. This condition results from the separation of articular cartilage from subchondral bone

ANSWERS

1. ANSWER: B

SDHs are crescent in shape (see Figure 18.26) and are more common in patients with brain atrophy, including older adult and alcoholic patients, because the bridging vessels that cause these bleeds traverse greater distances in these patients. The bleed occurs between the dura and brain and is usually caused by acceleration-deceleration injuries. SDH is more common than epidural hematoma, occurring in up to 30% of patients with severe head trauma.

A biconvex-shaped density refers to an epidural hematoma. Most epidural hematomas result from a direct impact injury that causes a forceful deformity of the skull. An epidural hematoma is less likely in this patient because it is primarily a disease of the young and is rare in older adults and children younger than 2 years.

White densities in the cisterns and sulci suggest a traumatic subarachnoid hemorrhage. Subarachnoid hemorrhage is common in patients with severe head injury and is associated with early mortality. Severe head trauma is described as a GCS score of 8 or lower. This patient has a GCS score of 12, which makes this diagnosis less likely.

A normal head CT can be seen in patients with mild head injury, GCS score of 13 to 15, or severe head injury who have diffuse axonal injury that is often not apparent on initial injury. Given that this patient has moderate head injury based on his GCS score, these diagnoses are less likely.

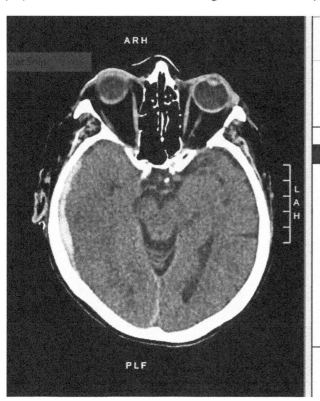

Figure 18.26 Head computed tomography.

Test-taking tip: When faced with a question that asks the most likely diagnosis, consider demographics (e.g., age, gender) and mechanism/situation to settle on the best answer.

2. ANSWER: C

Indications for emergent evacuation of an acute SDH include:

- An acute SDH with a thickness greater than 10 mm or a midline shift greater than 5 mm on CT scan regardless of the patient's GCS score
- A comatose patient (GCS score <9) if the GCS score decreases between the time of injury and hospital admission by 2 or more points
- A comatose patient who has asymmetric or fixed and dilated pupils on presentation
- A comatose patient whose intracranial pressure exceeds 20 mm Hg

Answer C is the only one that falls into these criteria.

Choices A and B are both of patients with mild to moderate head injury based on GCS who do not have findings on CT that would require emergent surgical evacuation.

The presence of an acute SDH in a patient on antiplatelet therapy is not an indication for emergent surgical evacuation unless the previously listed conditions exist. Antiplatelet therapy is, however, associated with delayed acute SDH, which is defined as an acute SDH that is not apparent on initial CT scan but appears on a follow-up CT. Seventy percent of these patients experience neurologic deterioration within 24 hours.

Test-taking tip: Even if you do not know the guidelines, this question can be figured out using clinical gestalt. The patient describe in C is the only critically injured patient with a worsening GCS.

3. ANSWER: C

This is a difficult question because all of the answers are potential findings with a basilar skull fracture. Typical findings include raccoon eyes (bilateral periorbital ecchymosis), conjunctiva hemorrhage, anosmia, Battle's signs (ecchymosis behind the ears), vision changes, cerebrospinal fluid rhinorrhea or otorrhea, step-off supraorbital edge, hearing loss, facial paralysis, and/or facial numbness.

Battle's sign, however, is the only physical exam finding that is 100% associated with basilar skull fractures.

The other three findings (raccoon eyes, conjunctival hemorrhage, and vision changes) are less specific and can be associated with other facial injuries, including facial fractures and direct ocular trauma.

Test-taking tip: If you are unsure of the answer, look for the one that is most dissimilar to the others. This is not a perfect rule but can be helpful.

4. ANSWER: D

This patient has suffered a concussion, which is the mildest form of TBI. It is defined by a transient alteration of neurologic function caused by nonpenetrating injury to the brain and characterized by normal imaging studies, if they are obtained. These patients should not return to sports until they are symptom free and have been cleared by their primary care provider or a specialist in concussion management.

A CT scan is not indicated in the patient if the PECARN decision rule for head injury in trauma is used. For ages 2 to 18 years, if the patient has a GCS score less than or equal to 14 or signs of a basilar skull fracture, then a CT of the head is indicated. Also, if the patients has one or more of the following, CT is indicated: repeated vomiting after the injury, loss of consciousness, significant mechanism (e.g., pedestrian vs. auto, fall from greater than 5 feet), or severe headache.

Given that this child does not have an acute injury requiring admission or specialty consultation, involving pediatrics would not be helpful.

Test-taking tip: With choices C and D, you have two opposites; this suggests that one of them is probably the correct answer.

5. ANSWER: D

This patient has a septal hematoma. Although a relatively rare injury, it is an important one to recognize because it can lead to significant morbidity, including abscesses, septal perforation, or saddle nose deformity, if left untreated.

Given the potential morbidity of a septal hematoma, immediate treatment in the ED with incision and drainage is the correct answer rather than referral to an ENT that might lead to delay in care and complications.

In adults, these injuries typically occur with significant facial trauma and nasal fracture, which might warrant further imaging, including a maxillofacial CT. However, in children, nasal septal hematoma may be found with minor nasal trauma, such as simple falls, collisions with stationary objects, or minor altercations with siblings, because their septum is thicker and more flexible. With a minor mechanism, such as in this case, advanced imaging is not warranted.

Nasal packing is not indicated in septal hematoma but rather is used in epistaxis that cannot be managed by less invasive treatment (e.g., direct pressure, topical agents).

Test-taking tip: Try to eliminate the answers that are most likely incorrect such as nasal packing (not used in this setting) and obtaining a CT (not usually indicated in minor trauma). This leaves you with an answer that requires action in the ED versus one that results in delay of care. Action in the ED will usually win out as the correct answer.

6. ANSWER: A

Orbital blowout fractures are usually the result of a direct blow to the orbit. This causes a sudden increase in the intraorbital pressure, which in turn causes decompression by fracture of one or more of the bounding walls of the orbit.

The inferior orbital wall (see Figure 18.27) is the most commonly injured in an orbital blowout fracture because it is the thinnest wall, followed by the medial wall. Fractures of the lateral and superior walls are uncommon.

Associated clinical findings with orbital blowout fractures include enophthalmos due to increased orbital volume; diplopia due to extraocular muscle entrapment; orbital emphysema, especially when the fracture extends into an adjacent paranasal sinus; and/or malar region numbness due to injury to the inferior orbital nerve.

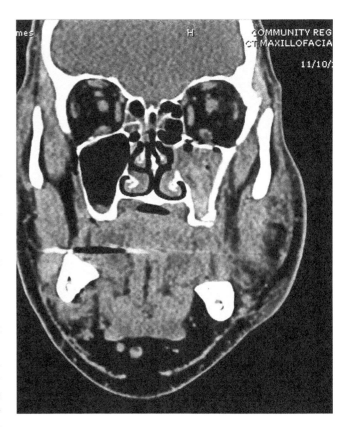

Figure 18.27 Head computed tomography.

Test-taking tip: This is a "you know it or don't" kind of question. If you don't know it, choose an answer and move on. You can perhaps mark it for review when you are done at the end of the test. Don't, however, let these kinds of questions get you stuck and waste your time.

7. ANSWER: A

The inferior orbital nerve is the most commonly injured nerve in an orbital blowout fracture. It courses within the bony floor of the orbit (the inferior wall), which is the wall most likely to fracture in this setting because of its relative thinnest compared with the other orbital walls.

The anterior-superior alveolar nerve runs in a canal in the anterior wall of the maxillary sinus, making injury to this nerve less likely in an isolated orbital blowout fracture.

The zygomatic branch of the facial nerve runs across the zygomatic bone to the lateral angle of the orbit, again making it less likely to be injured in a blowout fracture, where the inferior and medial walls are most likely to be injured.

The oculomotor nerve enters the orbit through the superior orbital fissure, again making it less likely to be injured with a blowout fracture.

Test-taking tip: Even if you do not know the anatomy and the correct answer to this question, you may be able to guess given the question is about an orbital blowout fracture and the only answer with "orbital" in it is the correct answer, A.

8. ANSWER: B

The clinical description of this patient presentation is consistent with a Le Fort II injury (Figure 18.28). A Le Fort II fracture is typically bilateral and pyramidal in shape. It extends superiorly in the midface to include fractures of the nasal bridge, maxilla, lacrimal bones, orbital floor, and rim. The nasal complex moves as a unit with the maxilla when the teeth are grasped and rocked.

A Le Fort fracture I is a transverse fracture separating the body of the maxilla from the pterygoid plate and nasal septum. The hard palate and teeth would move but not the nose.

A Le Fort III fracture, which is rare, involves craniofacial dissociation when the entire face is separated from the skull due to fractures of the frontozygomatic suture line, across the orbit, and through the base of the nose and ethmoids. With this fracture, the entire face shifts, with the globes held in place only by the optic nerves.

A Le Fort IV fracture is similar to a Le Fort III but with the frontal bone involve.

Test-taking tip: This is a "you know it or you don't" question. Questions regarding fracture classifications and types are common on emergency medicine standardized tests, so they are worth reviewing before the test.

9. ANSWER: B

This patient presents with a mandible fracture. Fractures of the mandible can result from any significant force, and because of the mandibles shape, multiple fractures may result from a single blow. This patient has overlying lacerations and mucosal tears suggesting an open fracture. Open mandible fractures require IV antibiotics that cover for oral flora, in this case, penicillin, and frequently require hospital admission. An oral maxillofacial surgeon should be consulted.

Choices A and B are not the most appropriate management of the patient because they do not involve IV antibiotics and consultation with a facial surgeon.

Le Fort Fracture Classification

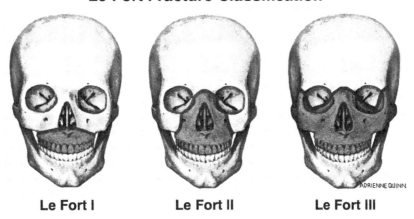

Le Fort I   Le Fort II   Le Fort III

Figure 18.28 Le Fort fracture classification.

Although obtaining a facial CT scan may help further characterize the injury and help discover occult injuries, it is not the most appropriate management.

Test-taking tip: When the question asks for the most appropriate management, it should clue you to think of what is the standard of care for that particular condition.

10. ANSWER: C

This patient presents with classic signs and symptoms of tension pneumothorax. He is hypotensive, tachycardic, and tachypneic; he does not have breath sounds over the left hemothorax; and his trachea deviates away from the affected side. The most appropriate initial management of this patient is needle decompression of the left side of the chest followed shortly by chest tube placement.

Tension pneumothorax is an emergency and is a clinical diagnosis, so a chest radiograph should not be obtained before treatment. A chest tube on the affected side is indicated but only after needle decompression, to convert the tension pneumothorax to a simple pneumothorax, has been performed.

The patient on initial presentation is speaking and has an intact airway, so he does not require emergent intubation.

Test-taking tip: With questions about the initial management of trauma, think of the primary survey and identifying and treating life threats.

11. ANSWER: C

In the absence of associated injuries, most patients with isolated sternal fractures who can achieve adequate pain control on oral medications can safely be discharged home.

Isolated sternal fractures, especially those only diagnosed on CT, are not a marker for blunt cardiac injury; therefore, a stat echocardiogram would not be indicated in this patient, nor would admission for cardiac monitoring. Without associated injuries and with normal vital signs, this patient does not require admission to a surgical service.

Test-taking tip: If one answer is opposite to all of the others (one suggests discharge home and the others point to further testing/admission), the answer that stands out as different from the others is probably correct.

12. ANSWER: C

This patient presents with a significant mechanism and a mildly displace sternal fracture on lateral chest radiograph. This should raise the clinician's level of concern for a cardiac contusion/blunt cardiac injury. Although there is no gold standard for the diagnosis of cardiac contusion, EKG is the most commonly recommended tool to screen for this injury. A normal EKG has an excellent negative predictive value (NPV) of greater than 95%. The addition of a negative troponin I to a normal EKG increases the NPV to almost 100%. Patient's with a normal EKG and negative troponin I do not need any further cardiac workup or monitoring.

Although cardiac CT may help to differentiate traumatic from ischemic injury, it is not a good initial screening tool. An echocardiogram can be a very useful tool to rule out structurally significant myocardial injuries but should not be used as a primary screening modality for blunt cardiac injury. A troponin alone without an EKG is not a sensitive screening tool.

Test-taking tip: This is a stable patient in whom you are trying to rule out an injury, so think least invasive and least expensive.

13. ANSWER: C

This patient has suffered a unilateral facet dislocation but exhibits no neurologic deficits and has no other associated injuries. Unilateral facet dislocations are considered stable and do not require urgent neurosurgical evaluation. This patient can be discharged with referral to neurosurgery.

In the absence of neurologic deficits suggesting underlying spinal cord injury, an MRI is not warranted. This patient has no clinical finding concerning for vascular injury in the neck (potential arterial hemorrhage from the neck/nose/mouth, cervical bruit, expanding cervical hematoma, or focal neurologic deficits), so a CTA of the neck is not indicated.

Test-taking tip: If one answer is opposite to all of the others (one suggests discharge home and the others point to further testing/admission), the answer that stands out as different from the others is probably correct.

14. ANSWER: A

Scapula fractures are very uncommon, representing less than 1% of all fractures. They are usually caused by high-energy trauma and should prompt suspicion for other associated injuries, including other associated orthopedic injuries (ribs, proximal humerus, and clavicle) and pulmonary injuries (pneumothorax, hemothorax, and contusions). The other fractures are not always associated with high-energy mechanisms or associated injuries.

Test-taking tip: You should be able to eliminate a spinal transverse fracture as an answer because it is distant from the lungs. Clavicle fractures are common low-mechanism injuries, which also makes it easy to exclude this answer. If you don't know the correct answer, this at least narrows the options down to two.

15. ANSWER: C

PCC is the most appropriate treatment at this time. This patient has an SDH on his CT. This is a life-threatening bleed, and his coagulopathy should be reversed as quickly as possible. In this case administering PCC is the best treatment. PCC is an inactivated concentrate of factors II, IX, and X, with variable amounts of factor VII.

Although PO vitamin K can help to reverse coagulopathy due to warfarin use, it does not reverse the coagulopathy quickly enough. In the setting of a life-threatening bleed, IV vitamin K can be given in conjunction with PCC.

Cryoprecipitate and platelets are not indicated in the treatment of life-threatening bleeds in patients on warfarin. Cryoprecipitate can be used in bleeding due to hemophilia A, and platelet replacement is indicated in patients with bleeding and significant thrombocytopenia.

Test-taking tip: This is a "you know it or don't" kind of question. If you don't know it, choose an answer and move on. You can perhaps mark it for review when you are done at the end of the test. Don't, however, let these kinds of questions get you stuck and waste your time.

16. ANSWER: D

This patient presents with stab wounds to the upper back and chest and is at high risk for a pneumothorax. Initial chest radiograph does not demonstrate a pneumothorax, but pneumothorax in stab wounds may be delayed for 4 to 6 hours. There is a 12% reported incidence of initially asymptomatic stab wounds to the chest that require delayed tube thoracostomy for hemothorax or pneumothorax. Therefore, this patient should not be discharged home but should be observed and a repeat chest radiograph obtained after 4 to 6 hours.

Given a normal chest radiograph and a patient in not significant distress, a tube thoracostomy does not need to be performed at this time. A needle decompression, which is the treatment for a suspected tension pneumothorax (hypotension, respiratory distress, and decreased breath sounds on the affected side) is also not indicated in this clinical setting.

Test-taking tip: The correct answer is predicated on correctly interpreting the imaging study as normal. There is a tendency to want to find radiographic abnormalities on imaging studies in test-taking situations. A normal study can also be informative.

17. ANSWER: D

Indications for ED resuscitative thoracotomy remain controversial, but some recommendations include penetrating torso trauma patients with less than 15 minutes of CPR, blunt trauma patients with less than 10 minutes of CPR, and patients in profound refractory shock due to trauma. Only the patient described in D presents with one of these indications.

The patient described in A is more consistent with a pneumothorax or tension pneumothorax for which needle decompression and/or tube thoracostomy would be the appropriate treatment.

The patient described in B was initially in shock but responded to resuscitation efforts so does not require ED resuscitative thoracotomy.

The patient described in C is outside of the time limits for ED resuscitative thoracotomy.

Test-taking tip: ED resuscitative thoracotomy is a heroic procedure that is not indicated in patients who have stabilized and that has limited value in patients with no signs of life.

18. ANSWER: D

The NEXUS cervical spine criteria are a decision rule that was created to avoid unnecessary cervical spine imaging. The NEXUS criteria are listed in Box 18.1.

Any patient who meets all of the criteria is deemed low enough risk to not have to undergo imaging of the cervical spine. Of the patients described, only D meets all the NEXUS criteria.

Box 18.1 NEXUS CERVICAL SPINE CRITERIA

- Absence of midline cervical tenderness
- Normal level of alertness and consciousness
- No evidence of intoxication
- Absence of focal neurologic deficit
- Absence of painful distracting injury

Test-taking tip: Decision rules are becoming more important in emergency medicine, so being aware of the most used (e.g., NEXUS, PECARN) rules is important.

19. ANSWER: C

This patient has a sucking chest wound on the right side, also called an open pneumothorax. These wounds result in a unidirectional flow of air into the pleural space during inspiration but do not allow air to escape during expiration because of tissue apposition surrounding the wound. If left untreated, these wounds can lead to a life-threatening tension pneumothorax.

The most appropriate initial treatment for this patient is a three-sided occlusive dressing. This dressing creates a one-way valve that allows air and blood to escape the wound, preventing reentry of air that can create a tension pneumothorax. After the dressing is applied, a chest radiograph should be obtained. A chest tube will also eventually need to be performed to treat the underlying pneumothorax.

Endotracheal intubation is not indicated in this patient initially because of a normal mentation and intact airway.

Test-taking tip: The wording of "most appropriate immediate management" suggests a potentially lifesaving therapy of which a chest radiograph is not. This helps to eliminate at least one answer if you are unsure of the correct answer.

20. ANSWER: C

The preferred site for a chest tube is the fifth intercostal space mid-axillary line. This is approximately the level of the nipple. The tube should go over the sixth rib to avoid the neurovascular bundle.

The second intercostal space, mid-clavicular line is a common site for a needle thoracostomy to be performed.

On expiration, the diaphragm rises to the fifth rib. Performing a tube thoracostomy at the sixth intercostal space would risk entering the peritoneum and causing injury to intraabdominal organs.

Test-taking tip: As long as you know the difference between a tube and needle thoracostomy, choice A should be easy to eliminate. Any procedure done on the chest wall is always over the rib to protect the neurovascular bundle. This leaves only two answers to choose from if you are unsure of the correct answer.

21. ANSWER: A

Radiography of the chest can be a valuable tool to screen for traumatic aortic rupture. A widened mediastinum, as seen in Figure 18.29, is the most sensitive sign and is found in the majority of aortic ruptures. Widened mediastinum, however, is not a very specific finding, and up to half of patients with blunt aortic injury do not have a widened mediastinum; thus, patients in whom there is a high suspicion of aortic injury should undergo a chest CT.

The possibility of blunt aortic injury should be considered in all patients who sustain a severe deceleration injury, especially patients involved in MVCs moving

in excess of 45 mph with evident of blunt force trauma to the chest.

First rib and scapular injuries are both suggestive of a high-energy mechanism and are associated with multiple other injuries, including pneumothorax, hemothorax, pulmonary contusions, cardiac injuries, and abdominal injuries. These fractures, however, are not sensitive for the diagnosis of blunt aortic injury.

A hemothorax on chest radiograph is not sensitive for an aortic injury; however, after tube thoracostomy placement, if there is a large initial rush of bright red arterial blood or significant ongoing losses, an aortic or other large vessel injury should be suspected, and the patient should be emergently transferred to surgery.

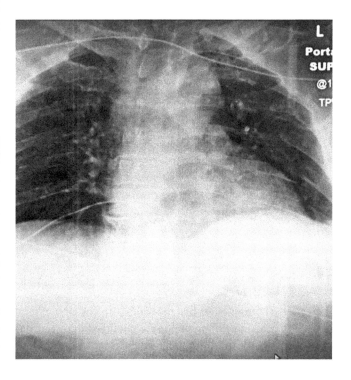

Figure 18.29 Chest radiograph.

Test-taking tip: Hemothorax is a relatively common finding after blunt chest trauma, and aortic injury is rare, so you should be able to eliminate this answer as a sensitive finding.

22. ANSWER: D

This patient presents with a mechanism and physical exam concerning for retrobulbar hematoma, or postseptal hematoma. This can lead to orbital compartment syndrome. An IOP higher than 40 mm Hg in the setting of trauma is considered an emergency, and a lateral canthotomy should be performed without delay. This should be performed by the emergency clinician unless there is immediate availability of an ophthalmologist.

CT of the orbits may be required to further delineate the injury and direct further treatment but is not an immediate, vision-saving modality.

The use of IOP-lowering agents such as IV carbonic anhydrase inhibitors, topical ß-blockers, α-agonists, and in some cases, IV mannitol may be indicated in this clinical setting before ischemia and vision loss occur. Oral carbonic anhydrase inhibitors (acetazolamide) are not indicated in this clinical setting, nor are analgesia and cool compresses alone.

Test-taking tip: Most appropriate immediate management suggests a life-, limb-, or in this case vison-saving procedure. Lateral canthotomy is the only answer of the four that meets this criterion.

23. ANSWER: A

This patient has a traumatic hyphema. Complications of a traumatic hyphema include corneal staining and elevated IOP. In patients with a traumatic hyphema, nonsteroidal antiinflammatory drugs (NSAIDs) should be avoided be these are antiplatelet agents and can lead to worsening bleeding.

Morphine is a reasonable agent to use in such patients if they have severe pain related to their injuries.

Topical and oral agents to decrease IOP may be indicated in these patients in consultation with an ophthalmologist.

Patients with uncomplicated hyphema can be discharged home with recommendations for gentle ambulation and head of the bed elevation. Admission is recommended for patients with hyphema greater that 50%, sickle cell trait, uncontrolled IOPs, and anticoagulated patients.

Test-taking tip: Acetazolamide and topical steroids are agents used to treat elevated IOPs, which is a complication of this pathology, so they can be eliminated as agents not to give.

24. ANSWER: D

This patient has suffered severe facial trauma as evidenced by the Le Fort III fracture. In addition to obtaining the appropriate consultation, this patient should also undergo blunt cerebrovascular injury screening (BCVI).

Both the Western and Eastern Trauma associations recommend patients with Le Fort II or III fractures undergo BCVI screening. A CTA of the neck is rapidly obtainable in most trauma centers and is the first-line test. However, a CTA can miss injuries, and in patients in whom there is a high degree of suspicion for injury, conventional arteriography should be obtained.

See Figure 18.28 for more detailed demonstration of the Le Fort classification.

CT of chest, abdomen, and pelvis is not indicated in this patient, who was only assaulted in the face and head and has no complaints or visible injury to the rest of his body.

Lethal complications have been reported after the insertion of a nasogastric tube after severe basilar skull fracture. It has thus been recommended that in the setting of basilar skull fracture and/or significant maxillofacial trauma, insertion of tubes in the nasopharynx should be avoided.

A soft tissue neck radiograph can be useful in a variety of clinical settings, including suspected epiglottitis, croup, retropharyngeal abscess, or airway foreign body. It does not have a role, however, in the setting of blunt head and neck trauma.

Test-taking tip: Choice A should be easy to eliminate given the clinical scenario, and most physicians have the picture of a nasogastric tube coiled in the brain burned into their memories, making choice B easy to discard.

25. ANSWER: D

The hangman's fracture, which involves traumatic spondylolysis of C2, occurs when the skull, atlas, and axis, functioning as a unit, are hyperextended as the result of an abrupt deceleration. As the name suggest, it was originally described in victims of hanging injury but in modern society is more commonly associated with head-on MVC.

All of the other fractures listed are considered stable.

A unilateral facet dislocation occurs when simultaneous flexion and rotation occur, causing the contralateral facet joint to dislocate. The superior facet rides forward and over the tip of the inferior facet, coming to rest within the intervertebral foramen. Because the facet is locked, this is a stable injury.

A clay shoveler's fracture, named for the fracture caused by the abrupt head flexion that clay miners might experience while lifting a heavy shovelful of clay, is an avulsion fracture of the spinous process. In modern society, this injury is seen with direct trauma to the neck or after sudden deceleration in an MVC that causes forced flexion of the neck. Because the injury only involves the spinous process, it is stable.

An isolated transverse process, similar to the clay shoveler's fracture, is stable.

Test-taking tip: If you have to guess, the name "hangman's fracture" might clue you to it being unstable because hanging can be a lethal mechanism.

26. ANSWER: A

This patient presents with a severe TBI after a fall. In patients with severe TBI, high-dose methylprednisolone is associated with increased mortality and is therefore contraindicated.

Mannitol can be administered at a rate of 0.25 to 1 mg/kg in patients with signs of progressive neurologic deterioration but is not associated with improved mortality or neurologic outcomes.

Levetiracetam can be used to prevent early posttraumatic seizures but is not associated with improved mortality.

Ketamine was classically thought to raise intracranial pressure, but that has not been found to be the case, and it can safely be used in patients with TBI.

Test-taking tip: Mannitol and levetiracetam are commonly used in head-injured patients so can easily be eliminated as the correct answer for this question.

27. ANSWER: C

SVT is the most common arrhythmia seen in TBI patients. Cardiac dysrhythmias in this setting are most often caused by high levels of circulating catecholamines. Ensuring adequate tissue perfusion is the primary goal in these patients, along with treating elevated intracranial pressure. The dysrhythmia will often resolve after these two issues are address.

A prolonged QT interval can be hereditary or can be acquired because of electrolyte abnormalities or the use of many common medications, including antibiotics, antihistamines, and antipsychotics. It is not associated with TBI.

First-degree atrioventricular block is defined as a prolongation of the PR interval beyond the upper limit of normal (0.02 second). It is often an incidental finding on EKG in asymptomatic patients and is usually benign. It is common in well-trained athletes but can also be caused by use of some medications, including calcium channel blockers and ß-blockers. It is not associated with TBI.

Ventricular tachycardia is the most common cause of sudden cardiac death in the United States and has many causes, the most common being cardiac ischemia. It can be seen in severe TBI but is not as common as SVT.

Test-taking tip: This is a "you know it or don't" kind of question. If you don't know it, choose an answer and move on. You can perhaps mark it for review when you are done at the end of the test. Don't, however, let these kinds of questions get you stuck and waste your time.

28. ANSWER: C

This patient presents with a mild head injury, defined as a GCS score of 13 to 15, after a fall. In any pediatric patient with blunt head trauma, the PECARN pediatric head injury rule should be applied. In patients younger than 2 years the following are high-risk criteria: GCS score <14, altered mental status (agitation, somnolence, repetitive questioning, or slow response to verbal communication), and palpable skull fracture. If any of those are present, then a noncontrast brain CT is indicated.

The following are considered low-risk criteria: nonfrontal scalp hematoma, loss of consciousness for less than 5 seconds, severe injury mechanism, and abnormal activity per parents. If any of these criteria are met, then consider a period of observation versus head CT.

This patient does not have any of these criteria, and therefore CT of the head is not indicated. A period of observation in the ED might be warranted, but admission is not required.

Seizure prophylaxis is not indicated in mild head injury but may be indicated in severe head injury.

Test-taking tip: Brush up on the clinical decision rules, such as PECARN, before the exam.

29. ANSWER: B

This patient has motor function associated with C5 (shrugging of shoulders), but nothing caudal to this, suggesting a cord injury at C6 (see Table 18.1).

Table 18.1 LEVEL OF SPINAL INJURY AND ASSOCIATED LOSS OF MOTOR FUNCTION

LEVEL	RESULTING LOSS OF MOTOR FUNCTION
C4	Spontaneous breathing
C5	Shrugging of shoulders
C6	Flexion at elbow
C7	Extension at elbow
C8–T1	Flexion of fingers
T1–12	Intercostal and abdominal muscles
L1–2	Flexion at hip
L3	Adduction at hip
L4	Abduction at hip
L5	Dorsiflexion of foot
S1–2	Plantar flexion of foot
S2–4	Rectal sphincter tone

Test-taking tip: Although memorizing all of the myotomes or dermatomes is probably not worth your time (unless you have a photographic memory), remember key ones (C4—breathing, C6—flexion at elbow, L1–2—flexion at hip, L5—dorsiflexion at hip) should get you close enough to get the right answer.

30. ANSWER: B

Aortic disruptions are life-threatening injuries that should always be suspected in any decelerating injury with significant energy. High-speed MVCs are the most common mechanism.

The most common site for aortic disruption or tear is the descending aorta at the isthmus just distal to the origin of the left subclavian artery. About 80% to 90% of aortic tears occur at this site.

Injuries at the other sites listed are less common but can occur. While injuries to the ascending aorta are less common, they are more likely to be lethal. Any patient in whom aortic injury is suspected should get a CT of the aorta if clinically stable and immediate cardiothoracic surgery consult.

Test-taking tip: This is a "you know it or don't" kind of question. If you don't know it, choose an answer and move on. You can perhaps mark it for review when you are done at the end of the test. Don't, however, let these kinds of questions get you stuck and waste your time.

31. ANSWER: C

This patient has a pulmonary contusion. A pulmonary contusion is a direct injury to the lung as a result of blunt trauma. Patients with pulmonary contusions can present with chest pain, tachypnea, contusion to the chest wall, hypoxia, and shortness of breath.

Chest radiograph classically shows ground-glass opacities, although this can be delayed. Areas of opacification on chest imaging within 6 hours of blunt trauma can be considered diagnostic of pulmonary contusion. CT is more sensitive for pulmonary contusions than chest radiograph and has shown these to be common in blunt trauma and a source of severe morbidity and mortality.

Aggressive fluid resuscitation should be avoided because this can lead to worsening lung injury. Neither steroids nor antibiotics are indicated in pulmonary contusion.

Aggressive respiratory therapy, which can include positive pressure ventilation, is the most appropriate treatment for this patient.

Test-taking tip: The patient is normotensive, so aggressive fluid resuscitation should be easy to eliminate as an answer. Steroids are never indicated in the initial management of trauma, leaving two possible answers to choose from.

32. ANSWER: D

This patient presents with minor chest trauma after an MVC. The NEXUS chest CT decision instrument is designed to identify patients who suffered blunt chest trauma but do not need advanced imaging. It is highly sensitive for clinically identifying the risk for major thoracic injuries and therefore for excluding patients who do not need advanced imaging.

The criteria are for advanced imaging are abnormal chest radiograph, rapid deceleration mechanism (fall >20 feet, MVC >40 mph), distracting painful injury, chest wall tenderness, sternal tenderness, thoracic spine tenderness, and scapular tenderness. If all of these are negative, then the rate of major thoracic injury is <1% and CT is not indicated. This patient has none of these findings, and thus CT is not warranted.

This patient has a GCS score of 15 with no loss of consciousness, so a head CT is not warranted, and given no other identifiable injuries, a consultation with a trauma surgeon is also not necessary.

Test-taking tip: Don't get fooled in a test-taking situation into believing something else has to be done. If the case scenario is low risk, sometimes less is better.

33. ANSWER: D

Immediate drainage of more than 1,500 mL of blood is a possible indication for urgent thoracotomy because it is suggestive of significant vascular injury. This is especially true in a patient in hemorrhage shock. Another potential indication is 200 mL drainage per hour for 3 hours.

The color of the blood is also important: dark, venous blood is more likely to cease spontaneously compared with bright arterial blood.

Test-taking tip: Operative management for hemothorax is relatively rare, so guessing the largest number is a safe bet.

34. ANSWER: C

IOP measurement should be avoided in this patient because he likely has an open globe injury as evidenced by the irregularly shaped pupil and severely decreased vision in the affected eye. Increased pressure on the globe that may be created by attempting to measure pressures may worsen the injury. Broad-spectrum antibiotics should be administered to patients with an open globe injury.

Although there was initially concern that ketamine increases IOP, which would be contraindicated in this patient, more recent evidence suggests that clinically this is not the case, and if this patient needed to be intubated or sedated it could be used.

A fluorescein exam is safe in this patient and, if performed, may show Seidel's sign, which is considered diagnostic of an open globe injury.

Test-taking tip: The picture is of an open globe injury, which should raise the concern for avoiding increased IOP. Antibiotics and fluorescein do not do this so can easily be eliminated as the correct answer.

35. ANSWER: C

In hemodynamically unstable patients with blunt abdominal trauma, bedside ultrasound (when available) is the initial diagnostic modality of choice to identify the need for emergent laparotomy.

While CT of the abdomen and pelvis with IV contrast is the noninvasive gold standard for diagnosing abdominal injuries, it is not indicated or appropriate in unstable patients.

KUB is plain film radiographic imaging. While this modality may reveal some findings (such as subdiaphragmatic free air, bony injuries, or radiopaque foreign bodies), it is not the initial preferred imaging modality in the emergent setting.

DPL is 98% sensitive in determining intraabdominal bleeding or bowel injury that may require immediate laparotomy and should be considered in an unstable patient if FAST exam is not available, difficult to perform, or inconclusive. DPL is rapid to perform but is invasive and can miss diaphragmatic, retroperitoneal, or isolated hollow viscus injuries.

Test-taking tip: "Hypotensive" and "initial" are the key words in this question, indicating a fast bedside test that equals a bedside ultrasound/FAST exam.

36. ANSWER: C

Oral contrast is not essential to the evaluation of blunt abdominal trauma. While oral contrast has a theoretical advantage of improved identification of bowel injuries, pancreas injuries, and hematomas, it also has disadvantages. Disadvantages include vomiting, aspiration, and delayed diagnosis. Even with theoretical advantages, the sensitivity of CT does not differ significantly with or without oral contrast, and oral contrast is therefore not essential to the evaluation of blunt abdominal trauma.

Hemodynamically unstable patients with a positive FAST exam should go directly to the operating room for laparotomy.

IV contrast CT of the abdomen and pelvis (not IV, PO, and rectal contrast CT of the abdomen and pelvis) is the gold standard for evaluation of injuries in blunt abdominal trauma and has excellent sensitivity and specificity for intraabdominal injuries, particularly liver and spleen injuries. CT is less reliable in diagnosing bowel, mesenteric, pancreas, and diaphragmatic injuries.

DPL has a sensitivity of 98% for detecting intraabdominal injuries; however, DPL is not reliable in detecting bowel, diaphragmatic, and retroperitoneal injuries.

Test-taking tip: If you are unsure of the answer, you can eliminate choice A because unstable patients never belong in the CT scanner and choice D because DPL is rarely used anymore, leaving two answers to choose from.

37. ANSWER: C

Diaphragmatic injury is rare (0%–5% of patients with thoracoabdominal injury), may result from blunt or penetrating injuries, and is almost exclusively left-sided. Signs and symptoms are nonspecific, and delayed diagnosis may lead to herniation or to strangulation of abdominal contents.

Hiatal hernia refers to herniation of abdominal contents through the esophageal hiatus of the diaphragm and may be related to congenital malformations, surgical procedures, or in some cases, trauma.

Blebs (also known as bullae) are pulmonary lunacies often seen in lung disease. Ruptured blebs result in pneumothorax, not diaphragmatic injuries.

Pneumomediastinum (also known as mediastinal emphysema) is the presence of air or other gas in the mediastinum. Pneumomediastinum is categorized as spontaneous or traumatic. Traumatic pneumomediastinum can be the result of blunt or penetrating trauma, barotrauma from mechanical ventilation, or iatrogenic injury.

Test-taking tip: If you are unsure of the answer, you can eliminate hiatal hernia and ruptured bleb because they are not usually associated with trauma, leaving two answers to choose from.

38. ANSWER: A

Blunt injury to intestines can result from deceleration injuries and tearing of structures near a fixed point of attachment. Presence of a seat belt sign (linear ecchymosis of the abdominal wall) or presence of a lumbar distraction fracture (also known as a Chance fracture or transverse fracture through the vertebral body caused by flexion about an axis anterior to the vertebral column) may be associated with retroperitoneal and abdominal visceral injuries. Diagnosis may be difficult because injured structures may only have minimal bleeding, and early ultrasound and CT are often nondiagnostic. Observation and serial abdominal exams are indicated.

While orthopedics consult and treatment with thoracolumbosacral orthosis may ultimately be indicated for the Chance fracture, your more immediate next step should be evaluation of potential retroperitoneal and/or visceral injuries.

Evaluating for injuries with a DPL can identify intraabdominal bleeding/bowel injury that requires immediate laparotomy, is rapidly performed an d readily available, and has 98% sensitivity. DPL can miss significant retroperitoneal bleeding and isolated hollow viscus perforation and is contraindicated if there is indication for emergent laparotomy.

Emergent MRI is not indicated.

Test-taking tip: The key phrase in this questions is "most appropriate next step." You have identified an injury that needs management, which should allow you to narrow down the correct answer to A or B. Choice A is most appropriate because it is more important to manage possible life threats, such as occult intraabdominal injuries.

39. ANSWER: B

Your patient has blunt abdominal trauma and is hemodynamically unstable, an indication for immediate surgical consultation and laparotomy. The spleen and then the liver are the most commonly injured intraabdominal organs following blunt trauma. Your patient's left shoulder pain, known as Kehr's sign, is a classic symptom of splenic injury and is a result of diaphragmatic irritation from hemorrhage.

CT of the abdomen and pelvis with IV contrast is the noninvasive gold standard for the diagnosis of abdominal injury, but your patient is hemodynamically unstable and should go directly to the operating room for laparotomy and definitive treatments.

In a patient with blunt trauma and unstable vital signs, death may occur as a result of massive hemorrhage. It is inappropriate to wait for blood transfusion before definitive treatment.

Your patient is unstable and needs immediate laparotomy. It is not appropriate to delay care.

Test-taking tip: Unstable trauma patients need a surgeon, making B the clear choice.

40. ANSWER: C

With penetrating stab wounds, the liver is the most commonly injured organ, followed by the small bowel.

In gunshot wounds, the small bowel is the most commonly injured organ, followed by the colon and then the liver.

Test-taking tip: This is a "you know it or don't" kind of question. If you don't know it, choose an answer and move on. You can perhaps mark it for review when you are done at the end of the test. Don't, however, let these kinds of questions get you stuck and waste your time.

41. ANSWER: A

External tocodynamometric monitoring for a minimum of 4 to 6 hours of a potentially viable fetus is indicated for all pregnant patients evaluated for trauma, even those without obvious abdominal injury. If the patient has fewer than three contractions per hour during the initial 4-hour monitoring, she may be discharged home. If there are persistent contractions or uterine irritability, fetal monitoring may be extended to 24 hours. If there is evidence of fetal distress or uterine irritability during the initial assessment, then immediate obstetrician consultation should be obtained.

Serial abdominal exams may be indicated in patients after suffering abdominal trauma but are not enough in patients who have a potential viable fetus.

Pelvic examination after an ultrasound is obtained is indicated to determine placental location and to exclude placenta previa but would not be the next step or necessarily emergent. A sterile pelvic exam can identify injuries to the lower genital tract, vaginal bleeding, and rupture of amniotic membranes. Vaginal fluid with a pH of 7 is suggestive of amniotic fluid, and branch-like pattern (ferning) is suggestive of amniotic fluid.

A pregnant trauma patient with a potentially viable fetus, and even without obvious abdominal injury, should have 4 to 6 hours of external tocodynamometric monitoring and should not be discharged home without this monitoring even if they have appropriate follow-up and good return precautions.

Test-taking tip: This is a "you know it or don't" kind of question. If you don't know it, choose an answer and move on. You can perhaps mark it for review when you are done at the end of the test. Don't, however, let these kinds of questions get you stuck and waste your time.

42. ANSWER: D

While imaging studies should be minimized to avoid fetal exposure to ionizing radiation, never withhold imaging needed for appropriate maternal trauma management. Do not withhold critical maternal interventions or diagnostic procedures out of concern for potential adverse fetal consequences. Fetal exposure can be decreased by shielding the maternal abdomen and pelvis, and modified studies and dose-reducing techniques may be obtained.

Tetanus toxoid is a category C drug in all trimesters of pregnancy, but it is commonly accepted as safe and should be provided as needed. Tetanus antibiotics cross the placenta and can reduce the incidence of neonatal tetanus.

Fetomaternal hemorrhage is the entry of fetal RBCs into the maternal blood stream, and as little as 0.1 μL of fetal Rh-positive blood entering an Rh-negative mother's circulation can sensitize the mother and endanger the pregnancy (and future pregnancies). Rho(D) immunoglobulin should be administered to Rh-negative pregnant women with any abdominal trauma. There are two dose options: 50 mcg IM for gestation £12 weeks and 300 mcg IM for gestation of ≥13 weeks.

A gravid uterus may compress the maternal inferior vena cava in the supine position and may put the mother at risk for "supine hypotension syndrome," with diminished venous return and decreased cardiac output. In an effort to minimize vena cava compression, all pregnant patients should be kept in the semi–left lateral decubitus position.

Test-taking tip: Words such as "always," "never," and "only" should clue you that this is probably not the correct answer. Absolute statements, such as these, are rarely true in life and in medicine.

43. ANSWER: A

Trauma is the leading cause of nonobstetric morbidity and mortality in pregnant women, with MVCs accounting for most blunt abdominal trauma, followed by falls and assault. Placental abruption can be seen in up to 5% of minor injuries and up to 50% of major traumatic injuries and is the second most common cause of fetal death (maternal death is the number one cause of fetal death).

During trauma, the elastic uterus deforms, and the inelastic placenta can shear from the uterine wall. The most sensitive clinical finding for placental abruption after trauma is uterine irritability (more than three contractions per hour). Other findings include abdominal pain, painful vaginal bleeding, and tetanic uterine contractions. Maternal complications of placenta abruption include disseminated intravascular coagulation and amniotic fluid embolism with the introduction of placental products into the maternal circulation.

Uterine rupture is rare (<1% of all injuries in pregnancy) and is more likely to be seen during the late second trimester and third trimester with direct impact on the uterus. Clinical findings are nonspecific and can include loss of palpable uterine contour, easily palpable fetal parts,

or abnormal fetal location on radiology studies. Fetal mortality rate is high.

Fetal tachycardia and vaginal bleeding are nonspecific and can be found with numerous injuries.

Test-taking tip: Fetal tachycardia and vaginal bleeding, as stated previously, are very nonspecific findings in the setting of trauma in pregnancy; they thus should be easily eliminated as an answer looking for the most sensitive clinical finding.

44. ANSWER: D

Perimortem cesarean delivery is a rare procedure because cardiac arrest is reported to occur in only 1 in 30,000 pregnancies. Indication for perimortem cesarean delivery is loss of vital signs in a pregnancy that is at (or near) the age of viability. Perimortem cesarean delivery is ideally performed at the 4-minute mark following onset of maternal cardiac arrest with delivery of the infant at 5 minutes. There should be no delay in performing the potentially life-saving maneuver because survival of the infant is directly related to the time elapsed from maternal cardiac arrest to delivery. CPR should continue during and after perimortem cesarean delivery to monitor the effects of cesarean delivery and resultant relief of physiologic aortocaval obstruction and to monitor for return of spontaneous maternal circulation.

While it is appropriate to ensure that you have adequate vascular access in a patient who is coding, in a pregnant patient, you should not delay delivery of a potentially viable infant. Infant survival is best when perimortem cesarean delivery is performed within 5 minutes.

A bedside FAST exam and ultrasound for fetal evaluation is not indicated in a case of maternal cardiac arrest and would delay attempts at a perimortem cesarean delivery.

It is appropriate to consider fluid resuscitation and blood transfusion in trauma patients who present with hemodynamic instability; however, this pregnant patient is actively coding, and you should not delay delivery of a potentially viable infant.

Test-taking tip: This is an extreme situation that calls for extreme measures of which the answer to perform a perimortem cesarean delivery fits best.

45. ANSWER: C

Pelvic fractures in older adults, particularly women, may occur from low-energy falls from standing or seated positions. CT may only be 77% sensitive for pelvic fractures (particularly posterior), and MRI should be considered for patients with pelvic pain and pain with weight bearing, even with negative CT imaging.

It is not appropriate to discharge a patient home with uncontrolled pain and inability to bear weight. Your patient needs additional imaging (MRI) for further evaluation.

While admission for pain control is reasonable, the most appropriate next step in management is a pelvic MRI for further evaluation of continued pain and inability to bear weight.

Again, discharge is not appropriate in a patient with uncontrolled pain and inability to bear weight. Despite negative radiographs and negative CT imaging, an MRI is indicated for further evaluation of pelvic fracture in this older adult, osteopenic female.

Test-taking tip: The picture of sending an older adult woman home on crutches should make it easy to exclude this answer, and sending a patient to a skilled nursing facility without a diagnosis should also raise the hair on the back of your next, leaving only two possible answers to choose from.

46. ANSWER: C

This patient is hemodynamically unstable with a pelvic fracture. Other sources of bleeding have been excluded with a negative FAST exam and negative CT scan. She should undergo angiography with embolization. Most bleeding from pelvic fractures is due to low-pressure venous bleeding; however, shock and death are generally secondary to arterial bleeding. The arteries most commonly involved are branches of the internal iliac system, with the superior gluteal and obturator artery being the most common. Up to 4 L of blood can be accommodated in the pelvis until vascular pressure is overcome by tamponade.

CT is the gold standard for evaluating pelvic injuries and is more sensitive than plain radiographs.

In pelvic fractures, hemorrhage is the primary cause of mortality. Your patient is hemodynamically unstable with a documented pelvic fracture. Your primary goal should be hemorrhage control with angiography.

Delayed death is often caused by sepsis from open fractures. It is reasonable to carefully inspect the skin over the posterior pelvis, gluteal area, perineum, vagina, and rectum to evaluate for open injuries; however, in this case, it is more important to control hemorrhage then to perform a pelvic exam.

Test-taking tip: The patient scenario is one of a patient in hemorrhagic shock. The next appropriate step is one to stop the bleeding, making it easy to eliminate B and D as correct answers.

47. ANSWER: B

Bladder injury occurs in about 2% of blunt abdominal trauma patients, with 70% to 97% associated with pelvic fractures. Direct blows to a distended bladder (bladder distention is often seen in alcohol-intoxicated patients), with high-energy mechanism, should raise your index of suspicion for bladder rupture.

Abdominal swelling from urine ascites and perineal or scrotal edema from urinary extravasation are common.

Bladder ruptures are classified as intraperitoneal (occurring at the superior dome of the bladder) and extraperitoneal (occurring at the inferior aspect of the bladder).

A cystogram is the gold standard imaging study in the diagnosis of bladder rupture.

Urethral injuries can be seen in 5% to 10% of pelvic fractures and may be associated with blood at the meatus but are not usually associated with abdominal swelling and scrotal edema

The ureter is the least frequently injured GU organ. Isolated ureteral injury is rare in trauma patients because the ureter is well protected in the retroperitoneum. The majority of ureteral injuries are caused by penetrating trauma. There are no specific history or physical exam findings for ureteral injuries, and they can easily be missed.

The kidneys are protected by adjacent structures but are suspended from the renal pedicle, and blunt trauma or rapid deceleration injuries may result in injuries including contusions, shattering of the kidney, and vascular injuries that may lead to necrosis.

Test-taking tip: The lower genitourinary findings, including blood at the meatus and scrotal swelling, should help you eliminate C and D as answers.

48. ANSWER: D

In blunt abdominal trauma with stable vital signs and gross hematuria, defined as >50 RBCs/hpf, an IV contrast CT of the abdomen and pelvis is indicated for diagnosis of renal or GU injury.

In the setting of blunt abdominal trauma and gross hematuria, you should have a high index of suspicion for renal or GU injuries. Your patient needs further evaluation with an IV contrast CT of the abdomen and pelvis. It is not appropriate to "do nothing."

Outpatient workup is not appropriate in this patient with blunt trauma and gross hematuria, although it may be appropriate in stable trauma patients with microscopic hematuria.

IV contrast CT of the abdomen and pelvis is the gold standard for assessing renal and GU trauma and is more sensitive and specific than an IVP.

Test-taking tip: The key to this question is realizing that a urinalysis with 75 RBCs/hpf represents gross hematuria. If you know this, then it is clear that the patient needs an immediate diagnostic test, which eliminates choices A and B.

49. ANSWER: A

Your patient hit her face on the bottom of the swimming pool, resulting in hyperextension of her neck. Her clinical findings are consistent with central cord syndrome. Central cord syndrome is the most common incomplete spinal cord lesion, caused by hyperextension. It is often seen in patients with preexisting osteoarthritic changes or cervical canal stenosis, making it more common in older patients. This hyperextension results in damage to the anterior spinal artery, which supplies the central portion of the spinal cord where motor fibers reside, resulting in weakness and numbness that are disproportionately greater in the arms than the legs.

Anterior cord syndrome is caused by flexion or extension with vascular injury of the anterior spinal artery or bony fragment injury and results in paralysis and loss of pain and temperature sensation. Position, touch, and vibration are preserved.

Brown-Sequard syndrome is the result of hemisection of the spinal cord, usually associated with penetrating trauma. This injury results in ipsilateral paralysis, loss of proprioception, and vibratory sensation. Contralateral loss of pain and temperature sensation is also seen.

Transient spinal shock refers to loss of muscle tone and reflexes seen after spinal cord injury. Duration of spinal shock is variable.

Test-taking tip: Brush up on your spinal cord syndromes before the exam because they are frequently tested.

50. ANSWER: C

The neck is defined by triangles, zones, and fascial planes. The anterior triangle (formed by the borders of the sternocleidomastoid, inferior mandible, and midline neck) contains the most vital structures and is further divided into the following horizontal zones:

Zone I: clavicles to the cricoid cartilage

Zone II: cricoid cartilage to the angle of the mandible

Zone III: angle of the mandible and base of the skull

Test-taking tip: Brush up on some basic anatomy before the test, especially as it is relevant to patient care.

51. ANSWER: B

In penetrating neck trauma, careful physical exam is more than 95% sensitive for detecting clinically significant vascular and aerodigestive injuries. Laryngotracheal injuries may present with stridor, dysphonia, air or bubbling in the wound, airway obstruction, hoarseness, subcutaneous emphysema, tracheal deviation, laryngeal edema/hematoma, and/or restricted vocal cord mobility.

Vascular injuries present with active bleeding, pulsatile or expanding hematomas, thrill or bruits, hypotension, or shock unresponsive to initial fluid therapy.

Pharyngoesophageal injuries present with odynophagia, dysphagia, hematemesis, blood in the mouth, saliva draining from the wound, and prevertebral air.

Test-taking tip: You should be able to easily eliminate A and C if you think about the anatomy of the neck.

52. ANSWER: B

Penetrating neck trauma may result in vascular injury and/or aerodigestive injuries. In a patient with penetrating neck trauma who is having painful swallowing, difficulty swallowing, blood in the mouth, saliva draining from the wound, or a trans-midline trajectory, you should have a high index of suspicion for pharyngoesophageal injury.

Esophagram or esophagoscopy should be expeditiously obtained because morbidity increases if repair is delayed by more than 24 hours. Combined esophagram and esophagoscopy have 100% sensitivity for pharyngoesophageal injury. Missed esophageal injuries have a high morbidity and mortality (up to 50%).

CTA should be considered for evaluation of vascular neck injuries, not pharyngoesophageal injuries.

Bronchoscopy is more appropriate for tracheobronchial injuries.

Color-flow Doppler ultrasound is highly sensitive for detecting clinically important vascular injuries, but it cannot evaluate the aerodigestive structures of the neck.

Test-taking tip: The stem of the question points to an aerodigestive injury, which makes it easy to eliminate A and D as answers because these diagnostic modalities are used to evaluate vascular structures.

53. ANSWER: D

BCVI can result from cervical hyperextension and rotation or hyperextension during rapid deceleration, which can result in intimal dissections, thromboses, pseudoaneurysm, fistulas, and transections.

Catheter angiography is the gold standard for diagnosis of vertebral artery injury in blunt cervical trauma; however, it is invasive, time-consuming, and not readily available in most EDs.

While catheter angiography remains the gold standard for diagnosis of vertebral artery injury in blunt cervical trauma, CTA is readily available in most EDs and has excellent specificity (97%), and there is growing literature supporting use of CTA in the diagnosis of vertebral artery injury in blunt cervical trauma. In patients with injury identified by CTA, no confirmatory angiographic evaluation is indicated.

MRI has been gaining acceptance for evaluation of BCVI; however, sensitivity and specificity are lower than CTA, and MRI is not recommended as the sole screening tool for BCVI.

Duplex ultrasonography is noninvasive and inexpensive and has no contrast exposure; however, it is highly operator dependent, has limited views of zones I and III, and may miss small lesions.

Test-taking tip: "Gold standard" is the key phrase in this question, suggesting an order modality that might not be the most commonly used diagnostic study.

54. ANSWER: A

Vascular injuries are the leading cause of death in patients with penetrating trauma. Vascular injuries are present in up to 40% of patients with penetrating neck trauma with arterial injuries (predominately the carotid artery) accounting for 45% of penetrating neck vascular injuries. Venous injuries are found in up to 20% of patients with penetrating neck trauma.

Zone II (cricoid cartilage to the angle of the mandible) is the most commonly injured area (not zone I) and is easily accessed surgically.

Exposure and vascular control of injuries in zone I and zone III is more difficult, and most patients will undergo angiography and endoscopy to determine the need for operative intervention. Traditionally, zone II injuries undergo surgical exploration.

Wounds that are superficial to the platysma do not risk damage to vital structures of the neck; therefore, no imaging is required, and observation is appropriate.

Test-taking tip: The question presents a patient who is unstable and hemorrhage, which points to A as the correct answer.

55. ANSWER: D

Your patient has compartment syndrome from intraarterial injection of heroin.

The classic symptoms of compartment syndrome are pain/pain with passive stretching, paresthesias, and pallor, followed by paralysis and pulselessness later in the course.

Hand compartment syndrome, however, may not be associated with paresthesias, and assessing response to passive movement may make the diagnosis more difficult. Compartment pressure measurement in the small compartments of the hand may also be difficult, and diagnosis is typically made on a clinical basis.

Normal compartment pressure is <10 mm Hg. The delta pressure (the diastolic blood pressure minus the intracompartmental pressure) most commonly used to diagnose acute compartment syndrome is 30 mm Hg.

Clinical exam findings may be sufficient in the correct clinical setting to diagnose compartment syndrome. You do not have to have all classic findings (pain/pain on passive stretching, paresthesias, pallor, paralysis, pulselessness) to diagnose compartment syndrome, and in fact, paralysis and pulselessness are late findings of compartment syndrome. Timely diagnosis and fasciotomy is essential for limb salvage.

Compartment syndrome is not a diagnosis of exclusion. Laboratory testing and imaging are of no benefit in the diagnosis of compartment syndrome and may delay diagnosis, which may lead to permanent neuropathy and muscle necrosis.

Test-taking tip: Compartment syndrome is a limb-threatening condition, so it is easy to eliminate C as an answer because it states that this process is a diagnosis of exclusion (lots of tests and time delay).

56. ANSWER: A

Rapid and appropriate initial management of an amputated part is vital to salvage and preservation of function. Preservation of amputated parts is indicated whenever there is potential for replantation.

Appropriate care of the stump is as follows:

1. Remove jewelry and/or constrictive clothing
2. Irrigate the wound with normal saline
3. Wrap the wound with a pressure dressing
4. Apply a splint to prevent further injury and elevate

Appropriate care of the amputated part is as follows:

1. Remove all jewelry
2. Rinse the amputated part with saline solution
3. Wrap the amputated part in moist sterile gauze and place in a plastic bag or container. *Do not* immerse the amputated part in saline or hypotonic fluids. This may cause severe maceration and may make replantation technically more difficult.

4. Place the amputated part in a container and cool with separate containers of ice. *Do not* place the amputated part directly in ice.

Debridement and dissection should only be performed by the reimplantation team.

You should not clamp arterial bleeders. This may make reimplantation more difficult.

Test-taking tip: The procedures described in B and D are not commonly done in the ED for amputations so can easily be eliminated as potential correct answers.

57. ANSWER: C

High-pressure injection wounds (typically 2000–10,000 psi) are orthopedic emergencies. Despite often normal postinjection exams, areas may become edematous, pale, and tender and require surgical decompression and debridement.

Obtain an emergent orthopedics consultation, immobilize and elevate the affected extremity, update tetanus, and administer antibiotics.

While it is appropriate to update tetanus, this high-pressure injection wound may become ischemic, requiring surgical intervention, and discharge home is not appropriate.

Radiographs can provide valuable information regarding type of injection (such as radiopaque substance) and subcutaneous air. Immobilization is indicated. High-pressure injection injuries are orthopedic emergencies, and it is not appropriate to delay orthopedic consultation.

Again, high-pressure injection injuries are orthopedic emergencies, and definitive treatment includes surgical decompression and debridement. Admitting for observation alone is not enough.

Test-taking tip: Three answers (A, B, D) are similar to each other, suggestion a nonemergent condition. Only C stands out as a different answer, making it most likely the correct answer.

58. ANSWER: C

Chest compartment syndrome is seen with full-thickness burns of the anterior and lateral chest wall or circumferential full-thickness burns of the chest wall. This can lead to severe restriction of chest wall motion and increased peak inspiratory pressures and difficulty ventilating. An escharotomy is essential in relieving chest wall restriction. Because full-thickness burns are insensate and involve coagulation of vessels, no anesthesia is needed. A properly executed escharotomy releases the eschar to the depth of the subcutaneous fat only and results in minimal bleeding.

Perform an escharotomy of the chest by making incisions down the anterior axillary lines with cross-incisions at the junction of the thorax and abdomen.

The American Burn Association defines two requirements for the diagnosis of smoke inhalation injury: exposure to a combustible agent, and signs of exposure to smoke in the lower airway, below the vocal cords, by bronchoscopy. Treatment is supportive, and decreasing FiO_2 in a patient with hypoxia and smoke inhalation injury would not be recommended.

While cyanide poisoning should be considered in all inhalation injuries, hydroxocobalamin, not methylene blue, is the antidote for cyanide poisoning.

Carbon monoxide (CO)poisoning should also be considered in all inhalation injuries, particularly in enclosed areas; however, this clinical scenario is most consistent with chest compartment syndrome with circumferential full thickness chest wall burns and increased peak inspiratory pressure.

Test-taking tip: The combination of a full-thickness burn to the chest and an increased peak inspiratory pressure should point to you the correct answer.

59. ANSWER: B

The Parkland formula [4 mL × body weight (kg) × burn surface area (BSA) (kg)] is used to determine the amount of crystalloid for infusion in the first 24 hours in patients who present with partial-thickness and full-thickness burns. Half of the volume is administered in the first 8 hours, and the remaining half is administered over the next 16 hours.

The extent of burns can be determined by using the Rule of Nines, in which the head represents 9% and anatomic regions represent 9% or multiples of 9% of the total BSA.

In this case, each leg represents 18% (9% anterior and 9% posterior), for a total of 36% BSA.

4 mL × body weight (kg) × BSA (%)

4 mL × 90 kg × 36% = 12,960 mL

One-half of 12,960 mL is 6,480 mL therefore, 6,480 mL over the first 8 hours with the remaining 6,480 mL over the next 16 hours.

Test-taking tip: Brush up on some basic formulas, such as Parkland, that are used clinically before taking the test.

60. ANSWER: B

Burn depth has traditionally been described in degrees: first, second, third, and fourth degrees; however, classification based on need for surgical intervention has become the accepted nomenclature.

Superficial burns involve only the epidermal layer. Skin is red, painful, and tender, with no blistering.

Partial-thickness burns extend into the dermis and are further divided into:

A. *Superficial partial-thickness:* Involve the epidermis and superficial dermis and spare the deeper layers. Skin is blistered, and exposed dermis is red, moist, and painful. Scarring is minimal.
B. *Deep partial-thickness:* Involve the deep dermal layer. Skin is blistered. Exposed dermis is pale and white to yellow, and burned areas do not blanch. Absent capillary refill and pain sensation. May be difficult to distinguish from full-thickness burns. Scarring is common. Debridement and skin grafting may be needed.

Full-thickness burns involve the entire thickness of the skin, and all epidermal and dermal layers are destroyed. Skin is charred, pale, painless, leathery. Surgical repair and skin grafting is necessary.

Test-taking tip: This is a "you know it or don't" kind of question. If you don't know it, choose an answer and move on. You can perhaps mark it for review when you are done at the end of the test. Don't, however, let these kinds of questions get you stuck and waste your time.

61. ANSWER: A

Hydrofluoric acid is a corrosive inorganic acid often used in glass etching, electronic industries, and cleaning solutions. As fluoride ions complex with calcium and magnesium and in small, localized injuries, the main result is severe pain; however, large burns, inhalation injuries, or concentrated hydrofluoric acid exposure can lead to hypocalcemia, hypomagnesemia, hyperkalemia, cardiac arrhythmias, and death.

For minor exposures, like the one shown in the image, initial treatment consists of calcium gluconate gel to burned areas.

For poorly controlled pain, consider intradermal calcium, intraarterial calcium, or IV calcium (Bier block); for inhalation injuries, consider nebulized calcium; and for systemic toxicity (i.e., electrolyte abnormalities) and cardiac arrhythmias (such as prolonged QTc), treat with IV calcium.

This is not a thermal burn and does not require skin grafting.

Decontamination and copious irrigation with water (not normal saline) are recommended treatment for the majority of chemical burns with the exception of dry lime, elemental metals, and phenols. Water is not recommended for irrigation of dry lime, elemental metals, or phenol.

Phenol (carbolic acid) is moderately soluble in water, and irrigating with water can spread the chemical, causing increased absorption and toxicity. Polyethylene glycol (PEG) is used to remove phenol.

Test-taking tip: This is a "you know it or don't" kind of question. If you don't know it, choose an answer and move on. You can perhaps mark it for review when you are done at the end of the test. Don't, however, let these kinds of questions get you stuck and waste your time.

62. ANSWER: C

Chemical burns cause progressive tissue damage until the chemical is inactivated or removed. Acids damage tissue by coagulation necrosis. This process limits the depth of penetration of tissues.

Alkalis react with lipids and damage tissue by liquefaction necrosis. This process permits penetration of the chemical deep into the tissues until it is neutralized.

Exposure to alkali is more likely to produce deep disuse injury.

Wet cement is an alkaline substance that contains mainly calcium oxide followed by oxides of silicon, aluminum, magnesium, sulfur, iron, and potassium. When combined with water, an exothermic reaction converts calcium oxide to calcium hydroxide, a strong corrosive alkali.

Acetic acid (vinegar), hydrochloric acid, and sulfuric acid are acids that damage tissue by coagulation necrosis and have limited depth of penetration.

Test-taking tip: Wet cement is the only answer that stands out as different (all the others are acids) making it most likely to be the correct answer.

63. ANSWER: D

Urinary retention.

Cauda equine syndrome is an epidural compression syndrome that may be caused by intervertebral disk herniation, tumor, spondylosis, or inflammatory conditions and may present with low back pain (with or without radiation), weakness, sensory loss, decreased lower extremity reflexes, and bowel and/or bladder dysfunction.

Of all of these findings, the most common finding is urinary retention with or without overflow incontinence with a sensitivity of 90% and specificity of about 95%.

Treatment consists of emergent MRI and neurosurgical consultation.

Test-taking tip: This is a "you know it or don't" kind of question. If you don't know it, choose an answer and move on. You can perhaps mark it for review when you are done at the end of the test. Don't, however, let these kinds of questions get you stuck and waste your time.

64. ANSWER: B

S. aureus is the most common causative organism in all cases of osteomyelitis, including case of traumatic osteomyelitis after an open fracture.

Puncture wounds through tennis shoes have been implicated in pseudomonal osteomyelitis of the foot, but even in these cases *S. aureus* is more common.

Similarly, *S. paratyphi* is a consideration as a causative agent in patients with sickle cell disease, but *S. aureus* is still a more common cause in this patient population.

H. influenzae can cause osteomyelitis in children but is still less common than *S. aureus*, especially in vaccinated children.

Test-taking tip: *H. influenzae* and *Salmonella* infections are relatively rare and easy to eliminate, leaving two answers to choose from.

65. ANSWER: C

A Galeazzi fracture is a fracture of the distal third of the radius, usually shortened and displaced, with disruption of the distal radioulnar joint. It is more common in adults than children. The mechanism of injury is usually direct wrist trauma from a fall on outstretched hand (FOOSH), with the forearm in pronation. Clinically, there is often angulation of the radial forearm and mobility of the ulnar head.

A Colles fracture is a dorsally displaced radial metaphyseal fracture, also commonly caused by a FOOSH. It is the most common of all wrist fractures. On examination, the wrist will have the classic "dinner fork" or dorsiflexion deformity.

A fracture of the ulnar shift with associated radial head dislocation is referred to as a Monteggia fracture-dislocation. On examination, the forearm may appear angulated and shortened, and there are usually pain and swelling at the elbow.

A Smith fracture is also known as a reverse Colles and is a fracture of the distal radius with volar angulation of the distal fracture fragment. It can be caused by a FOOSH or direct blow to the dorsum of the wrist. The hand is palmarly displaced, creating a "garden spade" deformity.

The mnemonic MUGR (pronounced "mugger") can help you remember the difference between a Monteggia and a Galeazzi fracture: **M**onteggia—**U**lna fractured; and **G**aleazzi—**R**adius fractured.

Test-taking tip: Eponyms are commonly tested on standardized medical exams, so make time to review them as part of a study plan.

66. ANSWER: C

This is a Lisfranc injury, characterized by a fracture at the base of the second metatarsal or second cuneiform with dislocation of the lateral four metatarsals.

Direct trauma or hyperdorsiflexion of the joint between the midfoot and the forefoot (the Lisfranc joint) can result in this injury. It may result from a high-energy or low-energy mechanism and often results from an MVC, when the patient's foot is plantar-flexed as it presses the brake.

Common physical exam findings include significant foot swelling, tenderness over the tarsometatarsal (TMT) joint, and plantar ecchymosis.

There is significant morbidity associated with delay in treatment for this injury; thus, Lisfranc injures require orthopedic consultation in the ED. This injury requires ORIF to improve outcomes and reduce complications.

Test-taking tip: You can usually eliminate answers that have the word "always" or "never" in them.

67. ANSWER: B

Bennett and Rolando fractures are two intraarticular fractures of the thumb base resulting from an axial force acting on a partially flexed metacarpal.

A Bennett fracture is a fracture-dislocation in which the volar lip of the metacarpal base continues to articulate with the trapezium, while the remainder of the metacarpal is dislocated at the carpometacarpal joint. (The small volar fragment is held in place by the volar oblique ligament.)

A Rolando fracture is a comminuted fracture of the base of the thumb metacarpal, and the fracture fragments typically form a "Y" shape.

A Rolando fracture has a worse prognosis than a Bennett fracture.

Both of these fractures require a thumb spica splint and immediate outpatient hand service referral because they will most likely require ORIF. Neither requires emergent hand service consultation in the ED.

Test-taking tip: Eponyms are commonly tested on standardized medical exams, especially in orthopedics, so make sure to review them as part of a study plan.

68. ANSWER: D

Flexor tenosynovitis is commonly the result of a puncture wound on the volar surface of a digit, although this is not one of Kanavel's signs.

Kanavel's signs include diffuse fusiform swelling (tapering at both ends because of the course of the tendon sheath), finger held in slightly flexion, severe pain on passive extension, and tenderness along the course of the tendon sheath.

Treatment is IV antibiotics, update of tetanus as indicated, and consultation of the hand service for surgical incision and drainage.

Test-taking tip: Brush up on key signs and symptoms patterns (e.g., Kanavel's signs, Beck's triad) before the test.

69. ANSWER: A

SCFE is a condition that occurs in adolescent children around the age of 10 to 16 years. This condition is characterized by displacement of the capital femoral epiphysis from the femoral neck. It is more common in boys than in girls and often occurs in obese children.

The clinical presentation is slowly progressive and is usually atraumatic, or it may be associated with remote trivial trauma. The child will typically present with a painless limp or may have pain in the knee, thigh, groin, or hip. The hip will be adducted and externally rotated, and on exam, there will be limitation of internal rotation, abduction, and flexion.

Treatment is operative to stabilize the physis and avoid the potential complications of avascular necrosis of the femoral head and chondrolysis (narrowing of the joint space).

Test-taking tip: Brush up on common syndromes that commonly present to the ED.

70. ANSWER: D

This radiograph shows a perilunate dislocation. The radiolunate articulation is preserved, but the lunate is displaced and rotated volarly, with the other carpal bones located dorsally.

In a lunate dislocation, the lunate loses its articulation with the radius and is displaced and rotated volarly. The remainder of the carpal bones are displaced dorsally, and the articulation of the radius, capitate, and third metacarpal is preserved. Both a perilunate and a lunate dislocation result from forced hyperextension, such as a fall on an outstretched hand (FOOSH).

The most commonly injured ligament of the wrist is the scapholunate ligament, leading to a scapholunate dislocation. This is diagnosed when there is >3 mm of widening of the scapholunate space on radiograph.

More forceful trauma can lead to further ligament disruption, resulting in a lunate or perilunate dislocation, which are commonly associated with fractures of the

scaphoid or lunate. These injuries require emergent orthopedic hand consultation for possible ORIF.

De Quervain's refers to a noninfectious overuse syndrome resulting in pain on the radial side of the wrist with pinching or wrist movements.

Test-taking tip: Review the anatomy of the hand, especially the carpal bones and their fracture-dislocation patterns, because they are frequently tested.

71. ANSWER: C

This radiograph shows a posterior shoulder dislocation. Posterior dislocations are uncommon, accounting for fewer than 5% of all glenohumeral dislocations. A posterior dislocation can occur after a FOOSH with the arm held in flexion, adduction, and internal rotation or after a direct blow to the anterior aspect of the shoulder. Convulsive seizures due to either epilepsy or electric shock are associate with this type of dislocation.

A posterior dislocation is a commonly missed diagnosis because the radiographic findings can be subtle. Clinically, the patient will typically present with the arm held in adduction and internal rotation. Radiographically, the anterior-posterior view will show loss of the normal elliptical overlap of the humeral head and the posterior glenoid rim, as well as the humerus in internal rotation, the "lightbulb" or "rifle barrel" sign (as seen in this film). The axillary "Y" view is more diagnostic.

Posterior shoulder dislocations are less commonly associated with neurovascular injuries compared with anterior shoulder dislocations, which may result in injury to the axillary nerve and artery. Posterior shoulder dislocations, however, are more commonly associated with fractures, including fracture of the lesser tuberosity or neck of the humerus, fracture of the posterior aspect of the glenoid rim, and impaction fracture of the anterior aspect of the humeral head (reverse Hill-Sachs deformity), as well as injuries to the labrum and the rotator cuff.

Test-taking tip: This is a "you know it or don't" kind of question. If you don't know it, choose an answer and move on. You can perhaps mark it for review when you are done at the end of the test. Don't, however, let these kinds of questions get you stuck and waste your time.

72. ANSWER: B

A boutonnière deformity may result if the extensor mechanism overlying the PIP is damaged by a hyperflexion injury. The central extensor tendon attaches to the middle phalanx; thus, injury will disrupt extension of the PIP, but because the lateral bands of the extensor mechanism insert on the distal phalanx and remain intact, this will result in flexion at the PIP and extension of the DIP. There may be an associated dorsal chip avulsion fracture of the base of the middle phalanx. Treatment is to splint the PIP in extension for 4 to 6 weeks.

A mallet finger may also result from a jammed finger and refers to disruption of the terminal portion of the extensor tendon, which inserts into the distal phalanx and disrupts extension of the DIP. This may be associated with avulsion of the dorsal base of the distal phalanx. Treatment is to splint the DIP in extension for 6 weeks.

A gamekeeper's, or skier's, thumb results from forced abduction of the metacarpophalangeal (MCP) joint of the thumb and causes rupture of the ulnar collateral ligament. The patient will have tenderness along the ulnar aspect of the thumb and laxity on valgus stress of the MCP. Treatment of a partial tear involves a thumb spica splint, and treatment of a complete tear requires surgery to prevent chronic instability.

The volar plate is a thick ligament between the proximal phalanx and middle phalanx. This can be ruptured in a hyperextension injury of the finger. The patient will have swelling and tenderness over the volar aspect of the PIP and may have an associated avulsion fracture of the volar aspect of the middle phalanx. This is treated with splinting the finger in slight flexion.

Test-taking tip: This is a "you know it or don't" kind of question. If you don't know it, choose an answer and move on. You can perhaps mark it for review when you are done at the end of the test. Don't, however, let these kinds of questions get you stuck and waste your time.

73. ANSWER: C

This patient has physical exam findings suggestive of rupture to the anterior and posterior cruciate ligament. This should raise the clinical suspicion for a spontaneously reduced knee dislocation, especially given the high-velocity mechanism.

Popliteal artery injury is common in posterior knee dislocations and potentially limb-threatening. The exam must include evaluation of the popliteal pulse, pedal pulses, and ankle/brachial index (ABI). If there are obvious vascular deficits, the patient should go straight to the operating room, and if equivocal, a CTA should be obtained. There may also be injury to the peroneal nerve and, less commonly, the tibial nerve. Damage to the peroneal nerve will result in weakness of foot and ankle dorsiflexion (i.e., footdrop and weakness of toe extension). Damage to the tibial nerve will result in weakness of inversion and plantar flexion.

Although MRI may help to further characterize internal derangement to an injured knee that is not fractured, it is not usually emergently indicated in the ED.

CT without contrast may help to pick up occult fractures, but this is not the concern in this scenario.

Radiographs taken above and below a fractured joint may help to pick up missed injuries, but this patient does not have a fracture, so this is probably not indicated.

Test-taking tip: The key word in this question is "acute" management, suggesting a test that will discover an injury that may have significant morbidity. CTA is the only answer that fits this setting.

74. ANSWER: B

The earliest symptom in compartment syndrome is pain out of proportion to the injury associated with tense compartments. This is followed by the "5 Ps"—pain, pallor, paresthesias, paralysis, and pulselessness.

Compartment syndrome can result from trauma (fracture, crush injury, high-pressure injection injury, prolonged compression, hematoma) but may also result from other mechanisms, including infection.

The injury most commonly associated with compartment syndrome is a proximal tibial shaft fracture, and the anterior tibial compartment is most commonly involved. There are four compartments in the leg: anterior compartment, lateral compartment, superficial posterior, and deep posterior compartment. The anterior compartment contains the deep peroneal nerve, the anterior tibial artery and vein, the tibialis anterior muscle, and the extensor muscles of the foot. Associated findings of compression of the anterior compartment would be loss of sensation between the great toe and second toe and weakness of dorsiflexion of the great toe and foot.

A normal compartment pressure is 0 to 8 mm Hg. Compartment pressure >30 mm Hg is indication of injury, while a pressure >40 mm Hg is indication for fasciotomy.

Test-taking tip: Brush up on the clinical findings of common syndromes that present to the ED.

75. ANSWER: D

This is a Jones fracture, which is a transverse fracture of the fifth metatarsal at the level of the intermetatarsal joint. It is common in athletes playing running/jumping sports, when there is a transverse force applied to a plantar-flexed foot.

These fractures have a high incidence of nonunion and thus are managed either operatively or, if nondisplaced, conservatively in a non–weight-bearing cast for a minimum of 6 weeks.

In contrast, a pseudo-Jones or "dancer's" fracture is an avulsion of the base of the fifth metatarsal by the peroneus brevis tendon. This usually results from a plantar flexion/

inversion injury, as is common in an ankle sprain. Thus, tenderness at the base of the fifth metatarsal is part of the Ottawa ankle rules. This fracture heals well and needs only a rigid soled shoe (cast shoe).

Test-taking tip: Eponyms are commonly tested on standardized medical exams, especially in orthopedics, so make sure to review them as part of a study plan.

76. ANSWER: D

This radiograph shows displacement of the lateral mortise due to rupture of the deltoid ligament. Any time a medial malleolus fracture or injury to the deltoid ligament is suspected, a Maisonneuve fracture (fracture of the proximal third of the fibula associated with rupture of the deltoid ligament or fracture of the medial malleolus and disruption of the syndesmosis) must be ruled out. The associated proximal fibula fracture is shown in Figure 18.30. Any time a patient has medial ankle tenderness and swelling, an associated proximal fibula fracture must be ruled out.

The mechanism is usually eversion, not inversion, of the dorsiflexed foot in a high-intensity sport. This mechanism can result in a "high ankle sprain," which may be associated with rupture of the anterior tibiofibular ligament and injury of the syndesmosis. If there is a positive "squeeze test" or "dorsiflexion external rotation" test, this patient may need stress radiographs by orthopedics/podiatry to rule out

ligamentous instability. If weight-bearing films are possible, this will increase the sensitivity for ligamentous instability by showing displacement of the medial aspect of the mortise (increase in the width of the medial clear space).

The lateral ligament complex is usually injured by an inversion stress to the ankle.

Test-taking tip: Answers B and D are contradictory to each other, increasing the likelihood that one of them is the correct answer.

77. ANSWER: A

A nondisplaced spiral fracture of the distal tibial shaft is also called a "toddler's fracture" and is very common in ambulatory children with low-mechanism trauma. This injury is not suspicious for nonaccidental trauma. The fracture line may be difficult to see and may be mistaken for a nutrient vessel. Bony callus formation at follow-up confirms the diagnosis.

A "bucket handle" fracture, shown in Figure 18.31, is also called a metaphyseal "corner" fracture and results from intentional pulling and twisting. The shearing forces result in separation of the subperiosteal bone collar of the metaphysis, resulting in the disk-shaped fragment

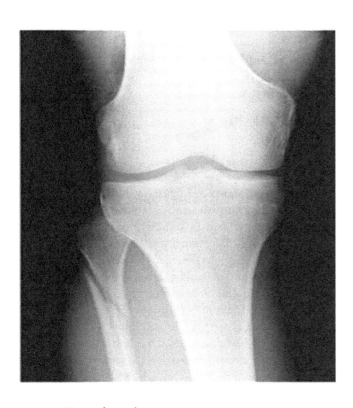

Figure 18.30 Knee radiograph.

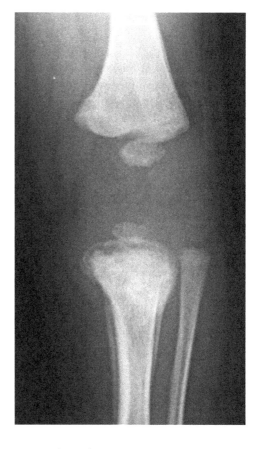

Figure 18.31 Knee radiograph.

described as a "bucket handle." This is very concerning for nonaccidental trauma, especially in a nonambulatory child.

The most common fractures in nonaccidental trauma are transverse or spiral diaphyseal fractures of the long bones in a nonambulatory child. The physician should maintain a high suspicion of nonaccidental trauma in any fracture in a nonambulatory child, in a new presentation of an old fracture, in a child with multiple fractures at different stages, and when the clinical history does not seem to fit the expected mechanism of injury.

Test-taking tip: This is a "you know it or don't" kind of question. If you don't know it, choose an answer and move on. You can perhaps mark it for review when you are done at the end of the test. Don't, however, let these kinds of questions get you stuck and waste your time.

78. ANSWER: D

Thoracic outlet syndrome is characterized by compression of the neurovascular bundle (brachial plexus, subclavian artery, and/or subclavian vein) as it courses through the thoracic outlet. Symptoms include pain, paresthesias/numbness (neurologic), swelling (venous), and arm ischemia (arterial). The syndrome may be associated with a cervical rib, muscular anomalies, or injury.

The most reliable test is the EAST. This is performed by having the patient raise the hands above the head and open and close the fist for 3 minutes. Inability to complete the test due to pain or paresthesias is a positive test. Adson's test evaluates specifically for arterial thoracic outlet syndrome (not neurologic or venous). In this test, both radial pulses are palpated while the patient turns the head from side to side. Loss of the radial pulse is a positive test. If conservative therapy (physical therapy, weight loss) fails, thoracic outlet decompression may be needed.

Adhesive capsulitis or "frozen shoulder" is characterized by limited range of motion of the affected shoulder and trouble with activities of daily living. On passive testing of external rotation, a sense of mechanical restriction of joint motion can often be appreciated.

Acute rotator cuff tears present with point tenderness over the site of the tear (the greater tuberosity). The drop-arm test, performed by passively abducting the arm to 90 degrees and asking the patient to hold the arm in this position, is positive with significant tears. Slight pressure on the distal forearm or wrist causes the patient to drop the arm suddenly.

Impingement syndrome of the shoulder is a spectrum of illness and is marked by progression of symptoms. The Hawkins-Kennedy impingement sign involves placing the arm into 90 degrees of flexion followed by internal rotation; the test is consider positive if the patient has pain with internal rotation.

Test-taking tip: This is a "you know it or don't" kind of question. If you don't know it, choose an answer and move on. You can perhaps mark it for review when you are done at the end of the test. Don't, however, let these kinds of questions get you stuck and waste your time.

79. ANSWER: B

This radiograph shows a Salter-Harris II fracture, which extends through the metaphysis. The Salter-Harris classification refers to physial, or growth plate, fractures. Salter-Harris II is the most common, representing more than 75% of growth plate fractures. The system classifies fractures from I to V, generally with I being the least complex and V being the most complex. Complications can include premature physial fusion and growth disturbance. A mnemonic to remember the classification is as follows:

S – slipped—across physis, or nothing seen radiographically = Salter-Harris I

A – above the growth plate—through growth plate and metaphysis = Salter-Harris II

L – lower than the growth plate—through growth plate and epiphysis = Salter-Harris III

T – through the growth plate—through epiphysis, growth plate, and metaphysis = Salter-Harris IV

R – rammed—growth plate is crushed = Salter-Harris V

Test-taking tip: Brush up on your Salter-Harris classifications because they are frequently tested on emergency medicine standardized tests.

80. ANSWER: D

This radiograph shows a large elbow effusion that presents with a posterior fat pad, which is always pathologic for an occult fracture, as well as an anterior sail sign. A normal elbow radiograph may have a small anterior fat pad, but a large anterior sail sign, as shown in this radiograph, indicates an elbow effusion. This can be the only radiographic abnormality seen with a radial head fracture, usually in adults, or a supracondylar fracture in children.

Test-taking tip: This is a "you know it or don't" kind of question. If you don't know it, choose an answer and move on. You can perhaps mark it for review when you are done at the end of the test. Don't, however, let these kinds of questions get you stuck and waste your time.

81. ANSWER: C

Finkelstein's test refers to ulnar deviation of the fisted hand and will reproduce the pain in de Quervain's tenosynovitis. De Quervain's tenosynovitis is an overuse inflammatory condition that causes pain on the radial side of wrist. This is due to inflammation of the abductor pollicis longus and the extensor pollicis brevis as they pass through the first dorsal compartment of the wrist. Treatment is with thumb spica splint, NSAIDs, or in severe cases, surgery.

Tinel's test, percussion of the median nerve at the wrist, and Phalen's test, maximal palmar flexion at the wrist, both refer to tests for carpal tunnel syndrome that have recently come under some scrutiny for not having adequate sensitivity or specificity.

Thompson's test is used to detect Achilles tendon rupture. If the foot does not plantar-flex when the calf is squeezed, this is a positive Thompson's test and is consistent with an Achilles tendon rupture.

Test-taking tip: Brush up on your musculoskeletal tests and signs because they are frequently tested on emergency medicine standardized tests.

82. ANSWER: D

When a child presents with pain and/or a limp, it is important to consider all of the diagnoses listed. Toxic (transient) synovitis is the most common cause of a painful hip in children, while septic arthritis is the most common cause of a painful hip in infants.

The patient with toxic synovitis is usually 3 to 8 years of age and presents with an acutely painful hip or knee and a limp. These patients are generally well-appearing but may have a slightly elevated temperature and erythrocyte sedimentation rate (ESR). They respond well to NSAIDs. This is, however, a diagnosis of exclusion, after a septic joint has been ruled out.

The patient with septic arthritis will typically present acutely ill-appearing, have a fever, and have an elevated ESR and white blood cell count. The most common organism overall is *S. aureus. Salmonella* is characteristic in patients with sickle cell disease. *Neisseria gonorrhoeae* should be suspected in adolescents.

The characteristic patient with SCFE is an obese adolescent male who presents with insidious onset of hip, groin, thigh, or knee pain.

The patient with Legg-Calvé-Perthes disease is typically 4 to 8 years old and presents with insidious onset of pain and limp due to idiopathic avascular necrosis of the femoral head. Temperature and ESR will be normal. If radiographs are normal and the patient cannot bear weight, consider obtaining an MRI because plain films may be normal early in the course of the disease.

Test-taking tip: This is a "you know it or don't" kind of question. If you don't know it, choose an answer and move on. You can perhaps mark it for review when you are done at the end of the test. Don't, however, let these kinds of questions get you stuck and waste your time.

83. ANSWER: D

This radiograph shows a Lisfranc injury, which is characterized by disruption of the TMT joint. The Lisfranc ligament connects the medial cuneiform to the second metatarsal and provides midfoot stability. This may or may not be associated with a fracture. In this case, it is not, and the radiographic abnormality is the increased space between the first and second metatarsals. Any time there is a fracture of the base of the second metatarsal (where the Lisfranc ligament attaches), a Lisfranc injury should be suspected. If the patient can tolerate a weight-bearing radiograph, this will help in making the diagnosis by making any space between the first and second metatarsals more evident. This injury needs urgent podiatry or orthopedic consultation to determine whether it will be managed conservatively (6 weeks in a non–weight-bearing cast) or operatively.

Test-taking tip: When one answer (urgent consultation) stands out for three similar answers (all weight-bearing immobilization methods), the different answer is probably correct.

84. ANSWER: C

This patient likely has a significant crush injury, based on mechanism, which is a relative contraindication to replantation because the tissues and neurovasculature are likely too severely damaged to undergo successful repair. That said, all digit amputations should be treated with rapid consultation with a hand surgeon. *All patients are candidates for surgical repair until the surgeon deems otherwise.* Tetanus and antibiotic prophylaxis should be given. The amputated part should be wrapped in moist gauze and placed in a clean, sealed plastic bag or specimen cup; then the sealed bag or cup should be placed in ice.

Some of the indications for replantation include amputation of the thumb at any level, amputation of multiple digits, virtually all pediatric amputations, and hand amputations through the palm and distal wrist. Some relative contraindications include severely crushed parts, amputations at multiple levels, and prolonged time of ischemia.

Test-taking tip: When one answers stands out as different from the others (run over by a tractor vs. all other minor mechanisms), it is probably the correct answer.

85. ANSWER: B

This is a Monteggia fracture, which is a fracture of the proximal third of the ulnar shaft associated with radial head dislocation. A Monteggia fracture is more common in children than in adults. It can be associated with a radial nerve injury. In pediatrics, there may be a bowing/plastic deformity of the ulna rather than a fracture associated with a radial head dislocation, so it is important to pay attention to the radiocapitellar line. It is very uncommon to see an isolated radial head dislocation in children (though it is common to see a subluxation of the radial head, i.e., nursemaid's elbow). Treatment in adults is ORIF; however, in children, it is usually closed reduction and immobilization.

A Galeazzi fracture is a fracture of the shaft of the radius with dislocation of the distal radioulnar joint. The ligaments of the inferior radioulnar joint are ruptured, and the head of the ulna is displaced from the ulnar notch of the radius.

A nightstick fracture is a fracture of the ulna, radius, or both. It is usually a defensive injury when a person uses the forearm to self-protect from a blow or a solid object.

Test-taking tip: You can eliminate choice A because its description of the fracture is not consistent with the radiograph. Study up on your fracture eponyms because they are commonly tested.

86. ANSWER: A

The Ottawa ankle rules include all of the above *except* A. The rules include tenderness along the *posterior* edge of the distal 6 cm of the medial or lateral malleolus, not the anterior edge. These rules have been validated by numerous clinical studies and provide guidelines for which patients do not need a radiograph of the ankle if they have none of the criteria.

Test-taking tip: Brush up on common rules such as Ottawa and NEXUS because they are commonly tested on emergency medicine standardized tests.

87. ANSWER: B

This radiograph shows a lateral tibial plateau fracture. The degree of depression and whether there is any associated ligamentous injury will help determine whether surgical management is indicated.

A tibial plateau fracture and any tibia or fibula fracture may be associated with compartment syndrome

Lateral tibial plateau fractures may be associated with a deep peroneal nerve injury; thus, the physician should examine and document sensation in the first dorsal webspace of the foot (between the great toe and second toe) and evaluate the patient's ability to dorsiflex the foot (rule out footdrop).

The most common complication is post-traumatic arthritis.

Test-taking tip: This is a "you know it or don't" kind of question. If you don't know it, choose an answer and move on. You can perhaps mark it for review when you are done at the end of the test. Don't, however, let these kinds of questions get you stuck and waste your time.

88. ANSWER: A

A nightstick fracture is a nondisplaced fracture of the ulnar shaft (it can also involve the radial shaft). A concomitant radial head dislocation (Monteggia fracture-dislocation) must be ruled out. A nightstick fracture may be associated with a radial nerve injury, and complications include nonunion.

A Colles fractures is of the distal radius with dorsal displacement and volar angulation, with or without an ulnar styloid fracture.

A Galeazzi fracture is a fracture of the shaft of the radius with dislocation of the distal radioulnar joint. The ligaments of the inferior radioulnar joint are ruptured, and the head of the ulna is displaced from the ulnar notch of the radius.

The Salter-Harris classification (I–V) refers to physial, or growth plate, fractures in children.

Test-taking tip: Brush up on your fracture eponyms because they are commonly tested on emergency medicine standardized tests.

89. ANSWER: C

With tenderness in the anatomic snuff box, one must assume that this patient has a scaphoid fracture. The scaphoid is the most commonly fractured carpal bone. Initial radiographs can be negative, so any patient with tenderness in the anatomic snuff box should be placed in a thumb spica splint and have repeat radiographs in 2 weeks. If at 2 weeks a fracture is still clinically suspected but the radiograph remains negative, MRI should be ordered.

This is an important injury not to miss because there is a high incidence of avascular necrosis owing to the poor vascularity of the scaphoid. This is especially true of injuries to the proximal portion of the scaphoid, which is the least well vascularized, because blood supply flows from the distal to the proximal portion of the bone.

Test-taking tip: This is a "you know it or don't" kind of question. If you don't know it, choose an answer and move on. You can perhaps mark it for review when you are done at the end of the test. Don't, however, let these kinds of questions get you stuck and waste your time.

90. ANSWER: B

A forearm fracture of both bones requires a significant amount of force; thus, these fractures are usually displaced. This usually requires ORIF. The most significant complication is compartment syndrome. Other complications include reduced ability to pronate and supinate, nonunion, and neurovascular injury.

Supracondylar fractures are most common in children between the ages of 5 and 10 years and area associated with nerve injuries, with the anterior interosseous nerve being the most commonly injured.

Monteggia fracture-dislocation is a fracture of the ulna diaphysis with anterior dislocation of the radial head. Complications include malunion, nonunion, synostosis, stiffness, and nerve palsy.

Galeazzi fracture-dislocation involves a fracture of the distal third of the radius with an associated dislocation of the distal radioulnar joint. Complications include malunion, nonunion, limited range of motion, and chronic pain.

Test-taking tip: Brush up on common causes of common presentations, such as compartment syndrome.

91. ANSWER: B

Thompson's test is performed with the patient prone and the knee flexed to 90 degrees. The calf is then squeezed, and the foot should passively plantar-flex. If there is no passive plantar flexion, this is a positive Thompson's test and indicates a complete tear of the Achilles tendon.

Thompson's test should be negative (the foot does passively plantar-flex with calf squeeze) with a gastrocnemius rupture.

Both an Achilles tendon rupture and gastrocnemius rupture occur with sudden contraction of the calf.

With a patellar tendon rupture, the patient will be unable to extend the leg or maintain a passively extended leg in extension. A patellar tendon rupture occurs with sudden contraction of the quadriceps, as occurs in jumping sports.

Test-taking tip: Brush up on your musculoskeletal tests and signs because they are frequently tested on emergency medicine standardized tests.

92. ANSWER: B

This is a torus fracture, which is an incomplete fracture characterized by buckling of the cortex. Children's bones are soft and pliable and tend to bend before they break.

A greenstick fracture is a fracture of a long bone in children where there is disruption of only one side of the cortex. Torus fractures are much more common than greenstick fractures.

A plastic deformity is when a bone bends but does not break. This usually occurs in the radius and ulna.

A Salter-Harris fracture is a fracture through the growth plate.

Test-taking tip: Torus fractures are subtle. Practice reading some pediatric radiographs before the test.

93. ANSWER: A

The most commonly injured nerve with a humeral shaft fracture is the radial nerve. The radial nerve supplies sensation for the first dorsal webspace of the hand and is responsible for thumb and wrist extension.

Choice B describes the median nerve function. Choice C describes the ulnar nerve function. Choice D is an incorrect answer and does not describe a particular peripheral nerve function.

Test-taking tip: Brush up on major nerve sensation and function.

94. ANSWER: B

This radiograph shows osteochondritis dissecans, an idiopathic process that occurs in adolescents and results in separation of a bone fragment from the articular cartilage. This bone fragment can result in a joint locking. Osteochondritis dissecans most commonly affects the *medial* condyle of the femur. It may also affect the elbow (at the capitellum) or the ankle (at the talus). Initial treatment is generally nonoperative and consists of immobilization and limited weight bearing.

Test-taking tip: This is a "you know it or don't" kind of question. If you don't know it, choose an answer and move on. You can perhaps mark it for review when you are done at the end of the test. Don't, however, let these kinds of questions get you stuck and waste your time.

19.

PROCEDURES AND SKILLS

Janak Acharya, Rimon Bengiamin, Nicholas Gastelum, Xian Li, and Fernando Macias

1. You are evaluating and planning to repair a 4-cm linear laceration on the forearm of a 24-year-old male. He informs you that the last time he had sutures, they used lidocaine and he developed a large red rash and swelling of his tongue that "they had to give me a shot in the leg for." Which of the following would be a reasonable alternative to use in this situation for local anesthesia?

    A. Bupivacaine
    B. Articaine
    C. Prilocaine
    D. Tetracaine

2. You receive a call from emergency medicine services (EMS) reporting that they are bringing in an otherwise healthy 3-year-old child from a primary care clinic. Reportedly, the child was undergoing a fairly extensive repair of multiple superficial lacerations. During the procedure the child began to complain of dizziness and numbness of the mouth and subsequently became unresponsive and had a tonic-clonic seizure. The patient is currently post-ictal but arousable. Heart rate (HR) is 130 bpm, blood pressure (BP) 60/40 mmHg, respiratory rate (RR) 15 breaths/min, oxygen saturation 99% on room air, and temperature 37° C. Fingerstick glucose is 126. EMS has established an IV line and is administering a 20-mL/kg bolus. You are concerned about possible systemic toxicity from local anesthesia. Which of the following is an appropriate antidote?

    A. Sodium bicarbonate
    B. Epinephrine
    C. Glucagon
    D. Lipid emulsion therapy

3. You are working in a small rural emergency department (ED) when EMS arrives with a 25-year-old female who suffered from a prolonged tonic-clonic seizure. She

arrives post-ictal, and her mother informs you that she has a ventriculoperitoneal (VP) shunt that has been in place since childhood. She was previously well until the past 3 days when she began complaining of nausea and a headache, which is unusual for her. Today she was more confused, and her mother called EMS after witnessing the tonic-clonic movements. Computed tomography (CT) scan reveals significant ventricular dilation. While you are waiting to get in touch with a neurosurgeon, your nurse informs you that the patient is now newly bradycardic with an HR in the 40s and is much less responsive. Which of the following statements is true with regard to tapping a VP shunt?

    A. Significantly elevated pressures >20 mm Hg suggest a proximal shunt occlusion
    B. Significantly elevated pressures >20 mm Hg suggest a distal shunt occlusion
    C. Accessing a VP shunt carries a high risk for iatrogenic meningitis
    D. Cerebrospinal fluid (CSF) infections can be ruled out by performing a routine lumbar puncture (LP) instead of accessing fluid from the shunt reservoir

4. You are managing a 32-year-old male intubated trauma patient who was involved in a high-speed motorcycle collision. He is intubated because of decreased mental status and has multiple injuries, including an open left tibia fracture that has been reduced and splinted. On re-evaluation you notice that the left foot seems to have become dusky in color. Removal of the splint does not seem to improve the color of the patient's foot. Which of the following would be an indication for emergent fasciotomy?

    A. Increased HR with passive flexion of the foot
    B. Compartment pressure >20 mm Hg
    C. Delta pressure <30 mm Hg
    D. Creatine kinase level >30,000 IU/L

5. You are managing a 45-year-old woman who has known cirrhosis due to hepatitis C. She arrives via EMS due to multiple episodes of vomiting blood and clot all morning. On arrival she is somnolent, and she proceeds to have two more episodes of large-volume hematemesis in the ED. You are concerned about her ability to protect her airway and proceed to intubate her. Despite aggressive treatment with crystalloid, blood products, and medications, she continues to have large volumes of blood come out of her oropharynx. Suspecting a variceal hemorrhage that is difficult to control, you elect to place a Minnesota tube. What is the most concerning complication of this procedure?

A. Infection
B. Gastric balloon rupture
C. Esophageal balloon rupture
D. Gastric balloon migration

6. You are re-evaluating a 65-year-old female patient who had a right internal jugular central venous catheter an hour ago to help with resuscitation for septic shock. Initial central venous pressure (CVP) on placement was 8 mm Hg, but now, an hour later, it has risen to 23 mm Hg. Which of the following is *not* likely to be a cause of an acute elevation of CVP?

A. Cardiac tamponade
B. Tension pneumothorax
C. Volume overload
D. Retroperitoneal bleeding

7. You are evaluating a 35-year-old wheelchair bound patient with a neurogenic bladder who had a suprapubic catheter placed 3 years ago due to chronic urinary retention. Since then, she has suffered from multiple urinary tract infections requiring multiple ED visits. Today she is brought in by her caretaker for concerns of signs of discomfort and decreased drainage from the catheter. Your nurse informs you that when attempting to replace the catheter, she is unable to remove it despite decompressing the balloon of the catheter. A bedside ultrasound reveals an inflated balloon despite attempting to remove the fluid from the inflation channel. You suspect that the balloon is not deflating appropriately and after clamping the catheter, cut the catheter proximal to the inflation channel without spontaneous decompression of the balloon. What is the next best step?

A. Overinflate the balloon with 20 mL sterile saline to allow for rupture and removal of catheter
B. Instill 5 mL of mineral oil into the inflation channel to allow for dissolving of the balloon to facilitate catheter removal

C. Inflate 1 mL of sterile saline into the balloon because it is likely unable to be removed because of balloon cuffing
D. Pass a guidewire along the inflation channel in an attempt to break apart obstructions within the inflation channel

8. You are evaluating a 45-year-old male with 3 days of left knee pain and swelling. He states he is no longer able to ambulate or bear weight on the knee and denies any trauma. His vital signs are BP 130/90 mm Hg, HR 86 bpm, RR 18 breaths/min, and temperature 38.4° C. Examination reveals a grossly swollen knee that is difficult to range because of pain. You perform an arthrocentesis because of concerns of a possible septic joint. Which of the following fluid analysis is highly suggestive of an infectious bacterial process?

A. Needle-shaped crystals that are negative birefringent
B. White blood cell (WBC) count >100,000 cells/μL
C. Polymorphonuclear neutrophils (PMNs) >75%
D. Synovial lactate <10 mmol/L

9. Which of the following sites is the most common for development of septic arthritis?

A. Hip
B. Great toe
C. Knee
D. Elbow

10. You are evaluating a 45-year-old female with a history of alcoholic cirrhosis who presents with 2 days of fever, abdominal pain, and increasing confusion. Vital signs include HR 110 bpm, BP 90/60 mm Hg, temperature 38.4° C, and RR 18 breaths/min. Her abdomen is distended with obvious ascites and is mildly tender diffusely. You suspect spontaneous bacterial peritonitis and prepare for a diagnostic paracentesis. Which of the following would be an absolute contraindication to performing this procedure?

A. International normalized ratio (INR) of 6
B. Platelets of $30 \times 10^3/\mu L$
C. Hypotension
D. Multiple dilated loops of bowel and suspect obstructive process

11. You are evaluating a 62-year-old female brought in by EMS for worsening abdominal pain. The patient has a history of hepatitis C complicated by cirrhosis. She states that over the past few days, she has had multiple episodes of diarrhea, sometimes mixed with mucus and blood, as well as an episode of vomiting. Her vital signs are HR 110 bpm, BP 110/65 mm Hg, temperature

38.8° C, and RR 16 breaths/min. On examination, her abdomen is distended but soft with a positive fluid wave, and there is diffuse tenderness in all quadrants but markedly worse in the left lower quadrant. A paracentesis reveals cloudy yellow fluid with 450 PMNs. The lab calls back with the Gram stain, which reveals polymicrobial growth on the stain. Which of the following is the next best step in the management of this patient?

A. Look for alternative source of infection because the patient does not meet criteria for spontaneous bacterial peritonitis at this time
B. IV antibiotics with admission for spontaneous bacterial peritonitis
C. IV antibiotics and CT scan of the abdomen and pelvis
D. Large-volume paracentesis

12. Which of the following patients should receive a head CT before LP for the evaluation of possible meningitis?

A. A 20-year-old male college student with 1 day of fever, headache, and scattered petechiae on the lower extremities
B. A 40-year-old female with 2 days of fever and headache and a platelet count of 25,000/μL
C. A 24-year-old female with a history of IV drug abuse and 2 days of fever and headache
D. A 55-year-old male with 4 days of fever, headache, vomiting, and new partial seizures involving the left arm

13. When evaluating a patient who is being considered for central venous access, which of the following is a complication that is seen with a left-sided approach of the internal jugular or subclavian vein but that can be avoided with a right-sided approach?

A. Pneumothorax
B. Catheter-related infection
C. Air emboli
D. Chylothorax

14. A 32-year-old pregnant female who developed sudden shortness of breath and an episode of syncope is brought in by EMS. Vital signs on arrival are HR 125 bpm, BP 85/60 mm Hg, RR 30 breaths/minute, temperature 36.5° C, and oxygen saturation 91% on a nonrebreather mask. She is confused and unable to tell you her gestational age but has a gravid uterus almost to the level of the xiphoid. On transition to the ED, the patient proceeds to become apneic and unresponsive and loses her pulses. Cardiopulmonary resuscitation (CPR) is started immediately. You decide in this patient to perform a perimortem cesarean delivery. Which of the following statements is true about this procedure and the anatomic changes of late pregnancy?

A. The purpose of a perimortem cesarean delivery is to save the child after maternal cardiac arrest
B. The procedure should be completed within 10 minutes of maternal arrest for the best chance at fetal survival
C. The purpose of a perimortem cesarean delivery is to improve maternal venous return
D. After dissecting to the peritoneum, the initial cut into the uterus should be along the superior half of the uterus

15. You are preparing to reduce a right femur fracture in a 60-year-old male involved in a motor vehicle collision (MVC). He is otherwise hemodynamically stable and has no other identified injuries. He weighs approximately 100 kg and received a total of 12 mg of morphine IV via EMS due to a prolonged transport time. He arrives sleepy but easily arousable to voice with HR 85 bpm, BP 145/90 mm Hg, RR 12 breaths/min, and an oxygen saturation 96% on 2-L nasal cannula. You are considering procedural sedation to allow for reduction of the femur fracture. Which of the follow medications would best allow for the patient to maintain spontaneous respiratory breathing but also sedation and analgesia?

A. Naloxone
B. Propofol
C. Ketamine
D. Midazolam

16. You are evaluating an agitated and combative patient brought in by police after he was found acting bizarrely in the street. He is screaming and requires five staff members to try and keep him in the bed without much success. You suspect excited delirium and work quickly to help control his agitation. Ketamine 5 mg/kg IM is administered, and after about a minute, the patient becomes more relaxed. While working on establishing IV access, your nurse informs you that the patient seems to have stopped breathing. You notice a patient who is sedated with obvious retractions of the chest wall without air movement of spontaneous respirations. What is the next best step in the management of this patient?

A. Obtain IV access
B. Administer naloxone 2 mg IM

C. Emergent endotracheal intubation

D. Positive pressure ventilation with jaw-thrust chin-lift maneuver

17. You are evaluating a 42-year-old male who was brought in from the homeless shelter after reportedly having a temperature there of 38° C. The patient arrives well-appearing and hemodynamically stable, but he does inform you that he has been off his HIV medication for quite some time and that this past week he has struggled with occasional frontal headaches. He has no evidence of neurologic defects, and a CT scan of the head is read as normal. You decide to perform an LP. The CSF color that returns is clear, opening pressure is 35 mm Hg H_2O. CSF WBCs are 105/mm³ (80% =monocytes), red blood cells (RBCs) are 30/mm³, and glucose is 50 mg/dL. This finding is most suspicious for which process?

A. Bacterial meningitis

B. Viral meningitis

C. Fungal meningitis

D. Guillain-Barré syndrome

18. You are evaluating a 34-year-old male with complaints of lower abdominal pain for the past day. He states that yesterday he inserted a plastic soda bottle into his rectum but has since been unable to retrieve it. He presents to the ED after worsening pain and inability to pass flatus or have a bowel movement. Rectal exam reveals a palpable smooth plastic object as well as some stool mixed with dark red blood. Abdominal radiograph reveals an outline of the foreign body along with some free air under the diaphragm. What is the next best step in the management of this patient?

A. Emergent surgical consult

B. CT scan of the abdomen and pelvis

C. Bedside removal of the foreign body

D. Ultrasound of the abdomen

19. You are placing a right internal jugular central venous catheter, and after completion of the procedure, your nurse informs you that there is difficulty with infusion of fluids through the catheter. You begin to suspect possible cannulation of the carotid artery. The patient has no identified neurologic deficits. Which of the following can be best used in the ED to detect arterial cannulation with a large-bore catheter?

A. Direct visualization

B. P_{CO_2} measurement compared with a venous sample

C. P_{O_2} measurement compared with an arterial sample

D. Compare blood color from catheter with an arterial sample

20. You are evaluating a 35-year-old male with a history of type 2 diabetes with 3 days of fever and pain when having a bowel movement. On exam, there is a large area of induration and redness along the 3-o'clock position of the rectum with surrounding erythema. Digital exam is difficult because of pain, and you are unable to pass a finger owing to fullness of the area of induration and patient discomfort. Which of the following is true about the management of this condition?

A. It can be managed with antibiotics alone

B. An incision and drainage should be performed in the ED

C. General surgery should be consulted

D. Urology should be consulted for emergent debridement

21. Which of the following is the correct management for the injury shown in Figure 19.1?

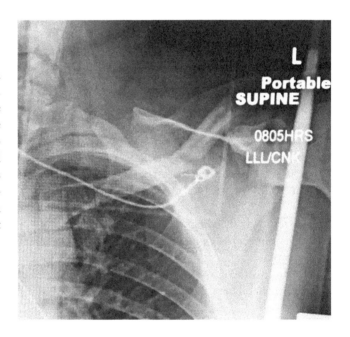

Figure 19.1 Chest radiograph.

A. Figure-of-eight splint

B. Sling

C. Coaptation splint

D. Posterior long arm splint

22. Which of the following has *not* been shown to reduce the incidence of positional headaches after LP?

A. Bed rest after the procedure

B. Needle design

C. Direction of the bevel during the procedure

D. Replacement of the stylet before needle removal

23. You are evaluating a 54-year-old male with a history of chronic obstructive pulmonary disease (COPD) who was brought in after a ground-level fall in which he fell face first onto the edge of the bathtub. Vital signs include HR 125 bpm, BP 100/50 mm Hg, RR 24 breaths/min, and oxygen saturation 88% on a non-rebreather mask. On examination he is agitated, with a Glasgow Coma Scale (GCS) score of 14 and evidence of a deformity along the bridge of the nose with deviation to the right. He has bilateral raccoon eyes and some dried blood at the mouth and nares. You feel some instability to the upper maxilla. He exhibits accessory muscle use and has breath sounds bilaterally, albeit with diffuse expiratory wheezing. Your nurse asks you if you would like to try the biphasic positive airway pressure (BiPAP) machine for his respiratory distress. Which of the following is an absolute contraindication for non-invasive positive pressure ventilation (NIPPV) in this patient?

A. Hemodynamic instability
B. Altered mental status
C. Facial fractures
D. Severity of respiratory distress

24. A 32-year-old female is intubated for respiratory failure due to severe asthma. The intubation goes smoothly with rapid sequence intubation but you are called to the bedside after about 10 minutes. The patient now has an HR of 154 bpm and a BP of 65/45 mm Hg. What is the next best step in the management of this patient?

A. Order a chest radiograph immediately
B. Disconnect the endotracheal tube (ET) from the ventilator
C. Administer 1-L normal saline IV bolus
D. Perform bilateral tube thoracostomy

25. Which of the following in *not* an absolute contraindication to nasal intubation?

A. Apnea
B. Epiglottitis
C. Basilar skull fracture
D. Recent nasal surgery

26. When performing a nasal intubation, which of the following procedures for advancement of the ET through the nares is correct?

A. Keep the bevel of the ET tube facing medially when advancing through the nares
B. Keep the bevel of the ET tube facing laterally when advancing through the nares

C. Lubricate the ET tube with lidocaine jelly for ease of passage and pain relief
D. The maximum size of ET tube that should be considered is a 6 mm

27. You are evaluating a 68-year-old male with a history of rheumatoid arthritis who was brought in from a nursing facility because of progressive shortness of breath over the past few days. He arrives in significant distress, speaking one-word sentences, and is hypoxic to 85% on his non-rebreather mask. A decision is made to proceed to intubation, but after administration of medications, you are unable to pass the ET. His rheumatoid arthritis has severely limited his neck range of motion, and you are unable to get a view of the cords at all because of his large tongue. There is a lot of difficulty with forming a mask seal owing to his large beard, and his oxygen saturation is now at 80%. What is the next best step in the management of this patient?

A. Calling for assistance
B. Positive pressure ventilation via BiPAP
C. Cricothyrotomy
D. Blind nasal intubation

28. In an adult patient, at what depth should one expect a bougie to get "held up" at the carina?

A. 20–30 cm
B. 30–40 cm
C. 40–50 cm
D. 50–60 cm

29. Which of the following is *true* about complications of arterial lines?

A. The rate of infection is higher in femoral arterial lines than radial arterial lines
B. Femoral artery pseudoaneurysms occur when the puncture is made too proximally
C. When suspected, pseudoaneurysms should be diagnosed by ultrasound
D. The femoral artery has the highest rate of thrombosis

30. Which of the following statements is *true* with regard to surgical airways?

A. Tracheostomy sites usually take about 1 month to mature
B. The majority of trachea-innominate fistulas develop >6 months after surgery
C. Cricothyrotomy can be considered in children >12 years of age
D. Tracheoesophageal fistula is most common within the first 7 days after surgery

31. You are evaluating an 8-year-old male brought in by EMS for severe anaphylaxis after eating peanuts. EMS providers have already given epinephrine and Benadryl IV en route, and the child still has significant angioedema with lip and tongue swelling. The lip and tongue swelling is so severe that the tongue is taking up the entire volume of the oropharynx. He is in significant respiratory distress with poor air movement, audible stridor, and oxygen saturation of 87% on a non-rebreather mask. What is the next best step in the management of this patient?

A. Blind nasal intubation
B. Direct laryngoscopy
C. Cricothyrotomy
D. Percutaneous transtracheal jet ventilation

32. You are evaluating a 35-year-old male who had his leg crushed in an elevator door about 6 hours ago. He states that he was doing well until about an hour before presentation when the soreness of his calf got unbearable and he was no longer able to walk on his leg. Radiographs show no acute fracture of the left leg, and there is an intact dorsalis pedis pulse. He is able to move his foot and toes, but you suspect impending compartment syndrome. What is the most sensitive finding before onset of ischemia in compartment syndrome?

A. Pain out of proportion to exam
B. Pain with passive stretch
C. Numbness
D. Loss of peripheral pulses

33. Which of the following is true about the pediatric airway?

A. Uncuffed tubes have a decreased incidence of postextubation stridor
B. Uncuffed tubes are thought to naturally seal at the level of the cricoid
C. Cuffed tubes are one of the main causes of laryngeal injury during intubation
D. Children older than 10 years should be intubated with uncuffed tubes

34. What is the recommended maximum dose of lidocaine with epinephrine when being used as a local anesthetic?

A. 3 mg/kg
B. 5 mg/kg
C. 7 mg/kg
D. 9 mg/kg

35. Which of the following is *not* an absolute contraindication for suprapubic catheter placement?

A. Pregnancy
B. Morbid obesity
C. Inability to palpate or visualize the bladder via ultrasound
D. History of pelvic radiation

36. A 68-year-old male with a medical history of metastatic lung cancer on chemotherapy presents to the ED with the chief complaint of shortness of breath and chest pain. Vital signs include BP 90/40 mm Hg, HR 110 bpm, RR 20 breaths/min, and oxygen saturation 94%. On physical exam the patient has jugular venous distention (JVD) and muffled heart sounds. The electrocardiogram (EKG) is nonspecific. The bedside ultrasound is shown in Figure 19.2. What is the most likely diagnosis?

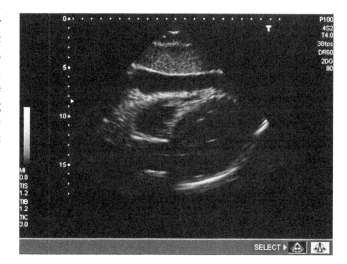

Figure 19.2 Ultrasound.

A. Poor global function
B. Right ventricular strain
C. Valvular dysfunction with regurgitation
D. Pericardial effusion with right ventricular collapse

37. A 28-year-old female presents after an MVC. She was wearing a seat belt and denies any head trauma or loss of consciousness. She complains mainly of abdominal pain. Her vital signs include BP 85/45 mm Hg, HR 110 bpm, RR 18 breaths/min, and oxygen saturation 96%. You decide to do a focused assessment with sonography for trauma (FAST) exam. On the pelvic view, shown in Figure 19.3, where is free fluid most likely to collect first? (Use labels on image to answer the question.)

A. A
B. B

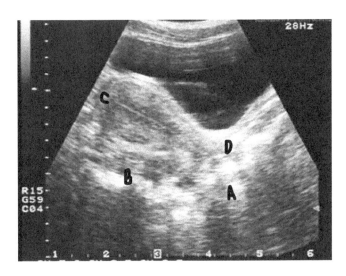

Figure 19.3 Ultrasound.

C. C
D. D

38. A 32-year-old female presents to the ED with chief complaint of abdominal pain and dizziness. She reports that she slipped and fell in the shower a few days ago and since that time has had left upper quadrant abdominal pain. Her vital signs are all normal, and the only pertinent findings on examination are a large ecchymosis to the left upper quadrant of the abdominal with localized tenderness but no rebound or guarding. You do an extended FAST (EFAST) exam, and some of the images from this are shown in Figure 19.4. What is the next appropriate step in the management of this patient, and what injury do you suspect?

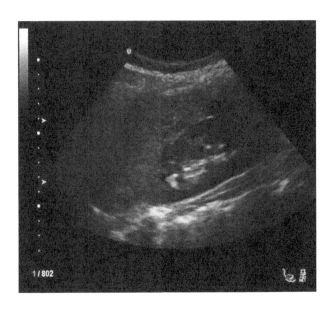

Figure 19.4A Ultrasound.

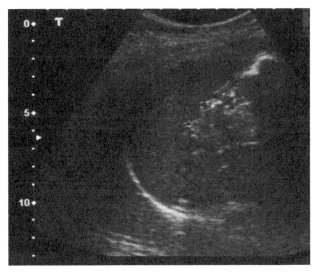

Figure 19.4B Ultrasound.

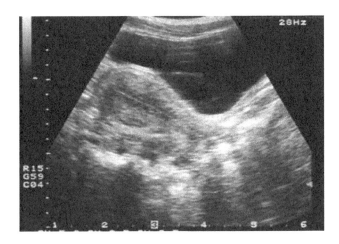

Figure 19.4C Ultrasound.

A. Discharge home for observation; renal contusion
B. CT scan; splenic injury
C. CT scan; small bowel injury
D. Labs; bladder injury

39. A 43-year-old female presents to the ED with chief complaint of pleuritic chest pain and shortness of breath. She recently returned from travel overseas. She is tachycardic, and her oxygen saturation is 92%. You suspect a pulmonary embolus, so you decide to do a bedside ultrasound of the heart as part of your initial evaluation. The image is displayed in Figure 19.5. Which cardiac window is this, and what other diagnosis will have this same finding?

A. Apical four-chamber view; mitral valve regurgitation
B. Subxiphoid view; pericardial effusion

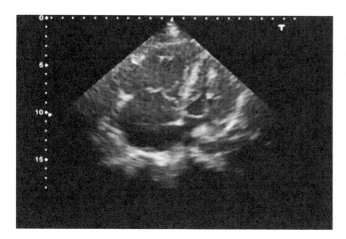

Figure 19.5 Ultrasound.

is one of the worst pains he has ever experienced. His vital signs are normal. After a full exam and sending some labs, you decide to evaluate his flank with ultrasound. One of the images you obtain is shown in Figure 19.7. What is the most likely diagnosis based on this image?

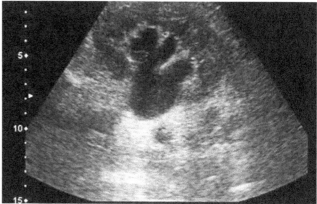

Figure 19.7 Ultrasound.

C. Apical four-chamber view; pulmonary hypertension
D. Parasternal short-axis view; cardiac ischemia

40. A 68-year-old male with history of hypertension presents to the ED with hypotension and abdominal pain. You are concerned that the patient may have an abdominal aortic aneurysm (AAA), so you decide to do a bedside ultrasound. You see the image shown in Figure 19.6. At what measurement would you call for surgical evaluation, and what is the proper way to obtain the measurement?

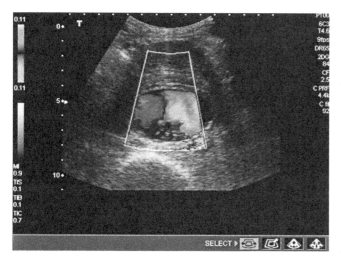

Figure 19.6 Ultrasound.

A. 3 cm measured outside wall to outside wall
B. 3 cm measured inside wall to inside wall
C. 5 cm measured outside wall to inside wall
D. 5 cm measure outside wall to outside wall

41. A 28-year-old male presents with the chief complaint of left flank pain. He reports that it started 2 days ago and

A. Simple renal cyst
B. Renal stone
C. Abscess
D. Hydronephrosis

42. A 40-year-old male is brought in by EMS after an altercation at a bar. The patient is lethargic and is intubated for airway protection. On your assessment you notice he has moderate facial trauma with right periorbital ecchymosis and swelling with slight exophthalmos. A retrobulbar hematoma and orbital fractures are noted on CT. After initial stabilization, what would be the indications to perform an emergent lateral canthotomy on this unconscious patient?

A. Evidence of retrobulbar hematoma alone is an indication for emergent canthotomy
B. Intraocular pressure (IOP) greater than 40 mm Hg along with an afferent pupillary defect
C. Severe proptosis
D. Suspected globe rupture

43. A 65-year-old female presents to the ED with the complaint of a headache. The headache is unilateral, right-sided, and retro-orbital, with associated nausea and vomiting. She has a history of migraine headaches, but this is different. She denies fevers or neck stiffness. Exam reveals a patient in moderate distress who prefers to keep her eyes closed, but she is neurologically intact. Her right eye shows injected sclera with a mid-dilated pupil and cloudy cornea. When using the Tono-Pen to confirm the diagnosis, which of the following can give a falsely elevated pressure reading?

A. Not calibrating Tono-Pen before use
B. Applying direct pressure on the globe when trying to help keep eyes open
C. Eye movement and accommodation during measurement
D. All of the above

44. A 20-year-old male presents to the ED with acute-onset left eye pain after leaving a movie theater. He reports nausea, vomiting, blurry vision, redness, and seeing halos around lights. You suspect acute angle closure glaucoma. Which of the following methods for measuring IOP is most accurate?

A. Applanation tonometry
B. Tono-Pen
C. Noncontact airpuff tonometer
D. They are equally accurate

45. A 20-year-old gravid female presents to your ED in active labor. A term male is delivered precipitously, and you notice he is apneic with an HR in the 40s. Resuscitation is initiated. He is successfully intubated but continues to have inadequate perfusion. Nurses are unable to obtain a peripheral IV line, and you do not have an appropriate-sized intraosseous (IO) line. What should be your next step to obtain vascular access?

A. Attempt a central venous catheter placement via femoral vein
B. Attempt a venous cutdown
C. Insert an umbilical vein catheter
D. Try to get a more experienced nurse to place a peripheral line

46. A 5-day-old female is brought in to your ED in cardiac arrest. The patient was successfully intubated by EMS, but they were unable to obtain vascular access. Which of the following is true regarding umbilical vein catheterization?

A. The umbilical vein can remain patent for about a week after birth
B. Umbilical vein catheterization is contraindicated in a patient with omphalitis
C. If the catheter enters the portal venous system, infusing hyperosmolar fluids can result in hepatic necrosis
D. All of the above

47. Which of the following is a *not* a likely complication of umbilical vein catheterization?

A. Hepatic necrosis
B. Air embolism

C. Splenic infarction
D. Cardiac perforation

48. A 3-year-old male is found by his parents unresponsive and apneic. On arrival, EMS finds the patient pulseless. Pediatric advanced life support (PALS) is initiated, and while the EMT is assisting ventilations, the paramedic attempts IV access unsuccessfully. What are the indications for IO access?

A. Administration of IV drugs or fluids commonly used during CPR
B. For routine IV fluid administration in an otherwise healthy child that is mildly dehydrated
C. For routine fluid maintenance after admission
D. For long-term antibiotics in a former IV drug abuser who has "no veins"

49. A 6-month-old female is brought in after an MVC. She is unresponsive, hypotensive, and tachycardic. No obvious active external bleeding is noted. Nurses are unable to obtain IV access, but you are able to obtain IO access. Which of the following can be given via an IO line?

A. Crystalloids such as normal saline or lactated Ringer's solution
B. Blood products
C. Dextrose solutions
D. All of the above

50. In which of the following patients would IO access be absolutely contraindicated?

A. An 8-year-old male patient in cardiac arrest with known osteogenesis imperfecta
B. A 3-year-old male patient in hypovolemic shock with burns to all possible cannulation sites
C. A 4-year-old male trauma patient with fractures proximal to possible cannulation sites
D. A 3-year-old male with known tetralogy of Fallot in cardiopulmonary arrest

51. A 35-year-old female with a history of lupus presents with dyspnea and syncope. She is hypotensive on presentation to the ED, with distended neck veins and muffled heart sounds, but her lungs are clear and equal bilaterally to auscultation. A newly enlarged heart is seen on chest radiograph. She is on a cardiac monitor and a non-rebreather mask, and nurses have established IV access. What is the next best step in the management of this patient?

A. Needle thoracostomy
B. Resuscitative endovascular balloon occlusion of the aorta (REBOA) placement through a right inguinal approach

C. Ultrasound-guided pericardiocentesis

D. Emergency dialysis

52. A 79-year-old male dialysis patient presents in pulseless electrical activity (PEA) arrest. The patient had a witnessed arrest, and resuscitative efforts have been ongoing for 10 minutes. Thus far, sodium bicarbonate, calcium chloride, and epinephrine have been given and bilateral needle thoracotomies performed without return of spontaneous circulation. What further treatment might this patient benefit from?

A. Calling the code because further intervention is futile

B. Emergency dialysis

C. 2 units of packed RBCs

D. Pericardiocentesis

53. What are the landmarks for performing a pericardiocentesis?

A. Second intercostal space mid-clavicular line

B. Fourth intercostal space mid-axillary line

C. 1 cm subxiphoid aimed to the left nipple

D. 2 cm subclavicular at the bend of the clavicle

54. In which of the following patients is the performance of an ED thoracotomy most indicated?

A. A gunshot wound (GSW) victim with no signs of life for 30 minutes who arrives in the ED in asystole

B. A blunt trauma victim who loses his pulses in the ED and is unresponsive to fluids and CPR

C. A patient with a widened mediastinum who goes into PEA arrest without a history of trauma

D. A GSW victim with a large head wound and no other visible injuries who loses pulses in the ED

55. Which of the following is *not* considered a sign of life in the context of indications to perform an ED thoracotomy?

A. Pupillary response

B. Movement of extremities

C. Cardiac electrical activity

D. Skin flushing

56. When delivering the heart from the pericardial sac during an ED thoracotomy, which structure is most likely to be injured?

A. Thoracic duct

B. Atrial appendage

C. Intercostal artery

D. Phrenic nerve

57. What landmarks are most commonly used for the placement of a tube thoracotomy?

A. Second intercostal space mid-axillary line

B. Second intercostal space mid-clavicular line

C. Fifth intercostal space mid-axillary line

D. Third intercostal space anterior axillary line

58. A 25-year-old male who has fallen 15 feet out of a tree presents with difficulty breathing and right-sided chest pain. On arrival to the ED, his has a GCS score of 15 but is in obvious respiratory distress. Initial vital signs are HR 130 bpm, BP 70/30 mm Hg, and SpO_2 80%. The patient has distended neck veins, poor movement of the right chest wall, crepitus to right chest wall, and decreased breath sounds over the right chest. The patient is on a monitor and a non-rebreather mask, and nurses are attempting IV access. What is the next best step in the management of this patient?

A. Rapid sequence intubation with rapid forceful ventilation

B. Seldinger technique tube thoracostomy over a guidewire at the right fourth intercostal space mid-axillary line

C. Needle thoracostomy at the right second intercostal space mid-clavicular line

D. Open chest tube placed at the right inframammary crease mid-axillary line

59. A 17-year-old male presents to the ED with the complaint of left-sided chest pain and shortness of breath after blowing up balloons for a party. His vital signs are HR 84 bpm, BP 124/70 mm Hg, and SpO_2 of 97%. His chest radiograph is shown in Figure 19.8. What is the most appropriate management for this patient?

A. Needle thoracostomy at the second intercostal space

B. Placement of a 36-French chest tube at the fifth intercostal space mid-axillary line using an open surgical technique

C. Discharge home without further management but with close follow-up with a primary care physician

D. Placement of an 18-French chest tube at the fourth intercostal space over a guidewire, using the Seldinger technique, and then attaching it to a Heimlich valve

60. An 83-year-old female presents with the complaints of weakness, dizziness, and chest pain. She has a GCS score of 15 and is speaking using full sentences. Her initial vital signs on presentation to the ED include HR 33 bpm and BP 70/palp mm Hg. Her EKG is shown in Figure 19.9. What is the next best step in the management of this patient?

A. Rapid sequence intubation
B. Biphasic cardioversion at 200 J
C. Atropine 1 mg IV push
D. Transcutaneous pacing

61. Which of the following patients meets emergent criteria for transvenous pacing in the ED?

A. A morbidly obese, hypotensive, and bradycardic male patient who has transcutaneous pacer pads in place but cannot get cardiac capture at maximal amperage
B. A cachectic female older adult in complete heart block who is hypotensive and bradycardic
C. A bradycardic hypotensive teenage patient who has overdosed on a calcium channel blocker
D. A normotensive but bradycardic patient with arteriovenous dissociation on EKG

62. What are the appropriate steps for transvenous pacing in the ED?

A. Sterile technique, femoral triple cordis placement, advance balloon deflated and inflate when "current of injury" tracing is present indicating atrial pacing, check balloon integrity
B. Sterile technique, internal jugular cordis placement, check pacer balloon, advance with balloon inflated until pacer spike is seen followed by a left bundle branch block tracing indicating ventricular

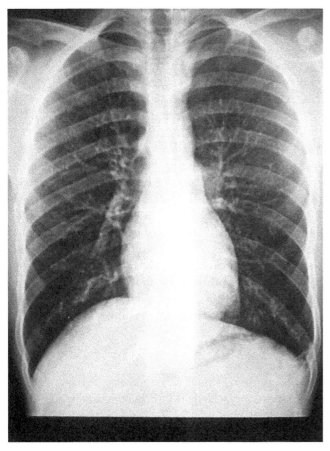

Figure 19.8 Chest radiograph.

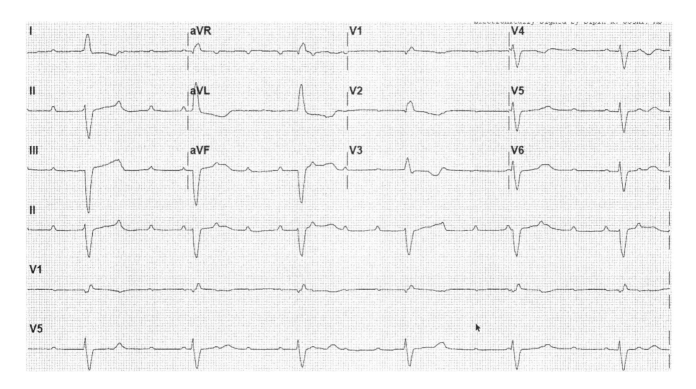

Figure 19.9 Electrocardiogram.

placement, lower amperage to lowest possible capture, deflate balloon

C. Sterile technique, subclavian cordis placement, advance pacer wire with balloon inflated 10 cm, withdraw pacer wire 1 cm, lower amperage to allow lowest possible capture

D. Sterile technique, internal jugular cordis placement, advance catheter with balloon inflated until "current of injury tracing" indicating ventricular placement, lower amperage to lowest possible capture setting, check balloon integrity with transthoracic ultrasound

63. Which of the following is *not* known to cause of orbital compartment syndrome?

A. Bony intrusion from fractures
B. Vitreous humor
C. Hematoma
D. Air

64. The goal of a lateral canthotomy is to reduce pressure within the orbit. By what mechanism does it accomplish this goal?

A. Release of blood from the retro-orbital space
B. Destruction of the canthal ligament, allowing the globe to fall into the back of the orbit
C. Destruction of the canthal ligament, allowing for iatrogenic proptosis
D. Release of vitreous humor, causing a reduction in IOP

65. Which of the following is a sign of orbital compartment syndrome?

A. Decreased IOP
B. Irregular papillary shape
C. Decreased retropulsion and "rock-hard" eyelids
D. Synechiae

66. A 50-year-old male with history of hepatitis C and alcohol abuse presents with abdominal distention and shortness of breath for 7 days. His initial vital signs include BP 140/80 mm Hg, HR 90 bpm, RR 14 breaths/min, oxygen saturation 98%, and temperature 37.7° C. Labs are drawn and are notable for a normal WBC count, brain natriuretic peptide (BNP), liver function tests (LFTs), and lipase. A bedside ultrasound is performed, of which one image is shown in Figure 19.10. During the examination, the patient had a negative sonographic Murphy's sign. Which of the following is the most likely diagnosis?

A. Acute heart failure
B. Chronic cirrhosis

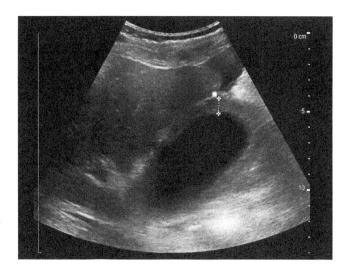

Figure 19.10 Ultrasound.

C. Acute pancreatitis
D. Acute cholecystitis

67. A 34-year-old male with history of injection drug abuse presents with an area of redness and swelling along the left forearm for 7 days. The patient does not recall how the process began. His vital signs are within normal limits. On physical exam, the left medial forearm is warm, erythematous, and tender to touch, without palpable fluctuance or crepitans. A high-frequency linear probe is placed over the affected area of the arm, and the image shown in Figure 19.11 is obtained. Which of the following is the next best step in management of this patient?

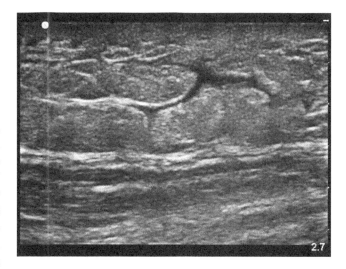

Figure 19.11 Ultrasound.

A. Consult surgery for foreign body removal
B. Consult surgery for possible necrotizing fasciitis

C. Incise and drain abscess, then discharge with oral antibiotics

D. Discharge with oral antibiotics

68. A 25-year-old female presents with intermittent lower abdominal cramping and vaginal bleeding. She states that she has had a recent positive home pregnancy test, and her symptoms started yesterday. Initial vital signs include BP 110/80 mm Hg, HR 80 bpm, RR 12 breaths/min, and oxygen saturation 99%. Labs are drawn and are unremarkable except for a serum β-human chorionic gonadotropin (β-hCG) level of 900 mIU/mL. You perform a bedside transabdominal pelvic ultrasound and obtain the image shown in Figure 19.12. What is the next best step in the management of this patient?

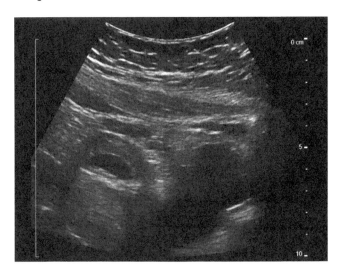

Figure 19.12 Ultrasound.

A. Discharge home with the diagnosis of intrauterine pregnancy and follow-up

B. Discharge home with instructions to follow up in 2 to 3 days for serial β-hCG level

C. Obtain a formal transvaginal ultrasound

D. Consult an obstetrician for an ectopic pregnancy

69. An 18-year-old male presents with left-sided chest pain and shortness of breath after an MVC. The patient is evaluated immediately on arrival in a trauma resuscitation bay with a supine chest radiograph, which was read as normal. Initial vital signs include BP 100/60 mm Hg, HR 100 bpm, RR 22 breaths/min, and oxygen saturation 92%. An EFAST is performed, and one of the images is shown in Figure 19.13. What diagnosis is this image most consistent with?

A. Pneumothorax

B. Hemothorax

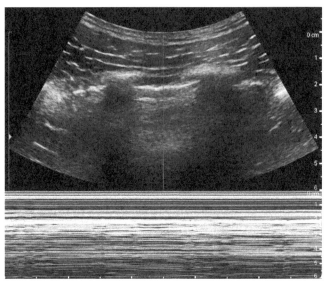

Figure 19.13 Ultrasound.

C. Normal findings

D. Pericardial effusion

70. A 44-year-old female presents with acute-onset upper abdominal pain. She reports that the pain started shortly after eating and has since resolved. The pain was worse over the right upper quadrant. She is afebrile, and her other vital signs are normal. Her labs, including complete blood count (CBC), chemistry 10 panel, LFTs, and lipase, are within normal limits. A limited abdominal ultrasound is obtained and is shown in Figure 19.14. What is the next best step in management of this patient?

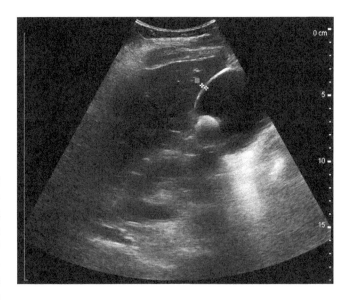

Figure 19.14 Ultrasound.

A. Admission for IV antibiotics

B. Outpatient referral for elective surgery

C. Consult gastrointestinal specialist for endoscopic retrograde cholangiopancreatography (ERCP)
D. Consult interventional radiology (IR) for percutaneous biliary drain

71. In which situation would placing vertical mattress sutures *not* be the best option for primary repair of a laceration?

A. A 45-year-old male construction worker who sustained a 3-cm linear forehead laceration when a metal beam struck him at work
B. A 65-year-old female with a 5-cm gaping laceration to the back of her neck sustained in an MVC
C. An 18-year-old male who sustained an 8-cm deep laceration to his posterior calf while playing soccer
D. A 35-year-old female with a 6-cm jagged, gaping laceration to her upper thigh sustained during a fall while hiking

72. A 23-year-old male presents to the ED with the complaint of right shoulder pain after falling on an outstretched hand while snowboarding. He is holding his arm in internal rotation and adduction, and he has pain with attempts at both active and passive range of motion. His radiograph is shown in Figure 19.15. What is the best way to manage this injury?

A. Reduction with scapular rotation
B. Reduction with the Milch technique
C. Reduction with the DePalma method
D. Reduction with the Stimson maneuver

73. A 3-year-old female is brought in by her mother with the complaint of left elbow pain and being unwilling to move her left arm. Her mother denies any history of trauma but states that earlier in the day, the child's two older siblings were swinging her between them by her arms. She has otherwise been well with no fever or other constitutional symptoms. On exam, she is well-appearing and has no obvious deformity, erythema,

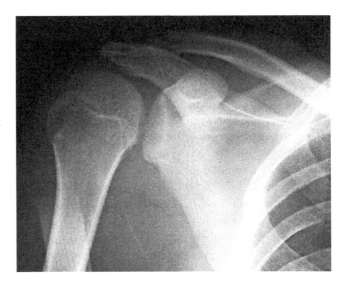

Figure 19.15 Shoulder radiograph.

or swelling to her left arm, but she refuses to move her left elbow and cries if you try to move it. What is the next most appropriate step in the management in this patient?

A. Discharge home with ibuprofen, ice, and rest
B. Obtain an elbow radiograph
C. Perform an immediate reduction
D. Set up to tap the elbow to evaluate for septic joint

74. A 4-year-old male is brought in by his father with a plastic bead in his right nares. It is unclear how long it has been there. Which of the following techniques is *not* recommended for removal of this foreign body?

A. Irrigation with warm water
B. Grasp the bead with alligator forceps
C. Place a catheter with a balloon behind the bead, inflate the balloon and apply gentle tension to remove the bead
D. Have the father perform the "kissing" technique whereby he occludes the left nares and blows into his son's mouth

ANSWERS

1. ANSWER: D

Lidocaine allergy is a potentially life-threatening reaction to a commonly used medication in most EDs. When its use is contraindicated, as in this scenario, physicians must seek alternative agents to use for local anesthesia.

Local anesthetics are generally separated into two groups, esters and amides, depending on their chemical makeup. When allergy is reported to a certain group (amides in this case), physicians should look to select an anesthetic in an alternative group.

The only ester in these options is tetracaine. In patients who report an allergic reaction to local anesthetics but cannot remember the specific name or class, there is a growing body of literature on using diphenhydramine as a safe alternative.

Test-taking tip: Although this is a recall question, a quick way to separate amides and esters is that amides all have two I's in the name while esters have one I.

2. ANSWER: D

While uncommon, systemic toxicity from local anesthesia must be considered in any situation in which patients develop central nervous system (CNS) or cardiovascular complications after administration of medications such as lidocaine. Emergency medicine physicians should be extremely prudent of this, especially during procedures in young patients, because overdose may occur even without accidental intravascular injection of anesthetics.

Early signs of local anesthetic toxicity generally affect the CNS and include lightheadedness, confusion, and circumoral numbness. As toxicity increases, it can precipitate tonic-clonic convulsions and CNS depression. Additionally, all local anesthetics can induce cardiac dysrhythmias and myocardial depression at high doses.

Lipid emulsion therapy (Intralipid) should be considered in patients suffering from hemodynamic instability or cardiovascular collapse after injection of local anesthetics. It is thought to improve cardiotoxicity by increasing clearance from cardiac tissue and possible reversing local anesthetic inhibition of myocardial fatty acid oxidation. Initial dosing is a 1.5-mL/kg bolus of 20% Intralipid followed by a 0.25- to 0.5-mL/kg/min infusion for 30 to 60 minutes if needed for refractory hypotension.

Sodium bicarbonate is used as an antidote for multiple common overdoses such as tricyclic antidepressants, salicylate, and toxic alcohols. Glucagon is a potential antidote for ß-blocker and calcium channel blocker overdoses. There are some concerns with using epinephrine for anesthetic toxicity because it could potentially provoke worsening dysrhythmias or exacerbate an ongoing arrhythmia.

Test-taking tip: Given the clinical scenario, it should be relatively easy to eliminate choices B and C, giving you two answers to choose from.

3. ANSWER: B

Accessing a VP shunt reservoir should generally be avoided by emergency medicine physicians without guidance from a specialist. However, there may be certain times when complications arise in settings where specialty backup is not available and patients are critically ill from elevated intracranial pressure (ICP), which may require emergent intervention, such as in the patient in this question.

Aside from normal measures to decrease ICP, such as hyperventilation and osmotic agents (e.g., mannitol, hypertonic saline), patients with VP shunts that are malfunctioning may be amenable to drainage directly from the reservoir. This is generally done under sterile conditions with a small-gauge butterfly needle inserted perpendicularly to the skin into the dome of a reservoir. The butterfly needle is attached to a manometer such as the one found in the LP kit, and fluid is allowed to drain out slowly.

If CSF fluid can be attained and pressures are elevated, this suggests an obstruction in the distal portion of the shunt. If fluid cannot be obtained, it is suggestive of a proximal shunt obstruction (more common). Care must be done to withdraw fluid slowly and to never aspirate directly from the reservoir because rapid decompression of CSF may induce subdural hemorrhage.

Although there is a known risk for infection from the procedure itself, the actual risk for causing a shunt infection from the procedure itself is <1%. Although literature is limited, neither LP on its own nor VP shunt evaluation can completely rule out infection in a patient. CSF infection is the largest cause of mortality in patients with VP shunts and is most common in the period after the procedure and in the very young and old.

Test-taking tip: When two answers have the same root (significantly elevated pressures >20 mm Hg), it is a pretty good guess that one of them is the correct answer.

4. ANSWER: C

Evaluation of possible compartment syndrome is challenging in patients who are obtunded or intubated. The patient in this question has a high-risk fracture for developing compartment syndrome.

Intercompartmental pressures should be evaluated with a device such as a Stryker needle. A delta pressure (diastolic

BP – compartment pressure) <30 mm Hg is highly suggestive of compartment syndrome and requires immediate consultation with a specialist. It is thought to be a more reliable measurement than isolated compartment pressures, although a compartment pressure >30 mm Hg is also highly suspicious for causing compartment syndrome.

Pain with passive range of motion is one of the earliest signs of impending compartment syndrome but would be difficult to assess in this intubated patient.

Rhabdomyolysis is a common complication in polytrauma patients, but an elevated creatine kinase level by itself is not diagnostic of compartment syndrome.

Test-taking tip: Because compartment syndrome is all about pressures, it helps to focus on the two answers that address pressures, helping you to narrow in on the correct answer.

5. ANSWER: D

Placement of a Minnesota (or Blakemore) tube is an uncommon but potentially life-saving procedure in patients with uncontrollable gastroesophageal hemorrhage. The tube is inserted similarly to an orogastric tube but uses a large inflatable gastric balloon as well as an esophageal balloon to tamponade a site of bleeding. After appropriate inflation of the gastric balloon and confirmation of the positioning, the tube is then placed on traction to allow for adequate pressure onto the bleeding sites.

Proximal migration of the gastric balloon into the esophagus can cause tracheal compression and respiratory distress or failure. For this reason a pair of scissors should be left at the bedside to cut the tubing should this be suspected.

Infection prophylaxis should be provided to all patients with suspected variceal bleed regardless if Minnesota tube placement is indicated.

Rupture of the gastric or esophageal balloon would cause loss of tamponade and require replacement of a new tube. Pain is a known side effect of this procedure because the inflated gastric tube can be quite uncomfortable for patients and adequate sedation is indicated.

Test-taking tip: Brush up on complications of procedures commonly performed in the ED.

6. ANSWER: D

CVP is an indicator of both central blood volume and the ability of the heart to move blood into the arterial system. While its monitoring may be useful in guiding resuscitation, it should probably not be used as the sole measurement in which to direct management of critically ill patients.

In general, conditions that cause hypovolemic or distributive shock will decrease CVP due to decreased central blood volume. Conditions such as right heart failure, cardiac tamponade, tension pneumothorax, and volume load all decrease the heart's ability to move blood into the arterial system and are generally associated with an increase in CVP.

Test-taking tip: In questions with the word *not*, you are looking for the answer that is different from the rest. Physiologically, retroperitoneal bleeding stands out as being different compared with the other three answer choices.

7. ANSWER: D

Suprapubic catheters are not uncommonly seen devices in the ED for patients who have contraindications for prolonged indwelling urethral catheters. The patient in this question has developed dysfunction of her suprapubic catheter as well as failure of the catheter balloon to deflate and facilitate removal of the catheter.

When troubleshooting catheter retention, one of the most common problems is balloon cuffing, whereby the balloon can be deflated but not removed. Either rapid aspiration of balloon contents or prior overdistention can cause the balloon to develop a shape that forms a hook and makes it unable to be removed.

Reinstilling a small amount (0.5–1 mL) of water can help reform the hook shape and facilitate removal. In this question, the balloon has failed to deflate at all and is not causing cuffing.

The first step is to rule out problems with the proximal inflation valve, which can be done by simply cutting the catheter proximal to the valve. If this does not deflate the balloon, the next step is to pass a small guidewire (such as that found in the central line kit) along the inflation channel to break apart any obstruction or debris that may have formed along the tract. Care should be taken to not rupture the balloon, whether mechanically (by overdistention or puncture with a wire) or chemically, because that can commonly result in direct bladder injury, intravesicular debris, or further complications.

If these interventions are unsuccessful, extraluminal rupture of the balloon should be done in consultation with a urologist.

Test-taking tip: This is a "you know it or don't" kind of question. If you don't know it, choose an answer and move on. You can perhaps mark it for review when you are done at the end of the test. Don't, however, let these kinds of questions get you stuck and waste your time.

8. ANSWER: B

Septic arthritis is a challenging and time-sensitive diagnosis with significant morbidity and mortality if missed by the emergency provider. It is a difficult diagnosis to make solely on physical exam and blood tests. Recent joint surgery within the past 3 months and cellulitis overlying a prosthetic joint are the two most suspicious clinical findings.

Providers are frequently left with the synovial fluid analysis to help make this diagnosis.

WBC counts >100,000 cells/μL and PMNs >90% are highly suspicious of an acute bacterial process. Synovial lactate >10 mmol/L is a promising test for diagnosing septic arthritis, although this requires further study. Negative birefringent needles are diagnostic of gout, although care must be taken as concomitant bacterial infection is possible. High RBC counts are more suggestive of hemarthrosis but can also be seen in ligamentous injury and traumatic taps.

Test-taking tip: Infection is all about WBCs and PMNs, allowing you to focus on these two answer choices.

9. ANSWER: C

Among native joints, the knee is the most common (about 50%) site of septic arthritis. This is followed by the hip, shoulder, ankle, elbow, and wrist. The great toe is the most common site for a gout flare. It is important to keep in mind that up to 20% of septic joints can be oligoarticular, involving multiple joints. Additionally, axial joints such as the sternoclavicular and sacroiliac joint may become infected in patients with a history of IV drug use.

Test-taking tip: Test takers can draw on their own experience to make an educated guess for this question as the knee is overwhelmingly the most common joint on which arthrocentesis is performed in the ED.

10. ANSWER: D

Paracentesis is a fairly common ED procedure for evaluating the cause of ascites or looking for possible infection of ascitic fluid. Absolute contraindications to the procedure include issues at the proposed puncture site such as overlying cellulitis, abdominal hernia, or visible vessels (caput medusae or superficial veins). Significant bowel distention and suspected abdominal adhesions are also contraindications to the procedure.

Uncorrected bleeding diathesis is a contraindication, but studies have shown the procedure being done safely in patients with INR levels <8 and platelets counts >20,000.

Hypotension by itself is not a contraindication to paracentesis, but it should be noted that patients undergoing large-volume paracentesis are at risk for postprocedural hypotension from intravascular volume depletion. It is important to keep in mind that if paracentesis is unable to be performed, spontaneous bacterial peritonitis should still be empirically treated in the high-risk patient.

Test-taking tip: While all of these answers would make this procedure higher risk than a routine paracentesis, only one would actually impede the provider from safely performing a paracentesis.

11. ANSWER: C

Most of the time, infection of ascitic fluid is due to spontaneous bacterial peritonitis, which is thought to occur when a small number of bacteria translocate into and colonize the ascitic fluid. It is diagnosed with the presence of >250 PMNs/mm, positive ascitic fluid culture, and no evidence of intraabdominal infection.

While this patient meets criteria based on paracentesis results, her history and examination (focal tenderness) are suggestive of secondary bacterial peritonitis. Secondary bacterial peritonitis is far less common than spontaneous bacterial peritonitis because it is the infection of ascitic fluid from an active surgical infection.

In this patient, the polymicrobial Gram stain is virtually diagnostic of a surgical cause of the patient's abdominal pain because spontaneous bacterial peritonitis is almost always caused by a single organism. Presence of a polymicrobial Gram stain should clue the provider to look further for an alternative cause of peritonitis, and patients with secondary bacterial peritonitis rarely get better with IV antibiotics alone.

Test-taking tip: This patient clearly has an infection that is related to her abdomen, based on the information provided in the stem, allowing you to eliminate choices A and D as potential correct answers.

12. ANSWER: D

The vast majority of patients who have findings concerning for meningitis can have LPs done safely without a CT scan.

Patients who would benefit from CT scan before LP include those who are immunocompromised, have a history of CNS disease, have had new-onset seizures within the past week, have a depressed level of consciousness, have papilledema, or have a focal neurologic deficit.

Only the patient in answer D meets one of these criteria with new partial seizures concerning for a possible mass lesion.

The patient in choice A has a story concerning for possible meningococcal meningitis and should have immediate administration of antibiotics and an LP. These management steps should not be delayed by obtaining a CT scan.

The patient in choice B should receive platelet transfusion before any procedures such as LP because of bleeding risk, but a CT scan is not necessary, nor is it necessary for the patient described in choice C.

Test-taking tip: LP is only potentially dangerous in patients in whom you are concerned about mass effect in the brain. This rule will help you to choose the correct answer.

13. ANSWER: D

When considering sites of central venous access, the preferred initial site is the right internal jugular vein because of its shorter and straighter course, decreasing the incidence of catheter malpositioning compared with the left internal jugular.

A unique complication that may occur during left-sided venous access is injury to the thoracic duct, which drains into the left subclavian vein, and this may result in a chylothorax.

Pneumothorax is a known risk that is greatest with subclavian vein access attempts. Catheter thrombosis, infection, and air emboli are all known complications of central venous access that can occur no matter the location of the access attempt.

Test-taking tip: Think about what could be different between a left-sided and right-sided approach in this procedure because the correct answer is an anatomic one.

14. ANSWER: C

A perimortem cesarean delivery is a procedure performed during maternal cardiac arrest in an effort to increase the chance of successfully resuscitating the mother with the additionally possibility of improving fetal survival. The primary goal is to improve venous return and cardiac filling pressures by relieving the uterine compression on the inferior vena cava.

Fetal survival and neurologic function have a precipitous decline after 4 minutes, making this a procedure that should be initiated quickly when its indication is recognized. Maternal respiratory function is altered in late pregnancy because there is physiologic narrowing of the upper airway during the third trimester and compression of the diaphragm because of the gravid uterus. The initial incision of the uterus should be a vertical incision along the lower half to avoid cutting into the placenta.

Test-taking tip: The rule of thumb with pregnant women is what is best for them is what is best for the fetus. This well help guide you to the correct answer.

15. ANSWER: C

There are a lot of medications at an emergency provider's disposal for procedural sedation. Ketamine has become an increasingly popular choice because of its large safety profile. It does not depress respiratory drive as much as most normal sedatives and also has a low risk for creating hypotension. Ketamine is not without side effects, though, because patients may still be at risk for central apnea, emergence reactions, and laryngospasm.

It is important to note that this patient is already experiencing the effects of the opiates given en route, and any additional agents should be given at a reduced dose, which can be increased after monitoring for effect.

Naloxone would reverse the mild respiratory depression this patient is experiencing from the morphine given en route but would not provide either sedation or analgesia for this patient.

Test-taking tip: Naloxone is a reversal agent for opioids that will not help with procedural sedation, allowing you to eliminate this as a potential answer.

16. ANSWER: D

The patient in this stem is likely suffering from laryngospasm as a result of ketamine administration. This side effect is reported in 1% to 2% of sedations in which ketamine is given. It is a spasm and closure of the vocal cords resulting in complete airway obstruction. If experienced or suspected, providers should act quickly to provide positive pressure ventilation with a bag-valve-mask and a peep valve, if available, because constant pressure with a good seal can break a laryngospasm.

If unsuccessful, providers should continue positive pressure ventilation and provide a painful stimulus to Larson's point bilaterally. Larson's point, located posterior to the earlobes between the mastoid process and the superior process of the rams of the mandible, is pressed on and lifted superiorly in the patient who is supine in bed. This generally allows for breaking of laryngospasm with one or two breaths.

If still unsuccessful, the next steps are administration of a mild sedative to attempt to relax the laryngospasm and, if that fails, intubation. It is not appropriate to establish IV access when this patient's respiratory problem has not been addressed. Naloxone is unlikely to have any effect on laryngospasm.

Test-taking tip: Brush up on common complications of medications administered in the ED.

17. ANSWER: C

The patient in this question has a history that is suspicious for possible intracerebral infection, namely cryptococcal meningitis. This fungal meningitis is primarily seen in immunocompromised individuals and presents with a slow and indolent timeline, making it sometimes hard to diagnose. In general, one the hallmarks of this infection is an elevated opening pressure.

This patient's CSF has an increased WBC count with a monocyte predominance that does not fit with bacterial meningitis. Viral meningitis should be considered, but given the history and elevated opening pressure, cryptococcal meningitis is of greater concern.

Guillain-Barré syndrome is a progressive ascending paralysis that is classically associated with a normal CSF WBC count with elevated protein (albuminocytologic dissociation).

Test-taking tip: The time course of the patient's symptoms allows you to eliminate choice A, and the lack of neurologic symptoms allows you to eliminate choice D, leaving you two answers to choose from.

18. ANSWER: A

The patient in this question has a rectal foreign body that has been impacted for a prolonged period of time and has caused a perforation. Although uncommon, perforation of the rectum or colon is a serious complication requiring emergent surgical consultation.

When unperforated, foreign bodies should be removed expeditiously to prevent prolonged trauma and possible progression to ischemic colon and perforation. Bedside removal can be attempted by the emergency provider for objects that are palpable on exam and have no sharp edges.

Evidence of perforation or peritonitis, presence of fragile objects (such as lightbulbs), sharp objects, broken glass, prolonged time since insertion, severe abdominal pain, and objects that are more than 10 cm proximal to the anal verge should involve surgical consultation.

Test-taking tip: Free air under the diaphragm is a surgical emergency until proved otherwise.

19. ANSWER: C

Arterial cannulation with a large-bore catheter is a rare but frightening complication of obtaining central venous access. If suspected, there are multiple techniques in which providers can attempt to identify possible arterial placement. Of the choices listed, direct visualization is the most reliable method, but this should only be done by a specialist in a controlled environment and should not be undergone in the ED.

The most reasonable option in the ED is P_{O_2} measurement compared with a known arterial sample. Measurement of P_{CO_2} will be unhelpful because values in venous samples will be similar to arterial measurements. Comparing of blood color is an option but may be challenging in critically ill patients or those in a shock state. Alternative options include transducing the catheter to look for a pulsatile waveform, which would confirm arterial placement.

Test-taking tip: Brush up on common complications of medications administered in the ED.

20. ANSWER: C

The patient has a history and exam concerning for a perirectal abscess. This condition is often highlighted by the history of pain with bowel movements and presence of redness and swelling around the rectum. While simple perianal abscesses may be drained in the ED by experienced providers, deeper perirectal abscesses are best managed in the OR with a surgeon.

Failure to drain and open these in a timely manner can lead to sphincter damage and incontinence. The presence of fever and the inability to examine a patient because of the degree of pain are both suspicious for deeper extension of the abscess, necessitating surgical consult and intervention.

Anorectal abscesses should not be managed with antibiotics alone.

Urology consult is sometimes required for Fournier's gangrene, a rapid and progressive soft tissue infection of the perineum that could potentially originate from an anorectal infection; however, this seems unlikely with this patient.

Test-taking tip: This is a "you know it or don't" kind of question. If you don't know it, choose an answer and move on. You can perhaps mark it for review when you are done at the end of the test. Don't, however, let these kinds of questions get you stuck and waste your time.

21. ANSWER: B

The midshaft clavicle fracture and scapula fracture shown in this image can be managed with a simple sling on the affected side as long as there is no evidence of neurovascular compromise.

Although historically, it was commonly treated with a figure-of-eight sling, recent studies have shown similar rates of healing with decreased patient discomfort when treated with a simple sling.

Coaptation splints can be used to treat midshaft humerus fractures that have no evidence of neuromuscular compromise, and posterior long arm splints are generally reserved for fractures involving the elbow and proximal forearm.

Test-taking tip: It should be easy to eliminate C and D as correct answers, leaving you two to choose from.

22. ANSWER: A

LP is a common ED procedure used to evaluate for a variety of potentially life-threatening causes of headaches. A recognized complication of the procedure is the post-LP headache, which is a common and potentially debilitating condition thought to result from a persistent CSF leak at the puncture site. This causes patients to have a severe positional headache, worse when trying to sit or stand up, that generally will begin 24 to 48 hours after the procedure.

Multiple factors help minimize the incidence of this complication, which sometimes results in need for repeat ED visits for a blood patch. These include smaller needle size (20–22 G), keeping the bevel perpendicular to the direction of the dura mater fibers, using a noncutting needle, and replacing the stylet before removing the LP needle.

It is also thought that the incidence of post-LP headaches should decrease with fewer LP attempts, although it has never been formally studied. Factors that have been traditionally thought to be risk factors for post-LP headache but have not borne out include the volume of CSF removed, bed rest after the procedure, increased hydration or IV fluids after the procedure, and whether the patient was supine or upright for the procedure.

Test-taking tip: This is a "you know it or don't" kind of question. If you don't know it, choose an answer and move on. You can perhaps mark it for review when you are done at the end of the test. Don't, however, let these kinds of questions get you stuck and waste your time.

23. ANSWER: C

NIPPV is a useful adjunct to the emergency provider's arsenal of interventions that can improve respiratory status and potentially avoid intubation. NIPPV is not appropriate for all patients, however, and the challenging patient in this question has multiple conditions that may make him a poor candidate for NIPPV.

The presence of a potentially unstable midface fracture is an absolute contraindication in this scenario because it introduces both the possibility of pneumocephalus and the inability to create an appropriate mask seal.

There are multiple other concerning features that this patient exhibits, including his tachycardia and relative hypotension, his agitation, and the severity of his respiratory distress, which suggest a high risk for failure of NIPPV, but none of these are absolute contraindications.

Test-taking tip: Brush up on absolute and relative contraindications to procedures commonly performed in the ED.

24. ANSWER: B

This patient has a history concerning for breath stacking from her obstructive lung disease. This results from unintended inability to inspire before complete exhalation of the preceding breath is completed, leading to increased intrathoracic pressure and eventually a collapse of systemic venous return.

The immediate way to relieve this process is to disconnect the patient from the ventilator, allowing for expiration of the retained air. Breath stacking can potentially be minimized or avoided with careful attention to ventilator settings in patients with obstructive lung disease. This is done by using smaller tidal volumes and low RRs to allow for a prolonged expiratory phase and permissive hypercapnia.

If this is ineffective, the next consideration would be an ET obstruction due to mucous plugging or a tension pneumothorax. It may be reasonable to pass a suction catheter to make sure the ET is patent because this can be done quickly before proceeding to evaluate and treat for a possible tension pneumothorax. While many patients with asthma and cold exacerbations are hypovolemic, it is a less likely cause of this patient's decline in hemodynamic status.

Test-taking tip: For patients in extremis, focus on the ABCs and think about life-saving interventions. This is a breathing problem, allowing you to eliminate A and C as potential answers.

25. ANSWER: D

There are certain instances in which nasotracheal intubation may be preferred. This is generally considered in patients in whom there are large intraoral masses (angioedema or tumor), severe trismus, or severe cervical spine disease or instability.

It is absolutely contraindicated in patients with apnea or impending respiratory arrest, suspected epiglottitis, midface instability, basilar skull fracture, or coagulopathy.

Relative contraindications include large nasal polyps, suspected nasal foreign bodies, recent nasal surgery, upper neck hematoma, history of epistaxis, and prosthetic heart valves.

Test-taking tip: Brush up on absolute and relative contraindications to procedures commonly performed in the ED.

26. ANSWER: B

After adequate topical anesthesia, the ET should be advanced with the bevel facing laterally such that the tube advances along the nasal septum and does not get caught on the turbinates.

Adequate anesthesia can be assisted by first placing a nasal trumpet, which can help introduce additional local anesthetic. The posterior pharynx can be further anesthetized by spraying lidocaine down the nasal trumpet before removing and introducing the ET. The ET itself should be lubricated with a water-soluble solution. While lidocaine jelly may seem like a good idea, there are reports of the jelly drying and obstructing the ET. It is always important to try to use the largest sized ET that fits; generally, in adults, this can go up to a 7-mm tube.

Test-taking tip: This is a "you know it or don't" kind of question. If you don't know it, choose an answer and move on. You can perhaps mark it for review when you are done at the end of the test. Don't, however, let these kinds of questions get you stuck and waste your time.

27. ANSWER: C

This challenging scenario highlights a patient with a pre-existing difficult airway that arrives in extremis, and as a provider, you are caught in a "can't intubate, can't ventilate" scenario. It is important to recognize this early because the decision should quickly be made to convert to a surgical airway by cricothyrotomy.

Trying to gather additional airway resources at this juncture is unlikely to be successful and may simply waste valuable time. Although calling for assistance is always reasonable, there is probably not enough time in this patient who is already severely hypoxic.

Blind nasal intubation needs to be done on a spontaneously breathing patient because it is unlikely to be successful on a paralyzed or apneic patient such as this one.

Test-taking tip: Knowing that you can't form a mask seal allows you to eliminate choice B, and knowing that apnea is an absolute contraindication to nasal intubation allows you to eliminate answer D, leaving you two answers to choose from.

28. ANSWER: B

A bougie is a useful airway adjunct for patients with difficult airways. After passing through the vocal cords, providers should feel for a characteristic click as it passes the tracheal rings.

Unfortunately, this is not always present, in which case the bougie should be advanced to see if it gets caught up at the carina, generally at a depth of about 30 to 40 cm in the normal adult. If the bougie is able to be continuously advanced past this depth without resistance, it is likely in the esophagus.

Test-taking tip: In general, with answers that involve a numeric answer, you can eliminate the extremes, leaving the two answers in the middle for you to choose from.

29. ANSWER: C

The most concerning complication for arterial lines is the development and potential rupture of a pseudoaneurysm, which is most common after arterial line placement in the femoral artery. It generally occurs within 5 to 6 days of arterial line removal and classically is a painful pulsatile mass with a thrill. When suspected, an ultrasound should be ordered for definitive diagnosis.

Infection rates seem equivalent for radial and femoral arterial lines. Femoral artery pseudoaneurysms occur when the puncture site is made too distally, at the level of the bifurcation of the femoral artery or below, because the vessel at this level lacks the fibrous wall that is usually necessary to help seal the puncture site.

Femoral artery thrombosis is rare because of its large vessel diameter.

Test-taking tip: Brush up on common complications of procedures commonly performed in the ED.

30. ANSWER: C

The only absolute contraindication for a surgical cricothyrotomy is age. While there is some debate about the lower end of the age spectrum in which cricothyrotomy can be considered (as young as 5 years), experts generally agree that the procedure is safe in patients older than 12 years.

Tracheostomy sites generally become mature 1 week after placement, but if a scenario occurs in which an exchange needs to be done in the ED soon after surgery, many experts recommend that the procedure be performed using bougie-assisted exchange.

Trachea-innominate fistula is a life-threatening complication that usually occurs within the first 3 weeks postoperatively, while tracheoesophageal fistula generally occurs more than 1 month after surgery.

Test-taking tip: This is a "you know it or don't" kind of question. If you don't know it, choose an answer and move on. You can perhaps mark it for review when you are done at the end of the test. Don't, however, let these kinds of questions get you stuck and waste your time.

31. ANSWER: D

The patient in this stem is having a severe anaphylactic reaction with angioedema causing respiratory failure. Having failed conventional therapies, one must move toward attempting to secure this airway, which is challenging given the obstructing angioedema.

Direct laryngoscopy will likely be impossible given the obstruction, and blind nasal intubation is not recommended in the crashing airway.

This patient would likely be best approached with percutaneous transtracheal jet ventilation in which a needle angiocath is inserted through the cricothyroid membrane such that a patient can be oxygenated and ventilated.

This provides more time to get help and establish a definitive airway, whether intubation by bronchoscopy or a surgical tracheostomy. Surgical cricothyrotomy may be considered but generally is reserved for patients older than 10 to 12 years.

Test-taking tip: Knowing that cricothyrotomy is not indicated in children this young allows you to eliminate this answer.

32. ANSWER: B

All of the answer choices fall within the spectrum of an evolving compartment syndrome. Generally, the initial finding that should alert the physician is pain in the affected limb out of proportion to exam.

Pain with passive stretching of the affected compartment is the most sensitive finding before onset of ischemia.

Paresthesias suggest ischemia to the nerve in the affected compartment. Paralysis is a late finding, and at this point, even with fasciotomy, full recovery becomes unlikely. Loss of peripheral pulses is a terminal finding that will generally lead to amputation because limb salvage is unlikely.

Test-taking tip: This is a "you know it or don't" kind of question. If you don't know it, choose an answer and move on. You can perhaps mark it for review when you are done at the end of the test. Don't, however, let these kinds of questions get you stuck and waste your time.

33. ANSWER: B

Historically, it has been taught that children younger than 8 to 10 years of age should be intubated with uncuffed ETs because of anatomic differences, while cuffed tubes may be used on older children and adults.

In adults, the narrowest portion of the airway is at the level of the vocal cords, but in children, it is more distal, at the level of the cricoid ring. It is thought that a properly sized uncuffed tube will seal naturally at the level of the cricoid ring.

The concept of cuffed tubes being unsuitable for pediatric airways is currently being challenged. There is no difference in postextubation stridor regardless of the type of tube used.

Oversized uncuffed tubes are the primary cause of laryngeal injury during intubation.

Test-taking tip: This is a "you know it or don't" kind of question. If you don't know it, choose an answer and move on. You can perhaps mark it for review when you are done at the end of the test. Don't, however, let these kinds of questions get you stuck and waste your time.

34. ANSWER: C

It is generally recommended that the highest dose of lidocaine with epinephrine that can be safely administered is 7 mg/kg. The recommended highest dose of lidocaine by itself is somewhere between 3 and 4.5 mg/kg.

The addition of epinephrine reduces systemic absorption, allowing for higher anesthetic concentration along nerves and prolonging blockade.

It is recommended to avoid using epinephrine near sites with an end-arterial blood supply such as fingers, toes, ears, penis, and nose.

Local anesthetic toxicity generally first presents as circumoral numbness, metallic taste, tingling, restlessness, and vertigo but can progress to seizures, coma, and cardiovascular collapse.

Test-taking tip: In general, with answers that involve a numeric answer, you can eliminate the extremes, leaving the two answers in the middle for you to choose from.

35. ANSWER: D

When evaluating a patient for placement of a suprapubic catheter, the only absolute contraindications are in pregnant patients and in scenarios in which the bladder is unable to be visualized by the provider using ultrasound.

Other relative contraindications include pediatric cases, coagulopathy, and situations in which the risks for pelvic adhesions are high, such as in patients with prior history of abdominal/pelvic surgeries and pelvic irradiation. Morbid obesity is not a contraindication as long as the provider can visualize the bladder with an ultrasound.

Test-taking tip: Brush up on absolute and relative contraindications to procedures commonly performed in the ED.

36. ANSWER: D

The case in this question is one of a hypotensive patient with chest pain. The ultrasound image shows a large pericardial effusion. The differential diagnosis for this is broad and includes the following:

- *Pericardial effusion.* This can result from trauma, ventricular rupture, cancer, or viral illness. Pericardial effusion can progress to pericardial tamponade, which results from right ventricular collapse resulting in poor filling of the heart. The patient develops hypotension, JVD, shortness of breath, and sometimes chest pain. Exam usually shows muffled heart sounds and JVD. This is the cause of this patient's presentation. The best bedside ultrasound view for visualizing this is either the parasternal long axis or subxiphoid view.
- *Poor global function.* This usually results from persistent cardiac injury. Patients develop congestive heart failure with occasional or persistent decompensation, including lower extremity edema, shortness of breath, chest pain, and JVD. EKG usually shows previous injury, and patients usually have a history of previous decompensation. The best bedside ultrasound view to evaluate global function and wall motion abnormalities is the parasternal short-axis view.
- *Right ventricular strain.* This alludes to a patient with a pulmonary embolus. Patients with pulmonary embolus generally present with sudden-onset pleuritic chest pain and shortness of breath. Sometimes patients will have a swollen leg and/or recent travel with possible deep venous thrombosis. The best bedside ultrasound cardiac view for evaluating for right ventricular strain is the apical four-chamber view. The left upper side of the screen displays a right ventricle that is larger than the left ventricle displayed on the right upper side of the screen, indicating right ventricular strain

Test-taking tip: To answer this question correctly, you do not need to interpret the image correctly because the question describes a classic picture of cardiac tamponade and Beck's triad (hypotension, muffled heart sounds, and JVD).

37. ANSWER: A

This question focuses on the longitudinal view of the pelvis in the FAST exam. Free fluid or blood appears as a jet-black stripe or area, similar in appearance to the bladder (sitting anterior to the uterus in the image above).

Area A, the area directly posterior to the cervix or the posterior cul-de-sac, is the most dependent part of the pelvis and where free fluid is most likely to collect first.

Area B is approximately one-third of the way up the uterine wall. Fluid that collects from the posterior cul-de-sac up to one-third of the way up the uterine wall is considered a small or physiologic amount of free fluid.

Area C is approximately two-thirds of the way up the uterine wall. Fluid that collects from the posterior cul-de-sac up to two-thirds of the way up the uterine wall is considered a moderate amount of free fluid.

If free fluid is seen up to area D, or all the way around the uterus, it is considered a large amount of free fluid. Any free fluid in the setting of trauma should prompt immediate surgical evaluation.

Test-taking tip: This is a "you know it or don't" kind of question. If you don't know it, choose an answer and move on. You can perhaps mark it for review when you are done at the end of the test. Don't, however, let these kinds of questions get you stuck and waste your time.

38. ANSWER: B

The images shown from the EFAST exam are normal; however, any patient with abdominal trauma and pain in the left upper quadrant should prompt concern for splenic injury. A negative FAST exam does not rule out splenic injury. Because the spleen is an encapsulated organ, a splenic injury can remain encapsulated, and ultrasound evaluation can appear normal. Definitive evaluation should be with CT scan.

It would be rare to make the diagnosis of renal contusion on an EFAST, and discharge home would not be appropriate without further workup.

It would also be rare to make the diagnosis of a small bowel injury on an EFAST, and although a CT scan might be indicated if this diagnosis were suspected, CT scan is also not very sensitive in making this diagnosis.

Lab tests might also be indicated but would not be helpful in making the diagnosis of a bladder injury.

Test-taking tip: In the setting of trauma, left upper quadrant pain should make you think of the spleen.

39. ANSWER: C

This is an apical four-chamber view, the best view for visualizing right heart strain, which can help increase suspicion for pulmonary embolus. The other diagnosis that will often show right heart strain is pulmonary hypertension. The critical finding that supports right heart strain is a right ventricle that is equal in size or larger than the left ventricle. In a dynamic image, you may also see paradoxical septal motion, which is a bowing of the septum toward the left ventricle indicative of a higher pressure in the right heart than the left.

Although subxiphoid views are good for visualizing pericardial effusions, this image does not show any fluid around the heart and is not a subxiphoid view.

The parasternal short-axis view is excellent for visualizing the left ventricle and assessing for wall motion abnormalities. A short-axis view is displayed below.

Test-taking tip: This is a "you know it or don't" kind of question. If you don't know it, choose an answer and move on. You can perhaps mark it for review when you are done at the end of the test. Don't, however, let these kinds of questions get you stuck and waste your time.

40. ANSWER: D

Any older adult patient with abdominal pain and hypotension in the ED should prompt evaluation of the abdominal aorta as part of the differential. Bedside ultrasound is a great tool for evaluation of AAA. Using a curvilinear medium-frequency probe or low-frequency probe on the midline abdomen, the aorta is visualized in the longitudinal and transverse views.

It is important to visualize the entire length of the aorta and obtain measurements throughout. Most aneurysms occur infrarenal and above the bifurcation in the iliac arteries. A normal measurement of the aorta is less than 3 cm.

When a measurement of 3 cm or larger is observed, the aorta meets criteria for AAA. The aorta is measured from outside wall to outside wall to take into consideration a thrombus that may be present, as displayed in the image. When an aorta measures 5 cm or larger, immediate surgical evaluation should be sought.

Test-taking tip: The image is not necessary to choosing the correct answer; rather, you need to know the criteria for an AAA on ultrasound and the indications for surgical evaluation.

41. ANSWER: D

This is a classic view of a kidney with hydronephrosis on ultrasound. The central jet-black fluid collection is indicative of moderate to severe hydronephrosis. Although this could be the result of a renal stone, there are no stones visualized, so we cannot exclude other reasons for obstruction such as prostatic hypertrophy, clot, or other anatomic issues.

A renal abscess would appear as a well-defined hypoechoic area within the cortex or in the corticomedullary parenchyma. You may also see internal echoes within and an associated diffusely hypoechoic kidney due to acute pyelonephritis.

Simple renal cysts would appear as well-marginated, thin-walled sacs of fluid on ultrasound.

Test-taking tip: This question relies on your ability to correctly interpret the ultrasound. Review some images that are key to making diagnoses in the ED before the test.

42. ANSWER: B

The orbit is a relatively confined space surrounded by bony walls with limited ability to expand. When trauma to the orbit occurs, causing an increase in intraorbital volume, such as with a retrobulbar hematoma, the increase in volume causes a rapid increase in pressure, leading to orbital compartment syndrome. Untreated orbital compartment syndrome can lead to ischemia of the optic nerve and retina and ultimately to vision loss in as short a time as 90 to 120 minutes.

In the awake patient, assessment of visual acuity, increased IOP, proptosis, and a relative afferent pupillary defect would indicate the need for emergent canthotomy.

In the unconscious patient, because you are unable to assess visual acuity, an IOP greater than 40 mm Hg, especially with a relative afferent pupillary defect, which indicates optic nerve ischemia, should prompt you to perform an emergent lateral canthotomy.

Test-taking tip: Brush up on indications for common procedures performed in the ED.

43. ANSWER: D

The Tono-Pen is a handheld electronic device that uses a small plunger to measure the resistance of the cornea when in contact. The cornea should be properly anesthetized before use, most commonly with a topical anesthetic such as proparacaine.

Despite anesthesia, patients will often require assistance in adequately opening their eyes. It is very important that when doing this you avoid applying direct pressure on the globe because this will cause a falsely elevated reading. This can be avoided by pressing the lids with your fingers against the bony rims of the orbit.

Proper equipment calibration is essential to avoid false-positive or false-negative results with any equipment used.

Eye movement and accommodation have been found to affect eye pressure measurements by as much as 5 to 10 mm Hg.

Test-taking tip: When one of the answer options is "all of the above," if two of the answers seem correct, that is most likely the answer, even if the other answer is questionable.

44. ANSWER: D

There are several techniques to measure IOP. Applanation tonometry measures the amount of force required to flatten a constant corneal area. It is considered the standard for measuring IOP and is mounted on most slit lamps.

The Tono-Pen is a handheld device that is relatively easy to operate and relatively accurate. It is easier to use on a supine patient who cannot sit up for a slit lamp exam.

The noncontact airpuff tonometer is a form of applanation tonometer that uses air to flatten the cornea instead of touching it. It does not require anesthesia.

All of these methods are all similarly effective in measuring IOP.

Test-taking tip: This is a "you know it or don't" kind of question. If you don't know it, choose an answer and move on. You can perhaps mark it for review when you are done at the end of the test. Don't, however, let these kinds of questions get you stuck and waste your time.

45. ANSWER: C

During a neonatal resuscitation, venous access for volume replacement and medication administration can be challenging. Retrospective studies have shown that obtaining peripheral IV access, central venous catheterization, or a venous cutdown can take significantly longer to achieve than IO or umbilical venous access.

IO has been shown to be faster than umbilical vein catheterization and has similar rates of success and complications.

Test-taking tip: Any answer that suggests a delay in performing a procedure during resuscitation is probably wrong.

46. ANSWER: D

The umbilical vein remains patent for about a week after birth and therefore can be used for access if necessary. Peripheral access is preferred in these cases if possible, but when not feasible umbilical vein catheterization may be attempted.

Absolute contraindications to umbilical vein catheterization include omphalitis, peritonitis, and necrotizing enterocolitis.

Although umbilical vein catheters can be used for central access, when placing one for emergency resuscitation, it is recommended to advance the catheter only about 1 to 2 cm beyond where good blood return is obtained. This is about 4 to 5 cm for a term infant. If advanced beyond that point, it is possible to enter the portal venous system, and if hyperosmolar fluids or medications are infused, it can lead to liver necrosis.

Test-taking tip: When one of the answer options is "all of the above," if two of the answers seem correct, that is most likely the answer, even if the other answer is questionable.

47. ANSWER: C

When placing an umbilical vein catheter during emergency resuscitation, it is recommended to advance the catheter only about 1 to 2 cm beyond where good blood return is obtained. This is about 4 to 5 cm for a term infant. If advanced beyond that point, it is possible to enter the portal venous system, and if hyperosmolar fluids or medications are infused, it can lead to liver necrosis.

Cardiac complications, including perforation, tamponade, and disorders of the heart rhythm, have been reported with umbilical vein catheterization. Usually, these are due to intracardiac placement of the catheter. To avoid this, there are standardized graphs to help determine the appropriate insertion length. If the graph is not available, you can estimate the approximate length by measuring the distance from the shoulder to the umbilicus and multiplying the result by 0.6. That should place the catheter above the diaphragm in the vena cava but below the right atrium.

Though rare, when removing the umbilical vein catheter, air embolism can occur if the infant generates intrathoracic pressure to draw air into the vein. This can happen with crying. When removing the catheter, immediately occlude the vein by either tightening a pursestring suture around the umbilical stump or applying pressure on or just cephalad to the umbilicus.

Other reported complications of umbilical vein catheterization include blood-borne infection, significant hemorrhage, and thromboembolic events. Splenic infarct has not been reported in the literature as a potential complication.

Test-taking tip: This is a "you know it or don't" kind of question. If you don't know it, choose an answer and move on. You can perhaps mark it for review when you are done at the end of the test. Don't, however, let these kinds of questions get you stuck and waste your time.

48. ANSWER: A

Obtaining vascular access during resuscitation can be both challenging and stressful, particularly in pediatric patients. IO access, first described in the 1930s, has been described as both a safe and effective means of accessing the vascular system and providing life-saving medications necessary for resuscitation. Furthermore, several studies have demonstrated that obtaining IO access is faster than peripheral IV access or venous cutdown in both adults and pediatric patients who are intravascularly depleted or during cardiac arrest.

IO access is recommended in both children and adults who need immediate resuscitation when IV access cannot be established rapidly and reliably. It is not routinely recommended during situations in which time is not a constraint. In the example given in the question, though it could be used to resuscitate a profoundly dehydrated pediatric patient in hypovolemic shock, the patient is only "mildly dehydrated," and therefore IV access should be attempted along with oral hydration if possible.

Though there is no specific time limit on how long an IO can be used, the risk for complications such as osteomyelitis increases after 24 hours. Most medications can be given via IO route, but this should not be used for routine administration of IV antibiotics in a patient who is not hemodynamically compromised. Central venous access through a peripherally inserted central catheter (PICC) line or central venous catheter is the preferred choice in in these patients.

Test-taking tip: Watch out for the use of words such as "routine." This commonly indicates something that can wait, and therefore it is likely the wrong answer in emergency medicine test questions.

49. ANSWER: D

Long bones are richly vascular structures with veins that drain the medullary sinuses in the bone marrow. They are able to accept large amounts of fluids and transport them into the central circulation rapidly. These veins supported by the bone matrix serve as noncollapsible veins during profound shock or cardiopulmonary arrest.

Most IV medications that are commonly used during cardiac arrest can be given via IO route. Studies have shown that these medications reach the central circulation at almost the same time and same concentration as when given by IV route.

Resuscitation fluids and blood products are also easily infused by IO route rapidly, with the size of the IO catheter being the rate-limiting factor. In the awake patient, infusions can be painful, so using preservative-free lidocaine before infusion is recommended.

Test-taking tip: When one of the answer options is "all of the above," if two of the answers seem correct, that is most likely the answer, even if the other answer is questionable.

50. ANSWER: C

A fractured bone or an extremity with known or suspected vascular injury is an absolute contraindications to IO cannulation. If IO access is placed in a fractured extremity, infused fluid will extravasate into the soft tissue. Not only will this not be effective, but it can also lead to compartment syndrome.

Though IO access in a patient with known osteogenesis imperfecta is associated with a higher risk for fracture because of brittle bones, it is only a relative contraindication.

Infections or burns to the affected cannulation site are also a relative contraindication but can be performed in life-threatening situations.

Patients with known right-to-left intracardiac shunts, such as those with tetralogy of Fallot, are at higher risk for cerebral fat or marrow embolisms. This is also a relative contraindication in life-threatening situations.

Test-taking tip: Brush up on absolute and relative contraindications of procedures commonly performed in the ED.

51. ANSWER: C

The patient's presentation in this case is classic for pericardial tamponade, with Beck's triad on physical examination and a newly enlarge cardiac silhouette on chest radiograph. Given how unstable this patient is, emergent bedside ultrasound-guided pericardiocentesis is indicated and could be life-saving.

Although this patient is hypotensive and has distended neck veins, her lung exam is not consistent with tension pneumothorax; thus, needle thoracostomy is not indicated.

REBOA is a novel and emerging management for the stabilization of ruptured AAA. Ruptured AAA typically presents with abdominal pain and hypotension, which is not consistent with this patient's presentation.

Although this patient is short of breath, her lung fields are clear to auscultation, and there is no other suggestion of fluid overload is the stem, making acute renal failure and the need for emergency dialysis unlikely.

Test-taking tip: Brush up on classic presentations in the ED such as Beck's triad and Cushing's triad.

52. ANSWER: D

This is a case of PEA arrest. Considerations for PEA arrest include hypoxia, hyperkalemia, hypokalemia, hypothermia, hypovolemia, hyper H+ (acidosis), thrombus from myocardial infarction or pulmonary embolism, tension pneumothorax, cardiac tamponade, toxins, or trauma.

Attempting to assess for reversible causes of PEA arrest is important, and in a dialysis patient in PEA arrest, electrolyte derangement and pericardial tamponade are high on the differential. Attempting a pericardiocentesis is the next most appropriate step because the patient has not responded to medications meant to reverse common electrolyte abnormalities in dialysis patients. Emergency dialysis is not indicated in pulseless, apneic patients.

Attempts to resuscitate this patient have only been ongoing for 10 minutes, so calling the code is probably not appropriate given the information provided in the stem.

The patient's presentation is not consistent with trauma, making hemorrhagic causes of his PEA arrest less likely, and thus transfusing packed RBCs in this situation is unlikely to be helpful.

Test-taking tip: Brush up on common mnemonics in emergency medicine including the H's and T's of PEA arrest.

53. ANSWER: C

The most common approach for a pericardiocentesis is 1 cm subxiphoid aimed to the left nipple. In patients who are pulseless and apneic, this procedure can be performed blindly, but it is more commonly performed using the guidance of an ultrasound.

The second intercostal space mid-clavicular line is a common location for a needle thoracostomy. Alternatively, the fourth or fifth intercostal space at the mid-axillary line may also be used for needle thoracostomy and for chest tube insertion. Two centimeters subclavicular at the bend of the clavicle is a common approach for subclavian line placement.

Test-taking tip: Brush up on the anatomy of procedures commonly performed in the ED.

54. ANSWER: B

Indications for ED thoracotomy in the setting of trauma include patients who have suffered penetrating trauma with less than 15 to 20 minutes of downtime; patients with blunt trauma with less than 10 minutes of down time; and patients with profound hypotension who are premorbid and unresponsive to fluids and other resuscitative efforts.

Though medical indications for emergency thoracotomy exist, such as ruptured descending dissection or descending aneurysm rupture, the outcomes in these cases are very poor, and no formal recommendations exist for the use of emergency thoracotomy in this patient population.

Test-taking tip: Brush up on indications for procedures commonly performed in the ED.

55. ANSWER: D

Signs of life associated with increased ED thoracotomy survival include pupillary response, spontaneous ventilation, presence of a carotid pulse, measurable BP, extremity movement, and cardiac electrical activity. Skin signs are not classically considered when making the decision to perform an ED thoracotomy.

Test-taking tip: Pupillary response and movement are clear signs of life, allowing you to exclude them as the correct answer.

56. ANSWER: D

Any of these structures might be injured during an ED thoracotomy; however, during the phase of the procedure when the heart is delivered from the pericardial sac, a pericardiotomy is done, and the phrenic nerve is most likely to be injured.

The phrenic nerve runs longitudinally along the pericardium and can be severed if the incision is not made anterior and longitudinal to its path. Some surgeons advocate for bluntly dissecting the pericardium to minimize the chance of injury to the phrenic nerve.

Test-taking tip: Brush up on the anatomy of procedures commonly performed in the ED.

57. ANSWER: C

The second intercostal space mid-axillary and third intercostal space anterior axillary lines are too high up in the axilla for chest tube insertion and risk injury of the vessels and nerves that run through that region.

The second intercostal space at the mid-clavicular is the classic landmark for needle thoracostomy placement but is not used for tube thoracotomy. Recently, given the large proportion of attempted needle decompressions that don't actually enter the chest pleural space, the fifth intercostal space at the mid-axillary line has become the favored site for both needle and tube thoracostomy. The risk for diaphragmatic injury is higher at this location, so it is recommended that the patient's chest be elevated to 45 degrees to prevent the diaphragm from riding high and being injured during tube placement.

Test-taking tip: Brush up on the anatomy of procedures commonly performed in the ED.

58. ANSWER: C

This patient exhibits the hallmark signs of a tension pneumothorax for which the next best step in treatment is a needle thoracostomy. After the tension pneumothorax has been decompressed, a tube thoracostomy can be placed at the fifth intercostal space mid-axillary line.

Rapid sequence intubation with forceful ventilation will worsen the tension pneumothorax and probably result in loss of pulses and cardiac arrest. This occurs because the pneumothorax will shift the mediastinum over and prevent venous return.

In patients with a tension pneumothorax, time is of essence, so placement of guidewire chest thoracostomy tube is generally too time-intensive to allow rapid resolution of the condition.

In patients at risk for imminent deterioration, even an open thoracostomy tube is too time-consuming. Therefore, the best answer is a needle decompression.

Test-taking tip: Distracting information can be used to mask the point of the question; try to think of what they are testing and get to the heart of the matter. The patient has a tension pneumothorax that needs to be fixed.

59. ANSWER: D

A spontaneous pneumothorax can occur at any age. Most commonly they are associated with asthma, smoking, breath holding, and tall stature.

This chest radiograph shows a left-sided pneumothorax.

A small pneumothorax (<2 cm) can reabsorb without intervention if the patient does not have symptoms and the pneumothorax is not expanding.

A tension pneumothorax, characterized by hypotension, distended neck veins, hypoxia, and absent breath sounds on the affected hemothorax, requires immediate needle thoracostomy and then chest tube placement.

A large pneumothorax, especially in the setting of trauma, requires placement of a large chest tube using open surgical technique.

A spontaneous pneumothorax larger than 2 cm requires drainage, but it can be done with a size 18-French chest tube at the fourth intercostal space. The smaller tube allows for the best cosmetic outcome in a stable patient. After decompression, it is possible for the pneumothorax to reaccumulate, so the chest tube should be attached to a Heimlich valve. When the chest tube is in place, many of these patients can be managed as outpatients.

Test-taking tip: Even if it is hard to correctly interpret the chest radiograph, this patient is not in extremis or even in distress, which helps you to eliminate A and B as potentially correct answers.

60. ANSWER: D

Unstable bradycardia requires emergent intervention; the challenge is choosing the appropriate intervention for the cause of the bradycardia. This patient, based on her EKG, is in complete heart block.

This patient has normal mentation and no evidence of airway compromise; thus, intubation is not necessary. Rapid sequence intubation could actually exacerbate the hypotension while not fixing the underlying problem.

Cardioversion also will not fix complete heart block and may convert the patient into ventricular fibrillation. Atropine usually does not increase the HR or improve perfusion because it only accelerates the atrial rate without conduction to the ventricle.

The only intervention that might improve the patient's condition is transcutaneous pacing. If capture is obtained, it can temporarily stabilize the patient until a transvenous pacer or permanent pacemaker can be place.

Test-taking tip: It should be easy to eliminate choices A and B, based on the information provided in the stem, leaving you two answers to choose from.

61. ANSWER: A

Transvenous pacing is an invasive and complicated method to pace a patient with an unstable bradydysrhythmia in the ED. The absolute indication for transvenous pacing is the unstable patient in whom transcutaneous pacing has failed. Other softer indications include patients that cannot tolerate transcutaneous pacing and situations in which sedation would further destabilize the patient.

The older adult patient with complete heart block who is hypotensive will likely respond to transcutaneous pacing. The teenager with a calcium channel blocker overdose needs appropriate medical management, including administration of antidotes such as high-dose glucagon.

Patients with hemodynamically stable bradycardia do not need immediate intervention but need monitoring and further testing. Permanent pacemaker placement may be the end result but does not need to happen emergently.

Test-taking tip: This is a "you know it or don't" kind of question. If you don't know it, choose an answer and move on. You can perhaps mark it for review when you are done at the end of the test. Don't, however, let these kinds of questions get you stuck and waste your time.

62. ANSWER: B

There is a learning curve to successful transvenous catheter placement, and it is a relatively rare procedure in the ED, making it a difficult procedure in which to maintain clinical competency.

Understanding the basic steps to placement is a good starting place. Internal jugular or subclavian cordis placement can be used to introduce the pacer wire, although many practitioners prefer the internal jugular approach.

It is important to check the pacer balloon before introduction into the cordis. The balloon will help the pacer wire float with venous flow into position. Position is determined by looking at the waveforms on a monitor, which confirm ventricular capture with pacer spikes followed by a left bundle branch block–type tracing.

Recently, ultrasound and fluoroscopy have been used in the ED to assist with placement confirmation.

Test-taking tip: The fact that B and D both mention the internal jugular location suggests that one of these is the correct answer, allowing you to eliminate the other two possibilities.

63. ANSWER: B

The orbit is a relatively closed compartment, and any space-occupying lesion can cause orbital compartment syndrome, leading to vision loss.

Bony fractures and concomitant edema can elevate eye pressures. Even edema alone without direct bony intrusion can cause elevated eye pressures and potential compartment syndrome.

The most common etiology is bleeding behind the globe, or retro-orbital hematoma.

Though rare, air from the sinuses pushed through the medial orbital wall causing orbital compartment syndrome has been described.

Vitreous humor from the globe would theoretically not increase orbital pressure because the volume within the orbit would be the same, making this the correct answer.

Test-taking tip: Vitreous humor naturally exists in the orbital compartment, making it different from the other three choices and the most likely answer.

64. ANSWER: C

The goal of a lateral canthotomy is to resolve the orbital compartment syndrome. This occurs by cutting the canthal ligament to allow the globe to move forward into a proptotic position. Given that there is pressure behind the globe in orbital compartment syndrome; canthal release will not allow the globe to fall back into the orbit.

The retro-orbital hematoma usually is coagulated and will not drain after lateral canthotomy. The vitreous humor already exists within the globe and does not increase the orbital pressure, making it a nonissue in orbital compartment syndrome.

Test-taking tip: Two answers involve destruction of the canthal ligament, suggesting that one of these answers is correct and allowing you to eliminate the other two options.

65. ANSWER: C

Afferent papillary defect, vision loss, proptosis, elevated IOP, rock-hard eyelids, and decreased retropulsion (pushing the globe back into the orbits) are all signs of orbital compartment syndrome.

After orbital compartment syndrome is confirmed, the lateral canthus is anesthetized with lidocaine with epinephrine. A hemostat can then be used to crush and devascularize the tissue. The lateral canthus is then incised with a blunt-ended scissor or scalpel. The canthal ligament can be then palpated and should feel like a guitar string. The canthal ligament is then ligated. Next, the inferior lid should be lifted into traction, and the inferior branch of that canthal ligament should be ligated. The superior branch should be left in place because the risk for injury to the lacrimal artery and other structures. Oculoplastics should then be consulted to repair the canthotomy electively for optimal cosmesis.

In the setting of orbital compartment syndrome, IOPs are elevated, not decreased.

Circumferential subconjunctival hemorrhage and irregular papillary shape can be a sign of globe rupture.

Synechiae are adhesions between the iris and the lens classically seen in iritis and uveitis.

Test-taking tip: Compartment syndrome always involves increased pressure, allowing you to easily eliminate choice A as a potential answer.

66. ANSWER: B

The bedside abdominal ultrasound demonstrates a thickened gallbladder wall greater than 4 mm. This finding, along with cholelithiasis, pericholecystic fluid, and a sonographic Murphy's sign (maximal tenderness over a sonographically identified gallbladder), is associated with cholecystitis.

Gallbladder wall thickening alone, however, is relatively nonspecific for cholecystitis and is associated with other conditions such as ascites, heart failure, pancreatitis, renal failure, and hypoalbuminemic states.

Though cholecystitis must be considered in patients with abdominal pain and a thickened gallbladder wall, it is unlikely in this scenario given the lack of gallstones and negative sonographic Murphy's sign, whose combined absence have a negative predictive value of 95%.

The most likely cause of the patient's symptoms of abdominal distention, shortness of breath, and ultrasound findings is ascites associated with long-standing liver disease given his history of hepatitis C and alcohol abuse.

The cause is less likely heart failure given a normal BNP and no history of heart disease. Pancreatitis is similarly unlikely given the lack of elevated lipase and abdominal pain, though it must be considered given the history of alcohol abuse.

Test-taking tip: This question requires correct interpretation of the ultrasound image provided. Brush up on some basic images common in the ED.

67. ANSWER: D

The image demonstrates "cobblestoning" of subcutaneous fat, consistent with cellulitis.

This pattern is created by hyperechoic subcutaneous tissue and fat being separated by hypoechoic edema in a reticular pattern. Because no discrete spherical or elliptical hypoechoic fluid collection concerning for abscess is identified by ultrasound, the most likely diagnosis is cellulitis. Therefore, the next best step in management would be to discharge the patient with oral antibiotics for treatment of uncomplicated cellulitis.

Though not demonstrated here, there have been cases of retained metallic foreign bodies among injection drug users who have broken the tip off hypodermic needles. In that instance, a linear hyperechoic structure would be seen on ultrasound.

Although cobblestoning may be seen on the periphery of soft tissue affected with necrotizing fasciitis, bedside ultrasound classically demonstrates "dirty shadowing" associated with subcutaneous emphysema. Furthermore, this patient is afebrile, appears well, and lacks other classic signs of necrotizing fasciitis, such as pain out of proportion and crepitus, making the diagnosis unlikely.

Test-taking tip: This question requires correct interpretation of the ultrasound image provided. Brush up on some basic images common in the ED.

68. ANSWER: C

The patient is presenting with lower abdominal cramping and vaginal bleeding in the setting of an early first-trimester pregnancy. Although the patient is hemodynamically stable, an ectopic pregnancy must be considered as part of the differential diagnosis.

A transabdominal ultrasound is performed that demonstrates a gestational sac consisting of a hypoechoic center (chorionic sac) surrounded by an echogenic ring (chorionic ring). This is one of first findings of an intrauterine pregnancy, seen at 4 to 5 weeks' gestation. However, no clear intrauterine pregnancy or yolk sac is identified within, making this an indeterminate study. This may be due to the lack of sensitivity with the transabdominal approach, thus requiring a transvaginal ultrasound for further evaluation.

The transvaginal ultrasound can identify most intrauterine pregnancies with β-hCG levels from 1,000 to 2,000 mIU/mL and in all patients with levels above 2,000 mIU/mL. If the transvaginal ultrasound still produces an indeterminate study, the patient should follow up for a repeat ultrasound and β-hCG in 48 hours. This is because the patient's β-hCG level is below the discriminatory zone of 1,000 mIU/mL, making the diagnoses of an very early intrauterine pregnancy, small ectopic pregnancy, and embryonic demise all possible.

Test-taking tip: This is a "you know it or don't" kind of question. If you don't know it, choose an answer and move on. You can perhaps mark it for review when you are done at the end of the test. Don't, however, let these kinds of questions get you stuck and waste your time.

69. ANSWER: A

The patient in this scenario is presenting with symptoms of left-sided chest pain and shortness of breath after an MVC, concerning for a traumatic pneumothorax.

The initial chest radiograph is read as normal; however, the patient was evaluated in the trauma resuscitation bay, and most likely the chest radiograph was obtained in the supine position. Supine chest radiographs will often miss a pneumothorax because they layer anteriorly.

By placing the ultrasound transducer over each anterior chest wall, the lung pleura are evaluated for normal sliding with respiration. This can either be visualized over time in the traditional B-mode (brightness or two-dimensional) or captured with M-mode (motion). In M-mode, one slice of the two-dimensional image is displayed over time.

If there is no motion below the lung pleural line due to a pneumothorax, the image remains static and a "barcode" or "stratosphere" sign is produced, as seen with this case.

In normal lungs, movement below the lung pleura produces a speckled pattern termed the "seashore" sign.

A hemothorax is identified by looking at the space above the diaphragm in the right upper and left upper quadrant views. Any hypoechoic fluid above the diaphragm in the setting of trauma would suggest the presence of a hemothorax.

A pericardial effusion is easily identified by examining for hypoechoic fluid surrounding the heart in subxiphoid or parasternal long-axis views.

Test-taking tip: You do not necessarily have to be able to correctly interpret the ultrasound. A patient with a normal chest radiograph after trauma but with persistent shortness of breath and hypoxia has an occult pneumothorax until proved otherwise.

70. ANSWER: B

The patient in this case presents with right upper quadrant abdominal pain with ultrasound imaging consistent with a large gallstone with posterior shadowing. The diagnosis of cholecystitis is unlikely given the lack of fever or leukocytosis. Furthermore, there is no obvious gallbladder wall thickening or pericholecystic fluid noted on ultrasound, which are findings concerning for cholecystitis.

If all of the findings suggestive for cholecystitis were present, then it would be appropriate to admit the patient for IV antibiotics along with a surgical consultation.

Because the patient's pain has improved and there are no other signs of biliary obstruction, such as abnormal LFTs or jaundice, outpatient referral for an elective cholecystectomy is appropriate.

An ERCP would be used in cases of gallstone pancreatitis, in which the patient would have an elevated lipase as well as persistent abdominal pain.

An IR-guided percutaneous biliary drain is used as a temporizing measure in critically ill patients with acute cholecystitis who cannot undergo surgery. This decision is typically made in collaboration with a surgeon.

Test-taking tip: Patients with resolution of their symptoms without intervention probably do not require emergent management.

71. ANSWER: A

The vertical mattress suture is a type of closure that is effective in closing deep wounds and wounds under tension. It also helps to provide eversion and opposition of superficial skin layers in areas such as the neck that tend to invert.

The disadvantage of this choice of wound closure is that it tends to creates more scarring than simple interrupted sutures and should not be used in cosmetically sensitive areas, such as the face.

Test-taking tip: The face is the only place that is different from the others, which are noncosmetic areas for wound closure.

72. ANSWER: C

The patient's presentation suggests a shoulder dislocation, and the radiograph shows the "lightbulb sign" whereby the head of the humerus is in the same axis as the humeral shaft, suggesting a posterior shoulder dislocation. Posterior shoulder dislocations are rare, accounting for 2% to 4% of all shoulder dislocations.

The most common method used to reduce posterior shoulder dislocations is the DePalma method, in which the affected arm is adducted and internally rotated with caudal traction applied. While maintaining traction and internal rotation, the medial aspect of the arm is pushed laterally, and then the arm is extended.

The other three techniques mentioned for reduction are used for anterior shoulder dislocations. Scapular rotation is performed with the patient in a prone position on the gurney. The affected arm hangs vertically off the edge of the gurney and weights (5–10 pounds) can be attached to the wrist. When muscular relaxation has occurred, reduction can be attempted by pushing the tip of the scapula medially. The Stimson method also involves laying the patient prone on a gurney with weights attached to the wrist, but no manipulation is attempted; rather, when the muscle spasm relaxes, the joint reduces spontaneously.

The Milch technique involves the provider standing on the affected side with the patient lying prone. The provider then places fingers on the affected shoulder, and to steady the displaced humeral head, the thumb pushes against it. The provider's other hand is then used to abduct and externally rotate the affected arm into an overhead position. The provider then pushes the humeral head back into the glenoid fossa.

Test-taking tip: There are many methods for shoulder dislocation reduction. Brush up on the common methods used in the ED.

73. ANSWER: C

This child's presentation is most consistent with a nursemaid's elbow, which is a subluxation of the radial head. It is most common in children between the age of 2 and 5 years and frequently occurs after traction on an extended arm.

When this injury is suspected, the best management is immediate reduction by manually supinating the forearm and flexing the elbow past 90 degrees or using hyperpronation of the forearm. The emergency practitioner can place the thumb over the radial head, and a palpable click may be felt with reduction. Success is measured by improvement in the child's pain and ability to resume using the arm.

A radiograph is not necessary when this diagnosis is suspected unless the mechanism of injury raises the concern for a fracture. Sending the patient home with just support measures and no reduction would not be appropriate management.

This patient does not have fever or other constitutional symptoms, nor is the joint erythematous or swollen, making septic joint a less likely diagnosis.

Test-taking tip: You can easily eliminate choice D, given the presentation described in the question.

74. ANSWER: A

The kissing technique, direct instrumentation with forceps (alligator or bayonet), and the use of a thin, lubricated balloon tip catheter are all well-described methods to remove nasal foreign bodies. Other well-described methods include direct instrumentation with a curved hook, cerumen loop, or suction catheter. Positive pressure ventilation, which is the desired effect of the kissing technique, can also be performed with a bag-valve-mask over the mouth if a parent is unwilling or unable to perform the kiss.

Irrigation with water, while a very successful technique in the removal of nonorganic materials from the ear, is not as useful in the removal of nasal foreign bodies and may actually push the object farther into the nares, making further attempts at removal more challenging.

Test-taking tip: Irrigation is good for ears but not for noses.

20.

EMERGENCY MEDICAL SERVICES, DISASTER MEDICINE, AND LEGAL ISSUES

Scott DeShields and Susan Woodmansee

1. A patient is brought in by emergency medical services (EMS) after sustaining a traumatic injury. The medics left his helmet on. Leaving the helmet on was:

A. Correct because the patient complains of numbness
B. Correct because the patient was injured during a football game
C. Incorrect because the patient does not complain of trouble breathing
D. Incorrect because the patient is awake

2. A patient is seen in a small rural emergency department (ED) for injuries related to a SCUBA diving incident that occurred in a high mountain lake. EMS plans to transfer the patient via air. The transferring physician:

A. Should keep the patient in her ED in the event of inclement weather
B. Must perform a tube thoracostomy for a pneumothorax before transport
C. Should not leave the ultimate decision of mode of transport to EMS and the receiving facility
D. Should intubate the patient before transport

3. Which of the following is *not* a generally accepted definition of a medical disaster?

A. Greater than 25 patients at one time to a well-staffed ED
B. Destructive effects that overwhelm the ability to meet the demand for health care
C. A sudden event of sufficient magnitude to require external assistance
D. An event that has a massive disruptive impact

4. Which of the following statements is correct regarding a patient in a mass casualty situation who is triaged as "black"?

A. The patient has no respiratory effort
B. The patient should receive no treatment
C. The patient is pregnant
D. The patient should be the first to be transported off scene

5. All of the follow statements about variola, a potentially serious biologic weapon, are true *except*:

A. The onset of debilitating symptoms is relatively fast
B. It is highly virulent
C. It can be transmitted in an aerosolized manner
D. It is not common

6. Which of the following is true regarding infections caused by *Bacillus anthracis*?

A. Gastrointestinal anthrax has a higher mortality rate than inhalation anthrax
B. *B. anthracis*, as a biologic agent, was first documented to have been used for warfare during World War I by Germany against the Allies
C. *B. anthracis* spores are unusual to find outside of bioweapons laboratories
D. *B. anthracis* spores are relatively easy to disburse

7. One reason that the ricin toxin, while potentially fatal, is considered to be less concerning as a biologic agent is that:

A. It is difficult to obtain
B. There is a readily available antidote
C. A conspicuously large quantity must be used
D. It is difficult to aerosolize

8. The presentation of a victim of a sarin gas attack is most similar to:

A. A victim of smoke inhalation from an office fire
B. An inadvertent ingestion of an organophosphate

C. A suicide attempt with an overdose of haloperidol
D. Cocaine toxicity

9. Which of the following pairs of decontamination conditions and treatments is not recommended?

A. Hot tar and petroleum jelly
B. Lithium metal and mild soapy water
C. Petrol and ethanol
D. Cyanoacrylate and acetone

10. Chlorine gas is preferred as a chemical warfare agent over other agents because:

A. It is highly toxic
B. It is easier to disperse
C. It is used to make routine industrial products like polyurethanes
D. It is hard to detect

11. A patient is brought to the ED following an explosion during the illegal manufacture of methamphetamine. The most likely injury that the patient will have sustained solely due to the blast is:

A. A pneumothorax
B. A long bone fracture
C. Barotrauma to the ear
D. Gastrointestinal bleeding

12. A nuclear reactor in the town where you work in as an emergency physician has a serious leak. In the first few hours and days after the incident, what are the most likely symptoms that patients will present with if they had significant radiation exposure?

A. Altered mental status
B. Nausea, vomiting, and diarrhea
C. High fevers and hypotension
D. Difficulty breathing

13. A patient is brought to a rural ED after being found in the rubble of a building that collapsed in an earthquake that occurred 2 days previously. He was pinned to the floor by a portion of wall that had fallen onto his legs. He complains of pain, numbness, and weakness to his bilateral lower extremities. He denies neck or back pain. The extremities are swollen and blistered. When deciding about transfer to a tertiary care center, the physician should consider which specialist the least important?

A. A nephrologist
B. A general surgeon
C. A neurosurgeon
D. A burn center

14. A patient who works in a food processing plant presents to the ED with a painful skin rash. The emergency provider suspects the correct culprit. The provider would be expected to elicit all of the following on history *except*:

A. He works with machinery in the plant that uses nonchemical technology to kill micro-organisms on apples
B. The pain has been continuous
C. There is erythema that comes and goes
D. He admits to "slacking off" sometimes when it comes to plant safety procedures

15. A 38-year-old male presents to the ED after suffering from a first-time seizure. The patient is accompanied by his wife, who is present during the entire ED encounter. On review of systems, the patient and his wife note that the patient had a fever and headache the day before the seizure. The patient is afebrile in the ED and currently denying any complaints, but the patient's wife says that he just isn't quite acting like his normal self. After normal labs return, the decision is made by the physician to perform computed tomography (CT) and lumbar puncture (LP) "just to be safe." The cerebrospinal fluid (CSF) is interpreted as normal, and the patient is discharged home. Two days later the viral cultures from the CSF are reported as positive for herpes simplex virus. When the physician calls the patient, the phone is answered by the patient's wife, who says that the patient is not home. How should the physician proceed?

A. Tell the patient's wife that it is very important for the patient to call back for test results at his earliest convenience
B. Tell the patient's wife that her husband has herpes encephalitis and that he needs to return to the ED immediately for admission and the initiation of treatment
C. Tell the patient's wife that the patient should return to the hospital immediately but that patient privacy laws prevent the disclosure of test results to anybody but the patient himself
D. Ask the wife when she expects the patient to return so that the physician can call back

16. A 63-year-old female presented to her gastroenterologist's office for a preoperative history and physical exam. The patient was scheduled to undergo a routine colonoscopy 2 days later. While in the exam room, the patient vomits twice and is noted by the staff to be pale in appearance. After measuring her blood pressure (BP) as 88/58 mm Hg, the patient is sent by ambulance to the ED. After the ED physician finishes her exam of the patient, she is told that the

patient's gastroenterologist is on the phone and would like to speak to the physician taking care of his patient. On the phone, the gastroenterologist says that he would like to give his version of events from his office that afternoon and to find out whether his patient will be able to undergo the upcoming scheduled endoscopy. How much information can the physician provide to the gastroenterologist?

A. She can only confirm that the patient is in the ED
B. She can confirm that the patient is in the ED and provide only the patient's location and general status
C. She can provide any pertinent information that would be relevant to the treatment being provided by the gastroenterologist
D. She can provide any and all patient information because the gastroenterologist is a physician and has a pre-existing relationship with the patient

17. A 58-year-old male is brought into the ED by ambulance. The patient had been watching TV with family 40 minutes prior when he suddenly stopped talking and was noted to be completely unable to move the right side of his body. The paramedic reports that the patient is a college professor with no past medical history and is currently taking no medications. The patient is awake on arrival but is still unable to speak despite his apparent ability to understand what is happening around him. He is also still unable to move the right side of his body but can answer yes/no questions by moving his head. After testing it is determined that the patient is within the necessary time window and is a potential candidate for thrombolytic therapy. With no family present yet at bedside, what is the best method to obtain informed consent for IV thrombolytic stroke treatment for this patient?

A. The physician can sign the consent along with a second physician, which will take the place of the patient's signature
B. There is no consent required because IV thrombolytics are the "standard of care" for acute thrombotic stroke in the absence of contraindications
C. The physician should wait for a family member or other surrogate decision maker to arrive so that consent can be given on behalf of the patient
D. The physician should have the consent discussion with the patient and allow the patient to make his own decision

18. A 17-year-old male is brought into the ED by paramedics after falling while trying to jump from a moving train onto the platform. He has a Glasgow Coma Scale (GCS) score of 12 on arrival with BP 80/

40 mm Hg and heart rate (HR) 128 bpm. Examination reveals a large scalp wound and a diffusely tender abdomen with free fluid visualized on the bedside ultrasound exam. The trauma team takes the patient to the operating room and fixes the scalp laceration as well as the liver laceration that was discovered on exploratory laparotomy. After waking up in the recovery room, the patient says that he never consented to the surgery and that he was going to sue everybody involved. What justification do the physicians have for not obtaining informed consent?

A. Therapeutic privilege
B. Emergency consent doctrine
C. Minor patient exception
D. Implied consent

19. A 16-year-old female presents to the ED with the chief complaint of pelvic pain. She says that she had sex with a new partner 1 week ago after finding out that her boyfriend was cheating on her. She has had a foul-smelling discharge for 3 days and burning with urination, and she is concerned that she might be pregnant. When the nurse asks where her parents are, the patient says that she is here alone and she does not want her parents to know that she is here. The nurse asks the physician how to proceed given that the patient is a minor. What is the best course of action?

A. The physician should treat the patient like any other female with similar complaints even though she is only 16 years old
B. The physician should tell the nurse to call one of the parents of the patient so that they can get consent to treat a 16-year-old minor
C. The physician should tell the patient that he doesn't feel comfortable treating her unless she gets an adult to accompany her during the ED visit
D. The physician should tell the patient that he can test her for pregnancy but that any further treatment would require parental consent

20. A 47-year-old female is brought into the ED by paramedics after being found on the ground outside of a liquor store. She was surrounded by beer bottles and has the odor of alcohol on her breath as the physician attempts to talk with her. The medics said that the patient tried to walk to the gurney by herself but that she was so unsteady on her feet that they had to assist her. As the physician tries to examine the patient he notices a 6-cm laceration to the top of her scalp, but she quickly becomes belligerent and tells the physician not to touch her. The patient will allow nurses to clean the wound, take her vital signs, draw blood, and transfer her to the CT scanner for a head CT. All of the patient's studies

are normal except for an elevated blood alcohol level. When the physician attempts to talk with the patient about closing her scalp wound, the patient mutters back in a slurred voice that she doesn't want the wound fixed. What is the best initial course of action?

    A. Discharge the patient because she is refusing wound closure and the rest of her exams are normal

    B. Chemically or physically restrain the patient just long enough to staple her wound closed

    C. Allow the patient enough time to become sober and then speak to her again about closing the wound

    D. Discharge the patient with clear instructions about keeping the wound clean and recommend a return to the ED in 2 days for a wound check and possible delayed closure

21. A 35-year-old female prisoner is brought into the ED by the prison staff after the patient had intentionally cut across her left arm multiple times with a razor blade. The prison guard who accompanied the patient to the ED described blood that was shooting from the inside of the patient's elbow and wrist before they were able to bandage her up and transport her. On arrival the patient's blood pressure is 86/48 mm Hg and HR is 121 bpm. She appears to have normal motor and sensation in the left hand and has normal capillary refill. The patient admits to cutting herself and says that she was just trying to get attention. She allows the physician to explore and repair her wounds. The patient's hemoglobin on arrival was 10.8, but after several hours in the ED the repeat hemoglobin is 6.2. The physician recommends a blood transfusion because the patient's blood pressure is still 88/54 mm Hg after 2 L of normal saline and the patient describes feeling lightheaded. Despite the physician's recommendations, the patient refuses the transfusion even though she clearly understands the risks and benefits explained to her. What should the physician do?

    A. Honor the wishes of the patient because she appears to have the capacity to make her own decisions

    B. Proceed with the transfusion because as a prisoner the patient no longer has any rights

    C. Have the guard sign the consent form and proceed with the transfusion because the prisoner is in his custody

    D. Discharge the patient because she is refusing care

22. A 73-year-old male walks into the ED with a chief complaint of headache and blurry vision. The symptoms started after walking out of his house into the bright sun. On exam, the patient is in moderate distress because of the pain in his head. The physician notes a "steamy" cornea with a mid-dilated pupil. The ED physician

calls the on-call ophthalmologist to come in to help treat the suspected acute angle closure glaucoma, but the ED physician is instead told to send the patient directly to the ophthalmology clinic. The ED physician is concerned about her obligations under the Emergency Medical Treatment and Labor Act (EMTALA) because she knows that the patient's emergency medical condition (EMC) has not been stabilized. What is the best advice for the ED physician?

    A. Discharge the patient to the ophthalmologist's office because EMTALA only applies to transfers

    B. Have the ED physician insist that the ophthalmologist come into the ED to treat the patient so that the EMTALA obligations will be satisfied

    C. Transfer the patient to another hospital that has an ophthalmologist who is willing to come into the ED to treat the patient

    D. Discharge the patient to the ophthalmologist's office because EMTALA allows for transfer of patients to an on-call provider's office when specialized equipment is available in the office

23. A 22-year-old G2P1 female at 39 weeks' gestation walks into the ED. She complains of abdominal cramping that she says feels like "labor pains." The pain started 30 minutes ago. She denies vaginal bleeding or fluid leakage and has no other complaints. On hearing the complaints from the triage nurse and noting the normal vital signs, the physician directs the nurse to have the patient go directly to Labor and Delivery without any additional ED treatment. Is this a violation of EMTALA?

    A. No; the patient is clinically stable, so EMTALA no longer applies

    B. No; Labor and Delivery is capable of performing a medical screening exam for purposes of EMTALA

    C. Yes; the patient presented to the ED, which requires the ED physician to perform a medical screening exam to determine whether there is an EMC

    D. Yes; the patient presented in labor, which by definition under EMTALA is an EMC that requires stabilization

24. An 11-year-old boy was the unrestrained passenger in a high-speed motor vehicle collision. He is brought in at 11 PM into the ED at a rural hospital where the ED physician is the only physician on the hospital grounds. The boy is resuscitated to the best abilities of the ED physician, and it is determined that the patient has a significant head injury. There are no neurosurgeons available on call, and the general surgeon says that she is willing to come in but that it will be at least 30 minutes and she's not sure if she can truly offer anything to this severely injured boy. The ED physician decides to intubate the patient and transfer him to the closest trauma center. As the paramedics are loading the patient, the patient begins to deteriorate. The paramedics ask the ED physician if she thinks the patient is stable for transfer under EMTALA. How should the physician proceed?

A. Keep the patient in the ED until she can get him stable enough for the paramedics to feel comfortable
B. Keep the patient in the ED until the general surgeon arrives and helps to determine whether the patient is stable for transfer
C. Get a CT scan of the patient's head, neck, chest, abdomen, and pelvis to help determine stability for transfer
D. Transfer the patient as soon as possible regardless of the patient being unstable because the only chance of the patient getting the necessary treatment is by getting him to the trauma center

25. A 48-year-old male from Cambodia presents to the ED with no complaints. The patient just moved to the United States and is requesting help in establishing a new local primary care physician. The patient had a list of medications that he brought with him from his home country. After spending much time trying to decipher what medications the patient was on, the ED physician discovered that the patient was being treated for tuberculosis, malaria, pertussis, and herpes. Which diseases should the ED physician be sure to report to the Centers for Disease Control and Prevention (CDC) and the local public health authority?

A. Tuberculosis, but not malaria, pertussis, or herpes
B. Tuberculosis and malaria, but not pertussis or herpes
C. Tuberculosis, malaria, and pertussis, but not herpes
D. Tuberculosis, malaria, pertussis, and herpes

26. A 23-year-old male arrives in the ED by private auto after his girlfriend found him bleeding and lying on the ground outside of a local bar. The patient says that he was jumped by two guys that he had never seen before. They broke several bottles over his head and proceeded to punch and kick him while he was down on the ground. The patient has several moderately complex lacerations to his face, and he initially demands that they be closed by a plastic surgeon. The patient is disruptive during his time in the ED, and his rude comments to the nurses make the entire staff want to expedite his discharge. The emergency medicine physician eventually closes up all of the lacerations after the patient acquiesces and then discharges the patient to the care of his girlfriend, who is willing to take the patient home. One week later, two

of the wounds became infected and required hospitalization for IV antibiotics. It was discovered that several small pieces of glass were retained in the wounds during closure. If the patient sues the ED physician, what standard of care will the physician be held to?

A. Reasonable care of an emergency medicine physician
B. Reasonable care of an emergency medicine physician of the same geographic locale
C. Reasonable care of a plastic surgeon because the patient requested closure by a plastic surgeon
D. Reasonable care of a physician who closes wounds as part of the physician's common practice

27. An ED physician is flying home from a medical conference when the flight attendant comes onto the overhead speaker asking for any physicians or other trained medical personnel to please report to the front of the cabin. The ED physician had been up late the night before, and rather than getting up to help, he put on his headphones and tried to fall asleep. As it turns out, the woman who required help died before the plane could reach medical care. Somehow the husband of the passenger who had died on the plane found out that there had been an ED doctor on the plane who refused to help his dying wife. What liability does the ED physician have if the widower files a lawsuit?

A. The physician will be liable because once he is aware that there is a person requiring medical assistance, a patient-physician relationship has been formed
B. The physician will not have any liability because he did not have an affirmative duty to help the woman
C. The physician will not have any liability because he never breached the standard of care because he never rendered any care
D. The physician will not have any liability because he was not the proximate or actual cause of the woman's death

28. An ED physician is following up on patients and finishing up her charting the day after a very busy night shift. One of the patients was a 43-year-old male who had presented with diffuse abdominal pain that had developed throughout the day. His labs were unremarkable except for a very slight leukocytosis and mildly decreased serum bicarbonate level. While in the ED he was repeatedly threatening to leave if he wasn't given more pain medication and said that he was going to call his lawyer. However, every time that the physician had walked past the patient, the patient was playing on his phone and appeared comfortable. The physician did not believe that the patient was having as much pain as described and made comments in the medical record that the patient was exhibiting

drug-seeking behavior. At the end of her shift, the ED physician decided to admit the patient to observation status because the patient insisted on his pain still being uncontrolled. The hospitalist admitted the patient as the ED physician was going home. In the hospitalist's history and physical exam chart, it was noted that the patient appeared distressed, had severe abdominal pain, and was peritoneal on exam. The surgery team was immediately consulted and took the patient to the operating room, where a perforated ulcer was discovered and repaired. How should the ED physician complete her chart when she now knows the actual diagnosis in a patient that she had a difficult interpersonal encounter with in the ED?

A. Complete the charting for the encounter as if she never knew the eventual outcome
B. Remove all mention of drug-seeking behavior when completing the chart because those comments would look very bad if the patient actually did file a lawsuit
C. Date and time the additional charting as an addendum so that it is clear that the documentation was taking place after the eventual diagnosis was made
D. Leave the chart exactly like it was when the physician left her shift so that nobody could accuse her of adding self-serving information after the fact

ANSWERS

1. ANSWER: B

In general, a helmet that is part of proper athletic protective wear (e.g., football, ice hockey) should be left on for transport to the ED because the helmet and shoulder pads are designed to maintain the cervical spine in a neutral position. There is no added benefit to removing the helmet in the field to place a rigid collar.

A patient with neurologic symptoms must be maintained in optimal cervical spine alignment. The helmet would be proper as part of athletic gear but would not be adequate if it were a motorcycle helmet. Motorcycle helmets do not have the same fit and are not worn with shoulder pads and therefore should be removed and replaced with a rigid cervical collar in the field.

Were the patient to have an airway emergency, any helmet would need to be partially or completely removed to address the emergent issue.

Depending on the helmet, an awake patient's helmet may be left on or removed.

Test-taking tip: If you can decide whether the medic's decision was correct or incorrect, you can leave yourself with only two answers to choose from.

2. ANSWER: C

A SCUBA-related accident may result in several different types of injuries, with decompression illness and air emboli as two of the most concerning. Following an understanding of Boyle's Law, decompression illness or the presence of air emboli can be exacerbated by high-altitude flight. Depending on the circumstances, the decrease in pressure may lead to a fatal outcome. The physician must communicate with the transferring agency when there is a concern for pressure-related problems. This may include fixed wing (that generally flies higher) versus helicopter, local geography, and so forth.

A small pneumothorax should not be at risk for expansion with low-altitude flight.

Ground transport should always be reconsidered if waiting for safe flying conditions would seriously delay care.

A decision to intubate should be based on the clinical presentation of the patient and the likelihood of decompensating during transport. The fact that the patient had a diving accident, on its own, is not an indication for intubation.

Test-taking tip: Little information is provided in this question about the patient's clinical condition, suggesting that the correct answer is not about clinical care, eliminating B and D as correct answers.

3. ANSWER: A

Generally, there is no specific number of patients accepted as a definition of a medical disaster because, depending on the locale and event, even a small number of patients may overwhelm a system (e.g., Ebola), whereas other locations may have the resources to handle large numbers of patients.

The other definitions listed are ones that have been developed by the American College of Emergency Physicians, the World Health Organization, and other emergency services organizations.

Test-taking tip: Three of the answers are very similar in their generality, suggesting they are correct, rather than the more specific answer.

4. ANSWER: A

"Black" is the lowest triage level because the patient sustained such devastating injures that, even if not now dead, death would be expected despite optimal medical treatment.

Triage algorithms, such as the simple triage and rapid treatment (START) algorithm (Figure 20.1), have providers assess for respirations and, if there are none, ask for an airway maneuver to be performed. If the patient does not have return of spontaneous respirations, the patient is triaged as "black."

A "black" triaged patient may or may not be dead yet when triaged. The patient may still have a pulse and cardiac activity but no respiratory effort. The patient may still receive comfort measures if feasible.

No currently used prehospital triage tools take into consideration whether patients in mass casualty incidents are pregnant.

Patients triaged as "black" are usually the last patients to be taken off scene. Immediate or "red" patients are patients with potentially treatable life-threatening injuries who should be transported off scene first.

Test-taking tip: This is a "you know it or you don't" kind of question. If you don't know it, choose and answer and move on. You can perhaps mark it for review when you are done at the end of the test. Don't, however, let these kinds of question get you stuck and waste your time.

5. ANSWER: A

Variola, the causative agent of smallpox, has an incubation period of 12 to 14 days, thus answer A is not correct.

All of the other statements about variola are correct. It is highly virulent with a reported mortality of 30%, and it is highly transmissible from person to person through saliva.

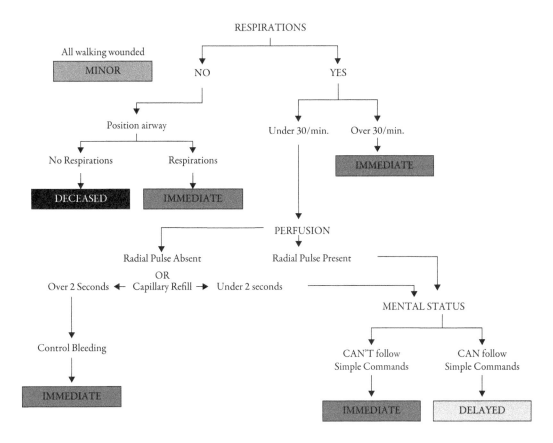

Figure 20.1 Simple triage and rapid treatment (START) algorithm.

Smallpox was declared officially eradicated in 1980, and outside of certain laboratory and health care workers, it is no longer a routine vaccination. The lack of prior infection or immunization increases the risk for and severity of disease to the general population after exposure.

Test-taking tip: Most emergency physicians have limited experience with biologic and chemical agents of warfare, but they are commonly tested. Study up on the basics of these agents before the test (Table 20.1).

Table 20.1 POTENTIAL OR KNOWN BIOLOGIC WARFARE AGENTS

AGENT	TYPE	WEAPONIZED	WATER THREAT	INFECTIOUS DOSE
Anthrax	Bacteria	Yes	Yes	6,000
Brucellosis	Bacteria	Yes	Probable	10,000
Tularemia	Bacteria	Yes	Yes	500,000
Shigellosis	Bacteria	Unknown	Yes	10,000
Cholera	Bacteria	Unknown	Yes	1,000
Salmonella	Bacteria	Unknown	Yes	10,000
Plague	Bacteria	Probable	Yes	500
Variola	Virus	Possible	Yes	10
Hepatitis A	Virus	Unknown	Yes	30
Cryptosporidiosis	Parasite	Unknown	Yes	130

6. ANSWER: D

The toxin is relatively easy to disburse and can be distributed through powder, sprays, food, and water. In 1979, several dozens of people living 4 km downwind from a bioweapons laboratory in the Soviet Union died because of improperly placed air filters. In 2001, five people died in the United States after being exposed to spores transmitted through the mail.

Inhalation anthrax is considered to be the deadliest form of anthrax. Without treatment, only 15% of patients will survive. With aggressive treatment, about 50% of patients will survive.

In World War I the Germans did not use anthrax directly as a biologic agent but rather used the spores to infect livestock that was to supply the Allies with food.

Unlike the smallpox virus that is only found in laboratories, anthrax spores can be found rather commonly in the natural environment.

Test-taking tip: Most emergency physicians have limited experience with biologic and chemical agents of warfare, but they are commonly tested. Study up on the basics of these agents before the test.

7. ANSWER: D

Ricin is a toxic protein from the castor plant that is difficult to process to a size smaller than 10 μm that would allow it to be aerosolized.

Ricin is derived from the ubiquitous castor plant, which can be found worldwide. The plant and seeds can also be purchased with little difficulty, and the ricin toxin can be manufactured without specialized equipment.

There is no antidote to ricin. Treatment is supportive care. Death is usually the result of multisystem organ failure.

Even a miniscule amount of ricin may be fatal. In 1978, a Bulgarian dissident died 3 days after being injected in the leg with a small capsule of ricin that came out of the end of an umbrella.

Test-taking tip: Most emergency physicians have limited experience with biologic and chemical agents of warfare, but they are commonly tested. Study up on the basics of these agents before the test.

8. ANSWER: B

Sarin is a nerve agent with properties similar to organophosphates. Sarin poisoning will present with cholinergic overdose-type symptoms including miosis, increased secretions, nausea, vomiting, diarrhea, bradycardia, seizures, coma, and death.

Victims of smoke inhalation may be exposed to cyanide. Cyanide interferes with oxidative phosphorylation. Cyanide poisoning can present with a wide variety of symptoms. While there is some crossover with the cholinergic symptoms, there are other symptoms of cyanide poisoning that are not seen with a classic cholinergic overdose, in particular metabolic acidosis. Also, while respiratory failure is seen in both cyanide and sarin, the mechanism of action is different.

A haloperidol overdose will normally cause an anticholinergic response, which often presents with dry mucous membranes, agitation, difficulty urinating, and tachycardia. In more severe cases, respiratory depression, severe hypotension, and coma may occur.

Cocaine will cause a sympathomimetic response, including tachycardia, agitation, diaphoresis, and mydriasis.

Test-taking tip: Most emergency physicians have limited experience with biologic and chemical agents of warfare, but they are commonly tested. Study up on the basics of these agents before the test (Table 20.2).

Table 20.2 CHARACTERISTICS AND EFFECTS OF CHEMICAL WARFARE AGENTS

AGENT	TOXIC EFFECTS
Nerve agents: Tabun Sarin Soman VX	Miosis, headache, hypersalivation, abdominal cramps, vomiting, bronchospasm, respiratory paralysis, convulsions
Blister agents: Mustard Lewisite	*Mustard:* Latent period of 6–8 hours, then redness, pruritus, pearl-like blisters, and necrotic lesions *Lewisite:* No latent period with development of pruritus, blisters, lung edema, and eye involvement
Choking agents: Phosgene Chloropicrin	Latent period of 6–8 hours followed by coughing, breathlessness, unrest, chest pain, and choking (in high concentrations, immediately deadly)
Blood agents: Hydrogen cyanide Cyanogen chloride	Dizziness, dyspnea, headache, cramps, seizures, respiratory arrest

9. ANSWER: B

Lithium metal reacts violently with water, causing an exothermic reaction that may result in a burn. Mineral oil or a similar oil should be used. An aqueous solution should only be employed after all metal has been removed.

Petroleum jelly may be used to remove *dry, cooled* tar. Mechanical abrasives should not be used because they may damage the skin.

Acetone may be used to remove cyanoacrylates (skin glues) on intact skin. An oil- or petroleum-based product should be used for the mucous membranes or around the eye.

A solution containing a small amount of ethanol can be helpful in removing a hydrocarbon.

Test-taking tip: This is a "you know it or you don't" kind of question. If you don't know it, choose and answer and move on. You can perhaps mark it for review when you are done at the end of the test. Don't, however, let these kinds of question get you stuck and waste your time.

10. ANSWER: C

Chlorine gas has widespread use in industry and manufacturing and therefore is readily available.

Nerve agents (such as sarin) and sulfur mustard gas are designated "schedule I" according to the international Chemical Weapons Convention because they have no legitimate use outside chemical weapons. Their use has been banned, and they are much more difficult to obtain in large quantities.

Chlorine gas is not highly toxic. It causes mucous membrane and pulmonary irritation and, in high, concentrations, causes death by asphyxiation. Sarin also causes death by asphyxiation but due to nervous system disruption and paralysis. It acts much more quickly, and far smaller amounts are needed to cause death,

All of the chemical weapon gases can be dispersed with equal ease.

Chlorine gas is yellow-green in color and has a distinctive odor. Sarin gas is much harder to detect because it is colorless and odorless.

Test-taking tip: Most emergency medicine physicians have limited experience with biologic and chemical agents of warfare, but they are commonly tested. Study up on the basics of these agents before the test.

11. ANSWER: C

The most common injury from a primary blast injury (PBI) is a ruptured tympanic membrane secondary to barotrauma.

Fractures may result from the "blast wave" but are not the most common injury encountered. The blast wave is a result of air that is superheated and compacted and delivers extremely high forces to a small area. Poorly compliant tissue, such as bone, is susceptible similarly to glass and concrete.

As opposed to a blast etiology, injuries from this type of explosion are much more likely to be the result of blunt trauma from being hit or from hitting a solid object, penetrating trauma from projectiles, crush injuries, burns, inhalation injuries, or toxin exposures.

The lungs and gastrointestinal tract can be injured as a result of stress or shearing forces due to blunt or penetrating trauma but are not usually affected by PBI.

Test-taking tip: This is a "you know it or you don't" kind of question. If you don't know it, choose and answer and move on. You can perhaps mark it for review when you are done at the end of the test. Don't, however, let these kinds of question get you stuck and waste your time.

12. ANSWER: B

People exposed to very high levels of radiation over a short period of time, as would occur in a radiation emergency, may develop acute radiation syndrome. Initial symptoms, which usually begin minutes to days after exposure, include nausea, vomiting, headache, and diarrhea. Patients may also have skin damage immediately after an exposure.

Typically, after the initial symptoms, people will feel healthy for a period of time and then will become sick again. These symptoms include loss of appetite, fatigue, fever, nausea, vomiting, diarrhea, and possible seizures and coma. Death during this stage is usually due to bone marrow suppression that leads to serious infection and bleeding.

Test-taking tip: Significant radiation exposure is also a situation that most emergency medicine physicians have little experience treating but that is frequently tested on standardized tests. Study up on radiation illness before taking the test.

13. ANSWER: C

The patient has neurologic symptoms (numbness and weakness), but these are most likely due to a crush injury, not an acute neurosurgical event such as spinal trauma or cauda equina.

The patient is at risk for an acute renal injury due to dehydration and the possibility of rhabdomyolysis and thus may need a nephrologist. The patient is also at risk for compartment syndrome of the legs due to the crush effect of the wall and may need the services of a general surgeon. This patient may also have suffered burns (electrical, chemical, or mechanical) to the extremities as evidenced by the blistering and may need care that can only be provided at a burn center.

Test-taking tip: Reading the question carefully will lead you to the correct answer. The question describes a patient only pinned to the floor by a wall on his legs and has no neck or back pain, making the need for a neurosurgeon unlikely.

14. ANSWER: B

The patient presents with a classic case of cutaneous radiation injury (CRI). CRI occurs after an exposure to a radiation source. It is not unusual for the injury to take several days to weeks to manifest. There may be erythema, blistering, desquamation, or ulceration. Commonly, the pain will be intermittent or a late manifestation and can be very difficult to treat. Similar to the pain, erythema associated with CRI is often waxing and waning.

The patient is at risk for CRI because he may have been exposed at work to radiation used in a food irradiator. Gamma radiation is commonly used to kill pests and extend the shelf-life of produce and other foods to make them safe for market. Accidental exposure to radiation can be due to several factors, including poor training, inadequate safety measures, ignorance, and theft.

Test-taking tip: Significant radiation exposure is also a situation that most emergency medicine physicians have little experience treating but that is frequently tested on standardized test. Study up on radiation illness before taking the test.

15. ANSWER: B

The purpose of the Health Insurance Portability and Accountability Act of 1996 (HIPAA) is to protect the privacy and security of Protected Health Information (PHI). In general, HIPAA limits the disclosure of PHI without the patient's prior authorization. However, disclosure of results to a patient's friends or family members is permissible under HIPAA if the physician determines that in his/her professional opinion that the patient would not object to the disclosure. In this case, the patient and his wife presented together to the ED, and both were active participants in the treatment process. Additionally, the diagnosis of herpes encephalitis is a potentially life-threatening diagnosis if not promptly treated. For both of these reasons, it is appropriate to provide the wife with the test results so that she can ensure a rapid return to the ED by her husband. In general, if there is a concern about how much information can or should be shared, go with the answer that provides for the best care for the patient in the most expeditious manner.

Choices A and D are not the best answer because it may not result in the timely notification to the patient of a life-threatening diagnosis.

Choice C is not the best answer because the physician can use his professional judgment to infer that the patient would not be opposed to the information being shared with his wife since she was a part of the entire ED visit and thus the patient's consent to disclosure can be inferred.

Test-taking tip: HIPPA and EMTLA are important laws that govern emergency care. Make sure you know the basics, both for your practice and for the test.

16. ANSWER: C

HIPAA is meant to help prevent the unauthorized disclosure of PHI. However, exceptions to the HIPAA limitations exist so that access to vital information isn't limited such that it can result in delayed patient care or other harm to the patient. Here, the gastroenterologist is calling the ED to provide an account of what happened in his office and to see if his patient will be able to undergo her scheduled procedure with him. As long as the requested PHI relates to the care provided by the requesting physician, direct patient authorization is not required.

Choices A and B are not the best answers because the gastroenterologist would be entitled to more than just location and general health status of the patient since the information that he is requesting is for the purpose of his future care of the patient.

Choice D is not the best answer because even though the gastroenterologist has a pre-existing physician-patient relationship, he would only be entitled to the information that is related to his care of the patient. "Any and all patient information" is broader than what the HIPAA exception allows for.

Test-taking tip: Sharing information that is pertinent about patient care between physicians is essential to the practice of quality medicine, making it easy to eliminate choices A and B.

17. ANSWER: D

In one of the original landmark informed consent cases, former Supreme Court Justice Benjamin Cardozo wrote that "Every human being of adult years and sound mind has a right to determine what shall be done with his own body." This forms the basis of the consent doctrine. Informed consent consists of a discussion between the physician and patient (or surrogate) and should involve the determination of capacity, a description of the diagnosis or condition, the proposed treatment including material risks and benefits, alternative treatments (including no treatment) with their material risks and benefits, and finally a verification of the discussion by a patient/surrogate signature. Even though this patient was unable to speak, it was clear that he was a high-functioning person who was still able to understand what was happening to him. For this reason, he should be the person for the physician to have the consent discussion with.

There is no legal basis for two physicians independently making a consent decision for a patient.

IV thrombolytics have potential risks and benefits that should be explained to a patient even if the physician feels like the administration of the medicine represents the best available therapy.

Waiting for a family member or other surrogate decision maker to arrive at the ED might delay treatment such that the best chance of improvement of the patient's symptoms is lost. Again, the patient in this instance is able to make his own decisions, and waiting for family to arrive is unnecessary.

Test-taking tip: The question clearly paints the picture of a patient competent to make his own decisions, making the correct answer obvious.

18. ANSWER: B

Informed consent is necessary to ensure that patients are free to decide what they will and won't allow to happen to their body. In general, informed consent should be obtained for any medical treatment or procedure in which there is a high likelihood of risk or complication or in which the severity of risk is high. Informed consent consists of a discussion between the physician and patient (or surrogate) and should involve the determination of capacity, a description of the diagnosis or condition, the proposed treatment including material risks and benefits, alternative treatments (including no treatment) with their material risks and benefits, and finally a verification of the discussion by a patient/surrogate signature. One commonly used exception to the informed consent in emergency medicine is the emergency consent doctrine. An emergency situation alleviates the need for informed consent when there is an immediate and imminent harm if the patient is not treated. This is the best exception to use for the situation described.

Therapeutic privilege refers to an antiquated mindset in which the physician is allowed to decide what is best for the patient. This is rarely applicable today, except in very limited situations in which revealing information to the patient would pose a serious psychological threat, such as suicide.

The fact that the patient is a minor does not relieve the physician from otherwise obtaining informed consent. It is the emergency situation that is controlling here.

Choice D is not the correct answer because implied consent refers to consent that is given through silence, inaction, or other circumstances that surround the situation. An example of implied consent occurs when a patient makes an appointment with her physician. The making of the appointment implies that she is willing to allow the doctor to examine and treat her. There is no implied consent in the situation described in the question.

Test-taking tip: The scenario in the question is clearly an emergent situation, pointing to the correct answer, "emergency consent doctrine."

19. ANSWER: A

In the United States, the 26th Amendment established the right to vote for those 18 years or older. This caused the majority of states to establish the age of majority as 18 years. This is the age at which it is recognized that a person is an adult capable of assuming control of their person, actions, and decisions. However, there are exceptions for consent to medical services in instances in which the patient is younger than 18 years. This includes legal distinctions such as a mature minor or emancipated minor. Most states also allow a minor to consent to medical treatment pertaining to pregnancy or sexually transmitted infections without the involvement of their parents. Because this patient is concerned about pregnancy and has symptoms consistent with a sexually transmitted infection, she should be treated the same as an adult female with similar complaints.

Test-taking tip: Only choice A is completely different from the other answers, suggesting that it is the correct answer.

20. ANSWER: C

The patient described did not have the capacity to give consent or refuse care. The elevated alcohol level in the setting of clinical intoxication (unsteady gait and slurred speech) demonstrates a lack of capacity to make decisions about her care. Since there was no friend or family member at the bedside to provide consent, the best strategy would be to allow the patient to sober up to the point that the physician could have an informed discussion of the risks, benefits, and alternatives to wound closure. To allow the patient to refuse wound closure and then discharge the patient while she is still clinically intoxicated would impose potential liability on the physician.

Discharging the patient is not the best choice because the patient has a wound that any reasonable person would want closed. The fact that the patient was refusing consent for closure while in a condition in which she lacked capacity should not provide reassurance to the physician. This discharge would be inappropriate.

The wound is not life-threatening such that it justified affirmatively acting against the patient's wishes to close the wound. If the physician feels that a delay could have realistically negatively affected the patient and that a reasonable person would consent to the procedure, then treatment could be justified. However, waiting for the patient to become sober is still the better answer.

Discharging an intoxicated patient who is not capable of making her own decisions is not a good idea. If she were sober and still refused wound closure, this plan might be reasonable, but the question asks for the best initial course of action.

Test-taking tip: Discharging a clinically intoxicated patient is never a good idea, allowing you to eliminate choices A and D.

21. ANSWER: A

Prisoners, like regular citizens, have a liberty interest protected by the Due Process Clause of the 14th Amendment to not be treated against their will. Just because a patient is also a prisoner does not mean that the patient has been stripped of all rights in regard to her decision making. The exceptions to this right to refuse medical treatment occur when the testing or treatment that is being refused by the prisoner would threaten the health and safety of the remaining prison population. This includes communicable diseases and treatable psychiatric illnesses. A prisoner may also be forced to accept treatment to protect against permanent injury, but this will often require a court order. Here, the patient's source of bleeding has been fixed and shouldn't pose a permanent risk. She still appears to be symptomatically anemic, but she is demonstrating the capacity to refuse consent to the blood transfusion. Her refusal should be honored.

It is not appropriate to proceed with the transfusion against the patient's will because even though the patient is a prisoner, she still maintains some basic rights, including the right to refuse medical treatment in situations such as the one described.

Prison guards have no legal right to provide consent for a patient.

Discharging the patient is not appropriate because even though she is refusing a blood transfusion, she is still hypotensive and symptomatic. Her symptoms should be treated with additional IV fluids and other measures to address her hypotension that she agrees to. She may even require an admission to the hospital for observation if her symptoms and hypotension do not resolve.

Test-taking tip: You can easily eliminate choice D because you should never discharge a hypotensive, symptomatic patient, leaving only three answers to choose from.

22. ANSWER: D

EMTALA generally requires that the stabilization of an EMC occur in the ED. If the ED physician needs the assistance of an on-call specialist to determine whether an EMC exists or for help stabilizing an EMC, that on-call specialist should do so in the ED. One exception to this rule is when a specialist has equipment in the office that might not be available in the ED. A common example of this situation is with ophthalmology. In this case it would be appropriate to discharge the patient to the ophthalmologist's office as long as there is assurance that the patient will be seen promptly in the office.

EMTALA does apply to transfers; however, under the definitions within EMTALA, a discharge is considered a transfer. As such, anybody who is discharged from the ED must also meet the requirements imposed under EMTALA.

Some specialists are actually better equipped to deal with the EMC in a private office where there is specialized equipment that is not available in the ED.

Transferring the patient to another ED would expose the transferring hospital to an investigation for an EMTALA violation. Here, the transferring hospital had an on-call ophthalmologist who was willing to treat the patient and help stabilize the EMC but preferred to do so in the private office. This is an acceptable practice under EMTALA.

Test-taking tip: HIPPA and EMTLA are important laws that govern emergency care. Make sure you know the basics, both for your practice and for the test.

23. ANSWER: B

Under EMTALA, a pregnant woman in labor is considered an EMC that can only be stabilized by the delivery of the fetus and the placenta. The woman described in the question may or may not be in labor, but that determination needs to be made through the medical screening exam. Most patients presenting to the ED require stabilization of any discovered EMC before being transferred outside of the ED. A pregnant woman in labor being sent to Labor and Delivery within the hospital is an exception to this rule. EMTALA allows for the medical screening exam of a patient with only a pregnancy-related complaint to be performed at Labor and Delivery, as in this scenario.

This patient appears to be in labor and is not considered to be medically stable under EMTLA. A medical screening exam is required to determine whether she truly is in labor. If she is in labor, vital signs are not the determinant of stability. The only way to stabilize the laboring patient under EMTALA is through delivery of the fetus and placenta.

Although the patient presented to the ED, the medical screening exam of a pregnant patient with a pregnancy-only complaint can have that screening exam performed at Labor and Delivery.

It is true that labor is an EMC requiring stabilization under EMTALA. However, the medical screening exam to determine whether the patient is in labor can be done at Labor and Delivery. This practice is within the bounds of EMTALA and would not be considered a violation.

Test-taking tip: If you can commit to whether or not this scenario is an EMTALA violation, it will limit your choices to two possible answers.

24. ANSWER: D

EMTALA requires the stabilization of any EMC before transfer. However, when the injury is incapable of being stabilized at the transferring facility, the best move is to proceed with the transfer to the center that might be able to provide the necessary treatment. This is the best option even though the patient has an unstable condition. The patient was determined to have a significant head injury, and there was nobody on call and available who was able to provide the necessary stabilizing treatments. In such a case, the best option is to try to expedite transfer to the trauma center.

Keeping the child in the ED to attempt to stabilize him is not appropriate because there is likely no intervention that can be done at this transferring hospital that will provide stabilizing treatment. The patient needs to be sent as soon as possible to the trauma center where there are resources (e.g., neurosurgery) to potentially handle such an injury.

The general surgeon on call has already stated that she doesn't think that she will be able to provide appropriate care for this patient. Waiting for the general surgeon will only delay the transfer to definitive care.

Obtaining CT scans at the transferring hospital will not help to stabilize the patient in any way. Discovering additional injuries that that will also require transfer to the trauma center will only serve to delay the transfer of the patient.

Test-taking tip: HIPPA and EMTLA are important laws that govern emergency care. Make sure you know the basics, both for your practice and for the test.

25. ANSWER: C

The lists of diseases reportable to health authorities varies from state to state. However, some diseases appear almost universally on all state lists. This includes diseases such as tuberculosis, malaria, pertussis, and other diseases that are highly infective, transmissible in blood, or congenitally transmitted. The CDC also publishes a list of diseases that are required to be reported to the CDC. Herpes is a viral infection that is so prevalent in the general population that it is not considered a reportable disease.

Test-taking tip: Knowing that herpes is quite common and the other diseases rarer should help point you to the correct answer.

26. ANSWER: A

When a physician faces a lawsuit for medical negligence, that physician will be held to the standard of what is reasonable for a physician of like or similar training to do under like or similar circumstances. Because this case involves an emergency medicine physician, she will be held to the standard of a reasonable emergency medicine physician.

Geography no longer plays a role in what is considered to be reasonable care. Before information became so easily disseminated and accessible, standards were considered to be different in different locations of the country. This is no longer the case.

The physician potentially being sued is an emergency medicine physician. The only way that the emergency physician would be held to the standard of a plastic surgeon would be if she held herself out as having training commensurate with a plastic surgeon, or if it were deemed that the wounds were beyond the scope of a reasonable emergency physician and she insisted on closing them anyway. Neither of those two situations applies to this case.

This physician does have specialized training in emergency medicine; therefore, she will be held to the standard of a reasonable emergency medicine physician, not just any physician who closes wounds as part of that physician's common practice.

Test-taking tip: This is a "you know it or you don't" kind of question. If you don't know it, choose and answer and move on. You can perhaps mark it for review when you are done at the end of the test. Don't, however, let these kinds of question get you stuck and waste your time.

27. ANSWER: B

While it may seem counterintuitive, a physician does not have a duty to assist in a medical situation on a plane, in a nearby auto accident, or in any other potential medical situation. The only time that a physician would have a duty to assist is if there was already a pre-established relationship between the physician and the potential patient (e.g., existing physician-patient relationship, caregiver, spouse, guardian), if there was a pre-existing duty (while on shift in the ED), or if the physician was the one responsible for the person being injured. Because this woman had no prior personal or special legal relationship with the physician, the physician does not have a legal duty to render medical assistance. This, however, does not mean that there wouldn't be an ethical or moral duty for the physician to assist.

This physician never had a duty to act and in fact did not act; therefore, a standard of care analysis would not be relevant. Similarly, causation will not be a debatable issue if there isn't already a legal duty to act imposed on the physician.

Test-taking tip: This is a "you know it or you don't" kind of question. If you don't know it, choose and answer and move on. You can perhaps mark it for review when you are done at the end of the test. Don't, however, let these kinds of question get you stuck and waste your time.

28. ANSWER: C

When charting on a patient after there is a bad outcome, adverse event, strained interpersonal relationship, or other difficult situation, there is a tendency by the physician to want to alter the medical record to make it appear more favorable toward the physician. This is always a terrible idea because any time an inconsistency or revision is discovered, it will be assumed to be self-serving and made with the intent of covering up what really happened. In such a case, it is still important to maintain complete documentation, but any additional information that is added to the chart should be done so with complete transparency. The best way to do this is to leave the initial chart as it originally was and to create a separate addendum that is dated and timed. Any additional information that is inserted into the chart can honestly be done through the addendum and will minimize any impressions of impropriety.

Documenting as though the eventual outcome is unknown is not ethical because the physician actually does know the outcome for this patient. Additionally, in the era of electronic medical records all entries are time-stamped, and it will be obvious that the additional charting occurred the following day.

Removing information from the chart after the fact to serve one's own interests will be easily discovered and will essentially be viewed as evidence of liability. Especially in cases that have the potential for a lawsuit or other administrative review, it is never a good idea to alter the chart to make it appear more favorable for the physician.

Leaving the medical record "as is" is not appropriate because the medical record should be an accurate representation of what occurred during the encounter. Here, the physician hadn't finished charting on this patient, and by not adding the remaining information she would be leaving the chart incomplete. The better option would be to complete the chart but to do so in such a way that it is obvious to the reader that the additions were made at a later time through a time-stamped addendum.

Test-taking tip: It should be easy to eliminate choice B as unethical and choice D an inappropriate because the chart must be complete, leaving only two answers to choose from.

LIST OF FIGURES

CHAPTER 20

INDEX